Carotenoids in Health and Disease

OXIDATIVE STRESS AND DISEASE

Series Editors

LESTER PACKER, PH.D.
ENRIQUE CADENAS, M.D., PH.D.

University of Southern California School of Pharmacy
Los Angeles, California

1. Oxidative Stress in Cancer, AIDS, and Neurodegenerative Diseases, *edited by Luc Montagnier, René Olivier, and Catherine Pasquier*
2. Understanding the Process of Aging: The Roles of Mitochondria, Free Radicals, and Antioxidants, *edited by Enrique Cadenas and Lester Packer*
3. Redox Regulation of Cell Signaling and Its Clinical Application, *edited by Lester Packer and Junji Yodoi*
4. Antioxidants in Diabetes Management, *edited by Lester Packer, Peter Rösen, Hans J. Tritschler, George L. King, and Angelo Azzi*
5. Free Radicals in Brain Pathophysiology, *edited by Giuseppe Poli, Enrique Cadenas, and Lester Packer*
6. Nutraceuticals in Health and Disease Prevention, *edited by Klaus Krämer, Peter-Paul Hoppe, and Lester Packer*
7. Environmental Stressors in Health and Disease, *edited by Jürgen Fuchs and Lester Packer*
8. Handbook of Antioxidants: Second Edition, Revised and Expanded, *edited by Enrique Cadenas and Lester Packer*
9. Flavonoids in Health and Disease: Second Edition, Revised and Expanded, *edited by Catherine A. Rice-Evans and Lester Packer*
10. Redox–Genome Interactions in Health and Disease, *edited by Jürgen Fuchs, Maurizio Podda, and Lester Packer*
11. Thiamine: Catalytic Mechanisms in Normal and Disease States, *edited by Frank Jordan and Mulchand S. Patel*

Related Volumes

Vitamin E in Health and Disease: Biochemistry and Clinical Applications, *edited by Lester Packer and Jürgen Fuchs*

Vitamin A in Health and Disease, *edited by Rune Blomhoff*

Free Radicals and Oxidation Phenomena in Biological Systems, *edited by Marcel Roberfroid and Pedro Buc Calderon*

Biothiols in Health and Disease, *edited by Lester Packer and Enrique Cadenas*

Handbook of Antioxidants, *edited by Enrique Cadenas and Lester Packer*

Handbook of Synthetic Antioxidants, *edited by Lester Packer and Enrique Cadenas*

Vitamin C in Health and Disease, *edited by Lester Packer and Jürgen Fuchs*

Lipoic Acid in Health and Disease, *edited by Jürgen Fuchs, Lester Packer, and Guido Zimmer*

Flavonoids in Health and Disease, *edited by Catherine Rice-Evans and Lester Packer*

Additional Volumes in Preparation

Phytochemicals in Health and Disease, *edited by Yongping Bao and Roger Fenwick*

Herbal Medicine, *edited by Lester Packer, Choon Nam Ong, and Barry Halliwell*

Carotenoids in Health and Disease

edited by

NORMAN I. KRINSKY
Tufts University
Boston, Massachusetts, U.S.A.

SUSAN T. MAYNE
Yale University School of Medicine
New Haven, Connecticut, U.S.A.

HELMUT SIES
Heinrich Heine Universität
Düsseldorf, Germany

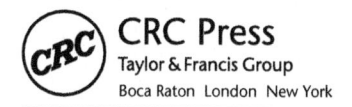

CRC Press
Taylor & Francis Group
Boca Raton London New York

CRC Press is an imprint of the
Taylor & Francis Group, an **informa** business

CRC Press
Taylor & Francis Group
6000 Broken Sound Parkway NW, Suite 300
Boca Raton, FL 33487-2742

First issued in paperback 2019

© 2004 by Taylor & Francis Group, LLC
CRC Press is an imprint of Taylor & Francis Group, an Informa business

ISBN-13: 978-0-8247-5416-7 (hbk)
ISBN-13: 978-0-367-39389-2 (pbk)

Library of Congress Cataloging-in-Publication Data
A catalog record for this book is available from the Library of Congress.

Visit the Taylor & Francis Web site at
http://www.taylorandfrancis.com

and the CRC Press Web site at
http://www.crcpress.com

Series Introduction

Oxygen is a dangerous friend. Overwhelming evidence indicates that oxidative stress can lead to cell and tissue injury. However, the same free radicals that are generated during oxidative stress are produced during normal metabolism and thus are involved in both human health and disease.

> Free radicals are molecules with an odd number of electrons. The odd, or unpaired, electron is highly reactive as it seeks to pair with another free electron.
> Free radicals are generated during oxidative metabolism and energy production in the body.
> Free radicals are involved in:
> Enzyme-catalyzed reactions
> Electron transport in mitochondria
> Signal transduction and gene expression
> Activation of nuclear transcription factors
> Oxidative damage to molecules, cells, and tissues
> Antimicrobial action of neutrophils and macrophages
> Aging and disease

Normal metabolism is dependent on oxygen, a free radical. Through evolution, oxygen was chosen as the terminal electron acceptor for respiration. The two unpaired electrons of oxygen spin in the same direction; thus, oxygen is a biradical, but is not a very dangerous free radical. Other oxygen-derived free radical species, such as superoxide or hydroxyl radicals, formed during metabolism or by ionizing radiation are stronger oxidants and are therefore more dangerous.

In addition to research on the biological effects of these reactive oxygen species, research on reactive nitrogen species has been gathering momentum. NO, or nitrogen monoxide (nitric oxide), is a free radical generated by NO synthase (NOS). This enzyme modulates physiological responses such as vasodilation or signaling in the brain. However, during inflammation, synthesis of NOS (iNOS) is induced. This iNOS can result in the overproduction of NO, causing damage. More worrisome, however, is the fact that excess NO can react with superoxide to produce the very toxic product peroxynitrite. Oxidation of lipids, proteins, and DNA can result, thereby increasing the likelihood of tissue injury.

Both reactive oxygen and nitrogen species are involved in normal cell regulation in which oxidants and redox status are important in signal transduction. Oxidative stress is increasingly seen as a major upstream component in the signaling cascade involved in inflammatory responses, stimulating adhesion molecule and chemoattractant production. Hydrogen peroxide, which breaks down to produce hydroxyl radicals, can also activate NF-κB, a transcription factor involved in stimulating inflammatory responses. Excess production of these reactive species is toxic, exerting cytostatic effects, causing membrane damage, and activating pathways of cell death (apoptosis and/or necrosis).

Virtually all diseases thus far examined involve free radicals. In most cases, free radicals are secondary to the disease process, but in some instances free radicals are causal. Thus, there is a delicate balance between oxidants and antioxidants in health and disease. Their proper balance is essential for ensuring healthy aging.

The term *oxidative stress* indicates that the antioxidant status of cells and tissues is altered by exposure to oxidants. The redox status is thus dependent on the degree to which a cell's components are in the oxidized state. In general, the reducing environment inside cells helps to prevent oxidative damage. In this reducing environment, disulfide bonds (S—S) do not spontaneously form because sulfhydryl groups kept in the reduced state (SH) prevent protein misfolding or aggregation. This reducing environment is maintained by oxidative metabolism and by the action of antioxidant enzymes and substances, such as glutathione, thioredoxin, vitamins E and C, and enzymes such as superoxide dismutase (SOD), catalase, and the selenium-dependent glutathione and thioredoxin hydroperoxidases, which serve to remove reactive oxygen species.

Changes in the redox status and depletion of antioxidants occur during oxidative stress. The thiol redox status is a useful index of oxidative stress mainly because metabolism and NADPH-dependent enzymes maintain cell glutathione (GSH) almost completely in its reduced state. Oxidized glutathione (glutathione disulfide, GSSG) accumulates under conditions of oxidant exposure, and this changes the ratio of oxidized to reduced glutathione; an increased ratio indicates oxidative stress. Many tissues contain large amounts of glutathione, 2–4 mM in erythrocytes or neural tissues and up to 8 mM in hepatic tissues. Reactive oxygen and nitrogen species can directly react with glutathione to lower the levels of this substance, the cell's primary preventative antioxidant.

Current hypotheses favor the idea that lowering oxidative stress can have a clinical benefit. Free radicals can be overproduced or the natural antioxidant system defenses weakened, first resulting in oxidative stress, and then leading to oxidative injury and disease. Examples of this process include heart disease and cancer. Oxidation of human low-density lipoproteins is considered the first step in the progression and eventual development of atherosclerosis, leading to cardiovascular disease. Oxidative DNA damage initiates carcinogenesis.

Compelling support for the involvement of free radicals in disease development comes from epidemiological studies showing that an enhanced antioxidant status is associated with reduced risk of several diseases. Vitamin E and prevention of cardiovascular disease is a notable example. Elevated antioxidant status is also associated with decreased incidence of cataracts and cancer, and some recent reports have suggested an inverse correlation between antioxidant status and occurrence of rheumatoid arthritis and diabetes mellitus. Indeed, the number of indications in which antioxidants may be useful in the prevention and/or the treatment of disease is increasing.

Oxidative stress, rather than being the primary cause of disease, is more often a secondary complication in many disorders. Oxidative stress diseases include inflammatory bowel diseases, retinal ischemia, cardiovascular disease and restenosis, AIDS, ARDS, and neurodegenerative diseases such as stroke, Parkinson's disease, and Alzheimer's disease. Such indications may prove amenable to antioxidant treatment because there is a clear involvement of oxidative injury in these disorders.

In this series of books, the importance of oxidative stress in diseases associated with organ systems of the body is highlighted by exploring the scientific evidence and the medical applications of this knowledge. The series also highlights the major natural antioxidant enzymes and antioxidant substances such as vitamins E, A, and C, flavonoids, polyphenols, carotenoids, lipoic acid, and other nutrients present in food and beverages.

Oxidative stress is an underlying factor in health and disease. More and more evidence indicates that a proper balance between oxidants and antioxidants is involved in maintaining health and longevity and that altering this balance in favor of oxidants may result in pathological responses causing functional disorders and disease. This series is intended for researchers in the basic biomedical sciences and clinicians. The potential for healthy aging and disease prevention necessitates gaining further knowledge about how oxidants and antioxidants affect biological systems.

The vital role of carotenoids in photosynthetic plants has been widely investigated for many years. Carotenoids synthesized in green plants are essential for the assembly, function, and stability of photosynthetic pigment–protein complexes. The light-harvesting function of carotenoids allows blue and green sunlight to be used for energy conversion. This involves energy transfer of carotenoid singlet excited states to nearby chlorphylls. Carotenoids also quench free radicals, which are produced in very high amounts by sunlight and are a product of metabolism in humans.

In recent decades the presence of carotenoids in our food supply and their role in human health have been of unprecedented interest. Some carotenoids are provitamin A precursors, and about a dozen carotenoids are found in human plasma, depending on diets rich in green fruits and vegetables, and yellow/red or yellow/orange vegetables. Fifty to sixty carotenoids are typically present in the human diet and several are found in human plasma, including α-carotene, β-carotene, lycopene, zeaxanthin, and lutein. Carotenoids are potent antioxidants and are known to affect many different cellular pathways. Zeaxanthin and lutein are accumulated in the fovea of the human eye and are thought to play a role in preventing damage to this region of the eye by blue light, an effect thought to be linked to age-related macular degeneration, the most common cause of irreversible blindness. Numerous epidemiological, interventional, and clinical human studies have been performed or are currently underway to elucidate more precisely the possible role of carotenoids and their stereoisomers and metabolites in human health and disease. The editors are to be congratulated on assembling chapters that address many of these topics in this timely publication.

Lester Packer
Enrique Cadenas

Preface

This volume is a collection of chapters by leading carotenoid researchers depicting the role or roles of carotenoids in human health and disease. The first multi-authored book on carotenoids, edited by Otto Isler of Hoffman-La Roche and published in 1971 (1), consisted of 12 chapters dealing primarily with different aspects of carotenoid chemistry. Only one chapter addressed the function of carotenoids (2). Since then, interest in carotenoids has shifted from the chemistry of this interesting class of compounds to their actions in plants, animals, and humans. We know that carotenoids have an important role in photosynthesis, and two excellent volumes devoted to this topic have been published (3, 4). However, there has not been a book devoted to the role of carotenoids in health and disease until this one. Although individual articles have been published in an attempt to present this material, sufficient information is now available to warrant publicaton of a comprehensive text. One of our reasons for compiling a volume devoted to carotenoids in health and disease was to put into a clear perspective the results of observational epidemiological studies, clinical studies, and intervention trials involving carotenoids that are continuing to this day. For example, what was intended to be an evaluation of the role of β-carotene in lung cancer prevention appears to have resulted in the demonstration of a unique relationship between high-dose β-carotene supplementation, smoking, and elevated cancer risk. This observation, which was totally unexpected, has led to new studies and observations to explain these unusual results.

But there is much more to carotenoids than β-carotene. Of the more than 600 carotenoids identified in nature, as many as 50, all of which may have differing biological activities, may be included in a typical human diet. This poses a serious challenge to investigators, particularly as they try to tease out the effects of individual carotenoids from the mixture that normally occurs in foods. Recent research has shown that risk of several chronic diseases is inversely related to the intake of dietary carotenoids. This deserves a very careful evaluation because carotenoids are a particularly widespread dietary component, thus if they are related to disease prevention, it should be relatively easy and inexpensive to alter the diets of individuals potentially susceptible to such diseases. These issues are addressed in several chapters in this volume.

Several carotenoids in addition to β-carotene deserve particular attention with respect to health and disease prevention. One is lycopene, the major pigment present in tomatoes and tomato products, which has been associated with a decreased risk of several cancers such as prostate cancer. In addition, the oxygen-containing (xanthophyll) carotenoids lutein and zeaxanthin (the major pigments in the macular region of primate eyes) have been proposed both as markers for age-related macular degeneration and as possible therapeutic agents to prevent this disease. For these carotenoids, clinical studies and intervention trials are underway to evaluate the validity of these relationships.

One may ask why a book is necessary for a class of compounds that have never been identified as being essential for humans. We are aware that no study has indicated that individuals placed on a completely carotenoid-free diet have experienced deficiency symptoms. But we may be well beyond deficiency symptoms when we deal with compounds such as the carotenoids or other families of plant products. There is compelling evidence that several of our dietary carotenoids exert profound effects on cellular processes when added to cell cultures at human physiological levels. Several chapters in this book describe these actions and give guidelines for what we may expect to find in humans. There are certainly strong suggestions that carotenoid intake is associated with 'good health.' But is this due to the carotenoids or to other components of the foods in which the carotenoids are present? We may be years away from answering this question, but we will do our best to present the current state of science in the field.

We are grateful to our authors for their contributions to the evaluation of carotenoids in human health and disease.

Norman I. Krinsky
Susan T. Mayne
Helmut Sies

REFERENCES

1. Isler O, Gutman H, Solms U. Carotenoids. Basel: Birkhäuser Verlag, 1971.
2. Krinsky NI. Function of carotenoids. In: Carotenoids. Isler O, Gutman H, Solms U, eds. Basel/Stuttgart: Birkhäuser Verlag, 1971: 669–716.
3. Young A, Britton G. Carotenoids in Photosynthesis. London: Chapman & Hall, 1993.
4. Frank HA, Young AJ, Britton G, Cogdell, R.J. The Photochemistry of Carotenoids. Dordrecht: Kluwer Academic, 1999.

Contents

Contributors

Demetrius Albanes, M.D. Division of Cancer Epidemiology and Genetics, National Cancer Institute, National Institutes of Health, Bethesda, Maryland, U.S.A.

Eileen Ang The University of Melbourne, Melbourne, Victoria, Australia

Arun B. Barua, Ph.D. Department of Biochemistry, Biophysics and Molecular Biology, Iowa State University, Ames, Iowa, U.S.A.

Paul S. Bernstein, M.D., Ph.D. Department of Ophthalmology and Visual Sciences, Moran Eye Center, School of Medicine, University of Utah, Salt Lake City, Utah, U.S.A.

Amy C. Boileau, Ph.D., R.D. Department of Regulatory Affairs, Abbott Laboratories, Columbus, Ohio, U.S.A.

Richard A. Bone, Ph.D. Department of Physics, Florida International University, Miami, Florida, U.S.A.

Ann Cantrell Department of Chemistry, Lennard-Jones Laboratories, Keele University, Keele, Staffordshire, England

Richard M. Clark, Ph.D. Department of Nutritional Sciences, University of Connecticut, Storrs, Connecticut, U.S.A.

Steven K. Clinton, M.D., Ph.D.   Department of Internal Medicine, The Ohio State University, Columbus, Ohio, U.S.A.

Michael Danilenko, Ph.D.   Department of Clinical Biochemistry, Faculty of Health Sciences, Ben Gurion University of the Negev and Soroka Medical Center of Kupat Holim, Beer-Sheva, Israel

John W. Erdman, Jr., Ph.D.   Division of Nutritional Sciences, Department of Food Science and Human Nutrition, University of Illinois, Urbana, Illinois, U.S.A.

Mario G. Ferruzzi, Ph.D.   Nestle Research Center, Lausanne, Switzerland

Harold C. Furr, Ph.D.   Craft Technologies, Inc., Wilson, North Carolina, U.S.A.

J. Michael Gaziano, M.D., M.P.H.   Divisions of Preventive Medicine and Aging, Department of Medicine, Brigham and Women's Hospital and Harvard Medical School, and Massachusetts Veterans Epidemiology Research and Information Center, VA Boston Healthcare System, Boston, Massachusetts, U.S.A.

Werner Gellermann, Ph.D.   Department of Physics and Dixon Laser Institute, University of Utah, Salt Lake City, Utah, U.S.A.

Wieslaw I. Gruszecki, Ph.D.   Department of Biophysics, Institute of Physics, Maria Curie-Sklodowska University, Lublin, Poland

David A. Hughes, Ph.D., R.Nutr., CertCRGCP   Nutrition Division, Institute of Food Research, Norwich, Norfolk, England

Norman I. Krinsky, Ph.D.   Department of Biochemistry, School of Medicine, and Jean Mayer USDA Human Nutrition Research Center on Aging, Tufts University, Boston, Massachusetts, U.S.A.

Mrinal K. Kundu, Ph.D.   Department of Chemistry, University of Basel, Basel, Switzerland

John T. Landrum, Ph.D.   Department of Chemistry, Florida International University, Miami, Florida, U.S.A.

Joseph Levy, Ph.D.   Department of Clinical Biochemistry, Faculty of Health Sciences, Ben Gurion University of the Negev and Soroka Medical Center of Kupat Holim, Beer-Sheva, Israel

Synnøve Liaaen-Jensen, Dr. techn., Dr. Sc. Department of Chemistry, Norwegian University of Science and Technology, Trondheim, Norway

Gordon M. Lowe School of Biological and Earth Sciences, Liverpool John Moores University, Liverpool, England

Julie A. Mares, Ph.D. Department of Ophthalmology, University of Wisconsin–Madison, Madison, Wisconsin, U.S.A.

Micheline M. Mathews-Roth, M.D. Channing Laboratory, Department of Medicine, Harvard Medical School and Brigham and Women's Hospital, Boston, Massachusetts, U.S.A.

Susan T. Mayne, Ph.D. Department of Epidemiology and Public Health, Yale University School of Medicine, New Haven, Connecticut, U.S.A.

Elizabeth C. Miller, M.S., R.D. Department of Internal Medicine, The Ohio State University, Columbus, Ohio, U.S.A.

Nora O'Brien, Ph.D. Department of Food and Nutritional Sciences, University College, Cork, Ireland

Tom O'Connor, Ph.D. Department of Food and Nutritional Sciences, University College, Cork, Ireland

Paola Palozza, M.D. Institute of General Pathology, Catholic University, Rome, Italy

Denise M. Phillip, Ph.D. School of Biological and Earth Sciences, Liverpool John Moores University, Liverpool, England

Cheryl L. Rock, Ph.D. Department of Family and Preventive Medicine, Cancer Prevention and Control, University of California, San Diego, La Jolla, California, U.S.A.

Robert M. Russell, M.D. Jean Mayer USDA Human Nutrition Research Center on Aging, Tufts University, Boston, Massachusetts, U.S.A.

Steven J. Schwartz, Ph.D. Department of Food Science and Graduate Program in Nutrition, The Ohio State University, Columbus, Ohio, U.S.A.

Howard D. Sesso, Sc.D., M.P.H. Divisions of Preventive Medicine and Aging, Department of Medicine, Brigham and Women's Hospital and Harvard Medical School, and Massachusetts Veterans Epidemiology Research and Information Center, VA Boston Healthcare System, Boston, Massachusetts, U.S.A.

Yoav Sharoni, Ph.D.   Department of Clinical Biochemistry, Faculty of Health Sciences, Ben Gurion University of the Negev and Soroka Medical Center of Kupat Holim, Beer-Sheva, Israel

Helmut Sies, M.D.   Department of Biochemistry and Molecular Biology I, Faculty of Medicine, Heinrich-Heine-Universität, Düsseldorf, Germany

Wilhelm Stahl, Ph.D.   Department of Biochemistry and Molecular Biology I, Faculty of Medicine, Heinrich-Heine-Universität, Düsseldorf, Germany

Guangwen Tang, Ph.D.   Carotenoids and Health Laboratory, Jean Mayer USDA Human Nutrition Research Center on Aging, Tufts University, Boston, Massachusetts, U.S.A.

T. George Truscott, Ph.D.   Department of Chemistry, Lennard-Jones Laboratories, Keele University, Keele, Staffordshire, England

Johannes von Lintig, Ph.D.   Institut für Biologie I, Universität Freiburg, Freiburg, Germany

Xiang-Dong Wang, M.D., Ph.D.   Nutrition and Cancer Biology Laboratory, Jean Mayer USDA Human Nutrition Research Center on Aging, Tufts University, Boston, Massachusetts, U.S.A.

Wolf-D. Woggon, Ph.D.   Department of Chemistry, University of Basel, Basel, Switzerland

Margaret E. Wright, Ph.D.   Nutritional Epidemiology Branch, Division of Cancer Epidemiology and Genetics, National Cancer Institute, National Institutes of Health, Bethesda, Maryland, U.S.A.

Andrew J. Young, Ph.D.   School of Biological and Earth Sciences, Liverpool John Moores University, Liverpool, England

1
Basic Carotenoid Chemistry

Synnøve Liaaen-Jensen
Norwegian University of Science and Technology, Trondheim, Norway

I. INTRODUCTION

This chapter deals with the chemical foundation for the other chapters in this book. For more detailed treatments reference is made particularly to comprehensive recent treatments, including the *Carotenoids* book series published by Birkhäuser, namely Vol. 1A, *Isolation and Analysis* (1); Vol. 1B, *Spectroscopy* (2); Vol. 2, *Synthesis* (3); and Vol. 3, *Biosynthesis and Metabolism* (4). Other useful references are the *Key to Carotenoids* (5) and the *Carotenoid Handbook* (6), giving structures and references to all known naturally occurring carotenoids. Whereas the former *Key* (5) is exhaustive, the new *Carotenoid Handbook* (6) gives a critical evaluation of published data and selected, recommended references to diagnostic evidence for established structures.

In this chapter selected carotenoid chemistry is treated that is relevant to the other topics covered in this book. Examples are chosen from carotenoids present in sources of importance in nutrition and health. Such sources include fruits, vegetables, algae, chicken, eggs, and fish. Furthermore, relevant to humans are the carotenoids in serum and retina.

II. CAROTENOIDS: GENERAL STRUCTURE

A. Structure and Properties

Carotenoids are usually yellow–red isoprenoid polyene pigments widely distributed in nature. The majority are tetraterpenes formally composed of eight

isoprene units, typically β-carotene (**1**). Also known are so-called higher
carotenoids with C$_{45}$ and C$_{50}$ (e.g., bacterioruberin, **2**) carbon skeletons.
Carotenoids with fewer than 40 C atoms are classified as C$_{30}$ carotenoids or
diapocarotenoids (actually triterpenes such as **3**), as apocarotenoids that are
formally in-chain oxidized carotenoids, or as norcarotenoids where carbon atoms
are formally removed from the skeleton. Hydrocarbons are referred to as
carotenes and oxygenated derivatives as carotenoids. Elements other than carbon,
hydrogen, and oxygen are not directly attached to the carbon skeleton in naturally
occurring carotenoids.

The most characteristic structural feature of a carotenoid is the conjugated polyene chain. The polyene chain represents a chromophore responsible for the characteristic colors, going from colorless (phytoene, **4**), to yellow
(4,4′-diaponeurosporene, **3**), orange (β-carotene, **1**), red (paprika pigment
capsanthin, **5**), pink (bacterioruberin, **2**) and blue with an increasing number of
conjugated double bonds. When associated with proteins as carotenoproteins
a dark blue color is obtained, as, for example, crustacyanin in lobster shells
(**7,8**). Unstable reaction intermediates such as carotenoid radical ions,
monocations and dications (**6**) absorb light in the near-infrared (NIR) region
(800–1000 nm) (**9**). The polyene chain is also responsible for the general
instability of carotenoids towards air oxidation, strong acids, oxidizing
reagents, heat and light, necessitating particular precautions during isolation
processes. Work with carotenoids must therefore take place under subdued light
in an inert atmos-phere (N$_2$) in the absence of strong acids and peroxides.

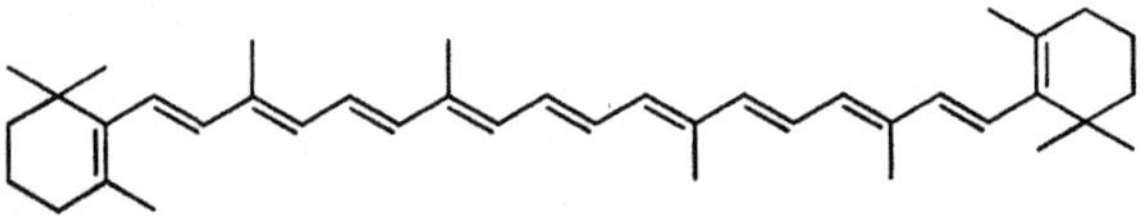

β-Carotene (**1**)

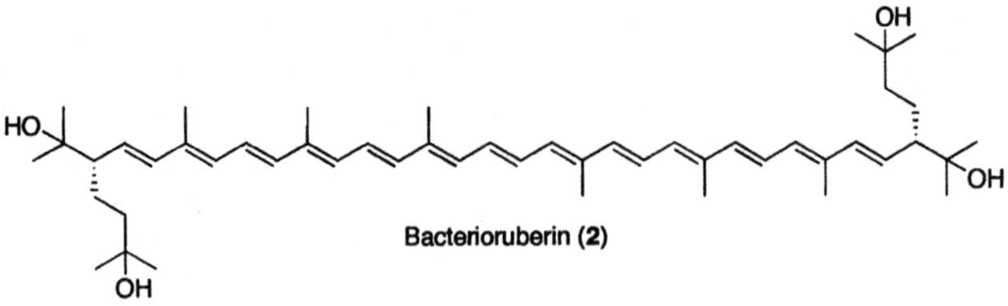

Bacterioruberin (**2**)

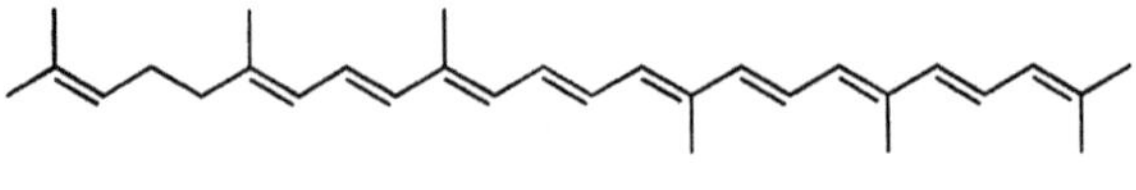

4,4′-Diaponeurosporene (**3**)

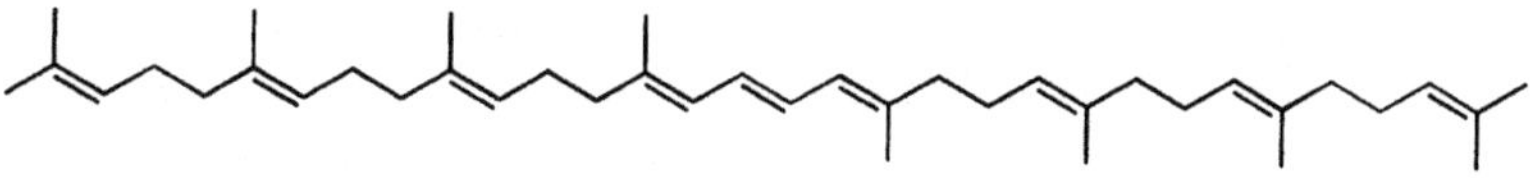

Phytoene (4)

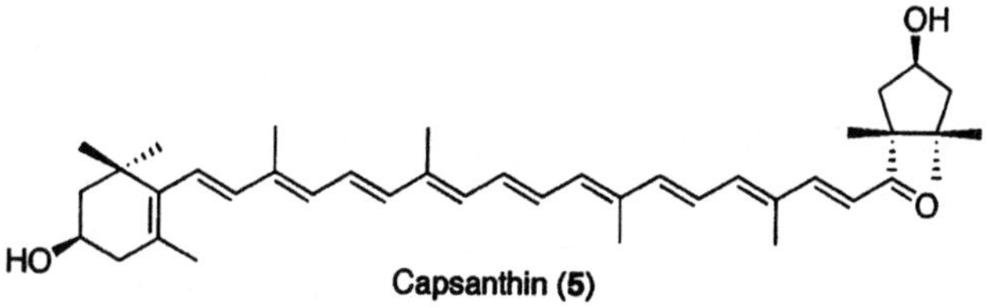

Capsanthin (5)

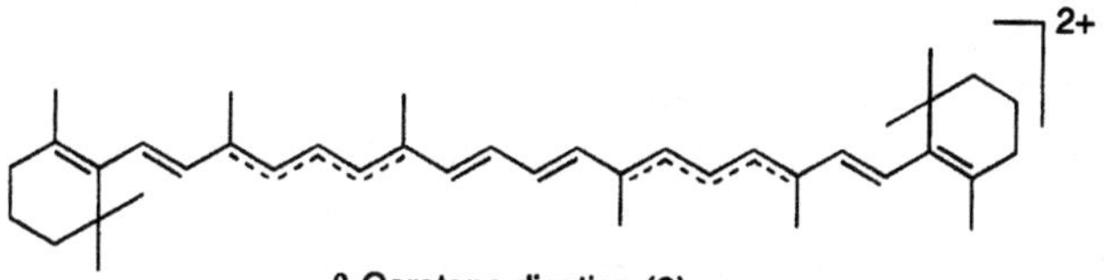

β-Carotene dication (6)

Furthermore the polyene chain is the basis for *cis-trans* isomerism, a very characteristic phenomenon in the carotenoid field, discussed in Part V.

Carotenoids may also contain acetylenic bonds and allenic bonds. Other functional groups in carotenoids are oxygen functions such as hydroxyl, methoxy, cyclic ethers, keto, aldehyde, carboxylic acids, lactones, acyl esters, glycosides, glycosyl esters, and sulfates. The reader is referred to the useful *Key to Carotenoids* (5) and the updated *Carotenoid Handbook* (6) for complete surveys. An example of a more complex structure is pyrrhoxanthin (7 *ex* dinoflagellates). It is a C_{38} norcarotenoid containing an acetylenic bond, an acyl ester (acetate), a butenolide-type lactone, cyclic ether (epoxide), and a secondary hydroxyl group.

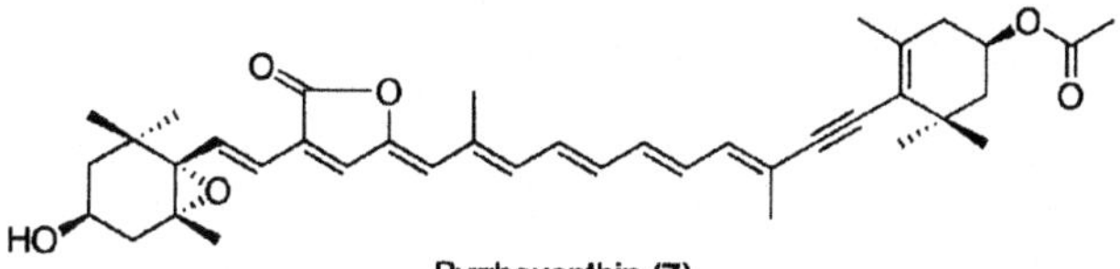

Pyrrhoxanthin (7)

Carotenoids that are important in health and nutrition have in general rather simple structures. Discussed in this chapter is particularly β-carotene (**1**), zeaxanthin, lutein, astaxanthin, lycopene, prolycopene, and neoxanthin.

It is the functional groups that are mainly responsible for the degree of polarity of the various carotenoids, as well as for their solubilities and chemical behavior.

B. Nomenclature

The approved numbering of the carotenoid skeleton is included for β-carotene (1) below. Most carotenoids have been assigned short trivial names useful in oral communication. In addition, IUPAC/IUB has published a semirational nomenclature system (10), defining the chemical structure in an unambiguous way, including the stereochemistry (three-dimensional structure) as treated below. In this system, β-carotene (trivial name) is β,β-carotene (semirational), thus denoting the two β end groups.

Examples of more complex rational names are fucoxanthin (8) present in Japanese algal food, and citranaxanthin (9) obtained from citrus fruits. Fucoxanthin (8) has several functional groups, including *sec.* and *tert.* hydroxyl, epoxy, keto, allene, and is a natural acetate. The R/S designation denotes the chirality (absolute stereochemistry) (see below). Citranaxanthin is a C_{30} apocarotenoid with an abbreviated carbon skeleton.

β-Carotene (1) with carbon numbers

Fucoxanthin (8)
(3S,5R,6S,3'S,5'R,6'R)-5,6-Epoxy-3'-ethanoyloxy-3,5'-dihydroxy-6',7'-didehydro-5,6,7,8,5',6'-hexahydro-β,β-caroten-8-one

Citranaxanthin (9)
5',6'-Dihydro-5'-apo-18'-nor-β-carotene-6'-one

It has been recommended that the semirational name should be given at least once in all carotenoid papers. Unfortunately, this has not been implemented in a consistent manner.

C. Occurrence

Carotenoids are synthesized de novo by all photosynthetic organisms, including phytoplankton, algae, higher plants, and phototrophic bacteria. In addition, they are produced by some other bacteria, yeasts, and fungi. Carotenoids are selectively absorbed in the various food chains, where they may undergo metabolic structural changes. For further information the reader is referred to chapters on occurrence (5,11,12) and on chemosystematics (4,11,12) elsewhere. Sources of carotenoids are also treated in Chapter 11 of this book.

III. ANALYSIS

In short the quantitative analysis of carotenoid mixtures involves suitable handling of the biological material; solvent extraction; optional saponification for removal of chlorophylls, fats, and so forth; chromatography on columns (large samples); thin-layer chromatography (TLC) and high-performance liquid chromatography (HPLC), taking the general precautions for work with carotenoids (1,2). This requires manipulations in an inert atmosphere or at reduced pressure, in subdued light, at the lowest possible temperature and in the absence of acids and of peroxides in the solvents. Quantification is based on known or approximate extinction coefficients for visible light absorption (1). Because exact extinction coefficients are frequently not known, e.g., for unknown components, for *cis* isomers (see Sec. IV), etc., caution should be made in quoting too exact results. The author discourages stating relative percentage composition with decimals.

General comprehensive treatments on isolation and analysis are available (1,2). Analysis of carotenoids in humans (Chapter 4) and HPLC analysis of human carotenoids (Chapter 5) are treated in detail in this book.

IV. SPECTROSCOPY

For comprehensive treatment of spectroscopic methods employed in studies of carotenoids, the reader is referred to a recent monograph (2). In the following the key information on carotenoid structure obtained by each of the most commonly used spectroscopic methods is considered.

A. Absorption Spectra in Visible Light

Electronic absorption spectra in the visible (VIS) region are indispensible for work on carotenoids. Carotenoids have strong light absorption (a high extinction coefficient) in visible light, and the VIS spectrum is used for quantitative determination of the carotenoid content in solutions. Exact extinction coefficients are available for most all-*trans* carotenoids. Extinction coefficients for *cis* isomers are generally lower and not readily available. Consequently, the content of *cis* isomers is frequently underestimated by using the extinction coefficient of the all-*trans* isomer. For unknown mixtures an approximate $A_{1\,cm}^{1\%} = 2500$ in hexane or acetone may be used.

The exact position of the absorption maxima and the spectral profile of the VIS spectrum provide most useful information. The absorption profiles are included for each structurally identified naturally occurring carotenoid in the new *Carotenoid Handbook* (6) and in a survey of algal carotenoids (13). The spectral fine structure may be expressed as %III/II (Fig. 1).

The length and type of chromophore and any conjugated carbonyl functions are reflected by the VIS spectrum. In entirely aliphatic systems (polyene chain not extending into terminal rings) the main middle λ_{max} increases in wavelength in hexane solvent from 397 nm (heptaene chromophore), 424 nm (octaene), 439 nm (nonaene), 454 nm (decaene), 472 nm (undecaene), 481 nm (dodecaene), to 493 nm (tridecaene) with the highest spectral fine structure for the nonaene system with nine conjugated double bonds.

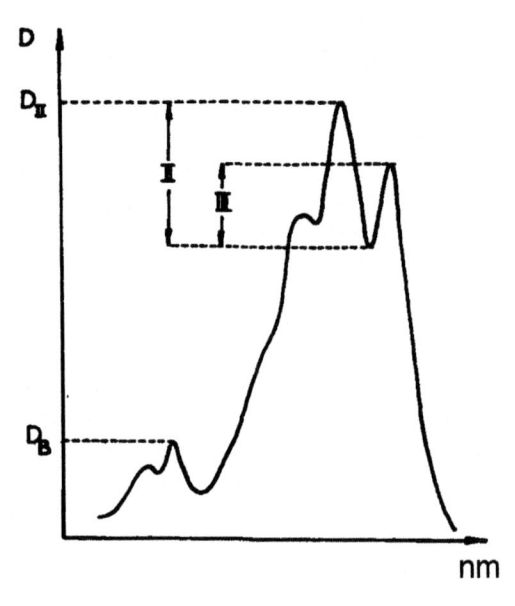

Figure 1 Explanation of terms used in expressions for describing the shape of the absorption spectrum in visible light (14).

Conjugated double bonds in the terminal rings contribute less to the bathochromic shift (to longer wavelength), and the spectral fine structure is reduced due to steric conflict between the ring and the polyene system. Conjugated carbonyl groups usually result in considerable reduction of spectral fine structure, particularly in a solvent such as methanol.

The presence of *cis* double bonds (see Sec. V) generally results in hypsochromic shifts (to lower wavelength), roughly by about 4 nm for one *cis* bond and more for two *cis* bonds. This change is accompanied by the appearance of a so-called *cis* peak at a position about 142 nm hypsochromically displaced from the longest wavelength maximum of the all-*trans* isomer in hexane solvent. For aliphatic systems the *cis* peak is double. The intensity of the *cis* peak may be expressed as $\%D_B/D_{II}$ (Fig. 1). The relative intensity of the *cis* peak increases toward the center of the carotenoid molecule in this manner *cis*-15 > *cis*-13 > *cis*-9.

During isolation work with carotenoids frequent recording of VIS spectra is recommended to monitor the stability.

B. Mass Spectrometry

Mass spectrometry (MS) is essential for the identification of carotenoids, requiring only microgram quantities. Of the various methods now available, electron impact remains the most common ionization method (2). By high-precision measurements the exact elemental composition is obtained. By common low-resolution measurements the molecular ion gives the molecular weight without decimal figures. The identification of the molecular ion should be supported by reasonable fragment ions such as M-92 and M-106 from the polyene chain and M-H_2O for carotenols. Detailed consideration of the fragmentation pattern of pure carotenoids provides useful structural information (2).

C. Nuclear Magnetic Resonance

Proton magnetic resonance (^{1}H NMR) may, in the hands of experts, serve as the single spectroscopic method for complete structural determination of a pure carotenoid, including relative stereochemistry. This requires the application of suitable two-dimensional methods now available, such as ^{1}H,^{1}H COSY, 2D ROESY, and HMBC techniques. In combination with ^{13}C NMR additional information is obtained. In modern structural studies of carotenoids, complete ^{1}H NMR and ^{13}C NMR assignments serve to prove the structure unequivocally. The position of *cis* bonds in carotenoids is readily established by ^{1}H NMR spectroscopy (2).

The structural result of a modern NMR analysis of a complex carotenoid, namely, the microalgal carotenoid pyrrhoxanthin (**7**), referred to in Sec. II as an

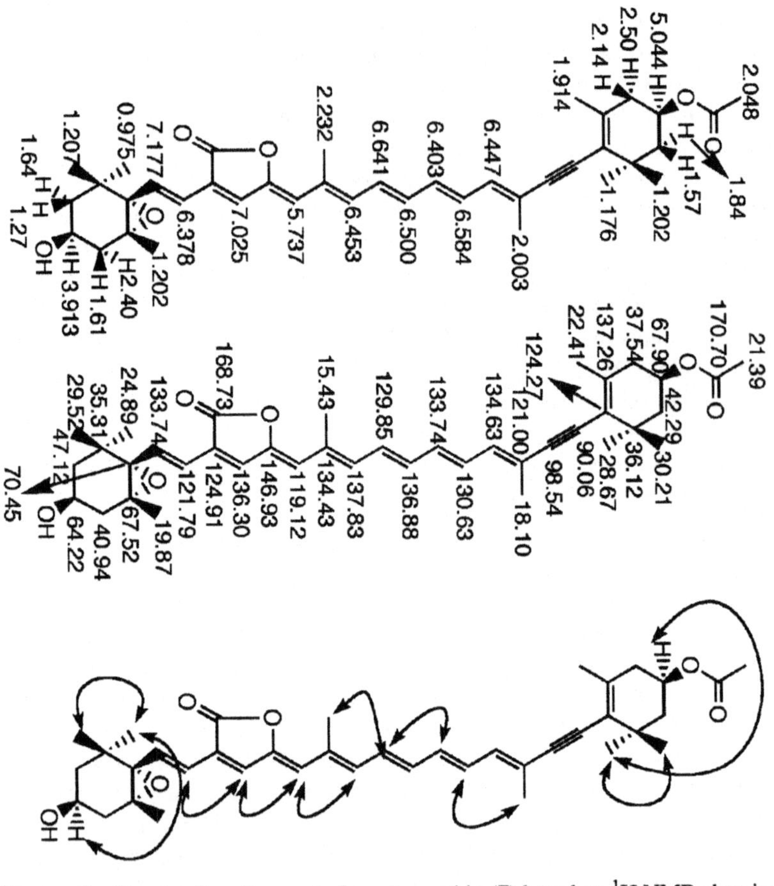

Figure 2 Structural assignment of pyrrhoxanthin (7) based on [^1]H NMR chemical shifts (top) and coupling constants, [^13]C NMR chemical shifts (middle), and 2D ROESY data (bottom) showing in-space interactions (15).

example of a carotenoid with complex structure, is illustrated in Fig. 2 (15). Further treatment is beyond the scope of this book.

D. Infrared Spectra

Infrared (IR) spectra, less commonly used nowadays, serve in structural determinations to identify functional groups, particularly different types of carbonyl functions, allenes, acetylenic bonds, and so forth, including functionalities such as sulfate that are not directly evident in NMR spectra.

E. Circular Dichroism

NMR spectroscopy serves to define relative configuration only. Absolute configuration (chirality; see Sec. VI) may in principle only be determined by direct comparison with a synthetic carotenoid of known stereochemistry or by X-ray analysis. Only some simple carotenoids have been successfully analyzed by X-ray spectroscopy due to problems in obtaining suitable crystals. However, certain key carotenoids have been degraded, and defined degradation products containing the chiral centers have been successfully studied by X-ray analysis and chiralities assigned.

Circular dichroism (CD) serves as a useful method for stereochemical correlation of carotenoids of known chirality with carotenoids under investigation. For a detailed treatment one can refer to a recent overview (2). The structural requirement for obtaining a CD spectrum is treated in Sec. VI. CD spectra can be obtained on microgram quantities of chromatographically pure carotenoids. Unfortunately, CD instruments are less available than the other spectrometers mentioned here.

It should be noted that for certain carotenoids exhibiting so-called conservative CD spectra (with several positive and negative maxima of high intensity, integrating to about zero), the presence of a *cis* bond results in mirror image CD. Hence, the presence of contaminating *cis* isomers causes problems. The intensity of the CD spectra is temperature dependent. Weak CD at room temperature is enhanced at a lower temperature ($-180°C$).

With reference to Sec. VI, enantiomeric carotenoids (with mirror image structures) exhibit mirror image CD spectra. Not all chiral centers influence the CD spectrum to the same extent. For instance, the absolute configuration of the 3'-hydroxy group of lutein (**10**) is not reflected in its CD spectrum, which is determined by the chiralities at C-3 and C-6'.

Lutein (**10**)

An additivy hypothesis, whereby the Cotton effect (CD contribution) of two chiral end groups in carotenoids of the same chromophore is additive (2,16), has been useful.

An example of conservative CD spectra is reproduced in Fig. 3, displaying (3S,3'S)-astaxanthin (**11**) and its enantiomer (**12**). The negligible CD of the in

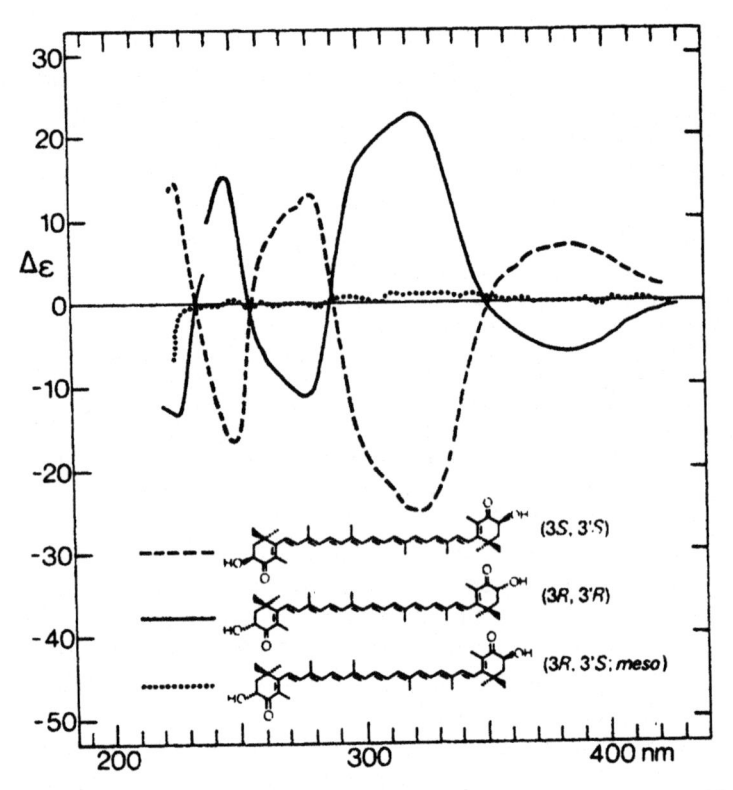

Figure 3 CD spectra in dichloromethane of (3S,3'S)-astaxanthin (**11**, – – – –), its enantiomer (3R,3'R)-astaxanthin (**12**, ———), and the (3R,3'S) *meso* form (**13**, ·········) (17).

principle optically inactive *meso* (**13**) form is also illustrated (17). For a closer treatment of chirality, see Sec. VI.

V. *CIS-TRANS* ISOMERISM

A. General Basis

Carbon–carbon double bonds located in cyclic parts of a carotenoid structure are in a sterically restricted position due to the ring system, e.g., the C-5,6 double bond in β-carotene (**1**) below. In principle each carbon–carbon double bond in the polyene chain of carotenoids may exhibit *cis* or *trans* configuration, as illustrated for lycopene (**14**) below. Some double bonds are called sterically hindered because the *cis* configuration leads to a sterically hindered configuration. While still referring to β-carotene (**1**), this is the case for the C-7,8, and the C-11,12 double bonds. This means that *cis* bonds are in practice formed under suitable conditions at C-9,10, C-13,14, the central C-15,15', and the C-13',14' and C-9',10' positions. Di-*cis* and poly-*cis* configurations are also possible but are energetically less favorable.

β-Carotene (1)

cis-Carotenoids differ from the parent all-*trans* isomer in VIS spectra, including the so-called *cis* peak (see Sec. IV), in adsorption affinity (HPLC, TLC), melting points, and solubility properties. *Cis* double bonds may also influence drastically the CD spectra of chiral carotenoids as mentioned in Sec. IV.

Assignment of *cis* configuration is based on VIS and NMR spectra or VIS/HPLC comparison with isomers obtained by total synthesis.

B. Nomenclature

According to the IUPAC nomenclature for carotenoids (10), the *cis-trans* convention is still used to denote the configuration of the polyene chain. *Cis* bonds have the largest substituents at each end of the double bond on the same side of the double bond. For a *trans* bond the largest substituents are on the opposite side. The more recent E/Z designation, based on the priority rules referred to for R/S absolute configuration in Sec. VI, may also be used and is unambiguous. In most cases *cis*-carotenoids have Z-configuration and *trans*-carotenoids E configuration. However, for in-chain substituted carotenoids, including pyrrhoxanthin (7), *cis* bonds represent the E-configuration.

C. Formation and Stability of *cis* Isomers

The generalization that all-*trans* carotenoids are usually the naturally occurring stereoisomer and the thermodynamically most stable one still holds, but with an increasing number of exceptions, e.g., the *Dunaliella* case discussed below. Bacteria living at extreme conditions frequently produce many *cis* isomers besides the all-*trans* carotenoid (18,19).

The *trans-cis* isomerization in solution is a facile process promoted by light, heat, and various catalysts. The common procedure is iodine-catalyzed stereoisomerization in light. Recently the application of diphenyldiselenide as an alternative catalyst has been explored for photochemical isomerization (20). This catalyst will at suitable conditions also isomerize allenic bonds (21), not further discussed here.

Detailed procedures for controlled *trans-cis* isomerization in the presence of iodine or diphenyldiselenide in appropriate solvents are available (20,21). The analysis is based on an HPLC instrument equipped with a diode array detector, allowing simultaneous recording of VIS spectra employing suitable columns. Irrespective of the starting isomer the same qualitative and quantitative equilibrium is reached. This is also the basis for reversibility tests, whereby an isomer is converted to the same equilibrium mixture, thereby confirming the parent all-*trans* carotenoid.

Iodine-catalyzed stereoisomerization leads to what was considered as a quasi-equilibrium defined by the conditions employed. However, since the application of diphenyldiselenide results in the same equilibrium, this is now considered to reflect the thermodynamic equilibrium (21).

In most cases, including common dicyclic carotenoids, the all-*trans* isomer is the dominating isomer in the thermodynamic equilibrium with lesser amounts of the *cis* isomers. This is, however, not the case for aliphatic carotenoids with very long polyene chains, for acetylenic carotenoids, and for so-called cross-conjugated carotenoids with in-chain aldehyde functions. Isomers with sterically hindered *cis* bonds, including prolycopene (**15**), are rare in nature, and are not encountered in this equilibrium mixture. Examples of such natural *cis* isomers, given below, include prolycopene (**15**) from a particular tomato variety, 9,9'-di-*cis*-alloxanthin (manixanthin, **16**) from old cultures of diatoms, and rhodopinal (**17**) from phototrophic purple bacteria.

Prolycopene (**15**, 7,9,7',9'-tetra*cis*-lycopene)

Manixanthin (**16**, 9,9'-di*cis*-alloxanthin)

Rhodopinal (**17**, 13-*cis*-rhodopin-20-al)

Since *cis* isomerization is such a facile process, *cis* isomerization inevitably occurs during the isolation and complicates the analysis of carotenoids. The *cis* isomers are in fact the most common isolation artifact, as discussed below in Sec. VIII.

D. β-Carotene

A detailed example for the analysis of *cis-trans* mixtures of β-carotene (**1**) can be found in (1). Whereas all-*trans* β-carotene (**1**) is the single geometrical isomer in most sources, the *Dunaliella bardawil (salina)* case deserves particular attention. In this green alga β-carotene (**1**) is produced in very large quantities as a so-called secondary carotenoid under extreme growth conditions (strong light and nitrogen deficiency). In this case the 9-*cis* isomer is the major isomer in addition to the all-*trans* isomer. The bent 9-*cis* isomer crystallizes less readily and is more soluble, which may offer advantages. The provitamin A activity is considered to be lower for the 9-*cis* than for the all-E isomer. For further comments, see Sec. VIII below.

9-*cis* β-Carotene (**1 b**)

E.   Lycopene

Lycopene (**14**) is a carotene with much current concern as to health aspects and prostate cancer (22). It is an entirely aliphatic carotene with a long conjugated undecaene (eleven) double-bond system, resulting in steric lability. The sterically unhindered mono-*cis* isomers (**14b–e**) are depicted below.

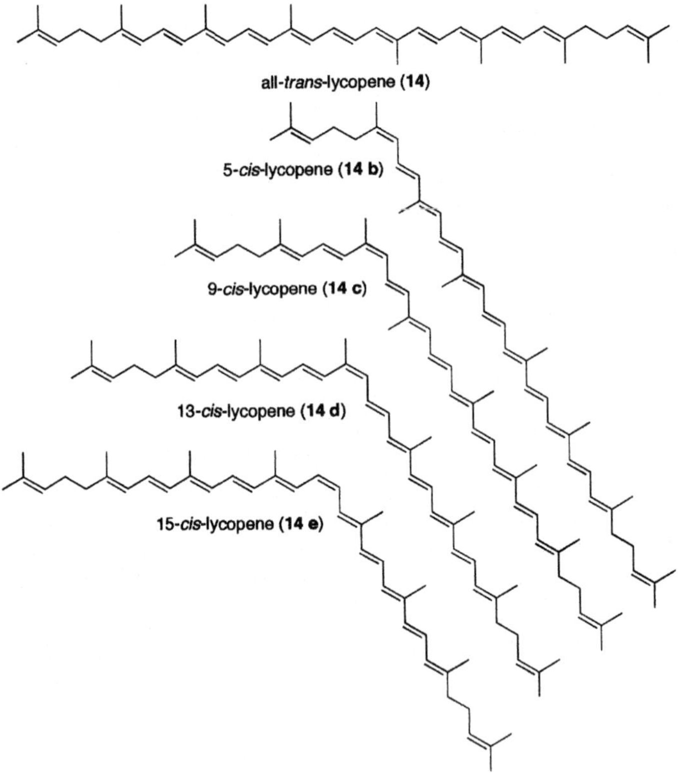

all-*trans*-lycopene (**14**)

5-*cis*-lycopene (**14 b**)

9-*cis*-lycopene (**14 c**)

13-*cis*-lycopene (**14 d**)

15-*cis*-lycopene (**14 e**)

The 5-*cis* isomer was overlooked until recently because of a difficult chromatographic separation from the all-*trans* isomer. Moreover, the all-*trans* and 5-*cis* isomers have identical VIS spectra and the *cis*-isomer with its terminal *cis* double bond has no characteristic *cis* peak.

However, the 5-*cis* isomer may now be successfully separated by HPLC analysis (23) and it now appears that when isomerized lycopene is present, the 5-*cis* isomer is always a dominating isomer besides the all-*trans*, e.g., in human blood (24).

In elegant synthetic work as many as 14 different *cis* isomers of lycopene (**14**) have been prepared by stereoselective total synthesis or isomerization and fully characterized by VIS spectra, HPLC, and NMR (23). This includes all sterically unhindered mono-*cis* isomers (**14b–e**) and the sterically hindered 7-*cis* isomer as well as several di-*cis* and tri-*cis* isomers and prolycopene (**15**). Prolycopene (7-*cis*, 9-*cis*, 7'-*cis*, 9'-*cis*) is naturally occurring in a particular tomato variety and has four *cis* bonds, two of which are sterically hindered.

An example of the state of the art is shown in an HPLC diagram (Fig. 4) of a lycopene mixture obtained by isomerizing all-*trans* lycopene (**14**) in refluxing heptane in the absence of catalyst and after filtration (24). The mixture consequently does not represent the thermodynamic equilibrium. In the particular

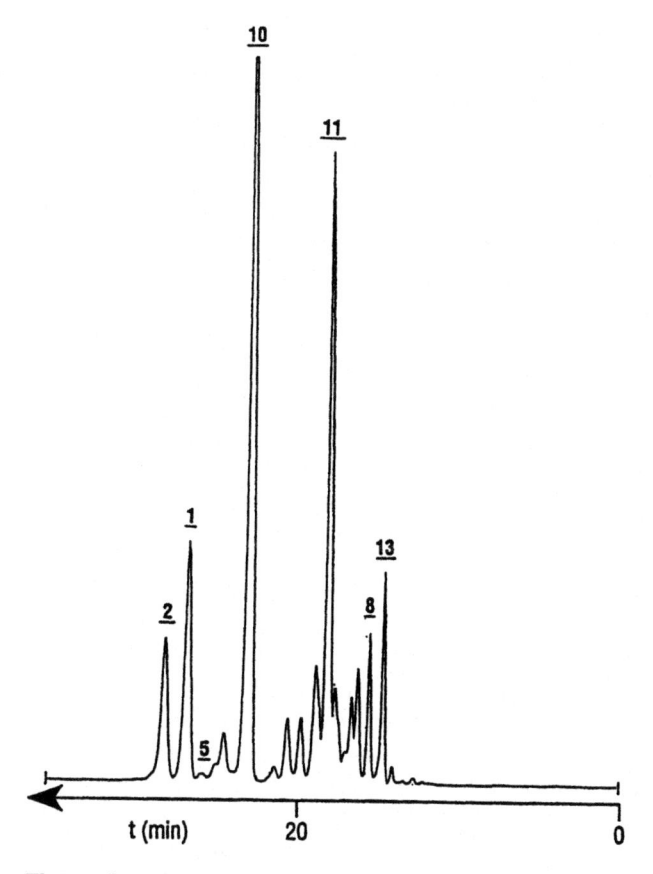

Figure 4 HPLC separation of a *cis-trans* mixture of lycopene on a Nucleosil 300-5 column developed with hexane containing 0.05% ethyldiisopropylamine (23). For peak identification, see text.

system developed for this HPLC separation the dominant mono-*cis* isomers [peak 2 = 5-*cis* (**14b**), peak 10 = 9-*cis* (**14c**), peak 11 = 13-*cis* (**14d**)] were well separated and exhibit shorter retention times than most of the di-*cis* isomers (peak 5 = 5,5'-di-*cis*, peak 8 = 9,9'-di-*cis*, peak 13 = 9,13'-di-*cis*). Peak 1 represents the all-*trans* (**14**) isomer.

VI. CHIRALITY

A. Definitions

We shall here define the terms chiral, achiral, chiral center, chiral carbon atom, chiral axis, enantiomer, *meso* form, diastereomer, epimer, racemization, and the requirements for optical activity and CD.

A chiral compound has a nonidentical mirror image. Thus, a sphere is not chiral because it is identical to its mirror image. It is achiral. The most popular example of a chiral subject is a hand. The right hand is the mirror image of the left hand. They are clearly not identical, as proved by trying to put a right-hand glove on the left hand.

The majority of the known carotenoids are chiral. The chirality is due to the presence of chiral centers, in most cases one or more chiral carbon atoms; for chiral axis, see below. A chiral carbon has four different substituents, e.g., H, OH, CH, CH_2.

The nonidentical mirror form is called an enantiomer. Enantiomers have identical physical properties, except for optical properties. Enantiomers can therefore not be separated by common chromatographic methods. A chiral chromatographic system (expensive columns) is required. Typical examples of enantiomers are the two astaxathins **11** and **12**, where the two chiral centers are both reverted (see Sec. IV.E). If only one chiral center is reverted in astaxanthin we have a special case, called a *meso* form (**13**). Since the two chiral centers in the the *meso* form are opposite we have a so-called internal compensation. This results in no optical activity of the *meso* form **13** in contrast to **11** and **12** which have opposite optical activities. Lack of optical activity also results for a 1:1 mixture of enantiomers. A process whereby a chiral center is converted to the opposite configuration (chirality) is called racemization.

Diastereomers contain two or more chiral centers. They differ in configuration at one or more, but not all chiral centers. Diastereomers have different physical properties and may in principle be separated upon chromatography.

Epimers represent a special case of diastereomers. In epimers only one chiral center has an opposite configuration. Typical examples of epimers are lutein (**10**) and epilutein (**18**) with opposite configuration at C-3' only.

Allenes (with two adjacent carbon–carbon double bonds connected by the same carbon), provided they are substituted in an appropriate way (two different

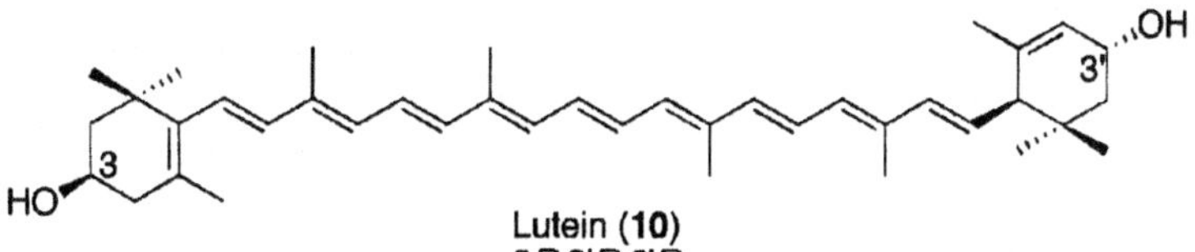

Lutein (10)
3*R*,3'*R*,6'*R*

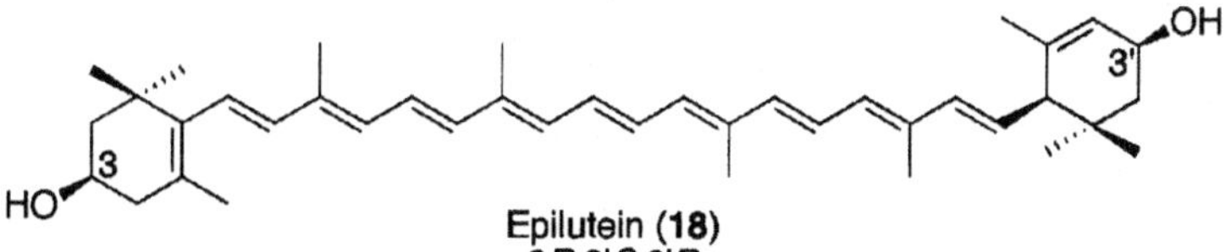

Epilutein (18)
3*R*,3'*S*,6'*R*

substituents at the two ends of the system), also represent a chiral center, actually a chiral axis. An example is neoxanthin (**19** and **20**) with different chirality for the allene in these two structures (hydrogen pointing up or down at the allene). Naturally occurring neoxanthin has structure **19**.

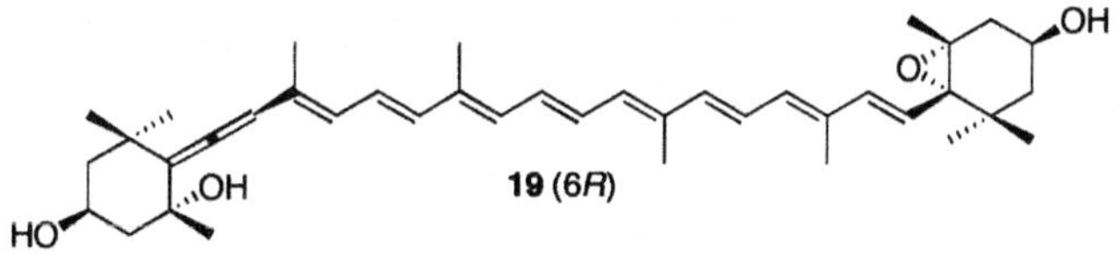

Neoxanthin, natural
3*S*,5*R*,6*R*,3'*S*,5'*R*,6'*S*

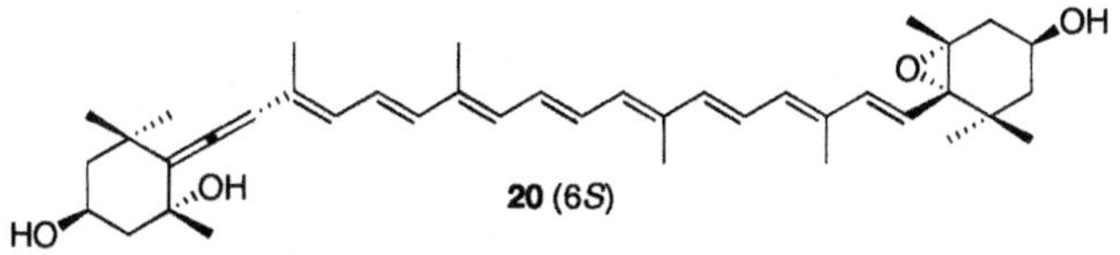

19 (6R)

Neoxanthin
3*S*,5*R*,6*S*,3'*S*,5'*R*,6*S*

20 (6S)

Optical activity can be measured by simple optical rotation, by optical rotatory dispersion (ORD) or by CD. For application of the CD method a substrate with a chromophore (unsaturated system) close to a chiral center is required. Carotenoids, containing a long polyene chain, lend themselves particularly well for this purpose; for CD, see Sec. IV E. Enantiomers have opposite CD curves, (Fig. 3), whereas diastereomers have less predictable CD spectra.

B. Nomenclature

Chirality is denoted by the symbols R and S according to the Cahn–Ingold–Prelog convention, involving priority rules for the four substituents at a chiral carbon atom, and looking at the direction you move when keeping the lowest priority substituent (usually H) in the back and going from the substituent with the highest to the next lowest priority. If it is clockwise you have R configuration, whereas an anticlockwise direction is denoted by S. Rules are defined for assigning R or S configuration to a chiral allene (25). R/S designation has already been given on carotenoid structures in Secs. IV and VI.

C. Examples

In the following are selected some particular carotenoid examples where chirality is important in a biological context.

1. Astaxanthin

Let us consider astaxanthin. Astaxanthin is present in all salmonid fishes, in various marine animals, as well as in some flowers. Astaxanthin is responsible for the pink color customers require from a healthy salmon. It was mentioned above that astaxanthin in principle can exist as three optical isomers, the 3R,3'R form **11**; its enantiomer, the 3S,3'S form **12**; and the optically inactive *meso* form, the 3R,3'S isomer **13**.

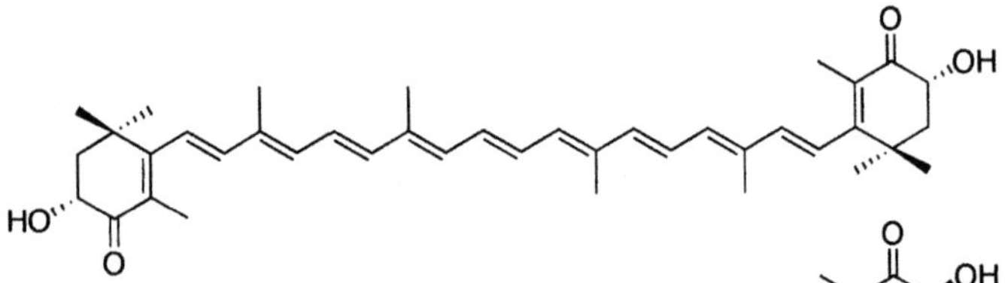

Astaxanthin (11)
3*R*,3'*R*

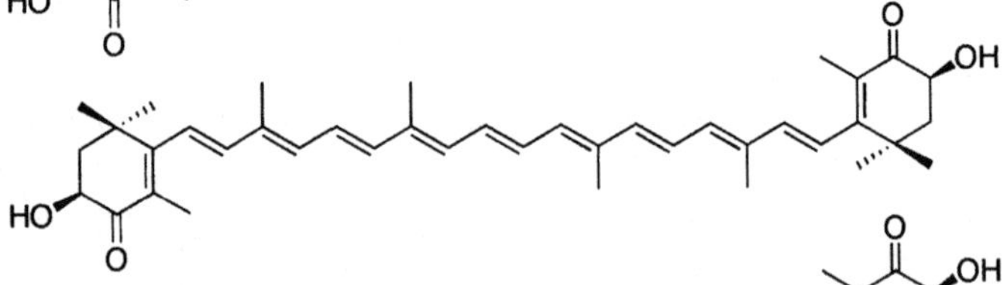

Astaxanthin (12)
3*S*,3'*S*

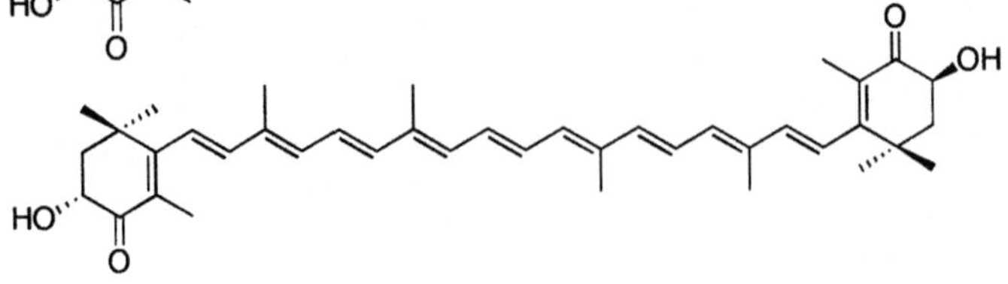

Astaxanthin (13)
3*R*,3'*S* (meso)

In red flowers (*Adonis annua*) the optically pure (3S,3'S) isomer **12** is present. At a time it was expected that carotenoids always were present in the biological material in pure optical form. When a nature-identical astaxanthin was desired by chemical synthesis for feed additive purpose upon salmon farming, it was anticipated that an expensive enantioselective synthesis of a single isomer was required. However, it turned out that in shrimp the three isomers occur naturally as a 1 : 2 (*meso* form) : 1 mixture. In salmon also the three isomers are present, but the ratio differs. Reported values are (3S,3′S) 75–85% of total astaxanthin, (3R,3′S, *meso*) 2–6% and (3R,3′R) 12–17% (26). Today the synthetic astaxanthin marketed is a 1 : 2 (*meso*) : 1 mixture, whereas that produced by the yeast *Pfaffia rhodozyma* is the optically pure (3R,3′R) isomer **11**. The third common source, the alga *Haematococcus* sp., provides the optically pure (3S,3′S) isomer **12**. It has been demonstrated that all three isomers are equally well resorbed by the fish and that no metabolic interconversion is observed in the flesh (27). It may also be mentioned that all three isomers are equally well bound in the blue crustacyanin astaxanthin complex present in lobster (28). Apparently a racemization process occurs in certain crustaceans including zooplankton on which the wild fish is feeding (26). The separation at the three astaxanthin isomers may be effected on a chiral HPLC column or after derivatization to diastereomeric camphanates on an achiral HPLC column (1).

2. Zeaxanthin

Our next example is zeaxanthin. The structure differs from astaxanthin only by lacking the two carbonyl groups in 4,4′ positions. Zeaxanthin has two chiral centers (C-3,3′) where the hydroxyl groups are located and may exist as the (3R,3′R) isomer **21**, the (3S,3′S) enantiomer **22**, and the (3R,3′S) *meso* form **23**.

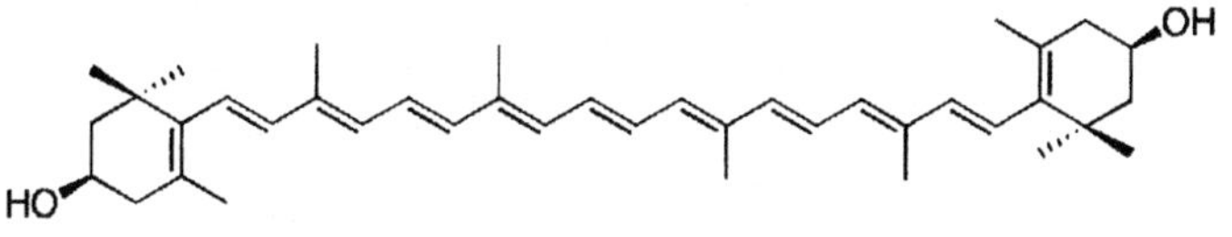

Zeaxanthin (21)
3R,3′R

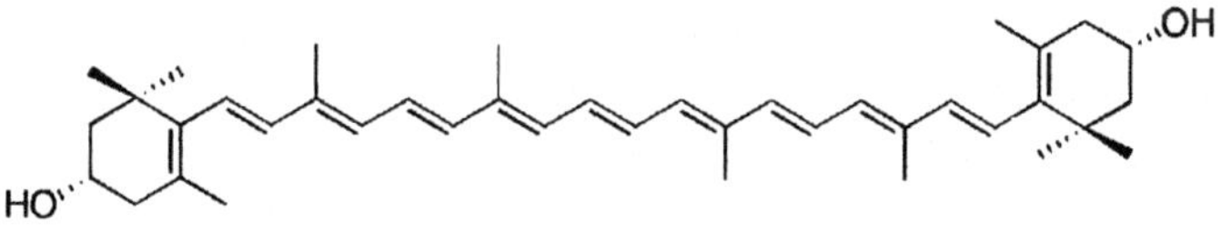

Zeaxanthin (22)
3S,3′S

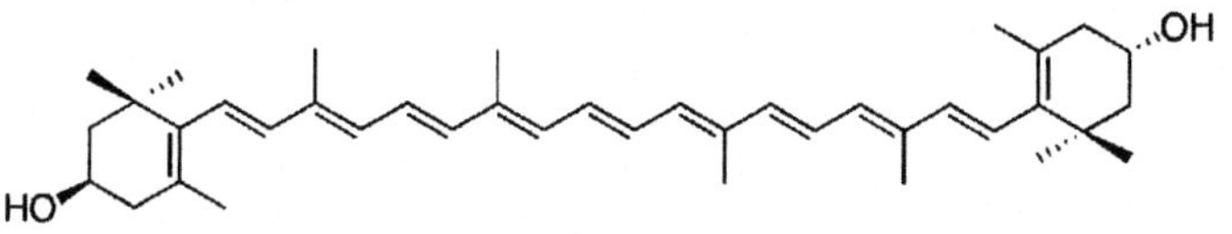

Zeaxanthin (23)
3R,3′S (meso)

In a mixture these three optical isomers are best separated after derivatization to diastereomeric carbamates on a common, achiral column. In nature the (3R,3′R) isomer **21** dominates by far, e.g., in maize and egg yolk, the (3S,3′S) isomer **22** is very rare, and the *meso* form (**23**) is occasionally encountered in animal sources, e.g., in human retina. The formation of the *meso* form in retina is tentatively formulated via lutein (**16**); see below.

3. Lutein

Let us proceed with a structurally more complex example, lutein. Lutein is a major carotenoid in all green leaves, in some various marine animals, and in human serum and retina.

Lutein has two different end groups with a total of three chiral carbons (C-3, C-3', and C-6'). Since each chiral carbon atom in principle can assume the (R-) or (S-) configuration, lutein can exist as eight different optical isomers, consisting of four pairs of enantiomers. Of two suggested systems for the denomination of the lutein isomers the systematic semirational, one is cited below (29).

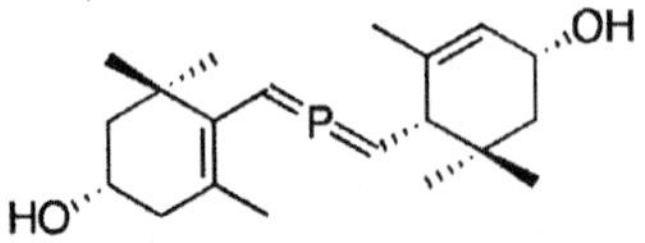

a
24 (3*S*,3'*R*,6'*S*)

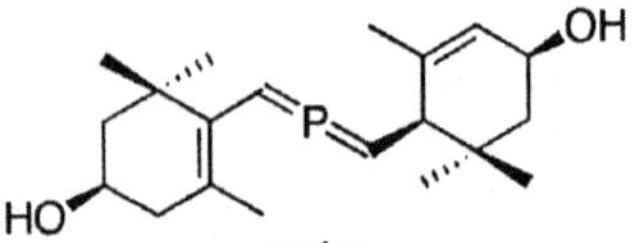

ent-a
18 (3*R*,3'*S*,6'*R*)

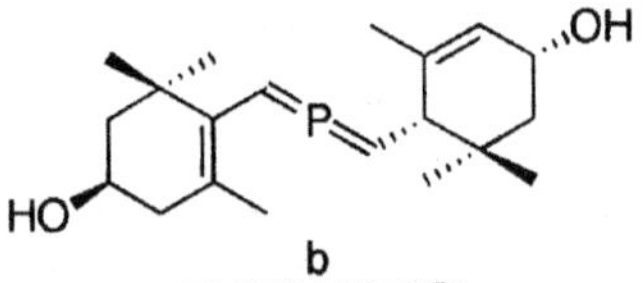

b
25 (3*R*,3'*R*,6'*S*)

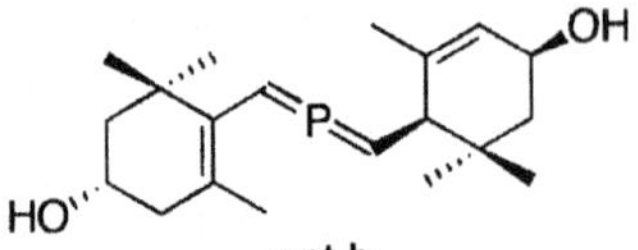

ent-b
28 (3*S*,3'*S*,6'*R*)

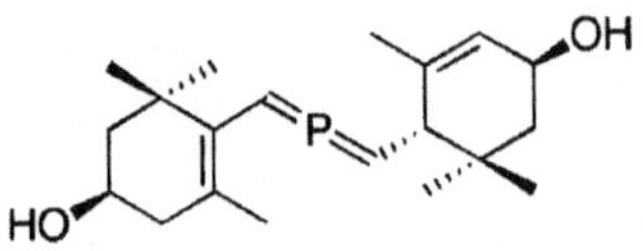

c
26 (3*R*,3'*S*,6'*S*)

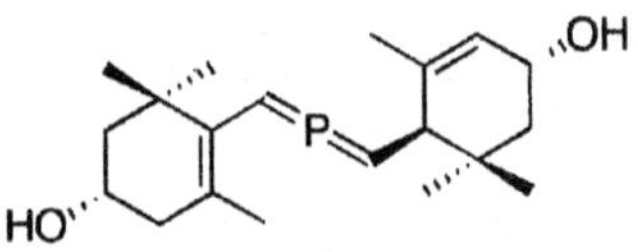

ent-c
29 (3*S*,3'*R*,6'*R*)

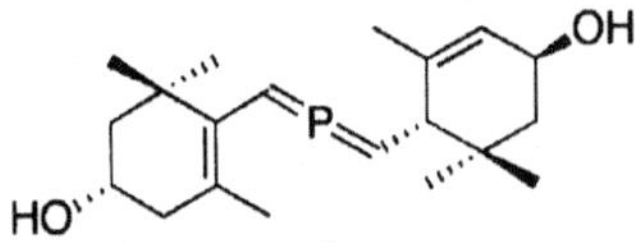

d
27 (3*S*,3'*S*,6'*S*)

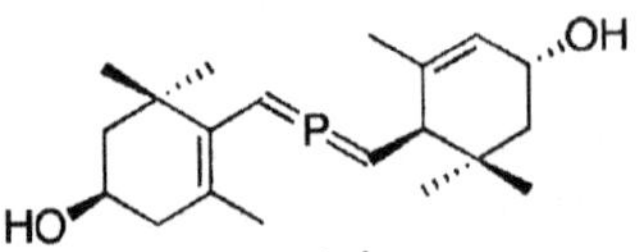

ent-d
10 (3*R*,3'*R*,6'*R*)

The common green leaf lutein is lutein ent-d (**10**) and the so-called epilutein from flowers of *Caltha palustris* is ent-a (**18**). Other alternatives are **24–29**. When mentioning lutein the chirality needs specification by the R/S nomenclature. It is interesting to note that five of these eight isomers have been claimed to occur in natural sources and six of them have been prepared by chemical synthesis (25). CD and ^{1}H NMR data are essential for the identification of the individual isomers. By ^{1}H NMR the C-3',6'-*trans* (hydroxy group and polyene chain on opposite side) or alternative *cis* relationship is readily established from relevant chemical proton shifts. It appears that lutein ent-d (**10**) and, to a much lesser extent, lutein ent-a (**18**) are synthesized de novo in nature, whereas the other lutein isomers are metabolic products in certain animals.

4. Neoxanthin

The structurally most complex carotenoid to be addressed here in conjunction with our consideration of chirality is neoxanthin. Neoxanthin has five chiral carbon atoms (C-3,5,3',5',6') and a chiral axis (the allene). All naturally occurring allenic carotenoids exhibit (R)-configuration for the allene, although the natural occurrence of (S)-allene at a time was claimed (30).

Of the several theoretically possible optical isomers of neoxanthin only the (3S,5R,6R,3'S,5'R,6'S) isomer **19** is encountered in nature (6R specifies the chirality of the allene). However, the allenic (6S) isomer **20** (see Sec. VI) has been prepared synthetically from the (6R) isomer by allenic isomerization in light, employing diphenyldiselenide as catalyst (21).

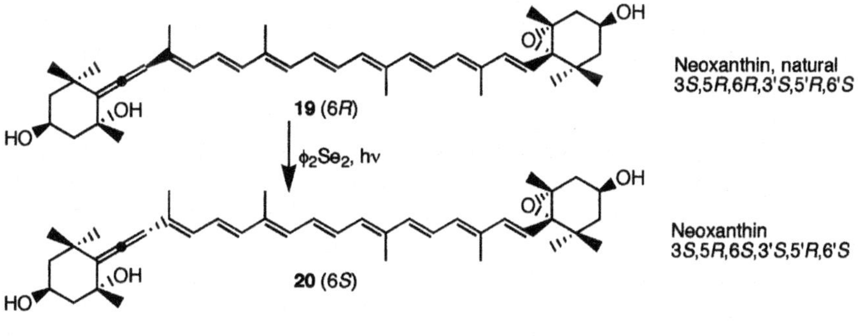

Neoxanthin, natural
3S,5R,6R,3'S,5'R,6'S

19 (6R)

ϕ_2Se$_2$, hv

Neoxanthin
3S,5R,6S,3'S,5'R,6'S

20 (6S)

The relative configuration between the 3'-hydroxy group and the epoxide is *trans* (on opposite sides of the ring) in neoxanthin (**19**) as in all other naturally occurring carotenoids with this particular structural element. The epoxide-furanoid rearrangement reaction is treated in Sec. VII.

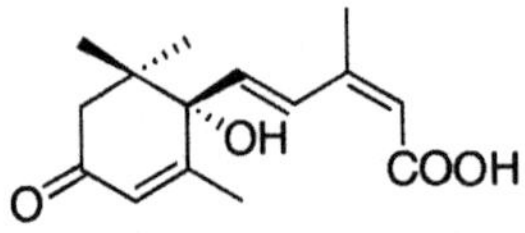

30
Abscisic acid

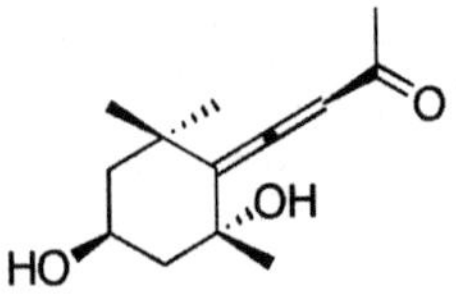

31
Grasshopper ketone

Epoxide carotenoids are abundant in fruits and flowers. The best source of neoxanthin (**19**) is spinach. Neoxanthin (**19**), as its 9′-*cis* isomer, serves in green leaves as the biosynthetic precursor of the growth hormone abscisic acid (**30**). The ant-repelling allenic grasshopper ketone (**31**) is also most likely a metabolic product of neoxanthin (**19**) (25).

VII. CHEMICAL REACTIONS

A. Partial Synthesis

Chemical reactions involving only functional group modifications are generally considered as partial syntheses of carotenoids. Examples are simple derivatization reactions such as acylation of carotenols or complex metal hydride reduction of ketocarotenoids. In such reactions the carotenoid skeleton is intact. However, some other simple chemical reactions that result in carbon skeletal changes may also be considered as partial synthesis, e.g., aldol condensation of carotenals with acetone to provide products of citranaxanthin (**9**) type with prolonged carbon skeleton, or oxidative cleavage of carotenoids to products with shorter carbon skeletons.

Derivatization reactions of carotenoids are still useful in characterization and identification of carotenoids, particularly in the absence of complete spectral data. Chemical reactions of carotenoids have been treated in detail elsewhere (31). This is also the case for microscale reactions useful for identification (1).

Three examples of partial synthesis are chosen here, which are relevant for topics treated in this book. The first example demonstrates the possible conversion of lutein (**10**) to epilutein (**18**) via the 3′-keto derivative **32**. Selective allylic oxidation provides the ketone **32** which by complex metal hydride reduction gives an approximate 1 : 1 mixture of lutein (**10**) and epilutein (**18**). Since these products are diastereomers they may be separated by chromatography. The keto derivative **32** has been encountered as a metabolite in both chicken and in eggs. Epimerization of lutein (**10**) in animal tissues to epilutein (**18**) is likely to occur by a similar set of enzymatic reactions.

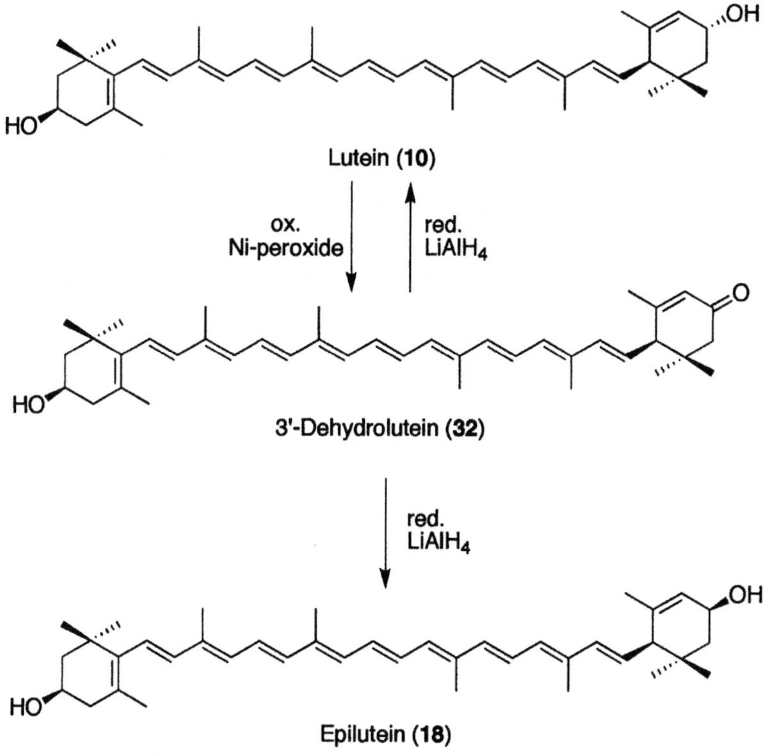

Lutein (**10**)

ox.
Ni-peroxide | red.
LiAlH$_4$

3'-Dehydrolutein (**32**)

red.
LiAlH$_4$

Epilutein (**18**)

The second example also deals with lutein (**10**), namely, its conversion to *meso*-zeaxanthin (**23**) by isomerization of the double bond of the ε ring into conjugation by means of strong base (33). Since this reaction does not influence the chirality of the C-3' hydroxy group, (3R,3'S, *meso*)-zeaxanthin (**23**) is obtained. The *meso* compound is in principle optically inactive, as has been verified in this case by lack of optical activity (no CD) (33). The technical conversion of lutein (**10**) *ex Tagetes* flowers to zeaxanthin is conducted by a process based on this reaction, and actually leads to *meso*-zeaxanthin (**23**).

The formation of *meso*-zeaxanthin in animal tissue is likely to proceed by a similar enzymatic reaction.

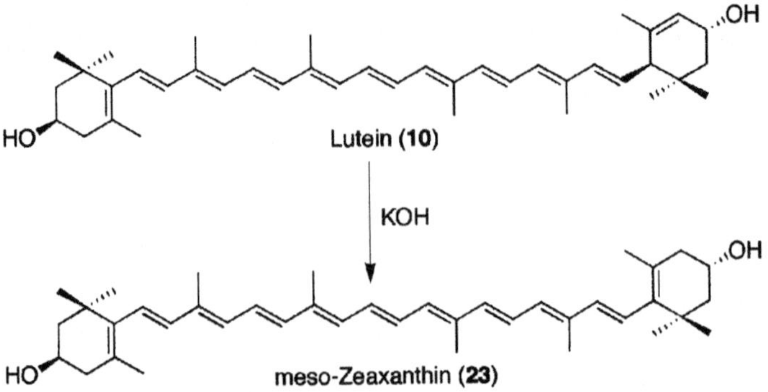

Lutein (10)

KOH

meso-Zeaxanthin (23)

The final example shows the reaction mechanism for epoxide-furanoid rearrangement of common carotenoid 5,6-epoxides of neoxanthin (19) type by the influence of weak acid.

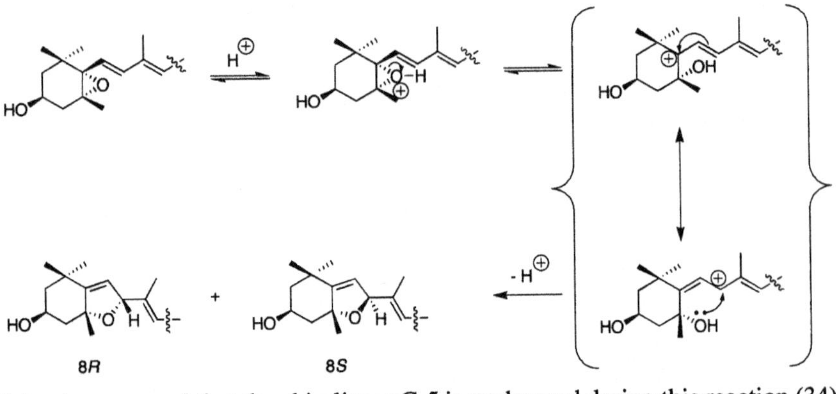

8R   8S

It has been proved that the chirality at C-5 is unchanged during this reaction (34). Since the reaction proceeds via a planar cation both C-8 diastereoisomers will result, in approximately the same amount. Like diastereomers in general, the two C-8 diastereomeric products may be separated chromatographically and characterized. Had this reaction occurred in nature via a stereospecific enzyme only one furanoid product would be obtained. Consequently, when two C-8 diastereomeric furanoid products are isolated upon analysis of a biological material it is taken as a strong indication that it deals with artifacts obtained by acid-catalyzed rearrangement of a natural carotenoid 5,6-epoxide during the isolation procedure (see Sec. VIII. B).

B. Total Synthesis

In contrast to the partial synthesis discussed above, the total synthesis of carotenoids is considered as a series of chemical reactions serving to build up the desired carotenoid skeleton with the functional groups in correct positions.

Formerly total synthesis of optically inactive carotenoids was considered satisfactory, even if chiral centers were present. However, today enantioselective synthesis with a single carotenoid product with the correct chirality at all chiral centers and correct configuration of all double bonds in the polyene chain is the ultimate goal. The art of total synthesis has been dealt with in extensive overviews (3,35). Highlights in the total synthesis of carotenoids may be illustrated by the total synthesis of several individual *cis* isomers of all-*trans* lycopene (**14**) (23), which is achiral, and total synthesis of (3*S*,5*R*,6*S*,3′*S*,5′*R*,6′*R*)-peridinin (**33**) with six chiral centers (36).

Peridinin (**33**)

VIII. SOME USEFUL LESSONS

A. Minimal Identification Criteria

In microscale isolation and analytical work a carotenoid is rarely identified by all spectroscopic data to the extent that an identification is unequivocal. Supplementary data by diagnostic chemical reactions may strenghten the identification. However, frequently identifications are based on HPLC data alone, which is not satisfactory evidence for a safe conclusion. A set of minimal identification criteria has been defined for a reasonably safe identification (1). These are:

1. VIS spectrum in one, preferably two, defined single solvents (for identification of the chromophore).
2. Chromatographic evidence in two defined chromatographic systems, preferably including HPLC (for establishment of relative polarity determined by functional groups), and direct co-chromatography with the authentic reference carotenoid.
3. Mass spectra of at least the quality giving the molecular ion and some supporting fragmentations, e.g., loss of toluene or xylene from the polyene chain, H_2O from carotenols, etc. (2).

These criteria may suffice for an achiral carotenoid. For determination of the absolute stereochemistry of chiral carotenoids, a combination of ^{1}H NMR and CD data is usually required.

If some of the above criteria are not fulfilled a tentative identification may in some cases be justified. In such a case the ending "-like" should be added. Thus, zeaxanthin-like would be an appropriate tentative identification of a carotenoid with β-carotene (1)–type visible spectrum and polarity compatible with a carotenoid diol in the absence of additional data.

B. Artifacts

The definition of carotenoid artifacts has been discussed (3). Artifacts are here considered as unwanted products of defined chemical structure arising during an unintended chemical reaction. Artifacts have conveniently been divided into two types as discussed in the following sections.

1. Pre-Extraction Artifacts

These may often be ascribed to improper handling of the biological material prior to extraction and are frequently overlooked. Included are enzyme-catalyzed reactions, acid-catalyzed reactions, and miscellaneous effects. The observation of chlorophyll degradation products in fresh extracts of photosynthetic tissues indicates that pre-extraction artifacts may be present.

2. Isolation Artifacts

Isolation artifacts are produced upon and after extraction by improper handling of the extracts. The type of reactions involved are light- and heat-induced reactions, acid-catalyzed reactions, base-catalyzed reactions, e.g., during saponification conditions, oxidations by air or peroxides (in ether solvent), reactions on active surfaces, thermal reactions, and miscellaneous effects. The most common artifacts are caused by *trans-cis* isomerization during the isolation procedure caused by exposure to daylight and slightly elevated temperature. In order to prove that a *cis* isomer is naturally occurring, fast extraction at low temperature followed by fast HPLC analysis in a suitable system is required (37). During standard isolation conditions some *trans-cis* isomerization is unavoidable.

Other very common artifacts are the so-called furanoxides or carotenoid 5,8-epoxides, formed from natural 5,6-epoxides such as neoxanthin (19) and peridinin (37) by the influence of weak acids, as shown in Sec. VII. The reaction leads to furanoid products with shorter chromophore. Since a new chiral center is created at C-8 both C-8 epimers (8R and 8S) are formed. These may frequently be separated chromatographically in approximately 4:6 ratio, thus representing evidence for the artifactual character of the products. Carotenoid epoxides are common in plant tissues, and precautions should be taken to avoid this complication during the isolation.

Another artifact is the base-catalyzed aldol condensation taking place with acetone and carotenals (aldehydes) during saponification conditions. The presence of acetone must be strictly avoided during saponification which by standard conditions are carried out in diethyl ether–ethanol containing about 5% sodium hydroxide. As an example the reaction of the C_{30} carotenal **34** with acetone leading to the methyl ketone citranaxanthin (**9**) is shown below, the natural occurrence of which may be questioned.

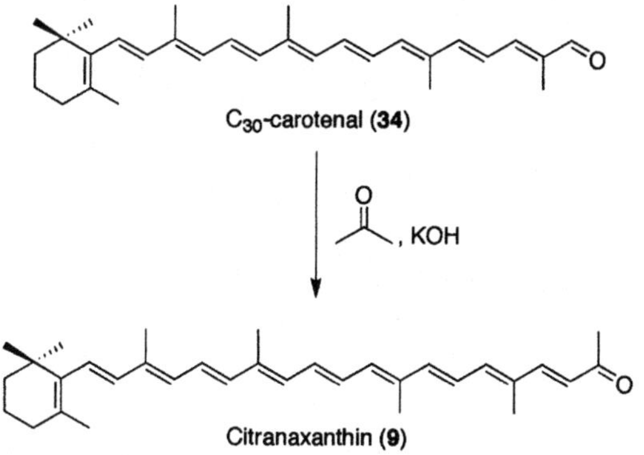

C_{30}-carotenal (**34**)

, KOH

Citranaxanthin (**9**)

Astaxanthin and its esters present in salmonid fishes readily undergo another base catalysed reaction of the α-ketol functional group with molecular oxygen (traces of air) at alkaline saponification conditions. This leads to the achiral enolised α-diketone astacene (**35**) shown below. Hence astaxanthin extracts should not be submitted to saponification conditions for removal of lipids.

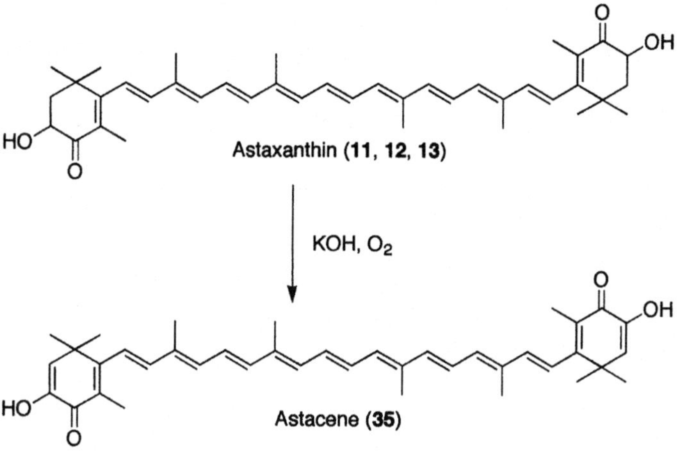

Astaxanthin (**11, 12, 13**)

KOH, O_2

Astacene (**35**)

Other reactions leading to particular artifacts have been treated elsewhere (3).

C. Natural Versus Synthetic

The term natural is rather magic in our days, in particular in relation to food and feed. Natural carotenoids may be considered as (37):

1. Carotenoids belonging to the biosynthetic pathways of living cells, or
2. Metabolic transformation products of such dietary carotenoids in animals

This definition does not require that a natural carotenoid was obtained by biosynthesis. Today nature-identical carotenoids may also be prepared by chemical synthesis, a fact of which people are frequently ignorant. Provided the chemical structure of a carotenoid obtained by chemical synthesis is identical in all respects, including stereochemistry, with that of a natural carotenoid, there is no difference between a natural and synthetic compound. However, in cases where chemical, including stereochemical, differences exist they are different. Let us consider two relevant examples as follows.

1. β-Carotene

The majority of natural sources contain the all-*trans* isomer as the dominant geometrical isomer as is the case for synthetic β-carotene (**1**). However, the green alga *Dunaliella bardawil* produces mainly the 9-*cis* isomer (**1b**). This means that there are different natural sources for the two isomers of β-carotene. The all-*trans* isomer (**1**) is also commercially available from chemical synthesis.

2. Astaxanthin

As outlined before astaxanthin can in principle exist as three different optical isomers (3S,3′S, *meso* and 3R,3′R). In marine organisms including salmonid fishes a mixture of these isomers (**11–13**) occur in varying proportion. This is mimicked in synthetic astaxanthin where the 1:2:1 ratio is fixed. It therefore may be argued on structural grounds, that the synthetic product is more similar to the marine animal case than other microbiological natural sources containing exclusively one of the three isomers (either 3S,3′S-astaxanthin in *Haematococcus* sp. or 3R,3′R-astaxanthin in *Phaffia rhodozyma*).

The lesson is that there may be no difference between a natural and a synthetic nature-identical carotenoid and that the term natural is a relative term to be used in connection with particular sources. For instance, a carotenoid that is naturally occurring only in a phototrophic bacterium is not natural relative to a human being.

REFERENCES

1. Britton G, Liaaen-Jensen S, Pfander H, eds. Carotenoids, Vol. 1A. Isolation and Analysis. Basel: Birkhäuser, 1995.

2. Britton G, Liaaen-Jensen S, Pfander H, eds. Carotenoids, Vol. 1B. Spectroscopy. Basel: Birkhäuser, 1995.
3. Britton G, Liaaen-Jensen S, Pfander H, eds. Carotenoids, Vol. 2. Synthesis. Basel: Birkhäuser, 1996.
4. Britton G, Liaaen-Jensen S, Pfander H, eds. Carotenoids, Vol. 3. Biosynthesis and metabolism. Basel: Birkhäuser, 1998.
5. Straub O. Key to Carotenoids, 2nd ed. Pfander H, ed. Basel: Birkhäuser, 1987.
6. Britton G, Liaaen-Jensen S, Pfander H, eds. Carotenoid Handbook. Compiled by Mercadante A, Egeland ES. Basel: Birkhäuser, 2003.
7. Zagalsky PF, Eliopoulos EE, Findlay JBC. The architecture of invertebrate carotenoproteins. Comp Biochem Physiol 1990; 97B:1–18.
8. Cianci M, Rizkallah PJ, Olazak A, Raftery J, Chayen NE, Zagalsky PF. The molecular basis of the coloration mechanism in lobster shell: β-crustacyanin at 3.2 Å resolution. PNAS 2002; 99:9795–9800.
9. Lutnaes BF, Bruaas L, Krane J, Liaaen-Jensen S. Preparation and structure elucidation of the charge delocalized β,β-carotene dication. Tetrahedron Lett 2002; 43:5149–5152.
10. IUPAC Commision of Nomenclature of Organic Chemistry and the IUPAC-IUB Commission on Biochemical Nomenclature. Nomenclature of carotenoids. Pure Appl Chem 1975; 41: 405–431.
11. Goodwin TW. The Biochemistry of the Carotenoids, Vol. 1, Plants, 2nd ed. London: Chapman and Hall, 1980.
12. Goodwin TW. The Biochemistry of the Carotenoids, Vol. 2, Animals, 2nd ed. London: Chapman and Hall, 1984.
13. Jeffrey SW, Mantoura RFC, Wright SW. Phytoplankton Pigments in Oceanography. Paris: UNESCO, 1997.
14. Liaaen Jensen S. The Constitution of Some Bacterial Carotenoids and Their Bearing on Biosynthetic Problems. Trondheim: Det Kgl. Norske Vitenskabers Selskabs Skrifter 1962, no. 8.
15. Englert G, Aakermann T, Liaaen-Jensen S. NMR studies on natural all-*trans* (9'Z, 11'Z)-(3R,3'S,5'R,6'R)-pyrrhoxanthin, an acetylenic C_{37}-skeletal nor-carotenoid butenolide. Magn Reson Chem 1993; 31:910–915.
16. Bartlett L, Klyne W, Mose WP, Scopes PM, Galasko G, Mallams AK, Weedon BCL, Szabolcs J, Tóth G. Optical rotatory dispersion of carotenoids. J Chem Soc C 1969; 2527–2544.
17. Müller RK, Bernhard K, Mayer H, Rüttimann A, Vecchi M. Beitrag zur Analytik und Synthese von 3-Hydroxy-4-oxocarotinoiden. Helv Chim Acta 1980; 63:1654–1664.
18. Rønnekleiv M, Liaaen-Jensen S. Bacterial carotenoids 52. C_{50}-carotenoids 22. Naturally occurring geometrical isomers of bacterioruberin. Acta Chem Scand 1992; 46:1092–1095.
19. Strand A, Shivaji S, Liaaen-Jensen S. Bacterial carotenoids 55. C_{50}-carotenoids 25. Revised structure of carotenoids associated with membranes in psychrotrophic *Micrococcus roseus*. Pure Appl Chem 1997; 69:2027–2038.
20. Strand A, Liaaen-Jensen S. Application of diphenyldiselenide as a new catalyst for photochemical stereoisomerization of carotenoids. Acta Chem Scand 1998; 52:1263–1269.

21. Refvem T, Strand A, Kjeldstad B, Haugan JA, Liaaen-Jensen S. Stereoisomerization of allenic carotenoids—kinetic, thermodynamic and mechanistic aspects. Acta Chem Scand 1999; 53:118–123.
22. Gerster H. The potential role of lycopene in human health. J Am Coll Nutr 1997; 16:109–122.
23. Hengartner U, Bernhard K, Mayer K, Englert G, Glinz E. Synthesis, isolation and NMR-spectroscopic characterization of fourteen (Z)-isomers of lycopene and of some acetylenic didehydro- and tetradehydrolycopenes. Helv Chim Acta 1992; 75:1848–1865.
24. Shierle J, Bretzel W, Bühler I, Faccin N, Hess D, Steiner K, Schüep W. Content and isomeric ratio of lycopene in food and human blood plasma. Food Chem 1997; 59:459–465.
25. Weedon BCL. Stereochemistry. In: Isler O, ed. Carotenoids. Basel: Birkhäuser, 1971:267–323.
26. Schiedt K. Absorption and metabolism of carotenoids in birds, fish and crustaceans. In: Britton G, Liaaen-Jensen S, Pfander H, eds. Carotenoids, Vol. 3, Biosynthesis and Metabolism. Basel: Birkhäuser, 1998:285–358.
27. Foss P, Storebakken T, Schiedt K, Liaaen-Jensen S, Austereng E, Streiff K. Carotenoids in diets for salmonids. 1. Pigmentation of rainbow trout with the individual optical isomers of astaxanthin in comparison with canthaxanthin. Aquaculture 1984; 41:213–226.
28. Renstrøm B, Rønneberg H, Borch G, Liaaen-Jensen S. Animal carotenoids 28. Further studies on the carotenoproteins crustacyanin and ovoverdin. Comp Biochem Physiol 1982; 71B:249–252.
29. Sliwka H-R, Liaaen-Jensen S. Partial syntheses of diastereomeric carotenols. Acta Chem Scand 1987; B41:518–525.
30. Liaaen-Jensen S. Stereochemical aspects of carotenoids. Pure Appl Chem 1997; 69:2027–2039.
31. Liaaen-Jensen S. Isolation, reactions. In: Isler O, ed. Carotenoids. Basel: Birkhäuser, 1971:61–188.
32. Liaaen-Jensen S, Hertzberg S. Selective preparation of the lutein monomethyl ethers. Acta Chem Scand 1966; 20:1703–1709.
33. Andrewes AG, Borch G, Liaaen-Jensen S. Carotenoids of higher plants. 7. On the absolute configuration of lutein. Acta Chem Scand 1974; 28B:139–140.
34. Eugster CH. Carotenoid structures, old and new problems. Pure Appl Chem 1985; 57:639–647.
35. Mayer H, Isler O. Total synthesis. In: Isler O, ed. Carotenoids. Basel: Birkhäuser, 1971:325–575.
36. Yamano Y, Ito M. First total synthesis of ($\pm$)-peridinin, ($\pm$)-pyrrhoxanthin and the optically active peridinin. J Chem Soc Perkin Trans I 1993; 1599–1610.
37. Liaaen-Jensen S. Artifacts of natural carotenoids—unintended carotenoid synthesis. In: Krinsky NI, Mathews-Roth M, Taylor RF, eds. Carotenoids Chemistry and Biology. New York: Plenum Publishing, 1989:149–184.

2
Carotenoids and Radicals; Interactions with Other Nutrients

Ann Cantrell and T. George Truscott
Keele University, Keele, Staffordshire, England

I. INTRODUCTION

A nutrient is defined as any substance that has nutritious qualities, i.e., that nourishes or promotes growth, and one that can be metabolized by an organism to give energy and build tissue. In this chapter a nutrient is assumed to be an amino acid, carotenoid, vitamin C, vitamin E, and other antioxidants such as polyphenols (Fig. 1 shows the structures of some important antioxidants discussed in chapter). While carotenoids, vitamin E, and vitamin C are often regarded as our most important dietary antioxidants, little is known of their possible interactions. The aim of this chapter is to discuss such interactions and to suggest how these may explain possible synergistic protective effects as well as how deleterious effects could arise. The carotenoids we consume, from our foods, food colorants, and possibly as dietary supplements, are thought to be antioxidants both by quenching singlet oxygen and by scavenging free radicals. This chapter concerns free radical reactions; readers interested in singlet oxygen may consult recent reviews (1,2) and the recent study of singlet oxygen quenching by carotenoids in liposomes (3).

Several dietary carotenoids may act as radical scavengers in vivo and hence their radical chemistry may be linked to disease prevention. However, the ability to scavenge free radicals is not in itself a sufficient prerequisite for an antioxidant. Currently, the chemistry of carotenoid/radical reactions is also generating wide interest. In photosynthesis, there is much debate on the role of β-carotene in the reaction centers as an electron carrier (4–8).

Autoxidation processes, such as lipid peroxidation, are associated with free radical chain reactions that involve peroxyl radicals (ROO$^\bullet$). Chain-breaking

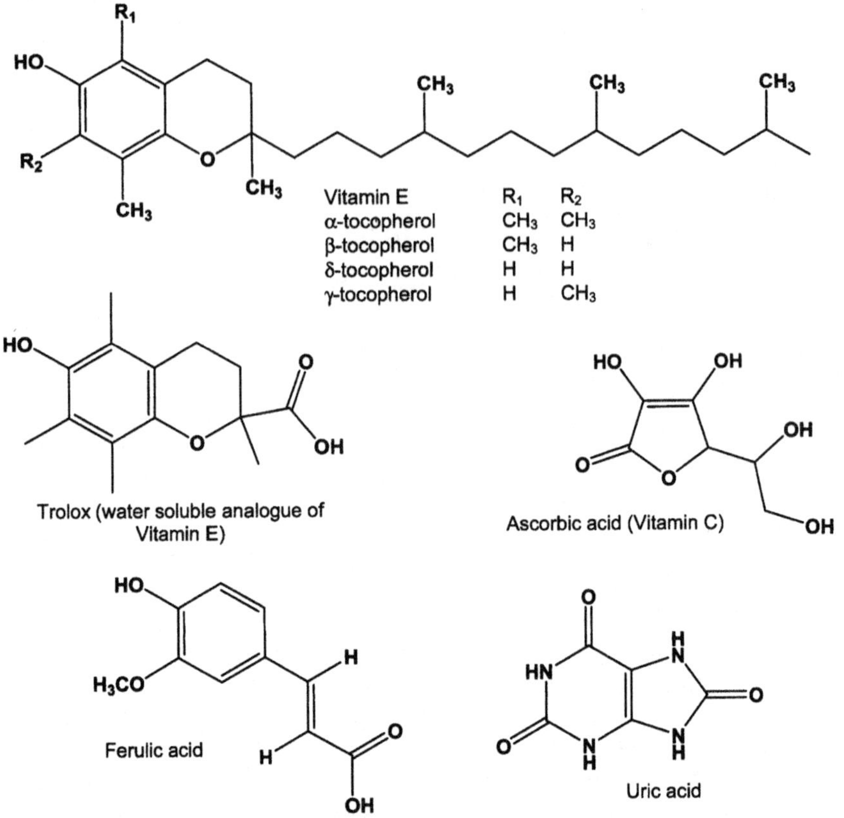

Vitamin E	R_1	R_2
α-tocopherol	CH_3	CH_3
β-tocopherol	CH_3	H
δ-tocopherol	H	H
γ-tocopherol	H	CH_3

Trolox (water soluble analogue of Vitamin E)

Ascorbic acid (Vitamin C)

Ferulic acid

Uric acid

Figure 1 Structures of some important biological antioxidants and the water-soluble analog of α-tocopherol.

antioxidants such as carotenoids (CAR) may impede such processes by rapidly and efficiently scavenging such free radicals (often by H-atom transfer; see Scheme 1.)

Initiator $+$ RH $\longrightarrow$ R$^{•}$	Initiation
R$^{•}$ $+$ O$_2$ $\longrightarrow$ ROO$^{•}$	Propagation
ROO$^{•}$ $+$ RH $\longrightarrow$ ROOH $+$ R$^{•}$	
ROO$^{•}$ $+$ ROO$^{•}$ $\longrightarrow$ PRODUCTS	Termination
ROO$^{•}$ $+$ CAR $\longrightarrow$ ROOH $+$ CAR$^{•}$	Inhibiton by CAR

Scheme 1

The resulting antioxidant-derived radical (CAR$^•$) must not be capable of propagating the chain reaction, i.e., it must not undergo H-atom abstraction reactions or react with oxygen to form another peroxyl radical. Such potentially deleterious reactions can be written as:

$$CAR^• + RH \longrightarrow CAR + R^• \tag{1}$$

$$CAR^• + O_2 \longrightarrow CAR\text{-}OO^• \tag{2}$$

Of course, if another species can efficiently remove the neutral radical, CAR$^•$, or other carotenoid radicals (e.g., the carotenoid radical cation CAR$^{•+}$), the deleterious reactions given above [Eqs. (1) and (2)] may be avoided.

Furthermore, carotenoid antioxidant activity depends on numerous other factors among which are the concentration and cellular distribution of the substance. Possibly related is that while early epidemiological studies have suggested a link between diets rich in carotenoids and a lower incidence of several serious diseases (9–11), subsequent epidemiological findings suggest little health benefits from dietary supplementation with β-carotene. There is even a possible deleterious effect in some subpopulations, such as heavy smokers (12,13).

Burton and Ingold (14) suggested that β-carotene reacts with peroxyl radicals via an addition reaction. They presented evidence that β-carotene functions as an effective chain-breaking antioxidant, but that under high oxygen pressures and at high β-carotene concentrations it can exhibit pro-oxidant behavior, possibly due to autoxidative processes. However, this work concerns oxygen pressures well above those of biological interest. A possibly related observation in a real-life situation concerns an interaction between dietary β-carotene and α-tocopherol (α-TOH) in muscles from chickens fed various levels of the two antioxidants (15). For a 15 ppm addition of β-carotene to the chicken feed, a significant antioxidant effect on fresh and cooked meats was noted, while a 50 ppm addition acted as a pro-oxidant. Most carbon-centered radicals react rapidly with oxygen to form peroxyl radicals (16). However, where the carbon-centered radical is resonance stabilized the reaction is reversible:

$$R^• + O_2 \longleftrightarrow ROO^• \tag{3}$$

The epidemiological evidence suggesting that diets rich in β-carotene are associated with a decreased incidence of many important diseases has been followed by claims that lycopene, the red pigment in tomatoes, is useful against cancer (particularly prostate cancer), atherosclerosis, age-related macular degeneration (ARMD), multiple sclerosis, and many other diseases (9–11). It is suggested that this may occur via prevention of lipid peroxidation. The claim that lycopene may offer protection against ARMD (11) is surprising because lycopene does not arise to any significant level in the eye; the carotenoids present in the macula of the eye are the xanthophylls, zeaxanthin, and lutein. These carotenoids may well protect against ARMD and cataract formation. The reasons for the selectivity of the hydroxy-containing carotenoids in the macular region of the eye, and a possible role for lycopene in reducing the onset of ARMD, is not clear but is discussed below. It must be emphasized that the reactions given in Scheme 1 and reactions associated with any lycopene radicals generated are likely to be similar to those of other carotenoids. Thus, the antioxidant/pro-oxidant properties of carotenoids, including lycopene, are not only dependent on how rapidly they scavenge different types of free radicals but also on the mode of reaction, and, consequently, the properties of the resulting carotenoid radicals (17–19).

Three reaction channels may be envisaged; electron transfer (producing the carotenoid radical cation), hydrogen abstraction (producing the neutral carotenoid radical), and addition (to produce the neutral radical adduct) (1,20,21) [Eqs. (4) to (6)].

$$CAR + ROO^{\bullet} \rightarrow CAR^{\bullet+} + ROO^{-} \qquad \text{Electron transfer} \qquad (4)$$

$$CAR + ROO^{\bullet} \rightarrow CAR^{\bullet} + ROOH \qquad \text{Hydrogen abstraction} \qquad (5)$$

$$CAR + ROO^{\bullet} \rightarrow (ROO\text{-}CAR^{\bullet}) \qquad \text{Addition} \qquad (6)$$

Hydrocarbon carotenoids such as lycopene and β-carotene are extremely hydrophobic molecules and hence they are found predominantly in lipophilic regions (22). The relative importance of the three reaction channels will depend on a number of factors including the nature of the reacting free radical and the structural features of the carotenoid (1,18), which will have a bearing on its location and orientation within the membrane (23). If the carotenoid is embedded deep within the membrane, then reaction 1 (electron transfer) will not be efficient because the nonpolar environment will not support charge separation. Electron transfer scavenging may be feasible for carotenoids such as zeaxanthin, which have polar substituents and can therefore span the membrane and possibly intercept radicals in aqueous regions at the cellular membrane surface. It is worth noting, however, that formation of radical cations of a range of carotenoids from reactions with free radicals has been observed in micellar media (24), in a quaternary microemulsion (25) and, very recently, in unilamellar dipalmitoyl phosphatidylcholine (DPPC) liposomes (26). This final example is interesting since it may be surprising to observe charge separation to produce radical cations in such a nonpolar environment.

There is some ambiguity as to the identity of the radicals formed following the reactions of carotenoids with different radical species. However, the spectral characteristics of radical cations and addition radicals have been identified. Carotenoid radical cations absorb in the near-infrared with peaks ranging from 820 nm for 7,7'-dihydo-β-carotene (77DH) to 950 nm for lycopene in methanol but these can vary depending on the environment studied (1,27). Radical adducts (e.g., CAR-ROO$^\bullet$) have peaks in the visible region (400–500 nm) and often may absorb in the region of the parent ground-state absorption (27,28). An unidentified absorption band (700–800 nm) is observed when carotenoids react with sulfonyl radicals, which decays to the radical cation (27). Reactivity with oxygen may be important when considering the consequences of producing carotenoid radicals. Carotenoid radical cations have been studied extensively and do not appear to react with molecular oxygen (29). However, the assignment and fate of the neutral carotenoid radicals, derived respectively from allylic H-atom abstraction (CAR$^\bullet$) and radical addition (R-CAR$^\bullet$), is less clear, and results have only been reported very recently (28). In this work El Agamey and McGarvey have given evidence for a lack of reactivity of carotenoid addition radicals toward oxygen based on a laser flash photolysis study of the reactions of carotenoids with acylperoxyl radicals in polar and nonpolar solvents. Furthermore, they point out that it is also unlikely that the neutral radical CAR$^\bullet$ reacts with oxygen [see also (30)]. Overall, therefore, it is important to consider the properties of the carotenoid radicals produced following reaction with oxidizing species and possible reactions that remove the carotenoid radicals.

II. PROPERTIES OF CAROTENOID RADICALS

The reactions of carotenoids with radicals such as the trichloromethylperoxyl radical (CCl$_3$O$_2^\bullet$) and hydroxyl radical (OH$^\bullet$) lead to the formation of carotenoid radicals as described above [Eqs. (4) to (6)], and it is the radical cations that have received the most attention. Other radicals produced have not been as extensively studied and information on these radicals is somewhat deficient; their properties are less well understood, although, as noted above, recently the formation of addition radicals from reaction of carotenoids with acylperoxyl radicals has been investigated (28). This section therefore mainly deals with carotenoid radical cations.

The fate of carbon-centered radicals such as carotenoid radical cations depends on their reactivity, which is governed by properties such as lifetime and redox potentials. The absolute oxidizing strength of the carotenoids gives a strong indication of how the carotenoid radical cations will react if "given" the opportunity.

The study by El Agamey and McGarvey not only characterized the radicals produced from the reaction of carotenoids with acylperoxyl radicals but also determined some of the radical properties. The addition radical (assumed to be an addition radical) produced from the reaction of 77DH with the phenylacetylperoxyl radical in hexane (with a peak at 455 nm) was observed to decay by first-order kinetics (the authors suggest that such a unimolecular decay could only result from a radical adduct, and that more complex kinetics would be observed for the decay of other radicals such as that produced via a hydrogen abstraction reaction or electron transfer) with a rate constant of $4 \times 10^3 \, s^{-1}$. This corresponds to a lifetime of 250 μs in hexane and its decay is proposed to occur through an intramolecular cyclization process (28). An addition radical (also assumed to be a radical adduct) produced from reaction of β-carotene and the trichloromethylperoxyl radical decays to the carotenoid radical cation with a rate constant of $1.8 \times 10^4 \, s^{-1}$ (lifetime 55 μs) (31). Such radical adducts appear to be less stable than the radical cations and therefore less likely to interact with other species.

Carotenoid radical cations have been studied in many environments by pulse radiolysis and have been shown to have relatively long lifetimes. They decay by second-order processes in pure organic solvents, but lifetimes can be estimated by using low doses to obtain their rates of decay. For example, in methanol they decay over hundreds of microseconds (32) whereas they have lifetimes of up to tens of milliseconds and their decay kinetics are more complex displaying many exponentials (this is ample time to undergo deleterious reactions with biological molecules) in heterogeneous environments such as micelles. In micellar environments, consisting of negatively charged, positively charged, or neutral micelles [sodium dodecyl sulfate (SDS), cetyl trimethyl ammonium bromide (CTAB), and Triton-X, 100 (TX-100) micelles, respectively] and calculations using two exponential decays, Edge et al. observed lifetimes of 7–16 ms and 40–100 ms in TX-100 and CTAB for β-carotene, canthaxanthin, zeaxanthin, astaxanthin, and lycopene; whereas in SDS micelles lifetimes of 600 ms were observed for canthaxanthin (33,34). In DPPC liposomes, the radical cations are also observed to have lifetimes of ms duration (26). This indicates that the environment has a large influence on the longevity of the carotenoid radical cations that may affect their reactivity. Such lifetimes in a lipid environment imply the opportunity for the radical cation to reorient itself within the membrane to facilitate reactions with biological substrates, which may lead to either damage or repair by aqueous species such as ascorbic acid (see below).

One other very important property is the one-electron reduction potentials of the carotenoids which is key to explaining the reactivity of carotenoid radical cations. Edge et al. (21) studied the relative redox potentials of a number of carotenoids. They determined the rate constants for electron transfer between various pairs of carotenoids in benzene using pulse radiolysis to generate the radical cation of one of the carotenoids in the pair [Eq. (7)] (Table 1).

$$CAR_1^{\bullet +} + CAR_2 \longrightarrow CAR_1 + CAR_2^{\bullet +} \tag{7}$$

Monitoring such carotenoid pairs gave the order of relative ease of electron transfer between the carotenoids studied so that the order from this study is astaxanthin > β-apo-8′-carotenal > canthaxanthin > lutein > zeaxanthin > β-carotene > lycopene, such that lycopene is the strongest reducing agent (the most easily oxidized) and astaxanthin is the weakest. They also showed that

Table 1 Rate Constants for Electron Transfer Between Pairs of
Carotenoids (CAR1 and CAR2)

Carotenoid radical cation ($CAR1^{\bullet+}$)	Rate constant ($\pm 10\%$)/10^9 dm^3 mol^{-1} s^{-1} for reaction with CAR2		
	LYC	β-CAR	ZEA
$ASTA^{\bullet+}$	9.2	8.0	4.6
$APO^{\bullet+}$	11.2	6.3	7.7
$CAN^{\bullet+}$	7.9	6.8	<1.0
$LUT^{\bullet+}$	5.2	<1.0	<1.0
$MZEA^{\bullet+}$	7.8	<1.0	—
$ZEA^{\bullet+}$	6.9	<1.0	—

lycopene quenches (i.e., reduces) the radical cations of all the xanthophylls
[Eq. (8)]:

$$XAN^{\bullet+} + LYC \longrightarrow XAN + LYC^{\bullet+} \tag{8}$$

This may explain the link between lycopene levels and the onset of ARMD,
although lycopene is not present in the eye.

The β-carotene one-electron reduction potential has been measured in
dichloromethane (35), and several other workers have also determined the redox
potentials of various carotenoids via cyclic voltametry and shown that lycopene
is the most easily oxidized (36,37). More recently, Edge and coworkers (38)
measured the absolute one-electron reduction potential (E^0 value) of β-carotene
in TX-100 micelles and extended this work to other carotenoids (34), i.e., they
determined E^0 for $CAR^{\bullet+}/CAR$. In both of these studies, the workers monitored
the reaction of the carotenoids with the tryptophan radical at various pH values
[this either involved generation of the tryptophan radical cation, $TrpH^{\bullet+}$, or its
neutral radical, $Trp^{\bullet}$, depending on the pH used, via pulse radiolysis; Equations
(9) to (10)]. The one-electron reduction potentials for tryptophan are well
established (Fig. 2 shows the reduction potential for tryptophan as a function of
pH) and therefore those of the carotenoids can be determined. The studies
followed equilibria of the type:

$$TrpH^{\bullet+} + CAR \rightleftharpoons CAR^{\bullet+} + TrpH \qquad (pH\ 4) \tag{9}$$
$$TrpH^{\bullet+} + H^+ + CAR \rightleftharpoons CAR^{\bullet+} + TrpH \qquad (pH\ 13) \tag{10}$$

In this study the authors showed that the redox potentials of β-carotene,
lycopene, zeaxanthin, lutein, and astaxanthin are all approximately the same
($E_0 \sim 1000$ mV) within experimental error. Although there is a trend with the
oxycarotenoids, canthaxanthin and astaxanthin, exhibiting higher oxidizing

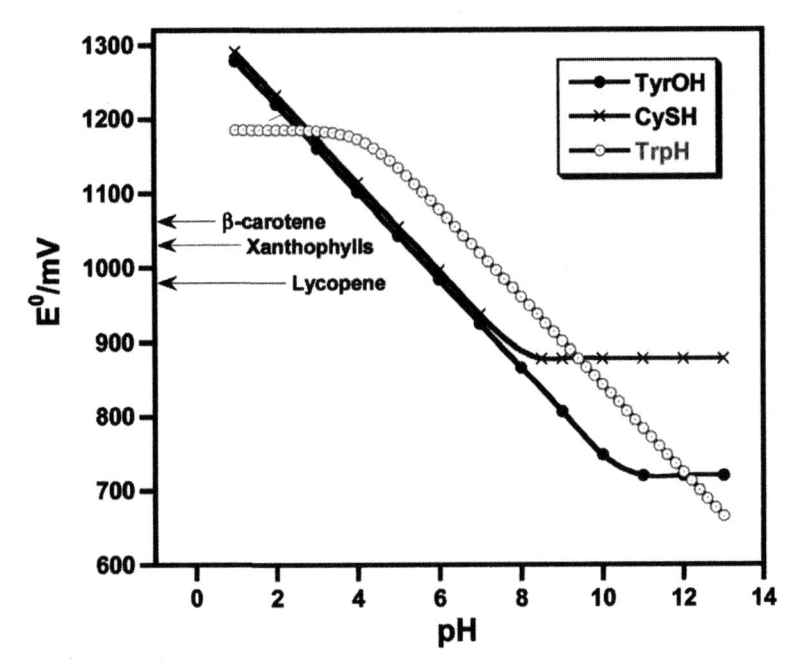

Figure 2 Known reduction potentials of amino acids, tryptophan, tyrosine, and cysteine as a function of pH. The position of the cartenoid reduction potentials obtained in Triton X-100 micelles (for xanthophylls and β-carotene) and Triton X-405/100 micelles (for lycopene) are also marked.

potentials than lycopene, with values of 1041, 1030, and 980 mV respectively (Table 2 gives the redox potentials obtained for the five carotenoids studied). The redox potentials were confirmed by using a dipeptide, TrpH-TyrOH. The initial product is TrpH$^{\bullet+}$ (formed via pulse radiolysis) and in the presence of carotenoid, the carotenoid radical cation is efficiently formed at pH 2 where TrpH$^{\bullet+}$ has a reduction potential of 1185 mV (Fig. 2). However, at higher pH values (where only TyrOH phenoxyl radicals arise), carotenoid oxidation is not observed.

Furthermore, recent work in our laboratory with shorter chain carotenoids (septapreno-β-carotene and 7,7'-dihydro-β-carotene with nine and eight conjugated double bonds, respectively) have shown an inverse trend toward higher redox potential with decreasing number of double bonds. The values obtained were 1075 and 1100 mV, respectively, for septapreno-β-carotene (SEPTA) and 77DH (unpublished results). Such trends correlate with studies of the reactivities of carotenoids according to their structure (39), e.g., reactivity in which the oxycarotenoids such as astaxanthin are more stable in the presence of

Table 2 One-Electron Reduction Potentials for the Carotenoid Radical Cations, Calculated from the Equilibrium with TrpH$^{\bullet+}$ in TX-100 Micelles

Radical cation	Reduction potential (V)
β-Carotene	1.06
Canthaxanthin	1.04
Zeaxanthin	1.03
Astaxanthin	1.03
β-Carotene[a]	1.03
Lycopene[a]	0.98

[a]Values in TX-405/TX-100 mixed micelles (34).

azo-initiated peroxyl radicals (AMVN and AIBN) and less reactive toward radicals such as the phenoxyl radical compared to lycopene and β-carotene (40). However, the carotenes may not necessarily be better antioxidants since they may be destroyed more quickly. In another study by Woodall, lycopene was destroyed the fastest but afforded the least protection against lipid peroxidation in egg yolk phosphatidylcholine (41). One further comment should be made on the reactivity of carotenoid radicals. It is well known that carotenoid radical cations do not react with oxygen but that at high pressures of oxygen and high carotenoid concentrations, β-carotene exhibits pro-oxidant behavior, as was discussed in the introduction (14). One explanation given for this phenomenon suggested that neutral radicals of β-carotene may react with oxygen to form carotenoid peroxyl radicals, which may propagate the chain reaction (14,42,43). However, recent work by El Agamey and McGarvey suggests that this is not efficient (28) and the neutral radicals CAR$^{\bullet}$ and ROO-CAR$^{\bullet}$ do not react with oxygen either (within the oxygen concentration range of 10^{-4}–10^{-2} M). Furthermore, they show no reaction with hydrogen donors such as linoleic acid (up to concentrations of 0.08 M) and therefore are unlikely to be involved in propagating chain reactions.

III. REACTION OF CAROTENOIDS WITH OTHER AMINO ACIDS

The reaction of carotenoids with tryptophan has already been discussed above, and carotenoids can repair the tryptophan radical cation. The phenoxyl radical $C_6H_5O^{\bullet}$ is a model of tyrosine. Its reaction with carotenoids has also been investigated (44). It has been suggested to react with β-carotene to give adduct formation and direct generation of the β-carotene radical cation. It was suggested (as is the case for the reaction with tryptophan) that the carotenoids may behave as antioxidants via repair of oxidized amino acids (1). On the other hand, the reaction of the carotenoid radical cation with the amino acids cysteine and tyrosine takes place at pH 7 (these amino acids are unable to oxidize the carotenoids β-carotene, zeaxanthin, astaxanthin, canthaxanthin, or lutein), with rate constants in the order of $10^4 \, M^{-1} \, s^{-1}$ and $10^6 \, M^{-1} \, s^{-1}$ for tyrosine and cysteine, respectively, in TX-100 micelles (34). The higher rate constant with cysteine suggests that other factors than redox potentials are important in the reactivity of carotenoid radical cations. In other words, carotenoids are capable of oxidizing cysteine and tyrosine at physiological pH:

$$TyrOH + CAR^{\bullet+} \longrightarrow CAR + TyrO^{\bullet} + H^+ \tag{11}$$

$$CySH + CAR^{\bullet+} \longrightarrow CAR + CYS^{\bullet} + H^+ \tag{12}$$

Such reactions are potentially harmful since, for example, there is the possibility of forming amino acid dimers and protein cross-links:

$$2TyrO^{\bullet} \longrightarrow \text{tyrosine dimers} = \text{protein cross-links}$$
$$= \text{protein damage} \tag{13}$$

Such reactivity of the carotenoids with tyrosine and cysteine may be predictive of their reactivity with other biomolecules whose reduction potentials are less than 1 V (Fig. 2), i.e., biomolecules that can be oxidized by $CAR^{\bullet+}$.

Much of the discussion so far has followed the properties of the carotenoid radicals (some of which can lead to deleterious effects), but little comment has been made about the possible repair mechanisms that may regenerate the parent carotenoids, other than the interactions of the various carotenoids. We now turn to the interaction of carotenoids with other nutrients, such as the water-soluble biomolecules vitamin C, ferulic acid, and uric acid, and the lipid-soluble molecule vitamin E.

IV. CAROTENOID RADICAL INTERACTIONS WITH VITAMIN C

Vitamin C (Fig. 1) is a water-soluble antioxidant that is claimed to reduce oxidative stress, although studies show either an inverse association (45) or no effect on cancer (46). Nevertheless, ascorbic acid can scavenge radicals and is thought to transfer radicals from the lipid phase to the aqueous phase via regeneration of lipid-soluble antioxidants. It has been shown to repair the radical cations of carotenoids, for example. Truscott and coworkers have shown that carotenoid radical cations are efficiently reconverted to the parent carotenoid by species such as vitamin C. The reaction has been observed in methanol, in

Table 3 Second-Order Rate Constants ($/10^7 \, M^{-1} \, s^{-1}$) for Repair of Carotenoid Radical Cations by Water-Soluble Biomolecules in Triton X Detergent Micelles

Carotenoid radical cation	Trolox[a]	Ascorbic acid[a]	Ferulic acid[a]	Uric acid[a]
β-Carotene	19	1.0	0.1	1.1
Lycopene	19	1.8	0.1	1.0
Astaxanthin	52	5.5	0.6	12.1
Canthaxanthin	47	4.3	0.5	1.0
Lutein	31	1.8	0.2	1.5
Zeaxanthin	26	1.5	0.2	1.0

Source: Ref. 50.

TX-100 (Table 3 gives the bimolecular rate constants) (47), and, more recently, in unilamellar liposomes of DPPC) (26), as shown in Figure 3.

$$CAR^{\bullet +} + AscH_2 \longrightarrow CAR + AscH^{\bullet} + H^+ \tag{14}$$

$$CAR^{\bullet +} + AscH^- \longrightarrow CAR + AscH^{\bullet -} + H^+ \tag{15}$$

Figure 3 shows the decay of the radical cation of monomer β-carotene in unilamellar liposomes (monitored at 920 nm, in the absence and presence of vitamin C). Quenching is clear even though the decay kinetics are somewhat complex. Analysis of the decay curves shows a good fit with two or more exponential decays in the presence of vitamin C and a single exponential decay in its absence. We interpret this as quenching of the β-carotene radical cation in the "outer" bilayer by vitamin C in the aqueous phase. However, the vitamin C cannot reach the "inner" bilayer(s) and hence the biphasic nature of the overall decay is due to these two or more environments of the β-carotene. In particular, these results suggest that β-carotene radical cation is able to interact with a water-soluble species even though the parent hydrocarbon carotenoid is probably entirely in the nonpolar region of the liposome. However, it must be remembered that the properties of the radical cations will be quite different from the parent carotenoid and may cause the molecule to move/reorientate to be nearer the aqueous phase of such cell membrane models. The repair of carotenoid radical cations by ascorbic acid is an efficient reaction and rate constants were obtained in unilamellar vesicles for β-carotene, zeaxanthin, and lutein of 11, 9.7, and $5.2 \times 10^6 \, M^{-1} \, s^{-1}$, respectively (26). These observations have led to the suggestion that the deleterious effects of β-carotene in heavy smokers are related to the generation of the β-carotene radical cation by, for example, $NO_2^{\bullet}$. The low levels of vitamin C found in the serum of heavy smokers would not quench the β-carotene radical cation and therefore promote the damage due to the relatively long-lived radical cation.

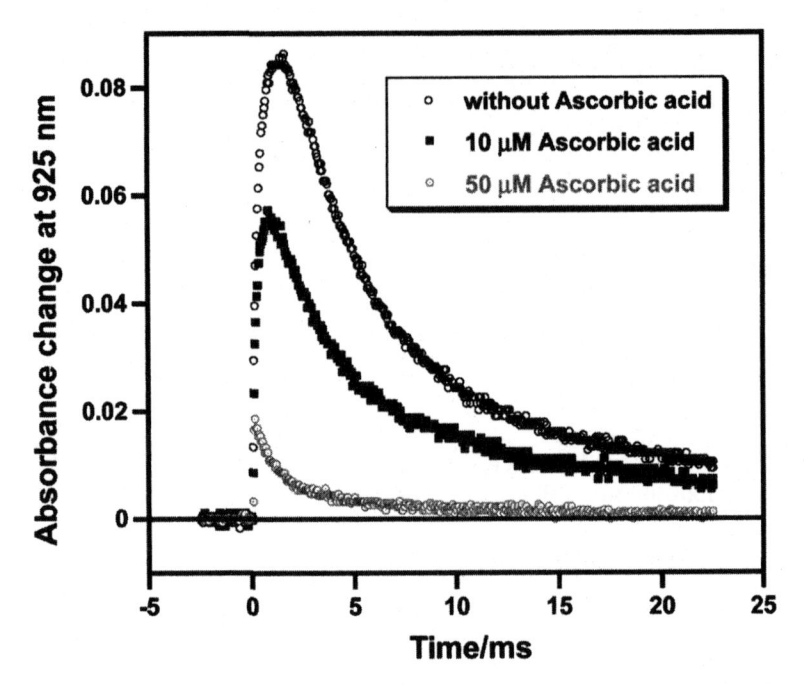

Figure 3 Quenching of β-carotene radical cation by ascorbic acid in DPPC unilamellar liposomes (monitored at 925 nm) (26).

The repair of carotenoid radical cations is at the expense of ascorbic acid and an ascorbate radical is produced. For example, the ascorbate radical will itself be repaired by glutathione or NADH, although at extremely high concentrations it may undergo deleterious reactions via Fenton chemistry (48).

V. CAROTENOID INTERACTIONS WITH VITAMIN E

Vitamin E encompasses α-TOH and its other isomers (Fig. 1). They function effectively as antioxidants as a result of the presence of the phenol group, which can undergo hydrogen abstraction reactions with peroxyl or carbon-centered radicals to produce a phenoxyl radical. Regeneration of vitamin E may occur through redox reactions with carotenoids, but ascorbic acid has also been shown to repair vitamin E radicals (49). These reactions have been studied by several workers (21,47,50) and are somewhat complex.

Truscott et al. showed that several carotenoids, excluding astaxanthin, are capable of repairing the radical cation of α-TOH in hexane (21) with subsequent generation of the radical cation of the carotenoid:

$$\alpha\text{-TOH}^{\bullet+} + \text{CAR} \longrightarrow \alpha\text{-TOH} + \text{CAR}^{\bullet+} \tag{16}$$

For astaxanthin (ASTA), the reverse reaction takes place and electron transfer occurs from the ASTA radical cation to α-TOH:

$$\text{ASTA}^{\bullet+} + \alpha\text{-TOH} \longrightarrow \text{ASTA} + \alpha\text{-TO}^{\bullet} + \text{H}^+ \tag{17}$$

The α-TOH$^{\bullet+}$ has an absorption peak at 460 nm, decays to the neutral radical in nonpolar environments (with an absorption maximum at 420 nm), and is much longer lived. This rapid deprotonation of α-TOH$^{\bullet+}$ to the neutral radical TO$^{\bullet}$ means that the reaction given above with the radical cation of α-TOH is not likely to be important in an in vivo situation. To investigate the interaction of carotenoid radical cations with vitamin E, however, a water-soluble analog known as Trolox (6-hydroxy-2,5,7,8-tetramethylchromane-2-carboxylic acid; see Figure 1) was used. Pulse radiolysis was used to generate the carotenoid radical cations in TX micelles and their decay monitored in the presence and absence of Trolox. Table 3 gives the rate constants for the reaction, which is a very efficient reaction for all the carotenoids. Thus, α-TOH may also reduce carotenoid radical cations in a polar environment (50).

It has been shown (51,52) that there is no reaction between α-TO$^{\bullet}$ and β-carotene, and it has also been clearly demonstrated (53) that for most carotenoids, including β-carotene, the reaction that occurs is:

$$\beta\text{-Carotene}^{\bullet+} + \alpha\text{-TOH} \longrightarrow \beta\text{-carotene} + \alpha\text{-TO}^{\bullet} + \text{H}^+ \tag{18}$$

A similar reaction has been reported for lycopene (LYC) (54) but, in contrast, LYC can reduce the δ-tocopheroxyl radical and slow formation of the LYC radical cation is observed

$$\text{LYC} + \delta\text{-TO}^{\bullet} \longrightarrow \text{LYC}^{\bullet+} + \delta\text{-TO}^- \tag{19}$$

In the same paper, an equilibrium was shown to exist between the LYC radical cation and the β- or γ-tocopheroxyl radicals:

$$\text{LYC}^{\bullet+} + \beta\text{-}/\gamma\text{-TOH} \longleftrightarrow \text{LYC} + \beta\text{-}/\gamma\text{-TO}^{\bullet} + \text{H}^+ \tag{20}$$

and an antioxidant hierarchy among the carotenoids and the homolog tocopherols was established (53,54).

In biological systems the interaction may be more complex and dose dependent as supported by the findings in poultry meat and frozen trout mentioned in the introduction (15). Differences in the protection of lipid membranes against oxidation for zeaxanthin and lutein have thus been attributed to differences in the organization of carotenoids in lipid membranes (55).

VI. INTERACTIONS WITH OTHER BIOMOLECULES

Other molecules present in our diet are also thought to act as antioxidants. These include phenolic compounds (other than vitamin E) such as hydroxycinnamic acids, including ferulic acid, which are widely distributed in plant tissue (56). They are found in many fruits and vegetables, and are formed from tyrosine or phenylalanine via the shikimate pathway. Ferulic acid has been shown to be a potent singlet oxygen quencher and possess a reduction potential of 595 mV (57). Again, it is the presence of the phenol moiety that bestows their radical-scavenging properties.

Uric acid is also a potent antioxidant that is a product of purine metabolism found in much higher concentrations than ascorbic acid. It has also been shown to have better protection against peroxynitrite anion in the presence of iron(III) ions (58). Uric acid was also shown to have a higher antioxidant activity than ascorbic acid (59).

We have studied the interaction of both the water-soluble antioxidants, ferulic and uric acid (uric acid is only slightly water soluble) with carotenoids in a micellar medium and found that ferulic acid is not as effective as ascorbic acid in the repair of carotenoid radical cations, whereas uric acid appears to be as effective if not more so. Table 3 gives the second-order rate constants for the repair of a number of carotenoid radical cations by ferulic, uric, and ascorbic acid. There may be many other compounds (60) that function as independent antioxidants, including other phytochemicals such as allium compounds (sulfur compounds derived from garlic and onions) and polyphenols (e.g., quercetin, catechin, etc., from alcoholic beverages) that may also function cooperatively via interactions with and repair of carotenoid radicals.

VII. STUDIES OF ANTIOXIDANT COMBINATIONS

It has been known for some time that combinations of antioxidants function better than lone antioxidants and that, for example, combinations have a cooperative effect on lipid peroxidation. Palozza and Krinsky observed a delayed AIBN-induced loss of microsomal tocopherols in the presence of β-carotene (61) and reported that carotenoids and vitamin E synergistically act as radical scavengers in rat liver microsomes (62). In the latter study there was an increase in α-TOH consumption in the presence of β-carotene, suggesting that α-TOH protects β-carotene. Terao et al. showed that δ-TOH enhanced the protective effects of β-carotene on photo-oxidation of methyl linoleate initiated by singlet oxygen (63). Other workers have demonstrated that combinations of carotenoids with γ-TOH are more effective in preventing hydroperoxide formation (64,65). These studies show that the pro-oxidant potential of carotenoids may be overcome by the presence of tocopherols. Combinations of β-carotene, vitamin E, and vitamin C have been shown to offer synergistic cell protection against species such as the peroxynitrite anion and nitrogen dioxide radical when compared with individual antioxidants (66).

An increase in risk of lung cancer among smokers who took β-carotene supplements was reported in the Alpha-Tocopherol, Beta-Carotene Cancer Prevention (ATBC) Trial (12) and among smokers and asbestos-exposed workers in the Beta-Carotene and Retinol Efficacy Trial (CARET) (67), but not among male physicians in the United States in the Physicians Health Study (only 11% of whom were current smokers), leading to confusion over the anti/pro-oxidant properties of carotenoids. Readers are referred to the chapter by Palozza in this book for a review of the in vitro and in vivo studies of the pro-oxidant effects of carotenoids. We mention a study by Russell (68) only. He has attempted to study whether there is a true hazard associated with β-carotene in control studies using the ferret that mimics the human tissue metabolism of β-carotene and has been used for studies of tobacco smoking and inhalation toxicology. In this study, ferrets were supplemented with physiological or pharmacological doses β-carotene, which were equivalent to 6 mg/day versus 30 mg/day in humans, respectively. The animals were exposed to cigarette smoke for 6 months. The data showed that in contrast with the pharmacological dose of β-carotene, a physiological dose of β-carotene in smoke-exposed ferrets had no detrimental effect and, in fact, may have afforded weak protection against lung damage induced by cigarette smoke. Further studies revealed an instability of the β-carotene molecule in the lungs of cigarette smoke–exposed ferrets. The authors proposed that oxidized β-carotene metabolites may play a role in lung carcinogenesis by a variety of mechanisms including acting as pro-oxidants and possibly causing damage to DNA. Furthermore, the ferret studies with high- and low-dose β-carotene in the presence of α-TOH and ascorbic acid (thereby stabilizing the β-carotene molecule) showed protective effects against smoke-induced squamous metaplasia in ferret lungs.

The photoprotective potential of the dietary antioxidants vitamin C, vitamin E, lycopene, β-carotene, and the rosemary polyphenol, carnosic acid, was tested in human dermal fibroblasts exposed to UV-A light (69). The authors concluded that vitamin C, vitamin E, and carnosic acid showed photoprotective potential, whereas lycopene and β-carotene did not protect on their own, although in the presence of vitamin E their stability in culture was improved, suggesting a requirement for antioxidant protection of the carotenoids against formation of oxidative derivatives that can influence the cellular and molecular responses.

Another study on skin (70) involved protection against erythema. Skin was exposed to UV light, and erythema observed as an initial reaction. When β-carotene was applied alone or in combination with α-TOH for 12 weeks, erythema formation induced with a solar light simulator was diminished from week 8. Similar effects were also achieved with a diet rich in lycopene. Ingestion of tomato paste corresponding to a dose of 16 mg lycopene per day over 10 weeks led to increases in serum levels of lycopene and total carotenoids in skin. At week 10, erythema formation was significantly lower in the group that ingested the tomato paste as compared to the control group. Thus, protection against UV light–induced erythema can be achieved by ingestion of a commonly consumed dietary source of lycopene. Such protective effects of carotenoids were also demonstrated in cell culture. The in vitro data indicated that there is an optimal level of protection for each carotenoid.

Combinations of antioxidants (β-carotene, vitamins C and E) also protect human cells against phototoxicity induced by porphyrins (UV irradiation leads to the formation of singlet oxygen and oxy radicals from porphyrins, which cause cell damage). Individual carotenoids were less effective than mixtures and the triple combination of β-carotene, vitamins C and E had an increased protection, suggesting that synergistic interactions occur (71). Thus, such antioxidant combinations may be protective against erythropoietic porphyria.

Stahl et al. (72) showed that combinations of carotenoids synergistically inhibited lipid peroxidation in multilamellar vesicles (as measured by formation of thiobarbituric acid reactive substances) and that the presence of lycopene or lutein is paramount to this observed synergism. An additive effect was observed for other combinations not including lycopene or lutein. Synergism was also observed on addition of α-TOH to the antioxidant mixture. The authors suggested the synergism may be a result of specific positioning of different carotenoids within the membrane.

The study of other antioxidant interactions may also be important. Pedrielli et al. (73) studied the interaction between flavonoids and α-TOH by oximetry in tert-butyl alcohol. In this solvent flavonoids are weak retarders of peroxidation of methyl linoleate initiated by AIBN. Quercetin and epicatechin were found to act synergistically with the chain-breaking antioxidant α-TOH. In chlorobenzene, a solvent in which flavonoids are chain-breaking antioxidants, quercetin and catechin each regenerated α-TOH, resulting in a co-antioxidant effect. The stoichiometric factor of the flavonoids as chain-breaking antioxidants in 1 : 1 mixtures with α-TOH was measured to be close to 1 for quercetin and slightly smaller for the catechins.

VIII. CONCLUSIONS

The radical cations of dietary carotenoids are rather easy to detect and study. Much is now understood concerning such radicals; they have been shown to be strong oxidants themselves (e.g., they are able to oxidise amino acids) and hence potentially detrimental. Regeneration of the carotenoid radical cation CAR$^{\bullet+}$ to the parent carotenoid CAR by water-soluble antioxidants such as vitamin C has also been observed and is speculated to be linked to detrimental effects of

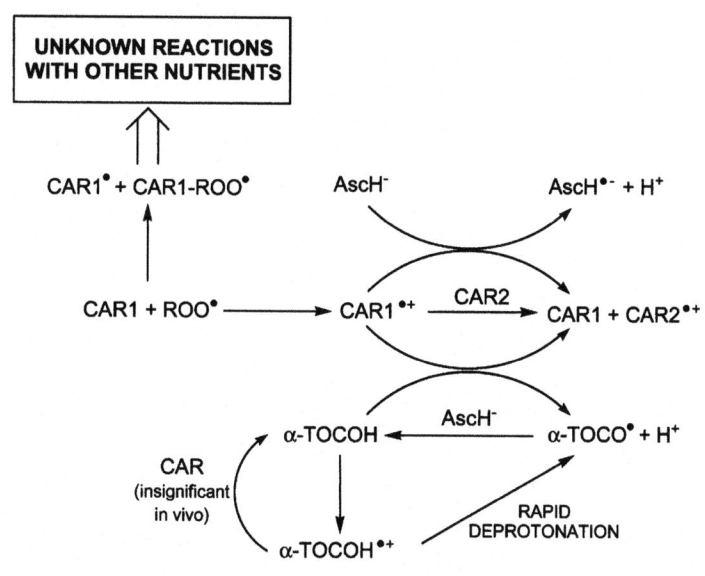

Figure 4 Interaction of carotenoid radicals with other nutrients, water-soluble vitamin C, and lipid-soluble vitamin E.

carotenoids when vitamin C is low. The interaction between tocopherol isomers and carotenoids is more complex and appears to depend on the precise tocopherol isomer; more work on this subject is needed. Figures 4 and 5 summarize the reactions of carotenoid radicals with other nutrients.

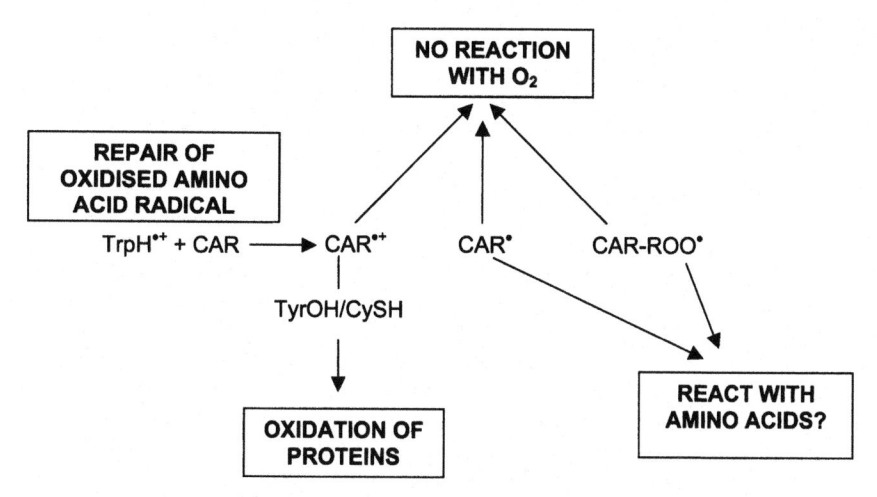

Figure 5 Potential antioxidant and pro-oxidant reactions of carotenoid radicals.

The other radicals of carotenoids (the neutral radical CAR• and addition radicals, such as [CAR-ROO]•) are difficult to study due to spectral overlap with the strong absorption bands of the parent carotenoid. As with carotenoid radical cations, they have been shown not to react efficiently with oxygen; hence, pro-oxidant chain reactions involving such a role for oxygen seem unlikely. Much is still to be learned about the properties of carotenoid neutral and addition radicals and of the interactions of these species with other nutrients.

ACKNOWLEDGMENTS

The authors thank the WCRF and the U.K. National Lottery Charities Board for financial support.

REFERENCES

1. Edge R, Truscott TG. Carotenoid radicals and the interaction of carotenoids with active oxygen species. In: Frank A, Young AJ, Britton G, Cogdell RJ, eds. The Photochemistry of Carotenoids, Dordrecht: Kluwer Academic, 1999:223–234.
2. Edge R, McGarvey DJ, Truscott TG. The carotenoids as anti-oxidants—a review Photochem Photobiol B: Biol 1997;41:189–200.
3. Cantrell A, McGarvey DJ, Truscott TG, Rancan F, Böhm F. Singlet oxygen quenching in a model membrane environment. Arch Biochem Biophys 2003;412:47–54.
4. Hanley J, Deligiannakis Y, Pascal A, Faller P, Rutherford AW. Carotenoid oxidation in photosystem II. Biochemistry 1999;38:8189–8195.
5. Vrettos JS, Stewart DH, de Paula JC Brudvig GW. Low-temperature optical and resonance Raman spectra of a carotenoid cation radical in photosystem II. J Phys Chem B 1999;103:6403–6406.
6. Rhee KH, Morris EP, Zheleva D, Hankamer B, Kuhlbrandt W, Barber J. Two-dimensional structure of plant photosystem II at 8-angstrom resolution. Nature 1997;389:522–526.
7. Steinberg-Yfrach G, Liddell PA, Hung SC, Moore AL, Gust D, Moore TA. Conversion of light energy to proton potential in liposomes by artificial photosynthetic reaction centres. Nature 1997;385:239–241.
8. Maniga NI, Sumida JP, Stone S, Moore AL, Moore TA, Gust D. Increasing the yield of photoinduced charge separation through parallel electron transfer pathways. J Porphyrins Phthalocyanines 1999; 3:32–44.
9. Blot WJ, Li JY, Taylor PR, Guo WD, Dawsey S, Wang GQ, Yang CS, Zheng SF, Gail M, Li GY, Yu Y, Liu BQ, Tangrea J, Sun YH, Liu FS, Fraumeni JF, Zhang, YH, Li B. Nutrition intervention trials in Linxian, China: supplementation with specific vitamin mineral combinations, cancer incidence and disease-specific mortality in the general population. J Natl Cancer Inst 1993;85:1483–1492.

10. Manson JE, Stampfer MJ, Willet WC, Calditz GA, Rosner B, Speizer FE, Hennekens CH. A prospective study of vitamin C and incidence of coronary heart disease in women. Circulation 1992;85:865–865.

11. Mares-Perlman JA, Brady WE, Klein R, Klein BEK, Bowen P, Stacewicz-Sapuntzakis M, Palta M. Serum antioxidants and age-related macular degeneration in a population based control study. Arch Ophthalmol 1995;113:1518–1523.

12. The Alpha-Tocopherol Beta-Carotene Cancer Prevention Study Group. The effect of Vitamin E and β-carotene on the incidence of lung cancer and other cancers in male smokers. N Engl J Med 1994;330:1029–1035.

13. Omenn GS, Goodman GE, Thornquist MD, Balmes J, Cullen MR, Glass A, Keogh JP, Meyskens FL, Valanis B, Williams JH, Barnhart S, Hammar S. Effects of a combination of β-carotene and vitamin A on lung cancer and cardiovascular disease. N Engl J Med 1996;334:1150–1155.

14. Burton GW, Ingold KU. β-Carotene: an unusual type of lipid antioxidant. Science 1984;224:569–573.

15. Ruiz JA, Pérez-Vendrell AM, Esteve-Garcia E. Effect of β-carotene and vitamin E on oxidative stability in leg meat of broilers fed different supplemental fats. J Agric Food Chem 1999;47:418–454.

16. Neta P, Huie RE, Ross AB. J Phys Chem Ref Data 1990;19: 413–513.

17. Rice-Evans CA, Sampson J, Bramley PM, Holloway DE. Why do we expect carotenoids to be antioxidants in vivo? Free Radic Res 1997;26:381–398 (and references therein).

18. Everett SA, Dennis MF, Patel KB, Maddix S, Kundu SC, Willson RL. Scavenging of nitrogen dioxide, thiyl, and sulfonyl free radicals by the nutritional antioxidant β-carotene. J Biol Chem 1996;271:3988–3994.

19. Martin HD, Ruck C, Schmidt M, Sell S, Beutner S, Mayer B, Walsh R. Chemistry of carotenoid oxidation and free radical reactions. Pure Appl Chem 1999;71: 2253–2262.

20. Polyakov NE, Kruppa AI, Leshina TV, Konovalova TA, Kispert LD. Carotenoids as antioxidants: spin trapping EPR and optical study. Free Radic Biol Med 2001;31:43–52.

21. Edge R, Land EJ, McGarvey DJ, Mulroy L, Truscott TG. Relative one-electron reduction potentials of carotenoid radical cations and the interactions of carotenoids with the vitamin E radical cation. J Am Chem Soc 1998;120: 4087–4090.

22. Britton G. Structure and properties of carotenoids in relation to function. FASEB J 1995;9:1551–1558.

23. Gruszecki WI. Carotenoids in membranes. In: Frank A, Young AJ, Britton G, Cogdell RJ, eds. The Photochemistry of Carotenoids, Dordrecht: Kluwer Academic, 1999:223–234.

24. Tinkler JH, Tavender SM, Parker AW, McGarvey DJ, Truscott TG. Investigation of carotenoid radical cations and triplet states by laser flash photolysis and time-resolved resonance Raman spectroscopy: observation of competitive energy and electron transfer. J Am Chem Soc 1996;118:1756–1761.

25. Adhikari S, Kapoor S, Chattopadhyay S, Mukherjee T. Pulse radiolytic oxidation of β-carotene with halogenated alkylperoxyl radicals in a quaternary microemulsion: formation of retinol. Biophys Chem 2000;88:111–117.

26. Burke M, Edge R, Land EJ, Truscott TG. Characterisation of carotenoid radical cations in liposomal environments: interaction with vitamin C. J Photochem Photobiol B: Biol 2001;60:1–6.

27. Mortensen A, Skibsted LH, Truscott TG. The interaction of dietary carotenoids with radical species. Arch Biochem Biophys 2001;385:13–19.

28. El-Agamey A, McGarvey DJ, Evidence for a lack of reactivity carotenoid addition radicals towards oxygen: a laser flash photolysis study of carotenoids with acylperoxyl radicals in polar and non-polar solvents. J Am Chem Soc 2003;125:3330–3340.

29. Simic MG. Carotenoid free radicals. Meth. Enzymol. 1992;213:444–453.

30. Chan, HW–S; Levett, G, Matthew, JA. Thermal isomerisation of methyl linoleate hydroperoxides. Evidence of molecular oxygen as a leaving group in a radical rearrangement J Chem Soc Chem Commun, 1978, 756.

31. Hill TJ, Land EJ, McGarvey DJ, Schalch W, Tinkler JH, Truscott TG. Interactions between carotenoids and the $CCl_3O_2^\bullet$ radical. J. Am. Chem. Soc 1995;117:8322–8326.

32. Edge R. Spectroscopic and kinetic investigations of carotenoid radical ions and excited states. PhD thesis, Keele University, 1998.

33. Edge R, Truscott TG. Carotenoids: free radical interactions. The Spectrum 2000;13:12–20.

34. Burke M, Edge R, Land EJ, McGarvey DJ, Truscott TG. One-electron reduction potentials of dietary carotenoid radical cations in aqueous micellar environments. FEBS Lett 2001;500:132–136.

35. Land EJ, Lexa D, Bensasson RV, Gust D, Moore TA, Moore AL, Liddell PA, Nemeth GA. Pulse radiolytic and electrochemical investigations of intramolecular electron-transfer in carotenoporphyrins and carotenoporphyrin quinine triads. Phys Chem 1987;91:4831–4835.

36. Liu D, Gao Y, Kispert LD. Electrochemical properties of natural carotenoids. J Electroanal Chem 2000;488:140–150.

37. He Z, Kispert LD. Electrochemical and optical study of carotenoids in TX100 micelles: electron transfer and a large blue shift. J Phys Chem B 1999;103: 9038–9043.

38. Edge R, Land EJ, McGarvey DJ, Burke M, Truscott TG. The reduction potential of the β-carotene$^{\bullet+}/\beta$-carotene couple in an aqueous micro-heterogeneous environment. FEBS Lett 2000;471:125–127.

39. Woodall AA, Wai-Ming Lee S, Weesie RJ, Jackson MJ, Britton G. Oxidation of carotenoids by free radicals: relationship between structure and reactivity. Biochim Biophy Acta 1997;1336:33–42.

40. Mortensen A, Skibsted LH. Importance of carotenoid structure in radical scavenging reactions. J Agric Food Chem 1997;45:2970–2977.

41. Woodall AA, Britton G, Jackson MJ. Carotenoids and protection of phospholipids in solution or in liposomes against oxidation by peroxyl radicals: relationship between carotenoid structure and protective ability. Biochim Biophys Acta 1997;1336:575–586.

42. Edge R, McGarvey DJ, Truscott TG. The carotenoids as antioxidants—review J Photochem Photobiol B: Biol 1997;41:189–200.

43. Edge R, Truscott TG. Prooxidant and antioxidant reaction mechanisms of carotene and radical interactions with vitamins E and C. Nutrition 1997;13:992–994.
44. Mortensen A, Skibsted LH. Kinetics of parallel electron transfer from β-carotene to phenoxyl radical and adduct formation between phenoxyl radical and β-carotene Free Radic Res 1996;25:515–523.
45. Bandera EV, Freudenheim JL, Marshall JR, Zielezny M, Priore JL, Brasure J, Baptiste M, Graham S. Diet and alcohol consumption and lung cancer risk in the New York State cohort (United States). Cancer Causes Control 1997;8:828.
46. Lippmann SM, Lee JJ, Sabichi AL. Cancer chemoprevenion: progress and promise. J Natl Cancer Inst 1998;90:1514.
47. Böhm F, Edge R, Land EJ, McGarvey DJ, Truscott TG. Carotenoids enhance vitamin E antioxidant efficiency. J Am Chem Soc 1997;119:621–622.
48. Halliwell B, Wasil M, Grootvels M. Biologically significant scavenging of the myeloperioxidase-derived oxidant hypochlorus acid by ascorbic acid. FEBS Lett 1987;213:15.
49. Bisby RH, Parker AW. Reaction of ascorbate with the α-tocopherol radical in micellar and bilayer-membrane systems. Arch Biochem Biophys 1995;317:170–178.
50. Burke M. Pulsed radiation studies of carotenoid radicals and excited states. PhD thesis, Keele University, 2001.
51. Valgimigli L, Lucarini M, Pedulli GF, Ingold KU. Does β-carotene really protect vitamin E from oxidation? J Am Chem Soc 1997;119:8095–8096.
52. Mortensen A, Skibsted LH, Willnow A, Everett SA. Reappraisal of the tocopheroxyl radical reaction with β-carotene: evidence for oxidation of vitamin E by the β-carotene radical cation. Free Radic Res 1998;28:229–234.
53. Mortensen A, Skibsted LH, Willnow A, Everett SA. Relative stability of carotenoid radical cations and homologue tocopheroxyl radicals. A real time kinetic study of antioxidant hierarchy. FEBS Lett 1997;417:261–266.
54. Mortensen A, Skibsted LH. Real time detection of reactions between radicals of lycopene and tocopherol homologues. Free Radic Res 1997;27:229–234.
55. Sujak A, Gabrielska J, Grudzinski W, Borc R, Mazurek P, Gruszecki WI. Lutein and zeaxanthin as protectors of lipid membranes against oxidative damage: the structural aspects. Arch Biochem Biophys 1999;371:301–307.
56. Hermann K. Occurrence and content of hydroxycinnamic acid and hydroxybenzoic acid in foods. Crit Rev Food Sci Nutr 1989;28:315–347.
57. Foley S, Navaratnam S, Land EJ, McGarvey DJ, Truscott TG, Rice-Evans CA. Sinlget oxygen quenching and the redox properties of hydroxycinnamic acids. Free Radic Biol Med 1999;26:1202–1208.
58. Spitsen SV, Scott GW, Mikheeva T, Zborek A, Kean RB, Brimer CM, Koprowski H, Hooper CD. Comparison of uric acid and ascorbic acid in protection against EAE, Free Radic Biol Med 2002;33:1363–1371.
59. Yousry MA, Naguib A. Fluorometric method for measurement of oxygen radical-scavenging activity of water-soluble antioxidants. Anal Biochem 2000;284:93–98.
60. Cooke MS, Evans MD, Mistry N, Lunec J. Role of dietary antioxidants in the prevention of oxidative DNA damage. Nutr Res Rev 2002;15:19–41.

61. Palozza P, Krinsky NI. The inhibition of radical-initiated peroxidation of microsomal lipids by both α-tocopherol and β-carotene. Free Radic Biol Med 1991;11:407–414.

62. Palozza P, Krinsky NI. β-carotene and α-tocopherol are synergistic anioxidants. Arch Biochem Biophys 1992;297:184–187.

63. Terao J, Yamauchi R, Murakami H, Matsushita S. Inhibitory effects of tocopherols and β-carotene on singlet-oxygen initiated photooxidation of methyl linoleate and soybean oil. J Food Proc Preserv 1980;4:79–93.

64. Haila KM, Heinonen M. Action of β-carotene on purified rapeseed oil during light storage. Lebensm Wiss Technol 1994;27:573–577.

65. Haila KM, Lievonen SM, Heinonen M. Effects of lutein, lycopene, annatto, and γ-tocopherol on autooxidation of triglycerides. J Agric Food Chem 1996; 44:2096–2100.

66. Bohm F, Edge R, McGarvey DJ, Truscott TG. β-Carotene with vitamins E and C offers synergistic cell protection against NOx. FEBS Lett 1998;436:387–389.

67. Omenn GS, Goodman GE, Thornquist MD, Rosenstock L, Barnhart S, Gylyscolwell I, Metch B, Lund B. The carotene and retinol efficacy trial (caret) to prevent lung cancer in high risk populations: pilot study with asbestos exposed workers. Cancer Epidermal Biomar 1993;2:381–387.

68. Russell RM. β-Carotene and lung cancer. Pure Appl Chem 2002;74:1461–1467.

69. Offord EA, Gautier JC, Avanti O, Scaletta C, Runge F, Kramer K, Applegate LA. Photoprotective potential of lycopene, β-carotene, vitamin E, vitamin C and carnosic acid in UVA-irradiated human skin fibroblasts. Free Radic Biol Med 2002;32:1293–1303.

70. Stahl W, Sies H. Carotenoids and protection against solar UV radiation. Skin Pharmacol Appl Skin Physiol 2002;15:291–296.

71. Böhm F, Edge R, Foley S, Lange L, Truscott TG. Antioxidant inhibition of porphyrin-induced cellular phototoxicity. J Photochem. Photobiol B Biol 2001;65:177–183.

72. Stahl W, Junghans A, de Boer B, Driomina ES, Briviba K, Sies H. Carotenoid mixtures protect multilamellar liposomes against oxidative damage: synergistic effects of lycopene and lutein. FEBS Lett 1998;427:305–308.

73. Pedrielli P, Skibsted LH. Antioxidant synergy and regeneration effect of quercetin, (−)-epicatechin, and (+)-catechin on α-tocopherol in homogeneous solutions of peroxidating methyl linoleate. J Agric Food Chem 2002;50:7138–7144.

3

Noninvasive Assessment of Carotenoids in the Human Eye and Skin

Paul S. Bernstein and Werner Gellermann
University of Utah, Salt Lake City, Utah, U.S.A.

I. INTRODUCTION

There is growing awareness that carotenoids may have an important role in the maintenance and promotion of good health and in the prevention of chronic disease (1). Much of this evidence derives from physiology studies that investigate carotenoid function in the tissues of interest or from epidemiological studies that relate various measures of carotenoid levels with disease status. The physiology studies normally employ quantitative analytical methods such as organic solvent extraction followed by high-performance liquid chromatography (HPLC) analysis to determine levels with high sensitivity and specificity, but they are invasive assessments requiring tissue biopsies or autopsy materials. Epidemiological studies generally rely on three means of assessment—dietary histories, serum carotenoid levels, and adipose carotenoid measurements—but these methodologies have many inherent weaknesses. Dietary assessment is an inexact science because it either relies on long-term subject recall via food frequency questionnaires or it employs short-term instruments such as food intake diaries that may not reflect long-term intake patterns. Recall bias can severely confound such assessments, and there may be large individual variations in carotenoid bioavailability. Serum and/or adipose levels of carotenoids are also commonly employed in these studies, but these are by definition invasive techniques since blood must be drawn or fat biopsies performed. The half-lives of carotenoids in the serum are measured in days, and in adipose tissues the half-lives are even longer, so that these levels are probably reasonable measures of medium- and long-term dietary intake, but they do not necessarily correlate well with levels in tissues, especially if saturable and specific uptake mechanisms are utilized. Thus, there has been considerable interest in the development of noninvasive means of assessment of carotenoid levels in accessible tissues. If reliable and repeatable, these noninvasive techniques can provide a convenient means to facilitate epidemiological inquiries on large populations. Likewise, these methods can prove invaluable in physiological and clinical studies since they can be used as repeated measures to monitor response to dietary or supplement interventions. This chapter will review the advantages and weaknesses of various noninvasive carotenoid assessment techniques used on the two most accessible human organs: the eye and the skin.

II. NONINVASIVE ASSESSMENT OF CAROTENOIDS IN THE HUMAN EYE

A. Overview of Carotenoid Function in the Eye

It has long been recognized that carotenoids may have an important role in ocular physiology. As far back as the 18th century anatomists noted that the primate fovea, the region of the retina responsible for high-resolution visual acuity, displayed a deep yellow coloration that they termed the "macula lutea" or "yellow spot" (2). In 1945, George Wald studied organic extracts of primate macular tissue and determined that the macular yellow pigment had spectroscopic and chemical features characteristic of xanthophyll carotenoids, ubiquitous plant derived carotenoids containing at least one oxygen atom along the core $C_{40}H_{56}$ isoprenoid carotene structure (3). Several decades later, Bone and Landrum preliminarily identified the macular carotenoids as lutein and zeaxanthin (4), and in a follow-up investigation, they were able to demonstrate the stereochemical nature of the macular pigment as a mixture of dietary (3R,3′R,6′R)-lutein, dietary (3R,3′R)-zeaxanthin, and nondietary (3R,3′S-meso)-zeaxanthin (5). They suggested that meso-zeaxanthin may be derived from a metabolic conversion in the eye from dietary lutein, and subsequent studies seem to confirm this hypothesis (6).

   Several groups have studied the distribution of lutein, zeaxanthin, and other carotenoids in the human and nonhuman primate eye using HPLC analysis or spectroscopic methods. In the foveal region of the retina, the concentration of lutein and zeaxanthin is enormously high, estimated to be in the range of 1 mM, by far the highest concentration of carotenoids anywhere in the human body (7). They are localized to the cone axons of the Henle fiber layer (8) or to the Müller cells of the fovea (9). The concentration per unit area declines rapidly with increasing eccentricity from the fovea, such that even a few millimeters away the retinal concentrations of lutein and zeaxanthin are approximately 100-fold lower than in the foveal center (10). At least a portion of these peripheral retinal carotenoids are associated with the photoreceptor outer segments (11,12). In the foveal area, the ratio of lutein to zeaxanthin and *meso*-zeaxanthin is in the range of 1 : 1 : 1, whereas in the periphery, lutein predominates over zeaxanthin by 3 : 1 and very little *meso*-zeaxanthin is present (13). In a comprehensive survey of all human ocular tissues, it is clear that uptake of lutein and zeaxanthin into the retina and the lens is highly specific since no other carotenoids except for a few closely related metabolites such as 3′-oxolutein and 3′-epilutein are detectable, whereas other ocular tissues contain a much more diverse carotenoid content similar to that of the serum (14). It is likely that the uptake of lutein and zeaxanthin into the retina (and possibly the lens) is mediated by saturable and specific xanthophyll-binding proteins (15). With the exception of the ciliary body, the total concentration of carotenoids per wet weight of tissue is generally lower than that of the peripheral retina.

The physiological role of the macular carotenoids has been the subject of considerable research interest. They are efficient antioxidants in a tissue composed of polyunsaturated lipids subject to significant oxidative stress from intense light and high oxygen levels (16,17). They absorb light with high efficiency in the 400-to 500-nm range, the region of the visible spectrum considered to be most phototoxic to the retina. Recent animal studies have indicated that lutein and/or zeaxanthin supplementation may provide protection in experimental models of retinal light damage (18). It is also possible that the macular carotenoids may help improve visual function by ameliorating chromatic aberration and haze caused by short-wavelength visible light (19).

The Eye Disease Case-Control (EDCC) study was the first large-scale study to provide epidemiological evidence that lutein and zeaxanthin may protect against age-related macular degeneration (ARMD), the leading cause of blindness among the elderly in the developed world. This study assessed participants' carotenoid levels through serum assays and food frequency questionnaires, and they reported that individuals who have high intakes of lutein and zeaxanthin have 43% lower rates of the wet form of ARMD (20,21). Subsequent studies by others have not confirmed such a large protective effect (22), but the EDCC data was compelling enough to launch a large-scale industry in the United States promoting supplements containing lutein and/or zeaxanthin to individuals at risk for visual loss from ARMD. The recent Age-Related Eye Disease Study (AREDS) has demonstrated that an antioxidant supplement combination containing high levels of zinc, vitamin E, vitamin C, and β-carotene can slow the progression of moderate ARMD (23), but no similar large-scale prospective interventional studies of lutein and/or zeaxanthin have been performed.

While the EDCC provided intriguing information, their carotenoid assessment methods, food frequency questionnaires, and serum analyses are indirect measures of the carotenoid status of the eye. It is of paramount importance to have data on the levels of carotenoids in the relevant tissue, the macula of the human eye. Supportive evidence was supplied by Bone and Landrum in a study in which macular and peripheral retinal carotenoid levels were measured by HPLC in postmortem specimens of donors with and without a known history of ARMD. They found that lutein and zeaxanthin levels were 38% lower in the macula of ARMD eyes relative to controls with no known history of ARMD (24). However, postmortem studies have significant limitations because historical information on clinical history and risk factors of the donors is generally unavailable. Thus, it is clear that noninvasive methods of assessment of macular carotenoid levels in living humans could be powerful tools in epidemiological research on AMD, and these methods would be expected to be very useful for monitoring studies of dietary and/or nutritional interventions designed to raise macular carotenoid levels.

B. Heterochromatic Flicker Photometry

The most commonly used method to measure macular pigment levels noninvasively in the human eye is the psychophysical technique known as heterochromatic flicker photometry (HFP). This technique was initially described by several investigators in the 1970s, and at that time it usually required rather extensive apparatus utilizing Maxwellian view optics, xenon arc lamps, and fixed optical tables (25,26). In recent years, newer versions using free-view (Newtonian) optics and simpler light sources such as light-emitting diodes or projector lamps have been described that allow for construction of portable flicker devices suitable for clinical studies at multiple sites (27,28). Since the details of the construction of modern HFP devices have been covered in these articles and in a recent review (29), the focus of this section will be on more general principles of the technique. Schematic diagrams of two types of HFP devices are given in Fig. 1.

HFP yields the concentration of carotenoids in the macula by determining the perceived optical density of the filtering effects of these yellow pigments at different wavelengths. The subject initially fixates on a spot of light rapidly alternating between a blue color near the absorption maximum of the macular pigment ($\sim$460 nm) and a green color in a region of the visible spectrum in which the macular carotenoid pigments do not absorb significantly ($\sim$540 nm). The subject adjusts the relative intensities of the blue and green lights until the sensation of flickering is minimized or eliminated. The subject then repeats the task using eccentric fixation on a region of the macula where the concentration of the macular pigment is assumed to be so low that its absorption of blue light is negligible. Typical eccentric fixation points are 4–9° from fixation

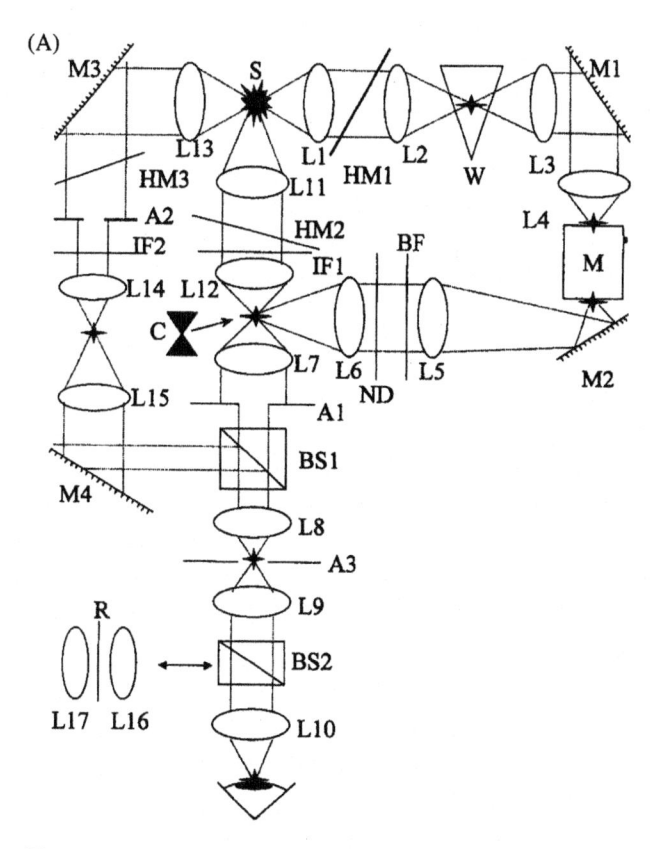

Figure 1 (A) A schematic of the optical system used to measure macular pigment optical density in Maxwellian view. A1–A3, Apertures 1–3; BF, blocking filters remove extraneous spectra from prism used within M; BS1 and BS2, beam splitters 1 and 2; C, flicker vanes with a first surface mirror used for alternating the standard and measuring stimulus; H1–H3, hot mirrors used to reduce heat transmission; IF1 and IF2, interference filters (used in conjunction with neutral density filters, ND1–ND3) render the standard and background stimulus monochromatic; L1–L17, planoconvex achromatic lenses; M, monochromator renders the measuring light monochromatic; M1–M4; right angle, first surface mirrors; R, reticle; S, xenon arc light source; W, wedge. (B) A schematic of the optical system used to measure macular pigment optical density in free view. A1 and A2, Apertures 1 and 2; BS, beam splitter; L1 and L2, planoconvex achromatic lenses; PC, photocell; H, hot mirror used to reduce heat transmission; S1 and S2, light sources; D1 and D2, optical diffusers. (From Ref. 27).

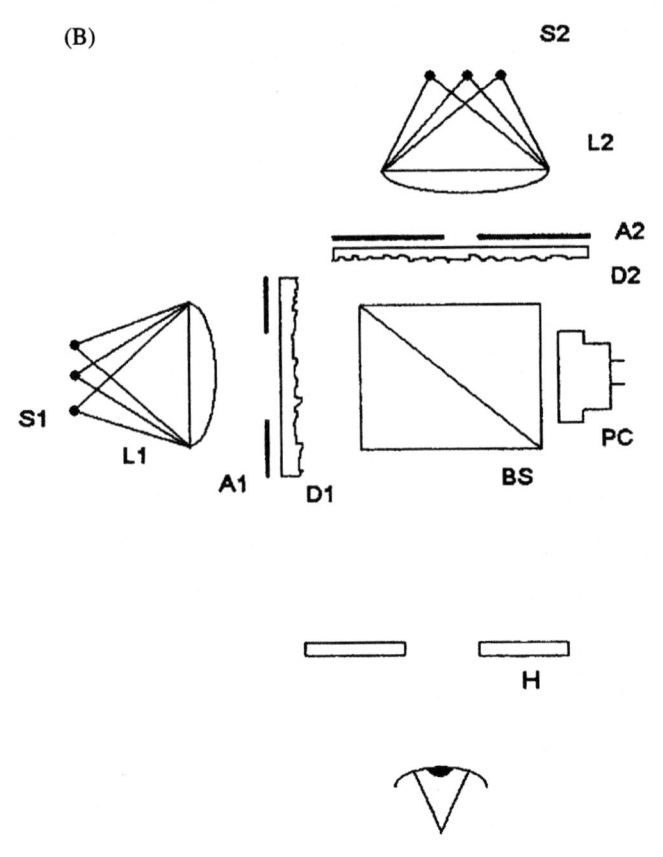

Figure 1 Continued.

(1.2–2.6 mm at the retinal surface). After repeated measurements using central and eccentric fixation, the perceived optical density of the macular carotenoids at the edge of the central flickering spot is calculated according to the following formula where macular pigment optical density (MPOD) is equal to the logarithm of the energy of blue light needed to minimize flicker at the test locus (B_{fov}) relative to the energy needed at the extrafoveal reference point (B_{ref}) (29):

$$\text{MPOD} = \log\left(B_{fov}/B_{ref}\right)$$

Some investigators utilize flickering spots of varying diameters to map out the macular pigment distribution at multiple points, typically along the horizontal meridian (30). Multiple wavelengths may be used in an attempt to recreate the macular pigment absorption curve to confirm that the subject is performing the task properly (31).

As with any psychophysical test, HFP relies on a number of assumptions. The subject must understand the assigned task and perform it with a high degree of attention to fixation, especially when working with an eccentric target. Thus, it is usually wise to provide adequate training to subjects and to confirm reliability by repetitive measurements at separate sessions. Despite extensive training, some subjects ($\sim$5%) never learn to perform HFP reliably, particularly when viewing the eccentric target, which is subject to perceptual (Troxler) fading (29). In our experience, elderly subjects tend to have more trouble performing HFP than younger subjects, especially if they have significant macular pathology.

Psychophysical macular pigment measurement requires that color perception be similar at the central and peripheral fixation sites. This is not a trivial problem because the distribution of the various types of photoreceptors varies considerably with increasing eccentricity (32). At the foveal center, there are no rod photoreceptors and no short-wavelength cones (S cones), but there is an abundance of medium-wavelength cones (M cones) and long-wavelength cones (L cones). Just outside of the foveal center, the density of rods and S cone rises, while the density of L cones and M cones drops precipitously. The S-cone peak density is within a 1 mm of the foveal center, whereas rod cell density peaks just outside of the macula at 5–7 mm of eccentricity. Thus, it is clear that color perception would not be expected to be the same at central and peripheral sites. HFP minimizes the contribution of S cones and rods by providing a blue background light to bleach these shorter wavelength pigments, and the flicker rate of the testing spot is higher than their critical flicker frequencies (29). This allows for the HFP task to be mediated primarily by the M-cone and L-cone systems. As long as the L/M ratio is invariant spatially, HFP should be valid. It appears this assumption is correct in young healthy individuals (33), but there is some evidence that with aging or macular pathology this assumption may not be correct (34).

HFP assumes that the carotenoid optical density at the eccentric fixation reference point is zero, and all other carotenoid optical density measurements are calculated relative to the zero point in order to correct for media opacities and interindividual differences in L/M cone ratios. If the reference point is not actually zero, then all other readings will be systematically underestimated. Therefore, it is important to make certain that the eccentric fixation point is far enough away from the foveal center in a region that no longer has substantial levels of carotenoids. It is known by HPLC studies that a low level of carotenoids is present throughout the peripheral retina (7,11,12), but the levels are generally low enough to be considered negligible when performing HFP unless the central concentration of carotenoids is also extremely low.

Numerous epidemiological HFP studies of macular pigment density have been published in recent years. Many of these investigations have focused on young healthy populations in order to ascertain correlations between macular pigment versus various putative risk factors for ARMD such as age, smoking, gender, iris color, body mass index, blood carotenoid levels, dietary carotenoid intake, etc. (35–38). Correlations have generally been of modest significance and sometimes even contradictory, due in part to the wide range of macular pigment levels in the population and the complex nature of carotenoid homeostasis, as well as differences in HFP methodologies between research groups. Relatively few HFP studies have been performed on patients with significant macular pathology, and these must all be interpreted with caution since some of the critical assumptions of HFP are undoubtedly violated in these subjects. The most notable of these studies demonstrated lower macular pigment levels in the clinically normal fellow eye of patients with unilateral exudative ARMD (38), whereas another group found that retinitis pigmentosa patients appear to have normal macular pigment levels (39).

HFP has also been employed in some small-scale dietary supplementation trials (40–42). In one of these studies, a steady rise in macular pigment optical density was seen in response to lutein supplementation after an initial lag period (40), whereas in other studies, responses to interventions with lutein supplements or dietary modification were quite variable, with some subjects showing no change at all despite several months of intervention (41,42). Possible explanations include poor subject compliance or the presence of saturated carotenoid binding sites in the macula. Also, since HFP measures macular carotenoid levels relative to a peripheral zero point, it is possible that a significant rise in carotenoids in the peripheral retina in response to supplementation could mask a response centrally.

As a subjective psychophysical test, HFP measurements can never be directly correlated with the "gold standard" of HPLC analysis of carotenoids in the macula. Thus, there has been considerable interest by some carotenoid researchers to develop objective optical methods to measure macular pigment noninvasively. These methods might require less reliance on subject training and attentiveness, and there is the potential to perform direct correlations with HPLC in human cadaver eyes or in animal model systems. These optical methods would be likely to have wider applications in subjects with significant macular pathology relative to HFP.

C. Reflectance Methods to Measure Macular Pigment

The first efforts to measure macular pigment objectively were photographically based reflectance techniques. Delori and colleagues took a series of fundus photographs using a variety of narrow-wavelength illumination filters (43). They found that photographs taken at 470 nm, near the absorption maximum of the macular pigment, exhibited a dark central spot corresponding to the peak of the distribution of the macular carotenoids. Other photographs taken at wavelengths longer than 500 nm showed a much less dense central spot that appeared to originate from increased foveal melanin density rather than macular carotenoids. Comparison of the on-peak versus the off-peak photographs allowed for a qualitative estimation of the macular carotenoids since it was assumed that other chromophores provide insignificant contributions to foveal absorbance. Quantitative assessments of macular pigment were not feasible due to limitations of the photographic technology at that time since subtle variations in subject alignment and flash intensity could lead to large picture-to-picture variations in exposure. Also, the filters used were probably not sufficiently monochromatic, and image digitization technology and registration algorithms were not adequately advanced.

More recently, with the advent of high-resolution digital fundus cameras and scanning laser ophthalmoscope (SLO) systems, there has been a resurgence of interest in this technology. Modern computing methods greatly simplify image registration and digital subtraction. Argon laser lines at 488 nm and 514 nm can be used for monochromatic on-peak and off-peak images, and confocal optics can be incorporated (44–46) (Fig. 2). The MPOD is then calculated according to the following equation where C_λ is a constant depending on the absorption coefficients of the macular pigment, and Ref values are the measured reflectances at the fovea and parafovea (14° outside the fovea) at 488 and 514 nm (46):

$$MPOD = C_\lambda{}^*[\log(Ref_{514,\,foveal}/Ref_{488,\,foveal})$$

$$- (Ref_{514,\,parafoveal}/Ref_{488,\,parafoveal})]$$

There are some limitations of this technology, however. The apparatus may be quite expensive, especially when they are custom modified SLO systems. As with HFP, it must be assumed that no other pigments anywhere in the optical path contribute significantly to relative absorbances on and off peak, and they are both subtractive technologies that require the carotenoid content of the periphery to be set to zero. More recently, it has been reported that relative changes of macular pigment distribution in response to lutein supplementation can be monitored using single-reflection SLO images with only 488 nm illumination (47).

A closely related technique called quantitative fundus reflectometry has been employed by several groups. In its typical form, the foveal region is illuminated successively with a series of narrow-bandpass filters on a rotating wheel, and reflected light is collected by a photomultiplier (48), video camera (49), or CCD camera (50) (Fig. 3). Then, using a sophisticated optical model, the average spectral contribution of the absorbance by macular carotenoids (D_{mac}) is calculated for the region illuminated according to the following equation, which determines the reflectance of the whole eye (R_{eye}) at various wavelengths (λ), taking into account the fixed spectral density of the nonaging lens ($D_{lens-na}$), the age-dependent spectral density of the aging lens (D_{lens-a}), the spectrally neutral scatter losses ($D_{medscat}$), the fixed spectral density of 24 mm of water

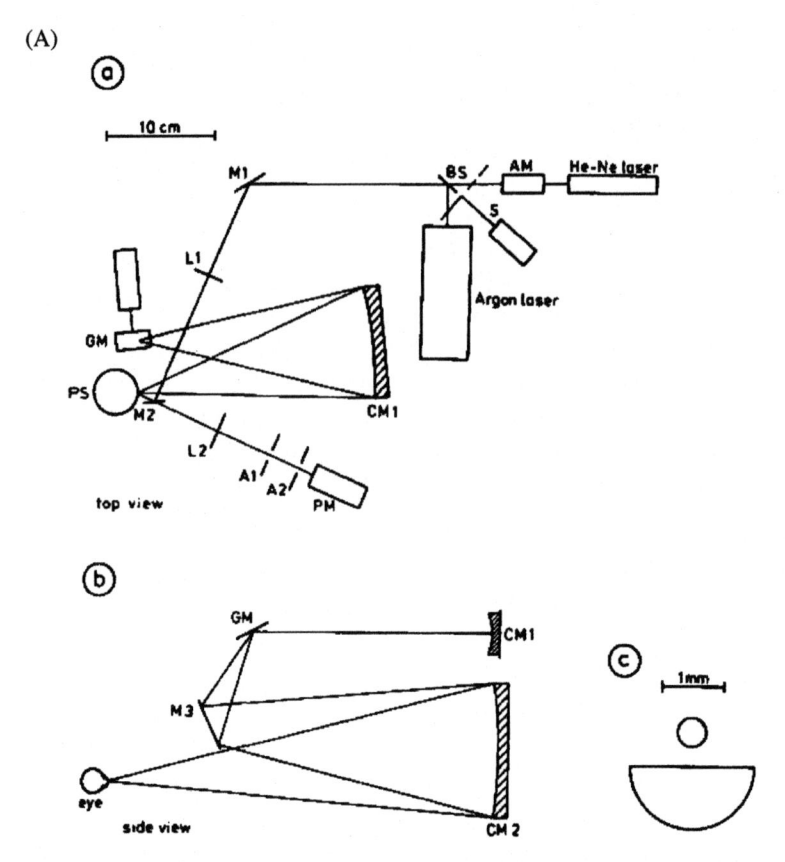

Figure 2 (A) Top view of a confocal SLO, drawn approximately to scale except laser and photomultiplier. AM, acousto-optic modulator; S, shutter allowing the Ar or He-Ne laser light; BS, beam splitter; M1, 2, 3, surface mirrors; L1 lens $f = 200$ mm, L2 lens $f = 40$ mm; PS, polygon scanner for horizontal deflection; GM, galvanometer mirror for vertical deflection; CM1 concave mirror $f = 218$ mm; CM2 $f = 356$ mm; A1, 2 apertures; PM, photomultiplier. (b) Side view of the SLO. (c) Dimensions of entrance and exit pupils in the plane of the subject's pupil. (From Ref. 44). B. Fundus reflectance maps at 488 nm (A) and 514 nm (B) made with a custom-built SLO. (C) Map of the sum of lens density and MP density, obtained by digital subtraction of log reflectance maps shown in (A) and (B). The bar at the left shows the coding of the density units from zero to 1.0. (From Ref. 45).

(B)

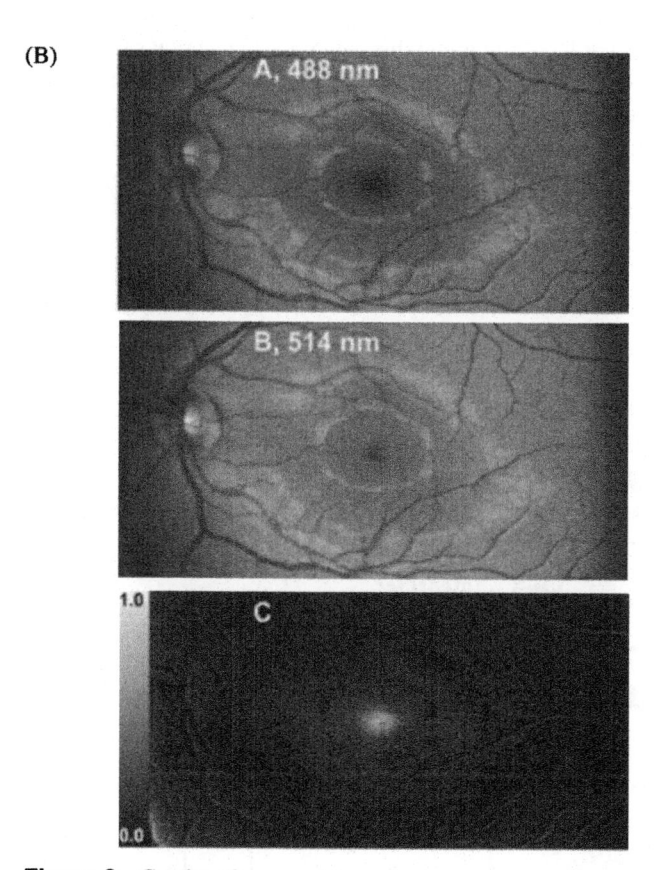

Figure 2 Continued.

representing the vitreous (D_{water}), the spectrally neutral reflectance of the inner limiting membrane (R_{ilm}), and the spectral reflectance of the photoreceptor layer (R_{recep}) (51):

$$R_{\text{eye}}(\lambda) = \{10^{[-2(D_{\text{lens-na}}(\lambda) + D_{\text{lens-a}}(\lambda) + D_{\text{medscat}} + D_{\text{water}}(\lambda))]}\}$$

$$* \{R_{\text{ilm}} + (1 - R_{\text{ilm}})^2 * 10^{[-2D_{\text{mac}}(\lambda)]} * R_{\text{recep}}(\lambda)\}$$

Since the sclera and the cone photoreceptor disks are the primary reflectors in this technique, the incident and reflected light must pass through multiple absorptive and reflective structures, making the optical model quite complex (Fig. 3), and it is unclear how much the model will have to be altered in the face of significant macular pathology. In its current form, image acquisition time is long enough that precise head alignment and fixation may be required.

Berendschot and colleagues have compared this technique to a digital subtraction SLO method in a lutein supplementation study (44). They found that SLO provided the most reliable data, and they estimated that macular pigment optical density rises in the range of 5% per month in response to 10 mg of daily lutein supplementation. More recently, this same group used reflectometry on an elderly cohort with normal maculae and compared them to a cohort with early

(A)

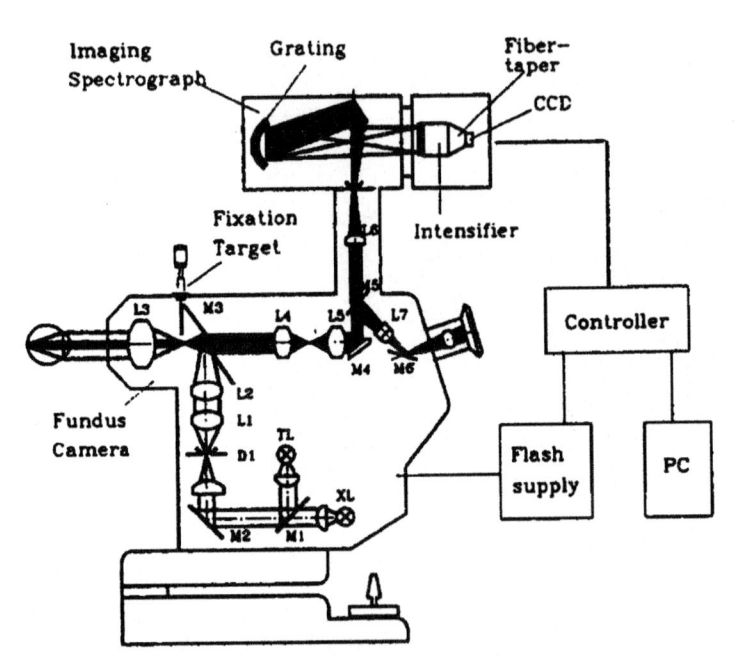

Figure 3   (A) Schematic of an imaging fundus reflectometer. TL, Tungsten halogen lamp; XL, xenon arc flash lamp; M, mirrors 1–6; L, lenses 1–7; D1, a slit-like field stop inserted into the illuminating beam of the camera for the duration of the measurement only. (From Ref. 50.) (B) Model of the optical reflectance of the fovea, with pathways through the receptor layer and reflections from the inner limiting membrane (ILM), the receptor disks, and the sclera. Reflectors (R) are indicated by horizontal lines. Absorbing pigments (D) are drawn as horizontal boxes. Cones are depicted as funnel-shaped objects. In the dark-adapted condition, the cones are filled with visual pigment. Light enters the eye from the top, as indicated by the downward-pointing arrow. Upward-pointing arrows represent light detected by the instrument, emerging from the eye after reflection from the different layers. Secondary reflections are assumed to be lost elsewhere. Only the reflection from the cone receptor disks is directional. (From Ref. 51.)

(B)

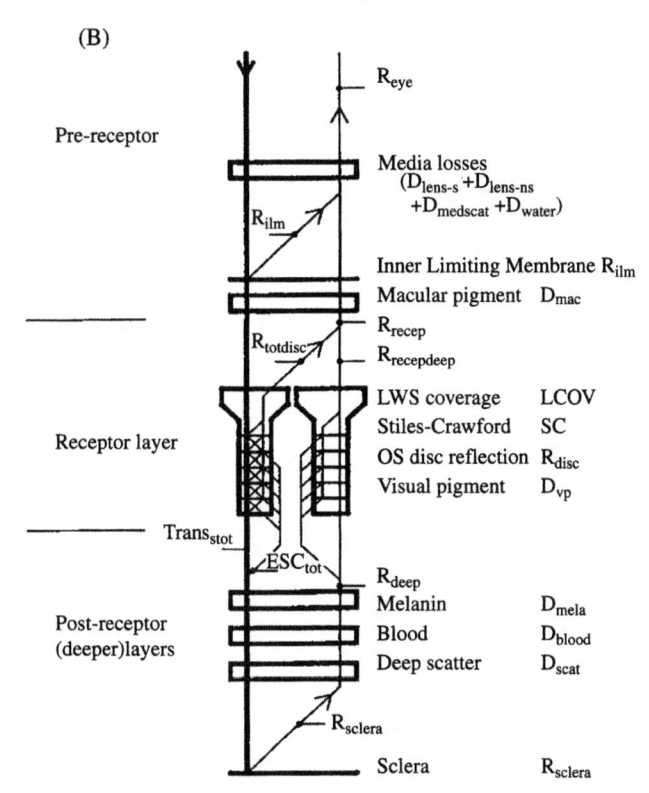

Figure 3 Continued.

age-related maculopathy (52). They could detect no difference in macular pigment levels between the two cohorts.

D. Lipofuscin Fluorescence Attenuation

Delori has developed a technique to measure macular pigment density based on attenuation of lipofuscin fluorescence originating from the retinal pigment epithelium (RPE) (53,54). The major fluorophore of lipofuscin is A2E, a compound formed by the condensation of two retinaldehyde molecules with phosphatidylethanolamine (55). A2E builds up with age in RPE cells in a more or less even distribution across the posterior pole of the eye (56). A2E has a fluorescence excitation spectrum that partially overlaps with the absorption spectrum of the macular carotenoids, and its emission spectrum is broad and at wavelengths well beyond the absorption of carotenoids (55). In Delori's technique, the foveal region is illuminated with two different wavelengths of near-monochromatic light, one within the absorption range of both the macular pigment and lipofuscin, and one within the absorption range of lipofusin alone (Fig. 4). The relative fluorescence under these two conditions is then compared incorporating appropriate correction factors for the quantum fluorescence efficiency at the two different excitation wavelengths at foveal and extrafoveal sites, and the mean peak macular pigment optical density preventing the excitation of lipofuscin fluorescence at the fovea D_{AF} (460) is calculated using the extrafoveal site as a zero point according to the following equation (54):

$$D_{AF}(460) = [1/K_{mp}(\Lambda_1) - K_{mp}(\Lambda_2)]^* \{ \log[F_P(\Lambda_1, \lambda)/F_F(\Lambda_1, \lambda)]$$
$$- \log[F_P(\Lambda_2, \lambda)/F_F(\Lambda_2, \lambda)]\}$$

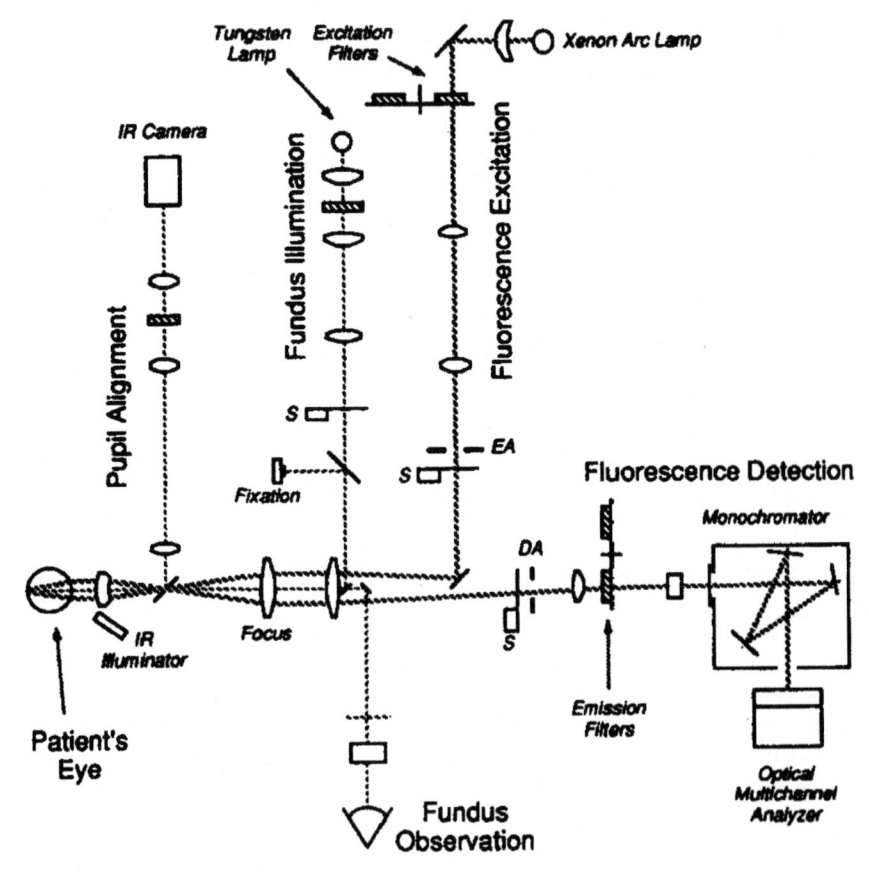

Figure 4 Optical diagram of a fundus spectrofluorophotometer. EA, confocal excitation; DA, detection apertures; S, shutters; IR, infrared. (From Ref. 53.)

In this model, the two excitation wavelengths Λ_1 (470 nm) and Λ_2 (550 nm) are in the high- and low-absorption ranges of the macular pigment, and the lipofuscin fluorescence is measured at the same emission wavelength λ (710 nm). F_F and F_P represent the autofluorescence of all layers located posteriorly to the macuular pigment at the fovea and perifovea (7° temporal to the fovea), respectively, and K_{MP} is the extinction coefficient relative to that at 460 nm. A critical but as yet unproven assumption of this technique is a requirement that no other fluorophores contribute significant fluorescence unless their spatial distributions precisely match that of A2E (54).

The lipofuscin fluorescence attenuation technique is not yet widely used. One report of a comparison versus HFP and reflectometry has been published that demonstrated reasonable correlations, although with some systematic differences (54). Studies on normal and ARMD subjects are reportedly in progress.

E. Resonance Raman Spectroscopy

All of the objective methods for assessment of carotenoids in the living human macula, as well as HFP, are based on the measurement of the characteristic absorption common to most carotenoids—a very high extinction coefficient of absorbance at around 460 nm and minimal absorbance beyond 500 nm. In 1998, Bernstein, Gellermann, and colleagues proposed a radically different method for objective measurement of carotenoids in the eye using resonance Raman spectroscopy (RRS) (57). This form of vibrational spectroscopy has now been developed for use in living human eyes. It has proven to be sensitive and very specific, and is well suited to large-scale screening of clinic populations (58–60).

When monochromatic light illuminates chemical compounds, the light scattered in all directions contains spectral information about quantized internal molecular vibrations. This process is known as Raman scattering, and it can be used to obtain a highly specific optical fingerprint of the molecules of interest. When analyzing the wavelengths of the scattered light with a spectrometer, one finds that most of the incident light is scattered at the same wavelength as the incident light. This light component, termed Rayleigh light, is due to elastic scattering in which no energy is exchanged between the light and the molecular vibrations, and it contains very little information about the scatterers; however, a small proportion of the incident light is shifted, in an inelastic Raman scattering process, to longer wavelengths by discrete light frequency shifts, termed Stokes shifts, which correspond exactly to the vibrational energies of the light-scattering molecules. Most carotenoids exhibit well-defined Raman spectra originating from vibrations of the common conjugated polyene backbone. For lutein and zeaxanthin dissolved in tetrahydrofuran (THF), these Stokes lines appear at 1525 cm^{-1} (C=C stretch), 1159 cm^{-1} (C—C stretch), and 1008 cm^{-1} (C—CH$_3$ rocking motions) (57,61). Ordinarily, the Raman scattering process is weak in intensity, requiring intense illumination, long acquisition times, and high sensitivity detectors, and in biological systems the spectra tend to be very complex due to the diversity of compounds present. This scenario changes drastically if the compounds exhibit absorption bands due to electronic dipole transitions of the molecules, particularly if these are located in the visible wavelength range. When illuminated with monochromatic light overlapping one of these absorption bands, the Raman-scattered light will exhibit a substantial resonance enhancement. In the case of the macular carotenoids, 488-nm argon laser light provides an extraordinarily high resonant enhancement of the Raman signals on the order of 10^5 (61). No other biological molecules found in significant concentrations in human ocular tissues exhibit similar resonant enhancement at this excitation wavelength, so in vivo carotenoid resonance Raman spectra are remarkably free of confounding Raman responses. Raman scattering is a linear spectroscopy, meaning that the Raman scattering intensity (I_S) scales linearly with the intensity of the incident light (I_L). Furthermore, at fixed incident light intensity, the Raman response scales with the population density of the scatterers $N(E_i)$ in a linear fashion determined by the Raman scattering cross section σ_R ($i \rightarrow f$) (a fixed constant determined by the excitation and collection geometries) as long as the scatterers can be considered as optically thin (59).

$$I_S = N(E_i)^* \sigma_R(i \rightarrow f)^* I_L$$

In vivo resonance Raman spectroscopy in the eye takes advantage of several favorable anatomical properties of the tissue structures encountered in the light scattering pathways. First, the major site of macular carotenoid deposition in the Henle fiber layer is on the order of only 100 μm thickness (8). This provides a chromophore distribution very closely resembling an optically thin film having no significant self-absorption of the illuminated or scattered light. Second, the ocular media (cornea, lens, vitreous) are generally of sufficient clarity not to attenuate the signal, and they should require appropriate correction factors only in cases of substantial pathology such as visually significant cataracts. Third, since the macular carotenoids are situated anteriorly in the optical pathway through the retina, the illuminating light and the back-scattered light never encounter any highly absorptive pigments such as photoreceptor rhodopsin and RPE melanin, while the light unabsorbed by the macular carotenoids and the forward- and side-scattered light will be efficiently absorbed by these pigments (59).

Initial ocular resonance Raman studies were performed on flat-mounted human cadaver retinas, human eyecups, and whole frog eyes using a laboratory grade Raman spectrometer and an argon laser. HPLC analysis was performed to confirm linearity of response, and the ability to achieve spatial resolution on the order of 100 μm was shown (57). An instrument suitable for clinical use in living humans and nonhuman primates was then developed (58,59) (Fig. 5). It consisted of a low-power argon laser that projected a 1-mm, 0.5-mW, 488-nm spot onto the foveal region through a pharmacologically dilated pupil for 0.5 s. One hundred eighty degree back-scattered light was then collected, and Rayleigh-scattered light was rejected through the use of high-efficiency bandpass filters before being routed via fiber optics to a Raman spectrometer and Peltier-cooled CCD camera interfaced to a personal computer equipped with custom-designed analysis software. Laser illumination levels on the retina were well within established safety standards. Living humans fixate on a suitable target to ensure alignment, while monkey experiments employed a video camera and red laser aiming beam to confirm foveal targeting. Using living monkey eyes, linearity of response at "eye-safe" laser illumination levels could again be established on this system relative to HPLC analysis of macular carotenoid levels after enucleation, and it was possible to rapidly measure a relatively large population of human volunteers (59,60). External calibration against lutein and zeaxanthin standard solutions in

(A)

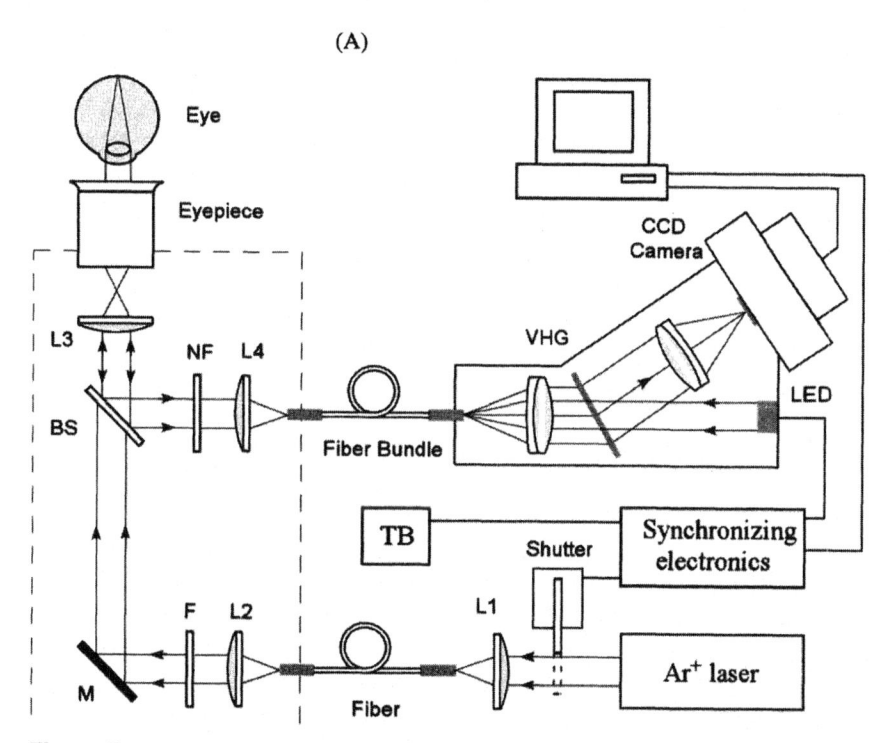

Figure 5 (A) Schematics of a fiber-based, portable Raman instrument for clinical applications. The instrument consists of an argon laser (*lower right*) for excitation, a light-delivery and collection module, a spectrograph (*upper right*), and electronics. The subject looks into the light module through an eyepiece and aligns his/her head position before a measurement. (From Ref. 59.) (B) and (C) Resonance Raman spectrum from a living human macula before (**A**) and after (**B**) subtraction of background fluorescence. (From Ref. 60.)

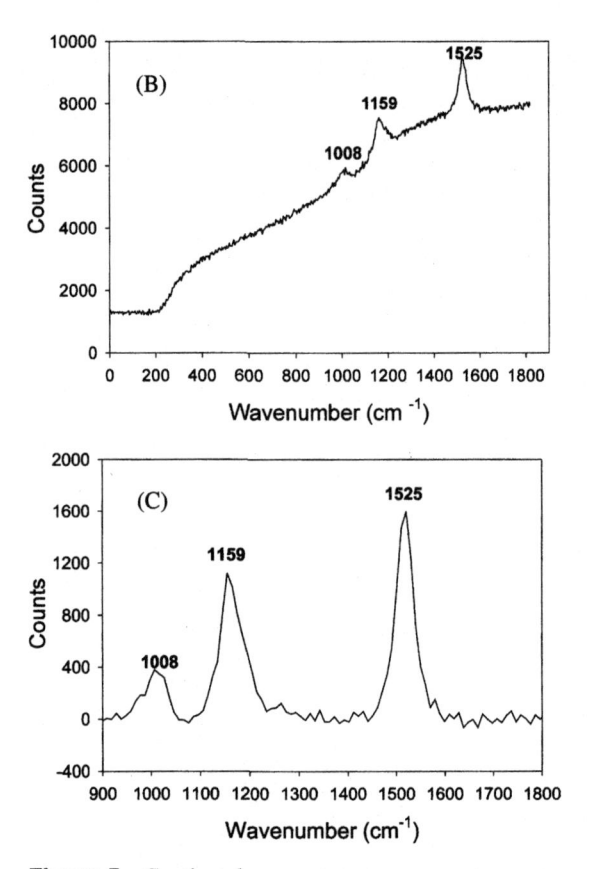

Figure 5 Continued.

1-mm-thick cuvettes showed that in vivo resonance Raman spectra of macular pigment were indistinguishable from in vitro standard spectra after fluorescence background correction had been performed (60). Detector response remained linear until optical densities of ~0.8, well past the amount expected to be encountered in the macula in the vast majority of subjects (60).

Initial experience with the resonance Raman scanner in a clinical setting revealed that it was sensitive, specific, and well accepted by the subjects. Intersession and intrasession repeatability was in the range of ± 10% (59,60), matching or exceeding other in vivo macular pigment measurement techniques, objective or subjective. Since the clinical version relies on foveal alignment on a fixation target, 20/80 or better acuity is ordinarily required. Subjects with dense media opacities such as visually significant cataracts or with poor pharmacological pupillary dilation (<6 mm) were generally excluded from studies since their readings may be artifactually low.

Surveying a large population of clinically examined normal individuals ranging from 21 to 84 years old, we found that there was an approximately 10-fold range of macular pigment in each decade and that there is a steady decline of average macular pigment readings with increasing age until the readings level off at a steady low level past age 60 (59). This decline cannot be explained by yellowing of the lens with age because nearly half of the elderly subjects had had prior cataract surgery and therefore had optically clear prosthetic intraocular lenses, but their macular pigment levels were consistently much lower than those of the young subjects with natural lenses. Macular carotenoids are 32% lower in ARMD patients who do not consume high doses of lutein supplements (≥ 4 mg/ day) regularly relative to age-matched controls who do not consume supplements (60,62). ARMD patients who had begun to consume high-dose lutein supplements regularly after their initial diagnosis of ARMD have levels in the normal range for their age. These findings are very supportive of the hypothesis that low macular carotenoid levels are a risk factor for ARMD and that macular pigment levels can be modified through supplements even in an elderly population with significant macular pathology.

Measurements made with RRS are not directly comparable to HFP since RRS in its current form measures *absolute* amounts of carotenoids in the *entire area* illuminated with the laser (57–59) whereas HFP measures perceived optical density *at the edge* of the illumination spot *relative* to a peripheral site (63). Nevertheless, an initial comparison study has been performed using HFP with 1.5° macular illumination versus RRS with a 1 mm laser spot (64). Baseline studies on 40 healthy individuals younger than 61 years revealed a highly significant correlation between the two methods, but intrasession and inter-session variability was much lower for RRS. Both methods displayed an inverse correlation with increasing age, but only RRS's decline was statistically significant, due in part to HFP's higher variability.

The next generation of ocular resonance Raman scanners will incorporate spatial mapping of macular carotenoid distributions. Using parallel CCD arrays and narrow-bandpass gratings, one tuned to the 1525 cm^{-1} C=C peak, and one off-peak just a few wavenumbers away, we recently developed a Raman instrument that is capable of producing a subtractive topographic pseudocolor map of macular carotenoid distributions at less than 50 μm resolution on human cadaver eyes (65) (Fig. 6). Efforts are underway to modify the instrument for use in living human eyes. The integral of the area illuminated in this imaging technique can be correlated with the previous single-spot resonance Raman method or with extraction and HPLC analysis. Initial employment of this mapping technique on human donor eyes reveals a remarkable variety of macular carotenoid distributions ranging from circularly symmetrical peaks to ridges to

A   B

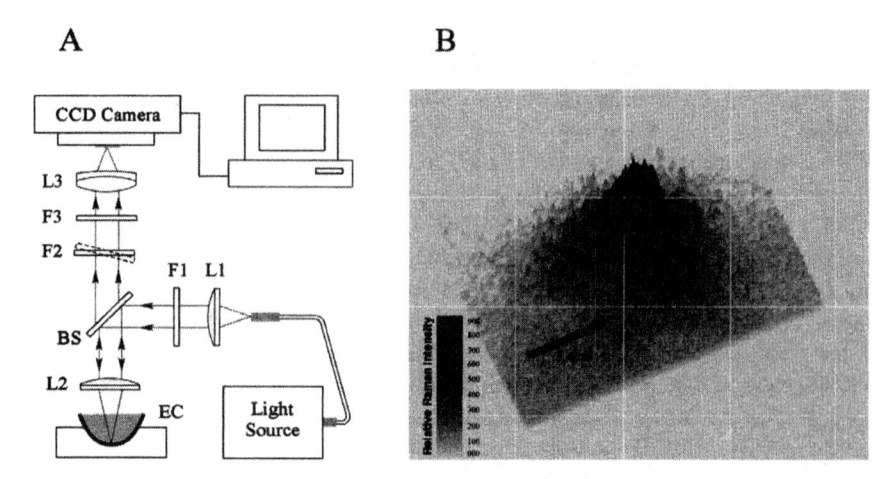

Figure 6 (A) Schematic diagram of resonance Raman apparatus for imaging an eyecup (EC). Lenses (L), filters (F), and a beam splitter (BS) are shown. F2 is an angle-tunable narrow-bandwidth filter. (B) Resonance Raman image of human eyecup showing a volcano-like distribution of the macular carotenoid pigment centered on the fovea. (From Ref. 65.)

volcano-like peaks with central depressions. There is also a wide range of peak widths at half-maximum, but it is clear that a 1-mm-diameter spot is sufficient to encompass the entire foveal peak of macular pigment in all eyes examined so far. It is anticipated that a similar instrument suitable for use in living human eyes will continue to provide new insights on the correlations of macular carotenoid levels and distributions with various macular pathological states.

III. NONINVASIVE ASSESSMENT OF CAROTENOIDS IN THE HUMAN SKIN

A. Overview of Carotenoid Function in the Skin

While only two carotenoids (lutein and zeaxanthin) are found in the human macula, all carotenoid nutrients found in human blood are also found in human skin. These are β-carotene, α-carotene, lycopene, lutein, and zeaxanthin, with the nonpolar lycopene and carotenes having much higher concentrations in this tissue relative to the xanthophylls lutein and zeaxanthin (66,67). Unlike the eye, at least a portion of lutein and zeaxanthin in the skin appears to be esterified to long-chain fatty acids (68). There is no evidence as yet that specific binding proteins are involved in carotenoid uptake and stabilization in this tissue.

Epidemiological and experimental studies show that a high dietary intake of foods rich in carotenoids could protect against many diseases besides macular degeneration, including cancer (69–71), cardiovascular diseases, and numerous pathological conditions linked to damage by oxygen-based free radicals (72,73). In the skin, carotenoids function as antioxidants scavenging free radicals (74), singlet oxygen (75,76), and other harmful reactive oxygen species (77) that are all formed as a by-product of normal metabolism and by excessive exposure of skin to ultraviolet (UV) light or sunlight.

When increasing the amount of carotenoids in the diet or consuming carotenoid-enriched supplements, these nutrients are initially accumulated in the lipoproteins in blood (78). The concentrations can be easily increased by 100% and higher. This increase in blood carotenoids then leads to an increase of carotenoid concentrations in all organs taking up lipoproteins, including skin. It has been shown that skin carotenoid levels are strongly and significantly correlated with carotenoid levels in plasma (66). As is found in plasma, dermal carotenoid levels are lower in smokers than in nonsmokers. β-Carotene levels in skin are known to increase with supplementation (79), and supplemental β-carotene is used to treat patients with erythropoietic protoporphyria, a photosensitive disorder (80). Supplemental carotenoids have also been shown to delay erythema in normal healthy subjects exposed to UV light (81–83). There is limited evidence that they may be protective against skin malignancies (67), but more research is needed to confirm these findings.

As with the eye, it would be useful to know skin carotenoid levels rather than just serum levels or dietary intakes. Skin biopsies are invasive, and HPLC analysis poses special challenges since distributions can vary from body region to body region. Skin also has much lower concentrations of carotenoids, and it has considerable amounts of fibrous tissue that must be broken down prior to analysis. Peng and colleagues reported a method using enzymatic predigestion with collagenase and pronase E that yielded reliable and reproducible results on skin biopsies as small as 28 mm^2 (66,84). Skin is an ideal target for noninvasive optical detection of carotenoids because it is readily accessible, is able to concentrate carotenoids, and shows a good correlation with plasma carotenoid status.

B. Reflectance Measurement of Carotenoids in Skin

Objective noninvasive optical methods to measure carotenoids are challenging since skin is a semiopaque tissue that is prone to considerable light scattering. Jungmann and colleagues developed a reflectometry-based system (85) that has been useful for monitoring relative changes in skin carotenoid content in small groups of volunteer subjects after supplementation (86). In this method, a region of the skin is illuminated with a 5-W halogen lamp via a fiberoptic reflection bundle, and the reflected light is analyzed between 350 and 850 nm using a spectrophotometer. This generates an uncorrected reflectance spectrum of the skin that is dominated by the spectrum of oxygenated hemoglobin with absorption maxima at 450, 540, and 570 nm. Estimation of the carotenoid levels in the skin is then performed using a nonlinear mapping procedure that links the initially recorded inhomogeneous reflection spectrum of the skin at discrete wavelengths (λ) to the absorption spectrum of a β-carotene solution in a cuvette. The basis for this estimation is the following equation in which $s(\lambda)$ is the unknown scattering coefficient of the tissue, k_0 (λ) is the background absorption, $c_i(\lambda)$ are the molar concentrations of the various tissue absorbers, $\varepsilon_i(\lambda)$ are their absorption coefficients, and $R_\infty(\lambda)$ is the skin reflectance (85):

$$(k_0 + \Sigma c_i + \varepsilon_i)/s = (1 - R_\infty)^2/(2^*R_\infty)$$

The degree of inhomogeneity can be calculated in this way, and a corrected spectrum can be obtained that is compensated for the heterogeneous distribution of carotenoids in the tissue and the unknown pathlength of the reflected light in the tissue. The spectrum is further corrected for the influence of other light absorption and scattering components on the skin reflectance spectrum using a partial component regression and a partial least-square multivariate algorithm to determine the deviation due to skin carotenoids. From this derived spectrum, an estimate of skin carotenoid concentration can be determined that is in the same range as reports using skin biopsies and HPLC analyses (86). They also found a significant correlation between baseline skin and serum carotenoid levels in a 12-week β-carotene supplementation study, and they were able to document an apparent rise in response to supplementation (86).

More recently, some of these same investigators have compared their reflectance method with measurements from a more commonly used Minolta Tristimulus Chroma Meter (87) (Fig. 7). In this technique, the colors of the measured skin surfaces are assigned numerical values (L^*, a^*, b^*) in color space, where L^* is the luminance quantifying the relative brightness ranging from total black ($L^* = 0$) to total white ($L^* = 100$), a^* is a value representing the balance between the reds (positive values) and the greens (negative values), and b^* is a value representing the balance between the yellows (positive values) and the blues (negative values). In agreement with the expected behavior for a substance that absorbs in the blue wavelength range, they found that the b^* values correlated with the carotenoid reflectance readings whereas the L^* and a^* values did not. Furthermore, skin carotenoid levels measured by either method correlated positively with minimal erythemal dose levels, an indication of resistance to UV-induced skin damage (87).

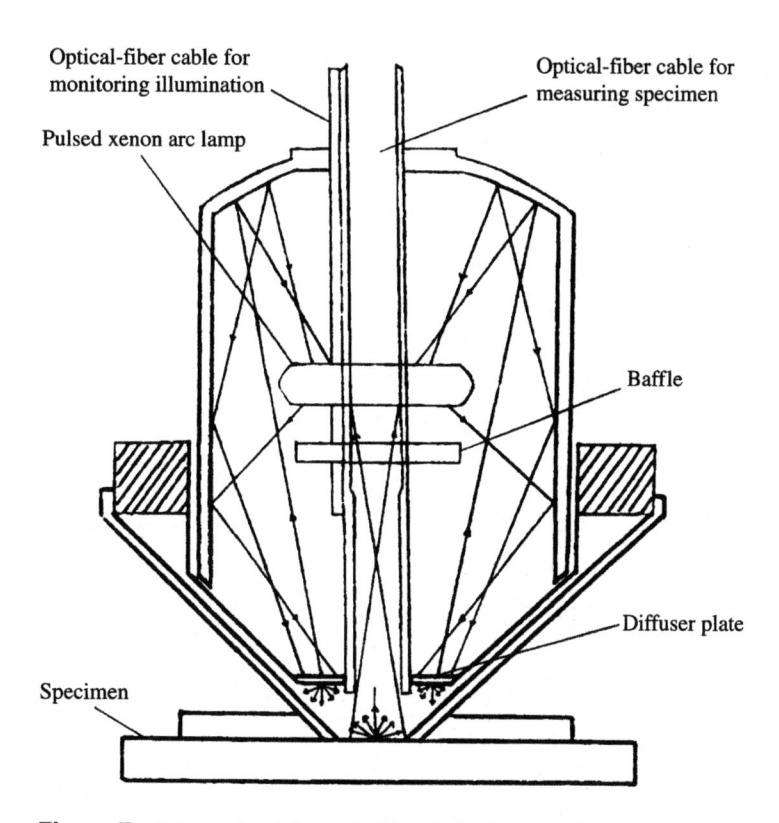

Optical-fiber cable for monitoring illumination

Pulsed xenon arc lamp

Optical-fiber cable for measuring specimen

Baffle

Diffuser plate

Specimen

Figure 7   Schematic of the optical head of a Minolta CR-300 Chroma Meter. A pulsed xenon arc lamp inside a mixing chamber provides diffuse, uniform lighting over the specimen area (8 mm diameter). Only the light reflected perpendicular to the specimen surface is collected by the optical fiber cable for color analysis. (Redrawn from http://www.minoltausa.com/).

C.   Raman Measurement of Carotenoids in Skin

Recently, we applied resonance Raman spectroscopy to carotenoid measurements in skin and oral mucosal tissue (67,88) (Fig. 8). This method is an appealing alternative to reflectance due to its high sensitivity and specificity that obviates the need for complex correction models. Also, this method allows one to measure absolute carotenoid levels in these tissues, so the method does not have to rely on induced concentration changes. Although absolute levels of carotenoids are much lower in the skin relative to the macula of the human eye, laser power can be much higher, and acquisition times can be much longer to

(A)

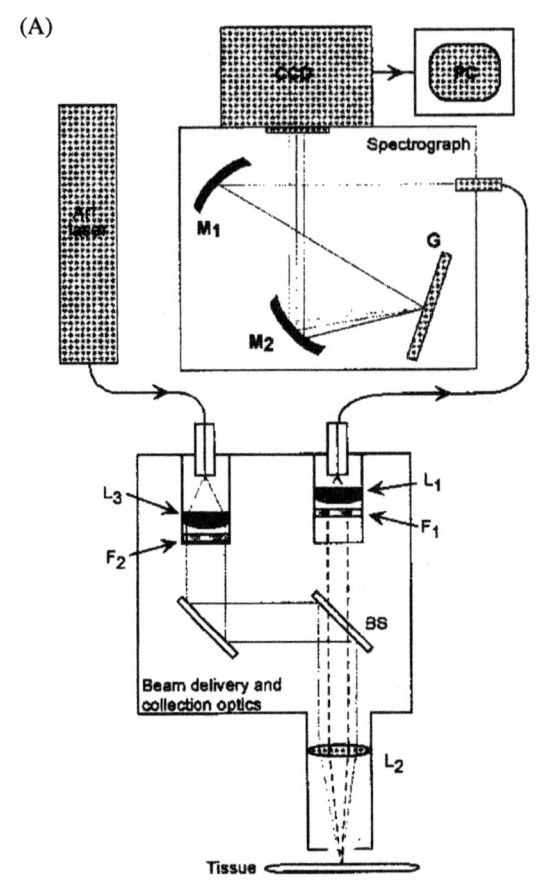

Figure 8   (A) Schematic of basic Raman scattering instrumentation used for detection of carotenoid pigments in human tissue. Excitation light from an argon laser is routed via optical fiber, beam expanding lens L3, laser bandpass filter F2, dichroic mirror BS, and lens L2 to the tissue. The Raman shifted back-scattered light is collimated by lens L2, directed through BS, filtered by holographic rejection filter F1, focused by lens L1 onto a fiber, and sent to a spectrograph. The wavelength-dispersed signals are detected by a charge-coupled detector CCD and displayed on a computer monitor PC. (B) Typical Raman spectra for human ventral forearm skin, measured in vivo. Illumination conditions: 488 nm laser wavelength, 10 mW laser power, 20 s exposure time, 2 mm spot size. Spectrum shown at top is spectrum obtained directly after exposure and reveals broad, featureless, and strong fluorescence background of skin with superimposed sharp Raman peaks characteristic for carotenoid molecules. Spectrum at bottom is difference spectrum obtained after fitting fluorescence background with a fifth-order polynomial and subtracting it from the top spectrum. The main characteristic carotenoid peaks are clearly resolved with good signal-to-noise ratio at 1159 and 1524 cm^{-1}. (From Ref. 67.)

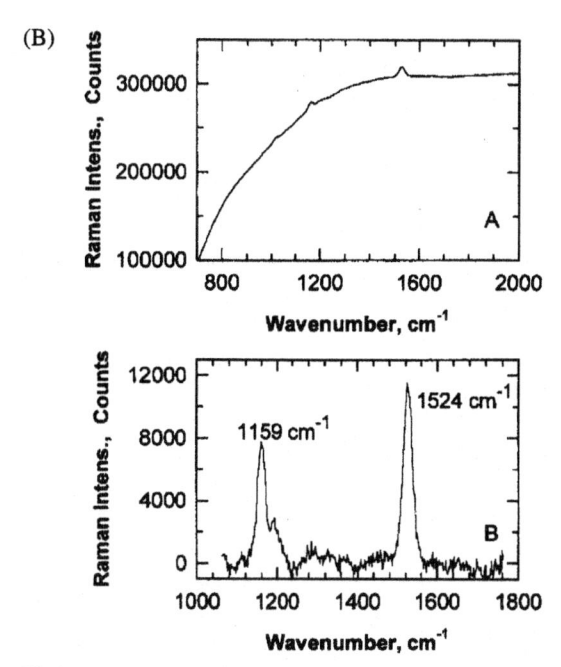

Figure 8 Continued.

compensate. Since the bulk of the skin carotenoids are in the superficial layers of the dermis (67), the thin-film Raman equation given in Sec. II.E is still valid. Background fluorescence of the tissue can be quite high, but baseline correction algorithms are still adequate to yield carotenoid resonance Raman spectra with excellent signal-to-noise ratios. The Raman method exhibits excellent precision and reproducibility (67,88). Deep melanin pigmentation likely interferes with penetration of the laser beam, so measurements are standardly performed on the palm of the hand where pigmentation is usually quite light even in darkly pigmented individuals. As with reflectometry, relatively high levels of skin carotenoids are measured by the Raman method on the forehead and on the palm of the hand, while other body areas are significantly lower (67,87). Quantitative validation studies to correlate skin Raman readings with HPLC analysis of biopsy specimens are in progress.

Measurements of large populations with the Raman device have demonstrated a bell-shaped distribution of carotenoid levels in the palm of the hand (89). Field studies have recently been carried out where a population of 1375 healthy subjects could be screened within a period of several weeks (90). Preliminary analysis of the data confirmed that smokers had dramatically lower levels of skin carotenoids as compared to nonsmokers. Furthermore, the study showed that people with habitual high sunlight exposure have significantly lower skin carotenoid levels than people with little sunlight exposure, independent of their carotenoid intake or dietary habits. When analyzed by a chemical assay based on urinary malondialdehyde excretion, an indicator of oxidative lipid damage, people with high oxidative stress had significantly lower skin carotenoid levels than people with low oxidative stress. Again, this relationship was not confounded by dietary carotenoid intakes that were similar in both groups. These observations provide evidence that skin carotenoid resonance Raman readings might be useful as a surrogate marker for general antioxidant status (89). Studies are also underway to determine whether low skin Raman measurements may be associated with increased risk of various skin cancers. Initial studies have demonstrated that lesional and perilesional Raman carotenoid intensities of cancerous and precancerous skin lesions are significantly lower than in region-matched skin of healthy subjects (67).

The larger number of conjugated carbon bonds in lycopene compared to the other carotenoids in skin produces an absorption band shift that can be used to measure lycopene independently of the other carotenoids (88). It is possible in this way to assess this carotenoid independently from the other dietary carotenoids. There is considerable interest in a specific role for lycopene in prevention of prostate cancer and other diseases (83,91), and a noninvasive biomarker for lycopene consumption would be of tremendous utility.

IV. CONCLUSIONS

Noninvasive assessment of carotenoids in the eye and skin has provided a wealth of data for the carotenoid research community, and additional epidemiological evidence in support of the role of carotenoids in preventing chronic disease is eagerly awaited. As these devices are further validated and as they enter common clinical usage, they are likely to have an important role in early diagnosis of individuals at risk for many debilitating disorders such as age-related macular degeneration and skin malignancies. Preliminary data suggest that these techniques will also be very promising for use in population studies, and employment of these technologies can be envisioned in case-control studies, large cohort studies, randomized diet intervention trials, and trials testing behavioral interventions at the population level. If this approach can be validated as a reproducible and valid biomarker of fruit and vegetable intake that is predictive of risk of chronic disease, then it is conceivable that these techniques could someday be used in routine nutritional surveillance and public health practice.

REFERENCES

1. Mares-Perlman JA, Millen AE, Ficek TL, Hankinson SE. The body of evidence to support a protective role of lutein and zeaxanthin in delaying chronic disease. Overview. J Nutr 2002;132:518S–524S.
2. Nussbaum JJ, Pruett RC, Delori FC. Macular yellow pigment, the first 200 years. Retina 1981;1:296–310.
3. Wald GL. Human vision and the spectrum. Nature (London). 1945;101:653–658.
4. Bone RA, Landrum JT, Tarsis SL. Preliminary identification of the human macular pigment. Vision Res 1985;25:1531–1535.
5. Bone RA, Landrum JT, Hime GW, Cains A. Stereochemistry of the human macular carotenoids. Invest Ophthalmol Vis Sci 1993;34:2033–2040.
6. Khachik F, de Moura FF, Zhao D-Y, Aebischer C-P, Bernstein PS. Transformations of selected carotenoids in serum, liver, and ocular tissues of humans and non-primate animal models. Invest Ophthamol Vis Sci 2002;43:3383–3392.
7. Landrum JT, Bone RA, Moore LL, Gomez CM. Analysis of zeaxanthin distribution within individual human retinas. Meth Enzymol 1999;299:457–467.
8. Snodderly DM, Brown PK, Delori FC, Auran JD. The macular pigment, I: absorbance spectra, localization, and discrimination from other yellow pigments in primate retinas. Invest Ophthalmol Vis Sci 1984;25:660–673.
9. JDM Gass. Müller cell cone, an overlooked part of the anatomy of the fovea centralis. Arch Ophthalmol 1999;117:821–823.
10. Landrum JT, Bone RA. Lutein, zeaxanthin, and the macular pigment. Arch Biochem Biophys 2001;385:28–40.
11. Sommerburg OG, Siems WG, Hurst JS, Lewis JW, Kliger DS, van Kuijk FJ. Lutein and zeaxanthin are associated with photoreceptors in the human retina. Curr Eye Res 1999;19:491–495.
12. Rapp LM, Maple SS, Choi JH. Lutein and zeaxanthin concentrations in rod outer segment membranes from perifoveal and peripheral human retina. Invest Ophthalmol Vis Sci 2000;41:1200–1209.
13. Bone RA, Landrum JT, Friedes LM, Gomez CM, Kilburn MD, Menendez E, Vidal I, Wang W. Distribution of lutein and zeaxanthin stereoisomers in the human retina. Exp Eye Res 1997;64:211–218.
14. Bernstein PS, Khachik F, Carvalho LS, Muir GJ, Zhao D-Y, Katz NB. Identification and quantitation of carotenoids and their metabolites in the tissues of the human eye. Exp Eye Res 2001;72:215–223.
15. Yemelyanov AY, Katz NB, Bernstein PS. Ligand-binding characterization of xanthophyll carotenoids to solubilized membrane proteins derived from human retina. Exp Eye Res 2001;72:381–392.
16. Bernstein PS, Katz NB. The role of ocular free radicals in age-related macular degeneration. In: Fuchs J, Packer L, eds. Environmental Stressors in Health and Disease. New York: Marcel Dekker, 2001:423–456. Reprinted in J Toxicol Cutan Ocular Toxicol 2001;20:141–181.
17. Beatty S, Koh H-H, Henson D, Boulton M. The role of oxidative stress in the pathogenesis of age-related macular degeneration. Surv Ophthalmol 2000;45:115–134.

18. Thomson LR, Toyoda Y, Langner A, Delori FC, Garnett KM, Craft N, Nichols CR, Cheng KM, Dorey CK. Elevated retinal zeaxanthin and prevention of light-induced photoreceptor cell death in quail. Invest Ophthalmol Vis Sci 2002;43:3538–3549.
19. Wooten BR, Hammond BR. Macular pigment: influences on visual acuity and visibility. Prog Retin Eye Res 2002;21:225–240.
20. Eye Disease Case-Control Study Group. Antioxidant status and neovascular age-related macular degeneration. Arch Ophthalmol 1993;111:104–109.
21. Seddon JM, Ajani UA, Sperduto RD, Hiller R, Blair N, Burton TC, Farber MD, Gragoudas ES, Haller J, Miller DT, Yannuzzi LA, Willet W. Dietary carotenoids, vitamins A, C, and E, and advanced age-related macular degeneration. JAMA 1994;272:1413–1420.
22. Mares-Perlman JA, Brady WE, Klein R, Klein BE, Bowen P, Stacewicz-Sapuntzakis M, Palta M. Serum antioxidants and age-related macular degeneration in a population-based case-control study. Arch Ophthalmol 1995;113:1518–1523.
23. Age-Related Eye Disease Study Group. A randomized, placebo-controlled, clinical trial of high-dose supplementation with vitamins C and E, beta carotene, and zinc for age-related macular degeneration and vision loss: AREDS Report No. 8. Arch Ophthalmol 2001;119:1417–1436.
24. Bone RA, Landrum JT, Mayne ST, Gomez CM, Tibor SE, Twaroska EE. Macular pigment in donor eyes with and without AMD: a case-control study. Invest Ophthalmol Vis Sci 2001;42:235–240.
25. Bone RA, Sparrock JMB. Comparison of macular pigment densities in human eyes. Vision Res 1971;11:1057–1064.
26. Werner JS, Wooten BR. Opponent chromatic mechanisms: relation to photopigment and hue naming. J Opt Soc Am 1979;69:422–434.
27. Wooten BR, Hammond BR Jr, Land RI, Snodderly DM. A practical method for measuring macular pigment optical density. Invest Ophthalmol Vis Sci 1999;40:2481–2489
28. Mellerio J, Ahmadi-Lari S, van Kuijk F, Pauleikhoff D, Bird A, Marshall J. A portable instrument for measuring macular pigment with central fixation. Curr Eye Res 2002;25:37–47.
29. Snodderly DM, Hammond BR. In vivo psychophysical assessment of nutritional and environmental influences on human ocular tissues: lens and macular pigment. In Taylor A, ed. Nutritional and Environmental Influences on the Eye. Boca Raton, FL: CRC Press, 1999:251–273.
30. Hammond BR, Wooten BR, Snodderly DM. Individual variations in the spatial profile of human macular pigment. J Opt Soc Am A 1997;14:1187–1196.
31. Werner JS, Donnelly SK, Kliegl R. Aging and human macular pigment density. Vision Res 1987;27:257–268.
32. Bernstein PS. Macular biology. In: Berger JW, Fine SL, Maguire MG., eds. Age-Related Macular Degeneration. St. Louis: Mosby, 1999:1–16.
33. Otake S, Cicerone CM. L and M cone relative numerosity and red–green opponency from fovea to mid-periphery in human retina. J Opt Soc Am A 2000;17:615–627.
34. Elsner AE, Burns SA, Beausencourt E, Weiter J. Foveal cone photopigment distribution: small alterations associated with macular pigment distribution. Invest Ophthalmol Vis Sci 1998;39:2394–2404.

35. Hammond BR Jr, Fuld K, Snodderly DM. Iris color and macular pigment optical density. Exp Eye Res 1996;62:293–297.
36. Hammond BR Jr, Curran-Celentano J, Judd S, Fuld K, Krinsky NI, Wooten BR, Snodderly DM. Sex differences in macular pigment optical density: relation to plasma carotenoid concentrations and dietary patterns. Vision Res 1996;36:2001–2012.
37. Bone RA, Landrum JT, Dixon Z, Chen Y, Llerena CM. Lutein and zeaxanthin in the eyes, serum and diet of human subjects. Exp Eye Res 2000;71:239–245.
38. Beatty S, Murray IJ, Henson DB, Carden D, Koh H, Boulton ME. Macular pigment and risk for age-related macular degeneration in subjects from a northern European population. Invest Ophthalmol Vis Sci 2001;42:439–446.
39. Aleman TS, Duncan JL, Bieber ML, de Castro EB, Marks DA, Gardner LM, Steinberg JD, Cideciyan AV, Maguire MG, Jacobson SG. Macular pigment and lutein supplementation in retinitis pigmentosa and Usher syndrome. Invest Ophthalmol Vis Sci 2001;42:1873–1881.
40. Landrum JT, Bone, RA, Joa H, Kliburn MD, Moore LL, Sprague KE. A one-year study of the macular pigment: the effect of 140 days of a lutein supplement. Exp Eye Res 1997;65:57–62.
41. Hammond BR, Johnson EJ, Russell, RM, Krinsky NI, Yeum K-J, Edwards RB, Snodderly DM. Dietary modification of human macular pigment density. Invest Ophthalmol Vis Sci 1997;38:1798–1801.
42. Burrows JL, Bernstein PS, Askew EW. [abstr PA065]. Serum and macular responses to antioxidant supplementation versus a carotenoid-rich dietary intervention in the elderly [abstr PA 065]. American Academy of Ophthalmology annual meeting abstracts on line. http://www.aao.org (accessed December 2003).
43. Delori FC, Gragoudas ES, Francisco R, Pruett RC. Monochromatic ophthalmoscopy and fundus photography. Arch Ophthalmol 1977;95:861–868.
44. van Noren D, van de Kraats J. Imaging retinal densitometry with a confocal scanning laser ophthalmoscope. Vis Res 1989;29:1825–1830.
45. Berendschot TT, Goldbohm RA, Klopping WA, van de Kraats J, van Norel, and Norren. Influence of lutein supplementation on macular pigment, assessed with two objective techniques. Invest Ophthalmol Vis Sci 2000;41:3322–3326.
46. Wustemeyer H, Jahn C, Nestler A, Barth T, Wolf S. A new instrument for the quantification of macular pigment density: first results in patients with AMD and healthy subjects. Graefe's Arch Clin Exp Ophthalmol 2002;240:660–671.
47. Schweitzer D, Lang GE, Beuermann B, Remsch H, Hammer M, Thamm E, Spraul CW, Lang GK. Objektive Bestimmung der optischen Dichte von Xanthophyll nach Supplementation von Lutein. Ophthalmologe 2002;99:270–275.
48. van Norren D, Tiemeijer LF. Spectral reflectance of the human eye. Vision Res 1986;26:313–320.
49. Kilbride PE, Alexander KR, Fishman M, Fishman GA. Human macular pigment assessed by imaging fundus reflectometry. Vision Res 1989;29:663–674.
50. Hammer M, Schweitzer D, Leistritz L, Scibor M, Donnerhacke K-H, Strobel J. Imaging spectroscopy of the human ocular fundus in vivo. J Biomed Optics 1997;2:418–425.

51. van de Kraats J, Bernedschot TTJM, van Norren D. The pathways of light measured in fundus reflectometry. Vision Res 1996;15:2229–2247.

52. Berendschot TT, Willemse-Assink JJ, Bastiaanse M, de Jong PT, van Norren D. Macular pigment and melanin in age-related maculopathy in a general population. Invest Ophthalmol Vis Sci 2002;43:1928–1932.

53. Delori FC, Dorey CK, Staurenghi G, Arend O, Goger DG, Weiter JJ. In vivo fluorescence of the ocular fundus exhibits retinal pigment epithelium lipofuscin characteristics. Invest Ophthalmol Vis Sci 1995;36:718–729.

54. Delori FC, Goger DG, Hammond BR, Snodderly DM, Burns SA. Macular pigment density measured by autofluorescence spectrometry: comparison with reflectometry and heterochromatic flicker photometry. J Opt Soc Am A 2001;18:1212–1230.

55. Sparrow JR, Parish CA, Hashimoto M, Nakanishi K. A2E, a lipofuscin fluorophore, in human retinal pigmented epithelial cells in culture. Invest Ophthalmol Vis Sci 1999;40:2988–2995.

56. Delori FC, Goger DG, Dorey CK. Age-related accumulation and spatial distribution of lipofuscin in RPE of normal subjects. Invest Ophthalmol Vis Sci 2001;42:1855–1866.

57. Bernstein PS, Yoshida MD, Katz NB, McClane RW, Gellermann W. Raman detection of macular carotenoid pigments in intact human retina. Invest Ophthalmol Vis Sci 1998;39:2003–2011.

58. Ermakov IV, McClane R, Gellermann W, Zhao D-Y, Bernstein PS. Resonant Raman detection of macular pigment levels in the living human retina, Optics Lett 2001; 26:202–204.

59. Gellermann W, Ermakov IV, Ermakova MR, McClane RW, Zhao DY, Bernstein PS. In vivo resonant Raman measurement of macular carotenoid pigments in the young and the aging human retina. J Opt Soc Am A 2002;19:1172–1186.

60. Bernstein PS, Zhao DY, Wintch SW, Ermakov IV, Gellermann W. Resonance Raman measurement of macular carotenoids in normal subjects and in age-related macular degeneration patients. Ophthalmology 2002;109:1780–1787.

61. Koyama Y. Resonance Raman spectroscopy. In: Britton G, Liaaen-Jensens, Pfander H, editors. Carotenoids, Vol. 1B, Spectroscopy. Basel: Birkhäuser, 1995: 135–146.

62. Bernstein PS. New insights into the role of macular carotenoids in age-related macular degeneration: resonance Raman studies. Pure Appl Chem 2002;74:1419–1425.

63. Werner JS, Bieber ML, Schefrin BE. Senescence of foveal and parafoveal cone sensitivities and their relations to macular pigment density. J Opt Soc A. 2000;17:1918–1932.

64. Wintch SW, Zhao D, Ermakov IV, McClane RW, Gellermann W, Bernstein PS. A double blind, placebo controlled, lutein supplementation study evaluating two macular carotenoid measurement methods: resonance Raman spectroscopy and heterochromatic flicker photometry [abstr 1744]. Association for Research in Vision and Ophthalmology (ARVO) annual meeting abstracts on line. http://www.arvo.org (accessed December 2003).

65. Gellermann W, Ermakov IV, McClane RW, Bernstein PS. Raman imaging of human macular pigments. Optics Lett 2002;27:833–835.

66. Peng Y-M, Peng Y-S, Lin Y, Moon, T, Roe DJ, Ritenbaugh C. Concentration and plasma-diet relationships of carotenoids, retinoids, and tocopherols in humans. Nutr Cancer 1995;23,233–246.

67. Hata TR, Scholz TA, Ermakov IV, McClane RW, Khachik F, Gellermann W, Persching LK. Non-invasive Raman spectroscopic detection of carotenoids in human skin. J Invest Dermatol 2000;115:441–448.
68. Wingerath T, Sies H, Stahl W. Xanthophyll esters in human skin. Arch Biochem Biophys 1998;355:271–274.
69. Clinton SK, Giovannucci E. Diet, nutrition and prostate cancer. Annu Rev Nutr 1998:18:412–440.
70. Cook NR, Stampfer MJ, Ma J, Manson JE, Sacks FM, Buring JE, Hennekens CH. Beta-carotene supplementation for patients with low baseline levels and decreased risks of total and prostate carcinoma. Cancer 1999;86:1783–1792.
71. Clinton SK. The dietary antioxidant network and prostate carcinoma. Cancer 1999;86:1629–1631.
72. Rao AV, Agarwal S. Role of antioxidant lycopene in cancer and heart disease. J Am Coll Nutr 2000;19:563–569.
73. Mortensen A, Skibstedt LH, Truscott TG. The interaction of dietary carotenoids with radical species. Arch Biochem Biophys 2001;385:13–19.
74. Böhm F, Tinkler JH, Truscott TG. Carotenoids protect against cell-membrane damage by the nitrogen dioxide radical. Nat Med 1995;1:98–99.
75. Foote CS, Denny RW. Chemistry of singlet oxygen. VIII. Quenching by β-carotene. J Am Chem Soc 1968;90:6233–6235.
76. Farmillo A, Wilkinson F. On the mechanism of quenching of singlet oxygen in solution. Photochem Photobiol 1973;18:447–450.
77. Conn PF, Schalch W, Truscott TG. The singlet oxygen and carotenoid interaction. J Photochem Photobiol B: Bio 1991;11:41–47.
78. Clevidence BA, Bieri JG. Association of carotenoids with human plasma lipoproteins. Meth Enzymol 1993;214:33–46.
79. Prince MR, Frisoli JK. Beta-carotene accumulation in serum and skin. Am J Nutr 1993;57:175–181.
80. Mathews-Roth MM, Carotenoids in erythropoietic protoporphyria and other photosensitive diseases. Ann NY Acad Sci 1993;691:127–138.
81. Stahl W, Heinrich U, Jungmann H, Sies H, Tronnier H. Carotenoids and carotenoids plus vitamin E protect against ultraviolet light–induced erythema in humans. Am J Clin Nutr 2000; 71:795–798.
82. Lee J, Jiang S, Levine N, Watson R. Carotenoid supplementation reduces erythema in human skin after simulated solar radiation exposure. Proc Soc Exp Biol Med 2000;223:170–174.
83. Giovannucci E. Tomatoes, tomato-based products, lycopene, and cancer: review of the epidemiologic literature. J Natl Cancer Inst 1999;91:317–331.
84. Peng Y-M, Peng Y-S, Lin Y. A nonsaponification method for the determination of carotenoids, retinoids, and tocopherols in solid human tissues. Cancer Epidemiol Biomark Prev 1993;2:139–144.
85. Jungmann H, Heinrich U, Wiebush M, Tronnier H. Der Einsatz der Reflektions-Spectroskopie in der Dermatologie am Beispiel des β-Carotins. Kosm Med 1996;1:50–57.
86. Stahl W, Heinrich U, Jungmann H, von Laar J, Schietzel M, Sies H, Tronnier H. Increased dermal carotenoid levels assessed by noninvasive reflection

spectrophotometry correlate with serum levels in women ingesting Betatene. J Nutr 1998;128:903–907.

87. Alaluf S, Heinrich U, Stahl W, Tronnier H, Wiseman S. Dietary carotenoids contribute to normal human skin color and UV photosensitivity. J Nutr 2002;132:399–403.

88. Ermakov IV, Ermakova MR, McClane RW, Gellermann W. Resonance Raman detection of carotenoid antioxidants in living human tissues. Optics Lett 2001;26:1179–1181.

89. Gellermann W, Ermakov IV, Scholz TA, Bernstein PS. Noninvasive laser Raman detection of carotenoid antioxidants in skin. Cosmetic Dermatol 2002;15:65–68.

90. Gellermann W, Ermakov I, Bernstein PS. Resonant Raman detectors for noninvasive assessment of carotenoid antioxidants in human tissue. In: Advanced Biomedical and Clinical Diagnostic Systems. Proceedings of the Society of Photo-Optical Instrumentation Engineers. 2003;4958:78–87.

91. Rao V, Heber D, eds. Lycopene and the Prevention of Chronic Diseases. Nutrition and Health Conference Report, Vol. 1, No. 1, Barcelona: Caledonian Science Press, 2002.

4

Methodology for Assessment of Carotenoid Levels in Blood Plasma and Plasma Fractions

Mario G. Ferruzzi
Nestle Research Center, Lausanne, Switzerland

Steven J. Schwartz
The Ohio State University, Columbus, Ohio, U.S.A.

I. INTRODUCTION

Associations between consumption of carotenoid-rich fruits and vegetables and health benefits have stimulated interest in measurement of carotenoids in biological matrices to best assess patterns of carotenoid consumption, bioavailability, and utilization in humans (1–5). As a result, methodologies have been developed and applied successfully to determination of carotenoid levels in a variety of human tissues including major organs such as liver and lung (6–8), prostate (9), lens and retina (10,11), buccal mucosal cells (12,13), cervical tissue (14,15), and blood plasma (6,14–23) and plasma fractions (24,25).

While a wealth of information may be gained by tissue analysis, it is circulating carotenoid levels that have been increasingly utilized in human studies as an indicator of carotenoid status. The diversity of circulating carotenoids was illustrated best by Khachik et al. (26) where 34 different carotenoids, including geometrical isomers, were resolved in extracts of human plasma. This diversity, combined with flexibility in sampling and opportunity for multiple sampling, makes blood plasma and corresponding plasma fractions a renewable and conveniently assessable tissue suitable for large clinical dietary interventions. Analysis of whole-blood plasma and plasma fractions offer a plethora of information to the researcher, including overall carotenoid status, carotenoid species and isomeric distribution, and plasma fraction distribution providing information on newly absorbed carotenoids.

As analytical methodology has evolved, so has its application to carotenoid analysis. No technique has had greater impact on the study of carotenoids than high-performance liquid chromatography (HPLC). Its versatility and reliability have allowed for wide application to every aspect of carotenoid research from horticultural to clinical studies. Early HPLC procedures for extracts of blood plasma allowed for separation and quantification of only a few carotenoids such as α-carotene, β-carotene, and lycopene (14,18). Total carotenoid levels were determined to be approximately 120 μg/dL, with lycopene and lutein/zeaxanthin being the most prominent (14). While these early methods were limited in comparison with today's technology, results have been consistent with more recent measurements where lycopene is the major circulating carotenoid, with lutein/zeaxanthin and β-carotene also representing significant portions of the overall circulating carotenoid pool (5,8,9,15,19). Yeum et al. (20) separated what may be considered a typical normal living human serum carotenoid profile including 13 carotenoid and carotenoid isomers in both men and women (Fig. 1 and Table 1).

Constant development and refinement of instrumentation and methodology has allowed for efficient, sensitive, and selective measurement of carotenoids

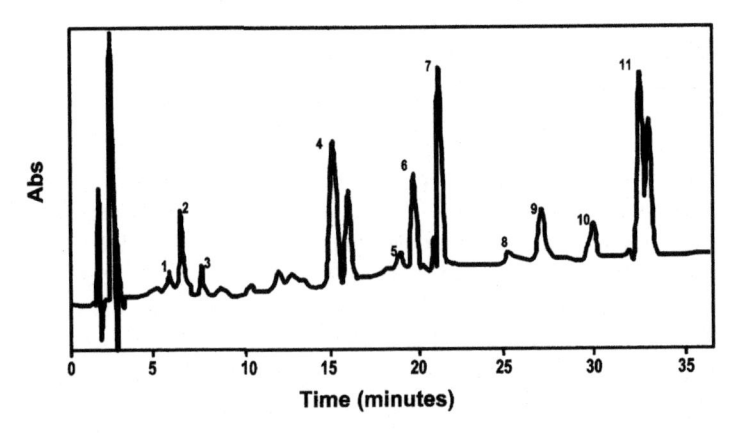

Figure 1   Reverse-phase C_{30} separation of 13 major carotenoid in human blood plasma as quantified by Yeum et al. (20). *Stationary phase*: 3 μm C_{30} carotenoid column (150 $\times$ 4.6 mm). *Mobile phase*: gradient elution using methanol/ methyl-*tert*-butyl ether/ water (83 : 15 : 2) and methanol/methyl-*tert*-butyl ether : water (8 : 90 : 2). One percent ammonium acetate was included in the mobile phases to enhance carotenoid recovery and separation. *Peak identifications*: 1 = lutein isomer; 2 = lutein; 3 = zeaxanthin; 4 = cryptoxanthin; 5 = 13-*cis*-β-carotene; 6 = α-carotene; 7 = all *trans* β-carotene; 8 = 15-*cis*-lycopene; 9 = 13-*cis*-lycopene; 10 = 9-*cis*-lycopene; 11 = all-*trans* lycopene.

Table 1 Concentration of 11 Carotenoid Species in Human Plasma[a]

Carotenoid	Young men	Young women	Older men	Older women
Lutein isomers	0.06 ± 0.01	0.08 ± 0.01	0.11 ± 0.02	0.07 ± 0.01
Lutein	0.22 ± 0.02	0.28 ± 0.03	0.38 ± 0.05	0.25 ± 0.03
Zeazanthin	0.03 ± 0.00	0.04 ± 0.01	0.05 ± 0.01	0.03 ± 0.00
Cryptoxanthin	0.34 ± 0.03	0.54 ± 0.09	1.04 ± 0.24	0.54 ± 0.11
13-*cis*-β-Carotene	0.03 ± 0.01	0.05 ± 0.01	0.09 ± 0.02	0.04 ± 0.01
α-Carotene	0.09 ± 0.01	0.18 ± 0.04	0.27 ± 0.07	0.20 ± 0.04
All-trans β-carotene	0.44 ± 0.07	0.80 ± 0.17	1.51 ± 0.41	0.78 ± 0.10
15-*cis*-Lycopene	0.01 ± 0.001	0.01 ± 0.001	0.01 ± 0.003	0.01 ± 0.00
13-*cis*-Lycopene	0.12 ± 0.02	0.10 ± 0.02	0.14 ± 0.02	0.09 ± 0.01
9-*cis*-Lycopene	0.07 ± 0.01	0.07 ± 0.01	0.08 ± 0.01	0.06 ± 0.00
trans-Lycopene	0.38 ± 0.05	0.37 ± 0.06	0.41 ± 0.06	0.28 ± 0.02

[a]Concentrations given in μmol/L.
[a]Adapted from Ref. 20.

present in various matrices, including blood plasma and plasma fractions. This chapter describes some unique and useful chromatographic techniques and specific methods of detection widely utilized in analysis of circulating carotenoid levels and other biological samples. While the focus will be on analysis of plasma carotenoids, a brief review of traditional liquid chromatography (LC) techniques will be provided. Finally, characteristic separations of extracts of blood plasma and plasma fractions will be used to illustrate the chromatographic resolution and sensitivity of these methods.

II. NORMAL-PHASE CHROMATOGRAPHIC METHODS

Initial HPLC methodology for carotenoid analysis focused on applications of normal-phase techniques combining a polar stationary phase such as silica, calcium hydroxide, and/or alumina with a nonpolar mobile phase such as hexane, petroleum ether, or acetone. Stewart and Wheaton (16) accomplished the first modern-type HPLC carotenoid separation by utilizing a stationary phase of magnesium oxide and zinc carbonate to separate carotenes and xanthophylls, respectively, with *n*-hexane and tertiary pentyl alcohol as the elution solvents. While this method demonstrated only a simple separation, normal-phase HPLC has been applied for a number of extremely complex carotenoid separations.

More recently, cyano-amino columns in combination with a mobile phase of n-hexane (95%) and ethyl acetate (5%) has been applied successfully to the separation of lycopene (21).

The real promise of normal-phase HPLC may be in its applicability as a separation mode for carotenoid geometrical isomers. Fiksdahl et al. (17) demonstrated the advantage of using normal-phase HPLC coupled with an ultraviolet and visible (UV-Vis) scanning spectrophotometer in the analysis of cis−trans carotenoid mixtures. Calcium hydroxide has specifically demonstrated excellent selective separation of acyclic and cyclic geometric carotenes and their isomers from a variety of matrices (22,23).

Major application of normal-phase methodology to analysis of circulating carotenoid levels has been limited by a lack of commercial availability, and inconsistency in column packing that results in variable retention times, peak areas, peak shape, as well as isomer resolution (23). However, excellent examples exist in the literature, including that of Van het Hoff et al. (24). In this method carotenoid concentrations in plasma and triglyceride-rich lipoprotein (TRL) fraction were determined using a Nucleosil 100 5CN column with n-heptane as mobile phase. UV-Vis detection was used to monitor concentrations of lycopene at 470 nm, β-carotene at 450 nm, and retinyl palmitate at 325 nm.

III. REVERSE-PHASE CHROMATOGRAPHIC METHODS

Reverse-phase HPLC methods have become much more prominent in carotenoid analysis due to the variety of commercially available stationary phases and packed columns. The most common of all stationary phases, octadecylsilane packing (C_{18}), was first described by Schmit et al. (25). C_{18} phases may be broadly divided into two categories important to consider in carotenoid analysis: monomeric and polymeric. When prepared from monochlorosilanes, C_{18} columns are said to be monomeric. Polymeric C_{18} columns are characterized by trichlorosilane cross-linkages between hydrocarbon chains. Furthermore, packing material may be endcapped to prevent adsorption of nonpolar compounds (23). Mobile phases for such reverse-phase systems typically are composed of polar solvent systems such as water, methanol, ethanol, and acetonitrile with organic modifiers such as chloroform, methylene chloride, tetrahydrofuran, and hexane determining the rate of elution. Presence of certain organic salts, such as ammonium acetate, further aid in resolution and recovery of carotenoids from the phase. It is often recommended that low concentrations of these salts (ammonium acetate and tetraethylamine, for example) be utilized when analyzing biological samples, such as plasma, which provides complex sample matrices limited in size and of low concentration.

Numerous carotenoid separation methods have been described using reverse-phase C_{18} columns. Vydac 218TP C_{18} columns (polymeric endcapped) have been extensively applied in carotenoid separation from plant material (27–29). Polymeric non-endcapped columns such as the Vydac 201TP have been extensively utilized and provide better separation of prominent carotenoids and geometrical isomers (28–31).

Wide availability, variety of columns, and ease of use have made C_{18} phases the most common phase in analysis of carotenoids in biological samples such as blood serum/plasma and plasma fractions. Numerous methods have been reported highlighting speed and reproducibility of these separations. A classic method was provided by Bieri et al. (14) to separate and quantify major plasma carotenoids. Methods developed by Craft et al. (32,33) have enjoyed wide application in plasma carotenoid analysis as they provide efficient and reproducible isocratic methodology measuring and quantifying approximately 90% of the plasma carotenoids present. More recent application of C_{18} technology to analysis of plasma carotenoids can be seen in the work of Lyan et al. (34) and El-Sohemy et al. (35). The latter method is particularly useful for resolving major serum/plasma carotenoids with a short 150 mm × 4.6 mm 3 μm Restek Ultra C_{18} column (Fig. 2). An interesting point to illustrate from Figure 2 is the inability of traditional C_{18} separations to baseline-resolve lutein and zeaxanthin species, resulting in reporting of total lutein + zeaxanthin. This lack of resolution often hampered the ability of early epidemiological studies to differentiate the importance of these two species. More recent methods were able to fully resolve these xanthophylls (36,37).

Numerous methods have been developed utilizing polymeric C_{18} column technology that provides excellent resolution between different carotenoid species. However, C_{18} methodology has been limited in the separation of carotenoid geometrical isomers. The importance of good isomer resolution is amplified when one considers that lycopene cis isomer species may represent up to 60% of total plasma lycopene (9,38). Lesellier et al. (30) described the superior resolution of carotenoid isomers provided by polymeric versus monomeric C_{18} columns for these analyses. β-Carotene and lycopene cis isomer levels have been reported based on C_{18} methods (33,34). While some success has been achieved in the separation of β-carotene isomers, resolution of lycopene isomers by C_{18} methodology is still an analytical challenge. Only basic resolution into isomeric fractions can be achieved by even the most advanced C_{18} technological methods. Lyan et al. (34) applied a Nucleosil C column and a Vydac C column in series to separate 22 carotenoid species, including improved resolution of major lycopene and β-carotene cis isomer species (Fig. 3). Resolution of lycopene isomers in plasma extracts by C_{18} was more recently improved by Böhm et al. (39) utilizing a Vydac 201TP54 column under subambient (9°C) temperatures resolving five major lycopene isomers in human plasma. While providing more satisfactory separations, these methods do not follow standard approaches and may be difficult to replicate

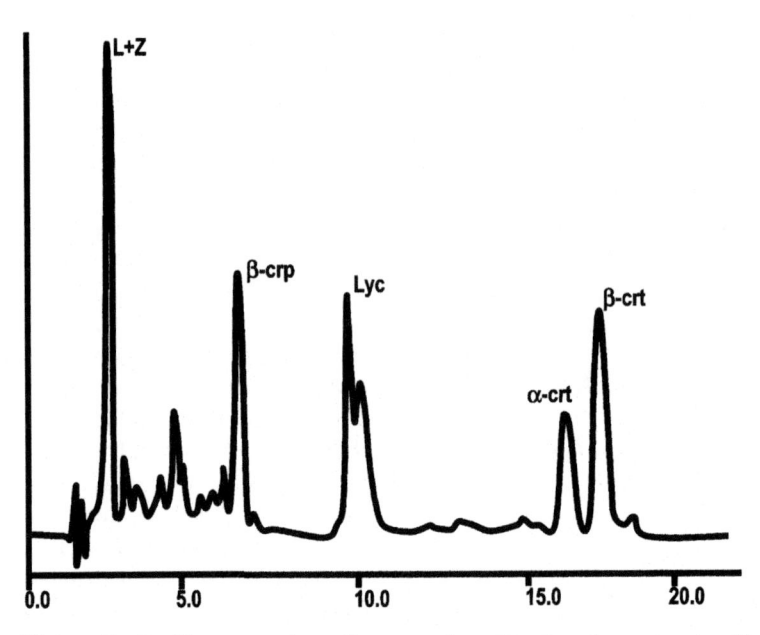

Figure 2 Rapid reverse-phase C_{18} separation of major plasma carotenoids. *Stationary phase*: 3 μm Resteck Ultra C_{18} column (150 mm × 4.6 mm) equipped with a trident guard column system. *Mobile phase*: (flow rate 1.1 mL/min) acetonitrile, tetrahydrofuran, methanol, and 1% ammonium acetate solution (68 : 22 : 7 : 3). Major peaks are identified on the chromatogram. Isomeric species were not identified. (Adapted with permission from Ref. 35.)

across research laboratories. More universal methodology was needed to further the understanding of carotenoid geometrical isomers' role in human health.

Development of a triacontyl (C_{30}) polymeric phase with high absolute retention and shape recognition of carotenoid molecules has enhanced carotenoid isomer separation (40). C_{30} columns are designed to have increased alkyl phase length, which has been directly linked to better isomer resolution. Effectiveness of this new stationary phase on mixtures of structurally similar carotenoids and their isomers has also been demonstrated (13,38,40,41). C_{30} column technology was found to be significantly more effective at carotenoid isomer separation than either Vydac 201TP54 or Suplex pkb-100 stationary phases (42).

Because of its unique resolving abilities, C_{30} technology has had wide application in analysis of biological extracts. Johnson et al. (43) applied C_{30} column technology for resolution of 9-*cis*-β-carotene isomers in extracts of human plasma and breast milk. Both Emenhiser et al. (9,41) and Yeum et al. (20) coupled the resolving ability of C_{30} technology with UV-Vis detection in separation and identification of major plasma carotenoids including predominant geometrical isomers (Figs. 1 and 4).

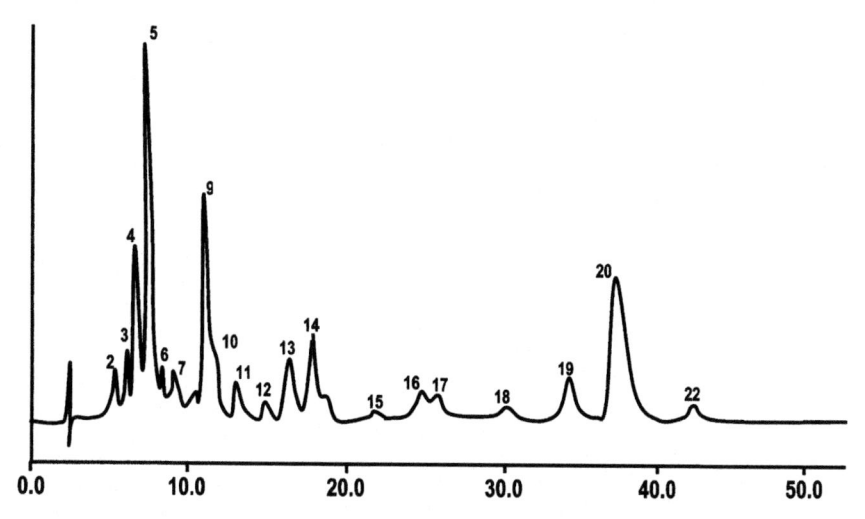

Figure 3 Reverse-phase C₁₈ separation of human plasma. *Stationary phase*: 3 μm Nucleosil in series with 5 μm Vydac TP254C and Hypersil guard column; detection at 450 nm; *Mobile phase*: (flow rate = 2 mL/min.) acetonitrile-methanol containing 50 mM acetate ammonium–dichloromethane–water (70 : 15 : 10 : 5, v/v/v/v). *Peak identifications*: 2 = unknown 1; 3 = unknown 2; 4 = unknown 3; 5 = lutein; 6 = zeaxanthin; 7 = unknown 4; 9 = unknown 5; 10 = unknown 6; 11 = unknown 7; 12 = unknown 8; 13 = β-cryptoxanthin; 14 = echinenone; 15 = unknown 9; 16 = *trans*-lycopene; 17 = *cis*-lycopene; 18 = *cis*-lycopene; 19 = α-carotene; 20 = β-carotene;; 22 = 13-*cis*-β-carotene. (Adapted with permission from Ref. 34.)

Further developments in alkyl-bonded stationary phases have resulted in the extended chain C₃₄. Bell et al. (44) synthesized such a phase by use of traditional polymeric synthesis as well as surface polymerization synthesis. Resulting columns were applied to mixtures of carotenoids and their isomers demonstrating increased selectivity toward certain cis isomers of both α- and β-carotene compared to both conventional C₁₈ and C₃₀ stationary phases. However, extended run times and lack of commercial availability have limited the ability to fully apply C₃₄ technology to the evaluation of biological samples including blood plasma and plasma fractions.

IV. HIGH-SENSITIVITY ANALYSIS

Carotenoid analyses are commonly performed by LC with UV and visible absorbance (UV-Vis) detectors operating at wavelengths of maximal absorption. Application of diode array detectors (DADs) provides additional spectral

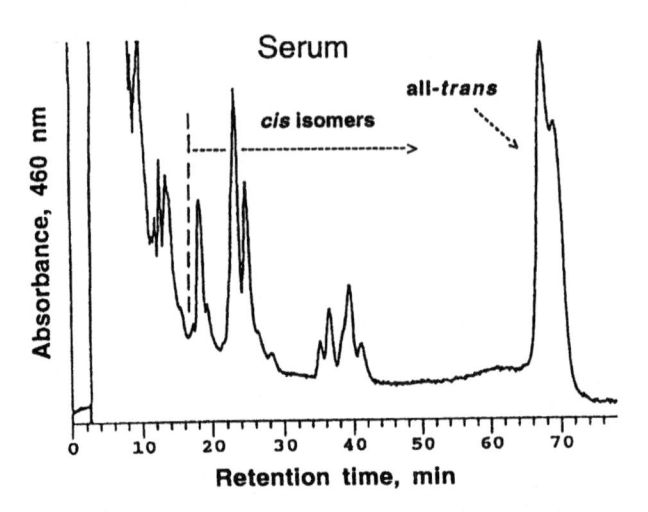

Figure 4 Representative chromatograms showing cis and trans isomers of lycopene from human serum. Separation was achieved on a C_{30} stationary phase with methanol and methyl-*tert*-butyl ether as elution solvents. Peaks eluting after 12 min were identified as isomers of lycopene. (Taken with permission from Ref. 9.)

information to facilitate component identification. However, these UV-Vis methods have limitations in detection and quantification of limited amounts of carotenoids often encountered in samples of limited size or plasma fractions with dilute carotenoid levels. Development of improved methodology to increase sensitivity and selectivity above that offered by traditional systems is critical to the extension of research and understanding of carotenoid absorption, distribution, and metabolism in humans.

HPLC methodology with postcolumn electrochemical detection (ECD) offers an alternative system based on oxidation and reduction properties of the electrochemically active carotenoids. Past studies have demonstrated that this type of detection provides a significant improvement in detection limits over UV-Vis methods for other electrochemically active compounds such as phenolics, tocopherols, and retinoids. These methods have typically focused on conventional single- or dual-channel electrochemical detectors (45–50). Using electrochemical methods, detection limits for carotenoids have been estab-lished at the femtomolar range representing a 10- to 1000-fold improvement in sensitivity relative to conventional UV-Vis absorbance detection methods (13,38,49).

Combination of ECD with the resolution capacity of C_{30} columns has perhaps provided some of the most useful separations of human serum with regard to our ability to expand the nature of traditional studies that rely on large

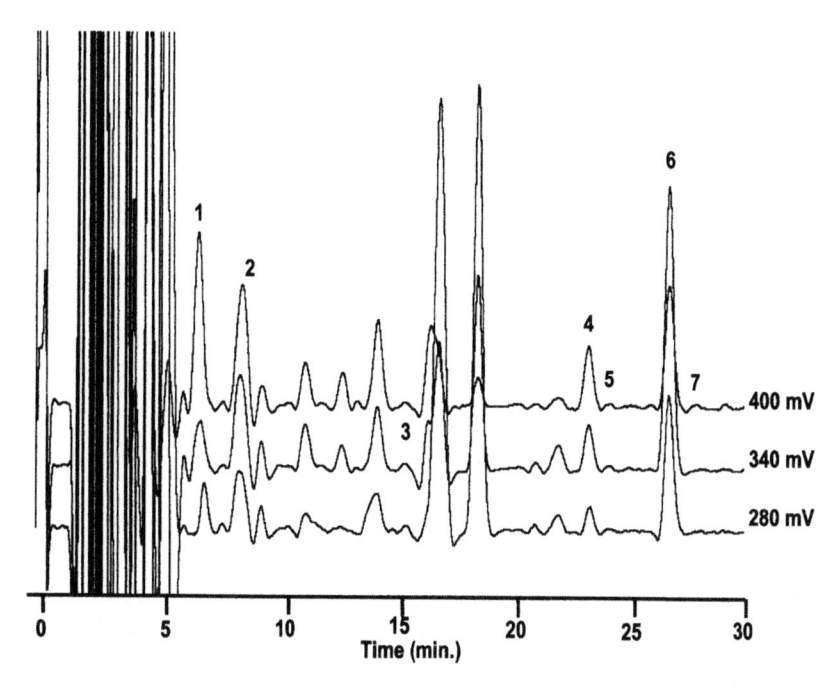

Figure 5 LC ECD C_{30} chromatogram of a 20-μL blood serum sample (20 nA full scale). Twenty-microliter aliquots of blood serum were deproteinized with incorporation of 100 μL of ethanol. Carotenoids were extracted as described by Ferruzzi et al. (13). Separations were achieved on a 3-μm C_{30} column prepared by National Institute of Standards and Technology (Gaithersburg, MD), using gradient elution with different concentrations of methanol-MTBE-ammonium acetate in reservoirs A (95:3:2) and B (25:73:2). *Peak identification*: 1 = lutein, 2 = zeaxanthin, 3 = β-cryptoxanthin, 4 = 13-*cis* β-carotene, 5 = α-carotene, 6 = β-carotene, 7 = 9-*cis*-β-carotene. (Taken with permission from Ref. 13.)

sample sizes. Figure 5 shows the resolution of major carotenoids from a 20-μL sample of blood plasma (13). Typically, much larger (about 200 μL) samples are common with LC methods utilizing conventional UV-Vis detection. Numerous carotenoids were identified in the serum sample including trans forms of lutein, zeaxanthin, β-cryptoxanthin, and α- and β-carotene and minor quantities of 15-*cis*-, 13-*cis*-, and 9-*cis*-β-carotene. Lycopene was not eluted in this separation but can be detected using LC-ECD. Figure 6 depicts isocratic LC-ECD separation of lycopene geometrical isomers from extracts of human blood plasma (38). An extended isocratic C_{30} method was applied in this study to maximize the resolution of lycopene isomers. This methodology clearly resolves 12 individual geometrical lycopene isomers present in human plasma and illustrates the

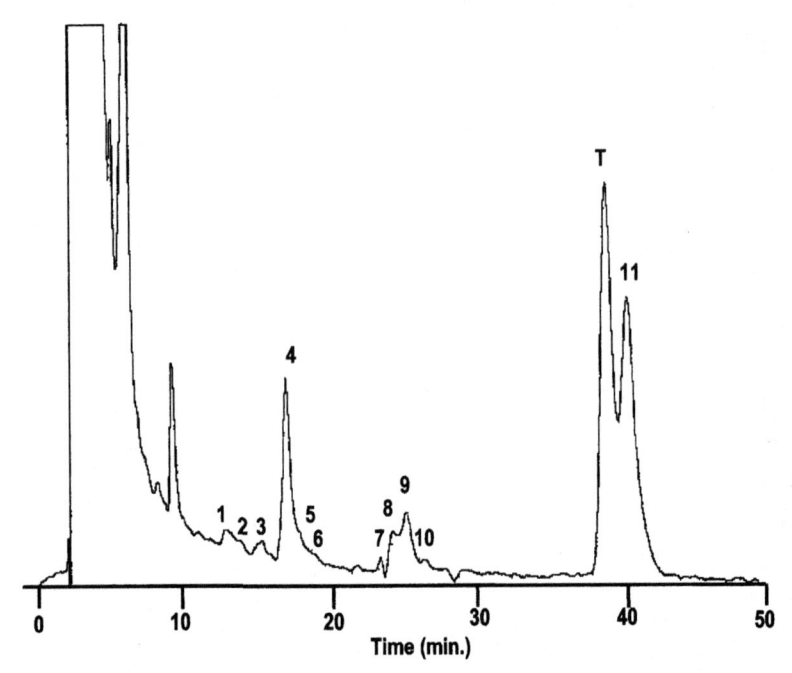

Figure 6 Isocratic C_{30} separation of a 50-μL sample of human blood serum. Depicted is channel 2 (320 mV), 20 nA full scale. Separations were achieved using an analytical scale, 250 mm × 4.6 mm i.d., 3-μm polymeric C_{30} column prepared at the National Institute of Standards and Technology (Gaithersburg, MD). Separations were achieved using an isocratic elution with a binary mobile phase of different concentrations of methanol-MTBE-ammonium acetate. Isocratic conditions were set at volume fractions 45% of reservoir A (95:3:2 volume fraction methanol-MTBE-1 mol/L ammonium acetate solution) and 55% of reservoir B (25:73:2 volume fraction methanol-MTBE-1 mol/L ammonium acetate solution) with a chromatographic run time of 50 min for all analyses. Peak identifications: T = *trans*-lycopene; 1–11 = *cis*-lycopene isomers. (Taken with permission from Ref. 36.)

abundance of *cis*-lycopene isomers in human plasma, approximately 60% of the total lycopene found in extracts (9).

Further enhancing the usefulness of the C_{30} ECD combination is incorporation of gradient separations. Separation of *cis*-lycopene isomers by gradient LC-ECD from blood plasma of patients consuming red Roma tomato and Tangerine tomato are shown in Figure 7a and b, respectively (38). Tangerine tomatoes (Golden jubilee and Tangela) have the capacity to biosynthesize several cis isomers of lycopene not commonly found in other varieties. The predominant carotenoid in Tangerine varieties is prolycopene, a tetra-*cis* isomer (7,9,7′,9′) of lycopene. The ability to both biosynthesize and accumulate a unique tetra-*cis*-lycopene isomer make the Tangerine tomatoes a potentially important tool for the study of *cis*-lycopene isomer absorption and metabolism in humans.

Similar lycopene isomer profiles were noted between samples separated by the isocratic method. The enhanced capability of gradient elution allowed for resolution of prolycopene from the blood plasma of patients consuming prolycopene from sauce produced from Tangerine tomato. Furthermore, two

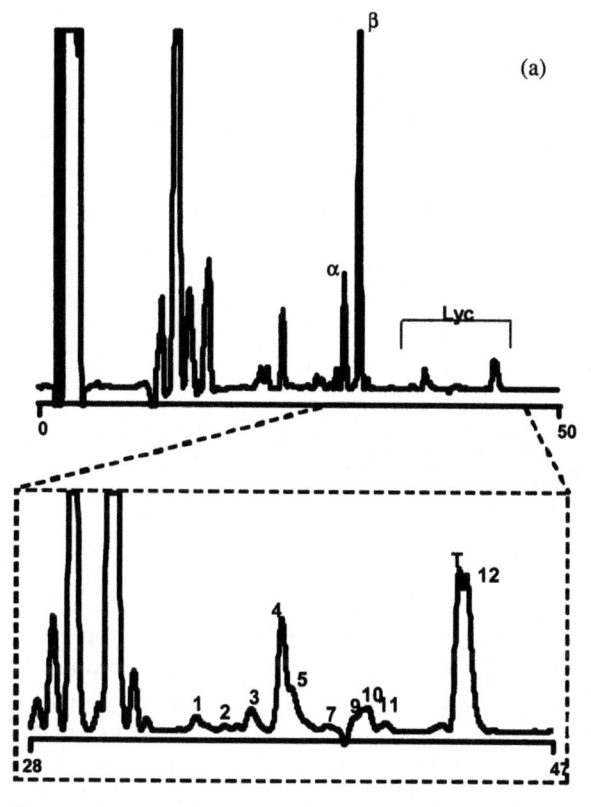

Figure 7   Representative lycopene isomer separation by gradient C_{30} LC-ECD from 100 μL human plasma of patients consuming sauce produced from (a) Roma and (b) Tangerine variety tomatoes. Separations were achieved using an analytical scale 250 mm × 4.6 mm i.d., 3-μm polymeric C_{30} column prepared at the National Institute of Standards and Technology (Gaithersburg, MD). Detection was performed on an eight-channel coulometric array detector. Channel 5 (440 mV) is depicted for both samples (20 nA full scale). Peak identifications: α = α-carotene; β = β-carotene; T = *trans*-lycopene; PL = prolycopene. Inset highlights *cis*-lycopene separation labeled 1–12. (Taken with permission from Ref. 38.)

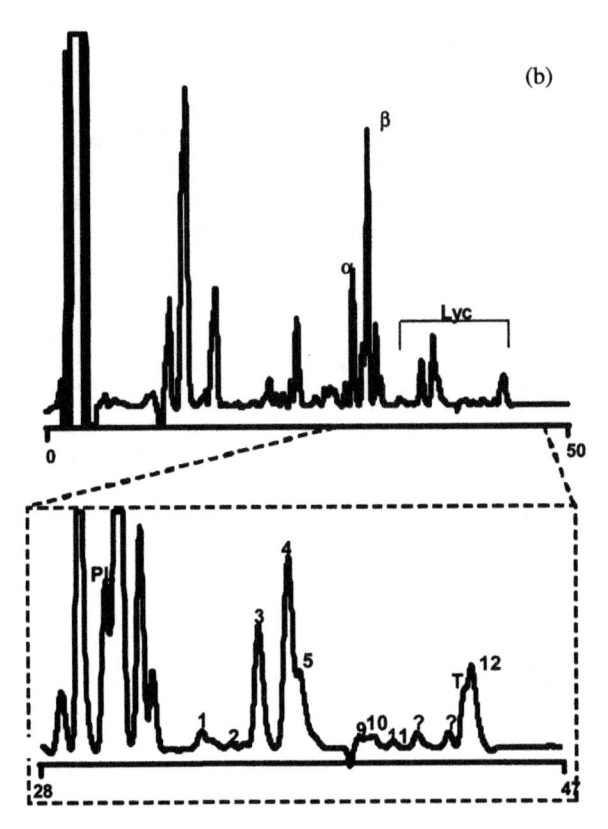

Figure 7 Continued.

unidentified peaks were noted in the plasma of patients consuming Tangerine tomato. In-line photodiode array detection revealed the UV-Vis absorbance spectra of these peaks to be similar to that of *trans*-lycopene and were absent in the native Tangerine tomato tissue. This may be evidence pointing to the possibility that these may also be minor lycopene isomers formed during food preparation, digestion, and/or absorption and distribution through the body. This gradient methodology offers a selective and sensitive method for the continued study of the relationship between *cis/trans* isomer ratio both in the diet, formed metabolically and present in human biological samples.

The sensitivity and resolution offered by the combination of C_{30} technology with ECD is perhaps best illustrated in the capacity of the method to accurately quantify low levels of dietary carotenoids and their isomers in the chylomicron fraction of plasma (51–52). Samples of plasma chylomicron fractions were drawn and isolated from subjects who consumed a representative salad containing approximately 44 g spinach, 44 g lettuce, 66 g shaved carrot, and 85 g tomatoes, along with a commercial soybean oil–based salad dressing (60 g). Blood samples (10 mL) were drawn at 0,3,6 and 9 hours following the consumption of the test meals. Following extraction, carotenoids were separated via a C_{30} gradient HPLC method and quantified by an eight-channel coulometric electrochemical array detector. Under the potential setting of 200–680 mV, all-*trans* carotenoids and several corresponding cis isomers were detected in all chylomicron samples at above the 1-fmol detection limit (Fig. 8). The enhanced sensitivity of this method allows for the direct comparison of bioavailable carotenoids in plasma chylomicron fraction as a function of subtle dietary manipulation and postconsumption time while facilitating a reduction in sample volume necessary for each blood collection. Application of this method has proven useful in the study of key factors influencing bioavailability of major carotenoids (52).

V. IDENTIFICATION

Separation and detection of carotenoid species must be followed by confident identification of the respective peaks. Analysis of carotenoids in biological matrices such as blood plasma offers an added level of complexity due to the complex nature of these extracts. Major techniques for identification include UV and visible absorption, mass spectrometry, and NMR.

A. UV-Visible

Generally, fat-soluble carotenoids are ideal for detection by UV-Vis absorbance due to their highly conjugated double-bond system that interacts with both UV and visible light (53). These strong interactions give rise to their strong yellow, orange, and red colors. Most carotenoids show a characteristic three peak or two peaks with a shoulder absorbance spectrum between 400 and 500 nm (54).

UV-visible detection is routinely accomplished with variable-wavelength detection at a wavelength of maximal absorption. A major advance was made with the introduction of the photodiode array detector (DAD). Multichannel photodiode array detection allows for simultaneous detection on multiple wavelengths giving rise to on-line UV-Vis spectra as a compound elutes from the LC column. Comparison of on-line spectra with that of known standards allows for rapid tentative identification of carotenoid species in complex biological matrices. DAD technology also allows for monitoring of multiple micronutrients, such as carotenes and retinoids, simultaneously.

Prior to development of DAD methods, creative techniques were applied for simultaneous detection. Aaran and Nikkari (55) used two single-wavelength

C30 LC-ECD traces

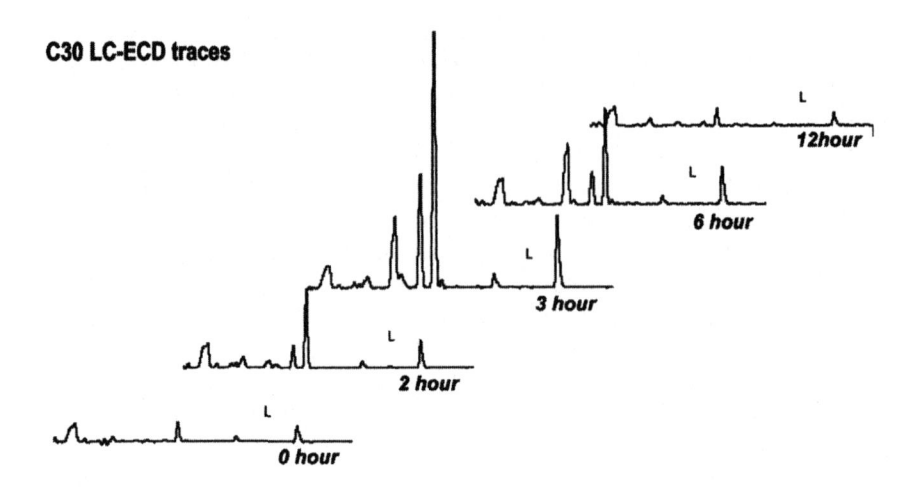

Change in chylomicron carotenoid content over time

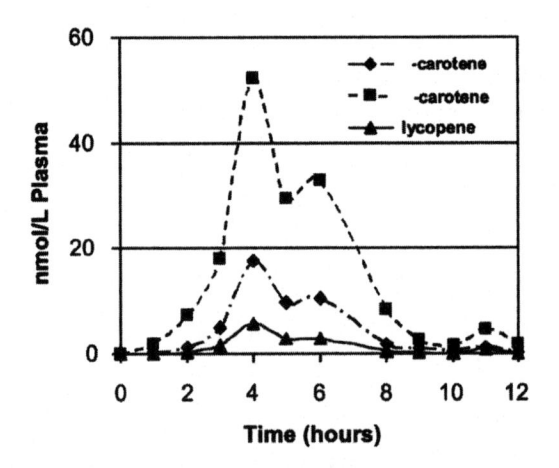

Figure 8 Time course of C_{30} ECD separation and detection of plasma chylomicron carotenoids for a single subject. Data depict plasma chylomicron carotenoid levels between 1 h and 12 h postconsumption of a standard test salad. Separations were achieved using an analytical scale 250 mm × 4.6 mm i.d., 3-μm polymeric C_{30} column prepared at the National Institute of Standards and Technology (Gaithersburg, MD). Detection was performed on an eight-channel coulometric array detector. Channel 5 (440 mV) is depicted for all samples (5 nA full scale). Peak identifications: $\alpha = \alpha$-carotene; $\beta = \beta$-carotene; T = *trans*-lycopene. *Inset depicts chylomicron carotenoid concentration versus time for the same time course.

detectors in series to monitor β-carotene, retinol, and α-tocopherol. A similar study by Comstock et al. (56) used a combination of UV-Vis and fluorescence detection. Sowell et al. (57) identified and quantified retinol, xanthophyll, carotenes, and retinyl esters in serum simultaneously using a multiwavelength detector. In recent years, numerous HPLC-DAD methods have profiled the same micronutrients using a simplified method with a single DAD detector (5,41,42,54,58–60).

B. Mass Spectrometry

Mass spectrometry (MS) offers a highly sensitive and selective detection system for carotenoid analysis by LC. While identification based on DAD detection remains tentative, data obtained from LC-MS add significant information aiding in confident identification of carotenoids (61). There have been numerous modes of LC-MS in recent years. Many of these modes differed in their interface and ionization methods. Some of the earliest methods of interfacing the LC system to the mass spectrometer include moving belt and particle beam combinations. While demonstrating early benefits, these methods had numerous shortcomings, including loss of chromatographic resolution, incomplete volatilization, pyrolysis, and inability to cover a complete carotenoid spectrum (61).

Development of an electrospray LC-MS method by van Breemen (62) demonstrated nonthermal ionization of carotenoid molecules as well as a high-sensitivity analysis (1–2 pmol limit of detection for lutein and β-carotene). Other modes of LC-MS include fast atom bombardment (FAB). FAB methods were a standard method used to work with thermally labile compounds. High-sensitivity analysis was also achieved in this mode (5 ng for lutein and 15 ng for α-carotene) (63), but this method remains less sensitive than newer ES techniques (61,64). More recently, tandem LC/MS-MS has been applied in highly sensitive analysis of lycopene isomers in blood plasma (65). With an on-column limit of detection of 11.2 fmol, this method offers a clear improvement and new opportunities in clinical investigations.

C. Nuclear Magnetic Resonance

Nuclear magnetic resonance (NMR) spectroscopy has been the classic technique for structural elucidation of newly discovered carotenoids (66). Low sensitivity and the need to obtain very pure samples in reasonable quantities (50–100 μg) has limited use of this technique for measurement and identification of carotenoids in blood and biological tissues. Laborious isolation procedures using semipreparative HPLC have been used to isolate purified carotenoid pigments for NMR experiments (60,67). NMR spectroscopy can be particularly useful to elucidate the geometrical configuration of E and Z isomers of carotenoids. Extensive studies reporting on the characterization and geometrical configuration of eight Z isomers of lycopene have been conducted (68). The advent of coupled HPLC-NMR has proven quite useful for the elucidation of carotenoid cis-trans isomeric structures, and this technique has been recently applied to the determination of lutein and zeaxanthin stereoisomers in spinach and in the retina (69). This method eliminates the need to isolate and purify large quantities of carotenoids that are sensitive to degradative reactions and provides a powerful tool for the unequivocal characteriztion of carotenoids in biological tissues.

VI. CONCLUSIONS

Development of new and more versatile analytical techniques continues to expand our ability to conduct basic research and understand the role of carotenoids in human health and disease prevention. Liquid chromatography has clearly become the method of choice for carotenoid analysis over the last 20 years. Application of traditional separation methods with UV-Vis detection has become commonplace in a carotenoid researcher's laboratory. The advent of more sensitive and selective analytical techniques (LC-ECD and LC-MS) allows for simplification of basic intervention studies and will further our understanding of the growing epidemiological evidence. With a continued focus on minimally to noninvasive but highly sensitive and selective methods, our abilities will further expand elevating carotenoid research to new levels.

REFERENCES

1. Giovannucci EL, Ascherio A, Rimm EB, Stampfer MJ, Colditz GA, Willett WC. Intake of carotenoids and retinoids in relation to risk of prostate cancer. J Natl Cancer Inst 1995; 87:1767–1776.
2. Giovannucci EL. Tomatoes, tomato-based products, lycopene, and cancer: review of the epidemiologic literature. J Natl Cancer Inst 1999; 91:317–331.
3. Su LCJ, Bui M, Kardinaal A, Gomez-Aracena J, Martin-Moreno J, Martin B, Thamm M, Simonsen N, van't Veer P, Kok F, Strain S, Kohlmeier L. Differences between plasma and adipose tissue biomarkers of carotenoids and tocopherols. Cancer Epidemiol Biomark Prev 1998; 7:1043–1048.
4. Mayne ST. Beta-carotene, carotenoids, and disease prevention in humans. FASEB 1996; 10:690–701.
5. Nguyen ML, Schwartz SJ. Lycopene: chemical and biological properties. Food Technol 1999; 53:38–45.

6. Schmitz HH, Poor CL, Wellman RB, Erdman JW. Concentrations of selected carotenoids and vitamin A in human kidney and lung tissue. J Nutr 1991; 121:1613–1621.
7. Schmitz HH, Poor CL, Gugger ET, Erdman JW. Analysis of carotenoids in human and animal tissues. Meth Enzymol 1993; 214:102–115.
8. Yeum KJ, Taylor A, Tang G, Russell RM. Measurement of carotenoids, retinoids, and tocopherols in human lenses. Invest Ophthalmol Vis Sci 1995; 36:2756–2761.
9. Clinton SK, Emenhiser C, Schwartz SJ, Bostwick DG, Williams AW, Moore BJ, Erdman JW. cis-trans Lycopene isomers, carotenoids, and retinol in the human prostate. Cancer Epidemiol Biomark Prev 1996; 5:823–833.
10. Peng YM, Peng YS, Lin Y. A non saponification method for the determination of carotenoids, retinoids and tocopherols in solid human tissues. Cancer Epidemiol Biomark Prev 1993; 2:139–144.
11. Peng YS, Peng YM, McGee DL, Alberts DS. Carotenoid, tocopherols, and retinoids in human buccal mucosal cells: intra- and interindividual variability and storage stability. Am J Clin Nutr 1994; 59:636–643.
12. Gamboa-Pinto AJ, Rock CL, Ferruzzi MG, Schowinsky AB, Schwartz SJ. Cervical tissue and plasma concentrations of alpha-carotene and beta-carotene in women are correlated. J Nutr 1998; 128:1933–1936.
13. Ferruzzi MG, Sander LC, Rock CL, Schwartz SJ. Carotenoid determination in biological microsamples using liquid chromatography with a coulometric electrochemical array detector. Anal Biochem 1998; 256:74–81.
14. Bieri JG, Brown ED, Smith JC. Determination of individual carotenoids in human plasma by high performance liquid chromatography. J Liq Chromatogr 1985; 8: 473–484.
15. Bui MH. Simple determination of retinol, α-tocopherol and carotenoids (lutein, all-trans-lycopene, α- and β-carotenes) in human plasma by isocratic liquid chromatography. J Chromatogr B 1994; 654:129–133.
16. Stewart I, Wheaton TA. Continuous flow separation by liquid chromatography. J Chromatogr 1971; 55:325–336.
17. Fiksdahl A, Mortensen JT, Liaaen-Jensen S. High-pressure liquid chromatography of carotenoids. J Chromatogr 1978; 157:111–117.
18. Katrangi N, Kaplan LA, Stein EA. Separation and quantitation of serum beta carotene and other carotenoids by high performance liquid chromatography. J Lipid Res 1984; 25:400–406.
19. Yakushina L, Taranova A. Rapid HPLC simultaneous determination of fat-soluble vitamins, including carotenoids, in human serum. J Pharm Biochem Anal 1995; 13:715–718.
20. Yeum KJ, Booth SL, Sadowski JA, Liu C, Tang G, Krinsky NI, Russell RM. Human plasma carotenoid response to the ingestion of controlled diets high in fruits and vegetables. Am J Clin Nutr 1996; 64:594–602.
21. Piretti MV, Diamante M, Bombardelli E, Morazzoni P. Anomalous behaviour of lycopene by HPLC on cyano-amino polar phase. Biomed Chromatogr 1996; 10:43–45.
22. Schmitz HH, Emenhiser C, Schwartz SJ. HPLC separation of geometric carotene isomers using a calcium hydroxide stationary phase. J Agric Food Chem 1995; 43:1212–1218.

23. O'Neil CA, Schwartz SJ, Catignani GL. Comparison of liquid chromatographic methods for determination of cis-trans isomers of β-carotene. J Assoc Off Anal Chem 1991; 74:36–42.
24. Van het Hof KH, de Boer BCJ, Tijburg LBM, Lucius BRHM, Zijp I, West CE, Hautvast JGAJ, Weststrate JA. Carotenoid bioavailability in humans from tomatoes processed in different ways determined from the carotenoid response in the triglyceride-rich lipoprotein fraction of plasma after a single consumption and in plasma after four days of consumption. J Nutr 2000; 130:1189–1196.
25. Schmit JA, Henry RA, Williams RC, Diekman JF. Applications of high speed reversed-phase liquid chromatography. J Chromatogr Sci 1971; 9:645–651.
26. Khachik F, Spangler C, Smith Jr. JC. Identification, quantifications and relative concentrations of carotenoids and their metabolites in human milk and serum. Anal. Chem. 1997; 89:1873–1881.
27. Saleh MH, Tan B. Separation and identification of cis/trans carotenoid isomer. J Agric Food Chem 1991; 39:1438–1443.
28. Bushway RJ. Determination of α- and β-carotene in some raw fruits and vegetables by HPLC. J Agric Food Chem 1985; 34:409–412.
29. Bushway RJ, Wilson AM. Determination of α- and β-carotene in fruit and vegetables by high performance liquid chromatography. Can Inst Food Sci Technol J 1982; 15:165–169.
30. Lessellier E, Marty C, Berset C, Tchapla A. Optimization of the isocratic nonaqueous reverse phase (NARP) HPLC separation of trans/cis - α- and β-carotenes. J High Res Chromatogr 1989; 12:447–454.
31. O'Neil CA, Schwartz SJ, Catignani GL. Comparison of liquid chromatographic methods for determination of cis-trans isomers of β-carotene. J Assoc Off Anal Chem 1991; 74:36–42.
32. Craft NE, Brown ED, Smith JC Jr. Effects of storage and handling conditions on concentrations of individual carotenoids, retinal, and tocopherol in plasma. Clin Chem 1988; 34:44–48.
33. Craft NE, Wise SA, Soares JH. Optimization of an isocratic high performance liquid chromatographic separation of carotenoids. J Chromatogr 1992; 589:171–176.
34. Lyan B, Azaïs-Braesco V, Cardinault N, Tyssandier V, Borel P, Alexandre-Gouabau MC, Grolier P. Simple method for clinical determination of 13 carotenoids in human plasma using an isocratic high-performance liquid chromatographic method. J Chromatogr B 2001; 751:297–303.
35. El-Sohemy A, Baylin A, Kabagambe E, Ascherio A, Spiegelman D, Campos H. Individual carotenoid concentrations in adipose tissue and plasma as biomarkers of dietary intake. Am J Clin Nutr 2002; 76:172–179.
36. Krinsky NI, Russett MD, Handelman GJ, Snodderly DM. Structural and geometrical isomers of carotenoids in human plasma. J Nutr 1990;120:1654–1662
37. Handelman GJ, Nightingale ZD, Lichtenstein AH, Schaefer EJ, Blumberg JB. Lutein and zeaxanthin concentrations in plasma after dietary supplementation with egg yolk. Am J Clin Nutr 1999; 70:247–251.
38. Ferruzzi MG, Nguyen ML, Sander LC, Rock CL, Schwartz SJ. Analysis of lycopene geometrical isomers in biological microsamples by liquid chromatography with coulometric array detection. J Chromatogr B 2001; 760:289–299.

39. Böhm V, Bitsch R. Intestinal absorption of lycopene from different matrices and interactions to other carotenoids, the lipid status, and the antioxidant capacity of human plasma. Eur J Nutr 1999; 38:118–125.

40. Sander LC, Sharpless KE, Craft NE, Wise SA. Development of engineered stationary phases for the separation of carotenoid isomers. Anal Chem 1994; 66:1667–1674.

41. Emenhiser C, Simunovic N, Sander LC, Schwartz SJ. Separation of geometric isomers in biological extracts using a polymeric C_{30} column in reversed-phase liquid chromatography. J Agric Food Chem 1996; 44:3887–3893.

42. Emenhiser C, Sander LC, Schwartz SJ. Capability of a polymeric C_{30} stationary phase to resolve cis-trans carotenoid isomers in reversed-phase liquid chromatography. J Chromatogr A 1995; 707:205–216.

43. Johnson EJ, Qin J, Krinsky NI, Russell RM. Beta-carotene isomers in human serum, breast milk and buccal mucosa cells after continuous oral doses of all-trans and 9-cis-beta-carotene. J Nutr 1997; 127:1993–1999.

44. Bell CM, Sander LC, Fetzer JC, Wise SA. Synthesis and characterization of extended length alkyl stationary phases for liquid chromatography with application to the separation of carotenoid isomers. J Chromatogr A 1996; 753:37–45.

45. Motchnik PA, Frei B, Ames BN. Measurement of antioxidants in human blood plasma. Meth Enzymol 1994; 234:269–279.

46. MacCrehan WA, Schonberger E. Determination of retinol, α-tocopherol, and β-carotene in serum by liquid chromatography with absorbance and electrochemical detection. Clin Chem 1997; 33:1585–1592.

47. MacCrehan WA, Schonberger E. Reversed-phase high-performance liquid chromatography separation and electrochemical detection of retinol and its isomers. J Chromatogr 1987; 417:65–78.

48. Ewing AG, Mesaros JM, Gavin PF. Electrochemical detection in microcolumn separation. Anal Chem 1994; 66:527–536.

49. Finckh B, Kontush A, Commentz J, Hubner C, Burdelski M, Kohlschutter A. Monitoring of ubiquinol-10, ubiquinone-10, carotenoids and tocopherol in neonatal plasma microsamples using high performance liquid chromatography with coulometric electrochemical detection. Anal Biochem 1995; 238:210–216.

50. De Leenheer AP, Nelis HJ, Lambert WE. Recent developments in the measurement of vitamin A carotenoids. Voeding 1992; 52:168–172.

51. Ferruzzi MG, Brown MJ, Nguyen ML, Cooper DA, White WS, Schwartz SJ. Application of a C_{30} HPLC-EC method to assess post-prandial carotenoid absorption from vegetables in humans. Experimental Biology Federation of American Societies for Experimental Biology, San Diego, CA, Apr 16–19, 2000.

52. Brown MB, Ferruzzi MG, Nguyen ML, Cooper DA, Eldridge AL, Schwartz SJ, White WS. The bioavailability of carotenoids is higher in salads ingested with full-fat versus fat-modified salad dressings as measured by using electrochemical detection. Am J Clin Nutr 2003. In press.

53. Ball, GFM. The fat-soluble vitamins. In: Nollet LML, ed. Food Analysis by HPLC. New York: Marcel Dekker, 1992.

54. Furr HC, Barua AB, Olson JA. Retinoids and carotenoids. In: De Leenheer AP, Lambert WE, Nelis HJ, eds. Modern Chromatographic Analysis of Vitamins, 2nd ed. New York: Marcel Dekker, 1992.

55. Aaran RK, Nikkari T. HPLC method for the simultaneous determination of beta-carotene, retinol and alpha-tocopherol in serum. J Pharm Biomed Anal 1988; 6: 853–857.

56. Comstock GW, Menkes MS, Schober SE, Vuilleumier J-P, Helsing KJ. Serum levels of retinol, beta-carotene, and alpha-tocopherol in older adults. Am J Epidemiol 1988; 127: 114–123.

57. Sowell AL, Huff DL, Yeager PR, Caudill SP, Gunter EW. Retinol, α-tocopherol, lutein/zeaxanthin, β-cryptoxanthin, lycopene, α-carotene, trans-β-carotene, and four retinyl esters in serum determined simultaneously by reversed-phase HPLC with multiwavelength detection. Clin Chem 1994; 40: 411–416.

58. Johnson EJ, Suter PM, Sahyoun N, Ribaya-Mercado JD, Russell RM. Relation between β-carotene intake and plasma and adipose tissue concentrations of carotenoids and retinoids. Am J Clin Nutr 1995; 62: 598–603.

59. Ben-Amotz A. Simultaneous profiling and identification of carotenoids, retinols and tocopherols by high performance liquid chromatography equipped with three-dimensional photodiode array detection. J Liq Chromatogr 1995; 18: 2813–2825.

60. Emenhiser C, Englert G, Sander LC, Ludwig B, Schwartz SJ. Isolation and structural elucidation of the predominant geometrical isomers of α-carotene. J Chromatogr A 1996; 719: 333–343.

61. van Breemen RB. Electrospray liquid chromatography–mass spectrometry of carotenoids. Anal Chem 1995; 67: 2004–2009.

62. van Breemen RB. Innovations in carotenoid analysis using LC/MS. Anal Chem 1996; 77: 299–304.

63. van Breemen RB, Schmitz HH, Schwartz SJ. Continuous-flow fast atom bombardment liquid chromatography/mass spectrometry of carotenoids. Anal Chem 1993; 65: 965–969.

64. Henry LK, Puspitasari-Nienaber NL, Jarén-Galán M, van Breemen RB, Catignani GL, Schwartz SJ. Effects of ozone and oxygen on the degradation of carotenoids in an aqueous model system J Agric Food Chem 2000; 48: 5008–5013.

65. Fang L, Pajkovic N, Wang Y, Gu C, Breemen RB. Quantitative analysis of lycopene isomers in human plasma using high-performance liquid chromatography–tandem mass spectrometry. Anal Chem 2003; 75:812–817.

66. Englert G. NMR Spectroscopy. In: Britton G, Liaaen-Jensen S, Plander H, eds., Carotenoids. Vol. 1B, Spectroscopy. Basel: Birkhauser, 1995: 147–260.

67. Khachik F, Steck A, Plander H. Isolation and structural elucidation of (13Z,13'Z,3R,3'R,6'R)-lutein from marigold flowers, kale and human plasma. J Agric Food Chem 1999; 47:455–461.

68. Hengartner U, Bernhard K, Meyer K, Englert G, Glinz E. Synthesis, isolation and NMR-spectroscopic characterization of fourteen (Z) isomers of lycopene and of some actylenic didehydro- and tetradehydrolycopenes. Helv Chim Acta 1992, 75:1848–1865.

69. Dachtler M, Glaser T, Kohler K, Albert K. Combined HPLC-MS and HPLC-NMR on line coupling for the separation and determination of lutein and zeaxanthin stereoisomers in spinach and in retina. Anal Chem 2001, 73:667–674.

5

Carotenoid Antioxidant Activity

Andrew J. Young, Denise M. Phillip, and Gordon M. Lowe
Liverpool John Moores University, Liverpool, England

I. INTRODUCTION

An antioxidant may be broadly defined as "any substance that when present at low concentrations compared to those of an oxidizable substrate, significantly delays or prevents oxidation" (1). Carotenoids are often regarded as dietary antioxidants, but how effective are they? Although more than 600 naturally occurring carotenoids have been identified (2), only 40 of these are ingested in the human diet, but fewer than 20, including both polar xanthophylls and apolar cyclic and acyclic carotenes from dietary sources, have been found in plasma and tissues (3,4). Trace levels of a number of carotenoid metabolites and potential oxidation products of dietary carotenoids (4), including, for example, 2,6-cyclolyopene-1,5-diols (5), anhydrolutein (6), and acycloretinol (7), have also been detected. Although a number of these oxidation products may be produced by interaction of carotenoids with reactive oxygen species (ROS) under controlled conditions (8,9; see below), their functional significance (if any) in biological tissues is not yet understood (see Ref. 10).

The potential roles played by dietary carotenoids in human disease prevention have only begun to be elucidated for a select few compounds in recent years. In general, carotenoids behave as effective antioxidants (e.g., as quenchers of singlet oxygen) in vitro and clear evidence exists from a majority of epidemiological studies that increased consumption of foods rich in β-carotene (and thereby increased plasma levels of β-carotene; 11,12) is associated with a reduced risk of lung and some other cancers (11; see Chapter 19). However, results from recent intervention studies [the Beta-Carotene and Retinol Efficacy Trial (13) and the Alpha-Tocopherol, Beta-Carotene Cancer Prevention Study (14)], have failed to demonstrate that carotenoids are protective in vivo. Indeed, the studies found that exposure of individuals taking supplemental β-carotene to "high-intensity" (15) cigarette smoke (or those individuals suffering from asbestosis, 16) increased lung cancer incidence. But why should β-carotene exhibit such procarcinogenic activity? Mayne and colleagues (16,17) and, more recently, Wang and Russell (18) highlighted a number of factors that may explain the apparent pro-oxidant behavior of β-carotene in these studies. These include the generation of relatively high amounts of deleterious oxidation products (see below) of β-carotene brought about by exposure to the ROS found in tobacco smoke or by metabolic processes via increased retinoic acid catabolism or interference with retinoid signal transduction (18).

This chapter reviews the current information concerning the ability of carotenoids to act as antioxidants in vitro and the mechanisms whereby these molecules function. The influence of the local environment on carotenoid function is discussed. We also review the evidence supporting a possible in vivo antioxidant role in humans.

II. REACTIONS AND REACTIVITY OF CAROTENOIDS

A. General Properties

Oxidative stress and free radical attack on biological structures are believed to be major factors in the initiation and propagation of the development of many degenerative diseases. Biomembranes rich in polyunsaturated fatty acids are particularly susceptible to the degradative process of lipid peroxidation (mediated by free radicals in particular). Carotenoids may function as chain-breaking antioxidants reducing lipid peroxidation of such vulnerable membranes. The ability of molecules such as carotenoids to act as antioxidants depends on a number of factors, including its structure and resulting chemical properties but also in relation to its location and form in biological tissues (see below). The antioxidant properties of carotenoids are primarily associated with their ability to quench singlet oxygen (19,20) and scavenge free radicals (21–24). In carotenoids the conjugated carbon double-bond system is considered to be the single most important factor in energy transfer reactions, such as those found in photosynthesis (25). It is this feature of the molecule that also permits the quenching of singlet oxygen ($^1O_2$). Interactions with other ROS produced in the body, including radicals such as superoxide ($O_2^{\cdot}$) and nonradicals such as hydrogen peroxide (H_2O_2), are dependent on other mechanisms (see below). While the electron-rich polyene chain of carotenoids is responsible for many of the properties of these molecules, it is also a prime target for attack by electrophilic compounds, contributing to the overall instability of these molecules. The antioxidant behavior of a carotenoid molecule (whether mediated by direct or indirect means) is dependent on its structure but also the nature of the oxidizing species itself.

B. Quenching of Singlet Oxygen by Carotenoids

The main mechanisms responsible for the quenching of $^1O_2$ by carotenoids involves direct energy transfer between these molecules. The lowest triplet energy level of β-carotene has been measured at 88 ± 3 kJ mol^{-1} (26). This compares to a value of 94 kJ mol^{-1} for $^1O_2$. In all solvents studied (27), $^1O_2$ is effectively quenched by carotenoids so long as the triplet state is low enough [reaction (1)], resulting in the formation of the carotenoid triplet state ($^3CAR^*$) which readily returns to the stable ground state dissipating excess energy as heat. Quenching constants for $^1O_2$ have been determined for a range of carotenoids in solution and reveal a close dependence between structure of the carotenoid and the ability to quench $^1O_2$ by energy transfer (19,20,27–30). Such quenching occurs near the diffusion-controlled limit. This is primarily governed by the length of the conjugated polyene chain and directly related to the energy of the low-lying triplet-excited states of these molecules. Other structural features, e.g., cyclization, may also affect rates of quenching as demonstrated by comparing rates for β-carotene and lycopene (both of which have 11 conjugated double bonds; see Table 1).

$$^1O_2^* + CAR \longrightarrow {}^3O_2 + {}^3CAR^* \tag{1}$$

In addition to the physical quenching of $^1O_2$, chemical quenching of $^1O_2$ by carotenoids can also occur, in which the quencher combines with oxygen or is oxidized and which leads to the destruction (bleaching) of the carotenoid molecule (29). Both chemical and physical quenching require a very close interaction between the carotenoid and $^1O_2$ molecules. In biological systems, a number of sensitizers can result in $^1O_2$ production, and the clinical use of β-carotene as an effective treatment for erythropoietic protoporphyria, in which $^1O_2$ is produced via sensitization of free porphyrins accumulated in the skin, is well established (31,32). Carotenoids such as β-carotene also serve to quench the triplet-excited state of many sensitizers, thereby preventing the formation of $^1O_2$ in the first place. The resulting carotenoid triplet dissipates its energy harmlessly as heat.

C. Free Radical Scavenging by Carotenoids

In the human body, a range of ROS are produced, including $^1O_2$, OH$^{\bullet}$, $O_2^{\bullet-}$, and H_2O_2 (1). The mechanisms and rate of scavenging of free radicals by carotenoids in solution is strongly dependent on the nature of the ROS itself (33). Carotenoids such as β-carotene are very reactive to peroxyl radicals but much less so to OH$^{\bullet}$

Table 1 Singlet Oxygen Quenching Rate Constants for Various Carotenoids (in Benzene)[a]

Carotenoid	Number of conjugated carbon–carbon double bonds	K_q ($\times 10^9$ M^{-1} s^{-1})
7,7'-Dihydro-β-carotene	8	0.3
Septapreno-β-carotene	9	1.38
8'-Apo-β-carotenal	9	5.27
Violaxanthin	9	16.0
Lutein	10	6.64
α-Carotene	10	12.0
9-cis-β-carotene	11	11.0
15-cis-β-carotene	11	11.0
Zeaxanthin	11	12.0
β-Carotene	11	13.0
Astaxanthin	11	14.0
Lycopene	11	17.0
3,4,3',4'-Tetradehydrolycopene	15	10.7
Decapreno-β-carotene	15	20.0
Dodecapreno-β-carotene	19	23.0

[a]All compounds are all-trans unless otherwise stated.
Source: Ref. 27.

and $O_2^{\bullet-}$ (21). The structure of the carotenoid molecule is also important, and the nature and position of substituent groups on the carotenoid molecule may directly affect its antioxidant ability. The reactivity of a number of carotenoids with ROS has been examined (34,35) and differences in reactivity between molecules shown to be related to differences in their electron density profiles. For example, the effect of keto groups at C-4 and C-4' in astaxanthin and canthaxanthin (which significantly alters their electron density profiles), or hydroxy groups at C-4 and C-4' in isozeaxanthin is to reduce the reactivity of these molecules by preventing hydrogen abstraction from these positions (34–36). The preferred sites for epoxidation of astaxanthin and canthaxanthin are different from that seen with β-carotene or zeaxanthin (35).

Carotenoids interact with free radicals in three main ways: electron transfer [reaction (2)], hydrogen abstraction [reaction (3)], and addition of a radical species [reaction (4)] (27,37). The mechanism and rate of scavenging is primarily dependent on the nature of the oxidizing species but less important is the structure of the carotenoid molecule (32). The nature of carotenoid–free radical interactions is discussed in detail in Chapter 3 and only an outline is provided here. Burton and Ingold (21) first proposed that β-carotene reacts with peroxyl radicals via an addition reaction [reaction (4)] and provided evidence that β-carotene can function as a effective chain-breaking antioxidant, at least at low partial pressures of oxygen (see below).

$$CAR + ROO^\bullet \longrightarrow CAR^{\bullet+} + ROO^- \qquad \text{electron transfer} \qquad (2)$$

$$CAR + ROO^\bullet \longrightarrow CAR^\bullet + ROOH \qquad \text{hydrogen abstraction} \qquad (3)$$

$$CAR + ROO^\bullet \longrightarrow ROOCAR^\bullet \qquad \text{addition} \qquad (4)$$

The antioxidant properties of carotenoids are thought to be dependent on the rate at which they scavenge different types of free radicals, the type of reaction involved, and the properties of any carotenoid radicals that may result (23,38,39). Potential (and likely) influential factors affecting the rates and mechanisms of these free radical reactions include the nature of the free radical and its environment (aqueous or lipid regions) as well as structural features of the carotenoid (23,35; cyclic or acyclic termini, polar or apolar end groups, redox properties), which not only alters their chemistry and hence reactivity but also governs their location and orientation within lipid bilayer structures (40) and even their tendency to self-aggregate in polar conditions (41). Lycopene, due to its open structure, is much more readily able to form a carbon-centered radical cation than β-carotene (34,38).

By comparison, interactions of carotenoids with reactive nitrogen species (RNS) are poorly understood. The capacity of a range of carotenoids to scavenge peroxynitrite both in solution and in isolated low-density-lipoprotein (LDL) in vitro has been studied (42). Xanthophylls (e.g., lutein and zeaxanthin) were less efficient scavengers of peroxynitrite than carotenes (e.g., β-carotene) in both systems. However, the activity of the xanthophylls was still comparable to that of well-known scavengers of peroxynitrite such as glutathione.

D. Partial Pressure of Oxygen

The antioxidant behavior of β-carotene is, in part, dependent on the partial pressure of oxygen (pO_2). Burton and Ingold (21) showed that at low pO_2, β-carotene acted as a chain-breaking antioxidant [consuming peroxyl radicals; Eq. (2)], while at higher pO_2 the carotenoid lost its antioxidant ability and actually exhibited prooxidant behavior due to autoxidation. This was demonstrated in solution using the trichloromethylperoxyl radical and β-carotene. At low pO_2, the β-carotene radical cation was readily formed, whereas in air and oxygen-saturated solutions a carotene radical adduct was also formed (22,43). This second species decayed to the relatively unreactive carotene radical cation. At low pO_2 this process consumes peroxyl radicals and the carotenoid acts as a chain-breaking antioxidant. At high pO_2 the carotenoid radical reacts with oxygen to produce a carotenoid peroxyl radical [autoxidation; reaction (5)], which is capable of acting as a prooxidant. Peroxidation is promoted in the presence of unsaturated lipid [reactions (6)–(7)]. The autoxidation of carotenoids is most pronounced at high concentrations of carotenoid (33). Indeed, whether carotenoids such as β-carotene, lutein, and lycopene act as an antioxidant or as a proxidant in human fibroblasts has recently been shown to be highly dependent on their cellular concentration (44). Optimal doses of each of these carotenoids required to protect the cells from UVB irradiation were very different.

$$CAR^{\bullet} + O_2 \rightarrow CAR\!\!-\!\!OO^{\bullet} \tag{5}$$

$$CAR\!\!-\!\!OO^{\bullet} + LH \rightarrow CAR\!\!-\!\!OOH + L^{\bullet} \tag{6}$$

$$L^{\bullet} + O_2 \rightarrow L\!\!-\!\!OO^{\bullet} \tag{7}$$

While such reactions have not yet been observed in vivo, it is appropriate to consider the possible physiological consequences of this as the different tissues and organs within the human body are very different in terms of distribution of pO_2; e.g., lung alveoli 100 mm Hg; venous blood 40 mm Hg, and blood in tissues 5–15 mm Hg (1). Concentration gradients for O_2 may exist within cells (1) and in tumors (45). A number of in vitro and in vivo studies have been performed at very high pO_2 (760 mm Hg), but while this might promote effective pro-oxidation of carotenoids it is essentially nonphysiological. It might therefore be expected that carotenoids may function differently in different parts of the body, so that they may, for example, be *less effective* antioxidants in the lung than in other tissues. It does not necessarily mean that the carotenoids will act as pro-oxidants. The relative effectiveness of carotenoids compared to that of other antioxidants, especially α-tocopherol, also depends on pO_2 (46). α-Tocopherol is much more effective as an antioxidant at high pO_2 but β-carotene is more effective at low pO_2. It can therefore be seen how these coantioxidants may act together to provide an effective defence against oxidation in different tissues.

E. Oxidation Products of Carotenoids

The different mechanisms by which carotenoids scavenge ROS may lead to a variety of carotenoid free radicals and adducts. These in turn determine the nature of the final reaction products. The potential harmful or beneficial effects of carotenoid oxidation products are an important consideration in assessing their biological effects. The structure of carotenoids, with its extensive conjugated double-bond system, means that the number and type of autoxidation products of molecules such as β-carotene may be very complex, especially as the sites for attack include the polyene chain as well as the β-ionone end groups. Identification of the reaction products resulting from the oxidation of molecules such as β-carotene and lycopene can, in theory, provide useful information on the type of oxidation reactions that have taken place; however, only a relatively small number of studies (primarily with β-carotene) have attempted to identify such products. These are summarized in Table 2. Inevitably the structure of the carotenoid molecule leads to a complex set of reaction products, although a pattern does emerge.

Table 2   Recent Studies that Have Identified the Oxidation Products of Carotenoids

Carotenoid	Oxidizing species	Main reaction products identified	Ref.
Lycopene	Peroxynitrite	Apocarotenals: 10′-apolycopenal, 8′-apolycopenal, 6′-apolycopenal Isomers: 13-*cis*-lycopene, 9-*cis*-lycopene	50
β-Carotene	AIBN	Apocarotenals: β-apo-15′-carotenal, β-apo-14′-carotenal, β-apo-14′-carotenal, β-apo-12′-carotenal, β-apo-10′-carotenal Apocarotenones: β-apo-13-carotenone Epoxides: β-carotene-5,6-epoxide, β-carotene-15,15′-epoxide[a]	8
β-Carotene	Dioxygen (ruthenium tetramesitylporphyrin catalyst/air)	Apocarotenals and apocarotenones: complete series observed Epoxides: β-carotene-5,6-epoxide (plus epoxides of apocarotenals) Isomers: 15-*cis*-β-carotene Others: $C_9,8'$-diapocarotene-dial, $C_{13},8'$-diapocarotene-dial	49
β-Carotene	AMVN	Epoxides: β-carotene-5,6-epoxide, β-carotene-5,6,5′,6′-diepoxide, β-carotene-15,15′-epoxide Isomers: *cis*-β-carotene-15,15′-epoxide	9,48

[a]Tentatine identification.
AIBN, azobisisobutylnitrile; AMVN, 2,2-azobis(2,4-dimethylvateronitrile).

The preferred sites of reaction in a carotenoid molecule are dependent on electron distribution and localization (35). El-Tinay and Chichester (47) first proposed that the β-ionone ring of β-carotene was especially prone to attack and that the initial product formed via oxidation would be β-carotene 5,6-epoxide. This product (and related epoxides including the furanoid 5,8-epoxide) is indeed commonly found (e.g., 9,48). More recent evidence (e.g., 8,49) suggests that epoxidation is not the only reaction and that multiple reactions can occur instead, perhaps simultaneously. In addition to the epoxides (mono- and di-5,6-epoxides and 5,8-epoxides, as well as in-chain epoxides), the principal oxidation products of β-carotene include a full range of in-chain cleavage products (β-apocarotenals and β-apocarotenones) and their epoxides. A number of studies have also observed the formation of a range of cis isomers formed from all-*trans* β-carotene and lycopene, particularly in the initial stages of oxidation or under mild oxidative conditions (49,50; G. Lowe and A. J. Young, unpublished data). Such isomerization is a feature of the quenching of excited triplet states of sensitizers and of $^1O_2$ (see Ref. (51)).

A procarcinogenic effect of the oxidative products mentioned above has been proposed (see Refs. (17) and (18)). For example, the binding of benzo[a]pyrene metabolites to DNA is promoted in the presence of oxidative products of β-carotene but inhibited in the presence of β-carotene itself (52). At high concentrations of carotenoid, high levels of oxidative products may be expected to form in the presence of ROS. Elevated levels of such oxidative products have been observed in vitro in the lung tissues from smoke-exposed compared to control ferrets (18,53). High levels of these products may also result in an acceleration of malignant transformation in lung tissues due to down-regulation of the RARβ gene (53).

The nature of the oxidizing species itself may have a marked influence on the reaction products found. For example, while Handelman et al. (8) observed a similar set of reaction products under both spontaneous and peroxyl radical–initiated autooxidation, use of hypochlorite or 2,2′-azobisisobutyronitrile (AIBN)-mediated oxidation produced a very different set of reaction products of β-carotene. It has been proposed that the pro-oxidant effects of carotenoids (or rather the lack of an antioxidant effect) may be due to their autoxidation (especially at high po$_2$; see above). The interaction of β-carotene with cigarette smoke (in a model system) yields 1-nitro-β-carotene and 4-nitro-β-carotene (as both *cis* and all-*trans* forms) with the former as the major product (54). The products of reactions (2) and (3) may react with molecular oxygen to yield peroxyl radicals (21). These species can partake in lipid peroxidation reactions, and therefore any alteration in concentration of the carotenoid or po$_2$ would influence the formation of carotenoid peroxyl radicals or carotenoid autoxidation. Increased peroxide values in the plasma and the liver of rats fed β-carotene have been recorded (55). However there is still a lack of direct evidence that the harmful effects of carotenoids in human diseases is related to their pro-oxidant effects.

III. REACTIONS OF CAROTENOIDS IN BIOLOGICAL SYSTEMS: INTERACTIONS WITH THEIR ENVIRONMENT

In biological systems carotenoids rarely, if ever, occur as free (monomeric) molecules "in solution." Rather they are predominantly found associated (often very tightly) with protein or lipoprotein structures, which may have a profound effect on the properties of the carotenoid molecule, affecting the way that these molecules function and may govern, at least in part, their interaction with ROS, for example. It should be remembered that carotenoids also directly influence their environment so that carotenoids generally bring about a degree of stabilization and are at the same time stabilized. Britton (35) and more recently, Young and Lowe (56) have discussed the role of a number of factors that may influence the antioxidant (or even promote pro-oxidant) activities of carotenoids in biological systems. These are (a) its structure (i.e., size, shape, and the nature, position, and number of substituent groups) and physical form (aggregated or monomeric, *cis* or *trans* configuration, etc.); (b) its location or site of action within the cell; (c) its potential for interaction with other carotenoids or antioxidants (especially vitamins C and E); (d) its concentration; and (e) the partial pressure of oxygen.

It is clear that the structure of a carotenoid molecule effectively dictates how these molecules are incorporated into, and may therefore subsequently affect or control, their local environment. For example, the solubility of carotenoids in aqueous solutions is generally extremely poor, effectively restricting them to the hydrophobic regions of biological systems. However, this behavior is greatly influenced by carotenoid structure so that different compounds (e.g., carotenes and xanthophylls) will be incorporated quite differently into membranes (40,56). Solubility is also affected by *cis/trans* isomerization (35).

The location of carotenoids within a cell will, of course, influence its free radical scavenging ability. Carotenoid reactions with different ROS may follow a completely different course in polar and/or apolar solvents (23,24,59–64), and differences in their behavior in different regions of a cell may therefore to be predicted. The nonpolar environment encountered by carotenes sitting deep within a membrane is unlikely to support electron transfer [reaction (2)] because charge separation will not be supported (D. McGarvey, personal communication). Thus, electron transfer scavenging may only be feasible for some xanthophylls that have polar substituents on each end group (e.g., diols such as zeaxanthin) and can therefore span or are held at the surface of a membrane, allowing them to intercept radicals in the aqueous phase at the membrane surface. β-Carotene is indeed less effective at preventing lipid peroxidation when exposed to a water-soluble peroxyl radical initiator in a liposomal environment, whereas zeaxanthin and β-cryptoxanthin effectively protected against both water- and lipid-soluble peroxyl radicals (34,36). Both β-carotene and zeaxanthin have the same number of conjugated carbon–carbon double bonds ($n = 11$) and behave essentially the same in solution (36), and differences in their antioxidant behavior could be attributed in this case to differences in their location and orientation within the lipid bilayer.

The orientation of a carotenoid molecule in a membrane is dependent on its structure and on the composition of the membrane itself (40). β-Carotene (and other carotenes such as lycopene) lie parallel with the membrane surface, deep within the hydrophobic core (63,64). In contrast, the diol zeaxanthin entirely spans the membrane and therefore reactions with its conjugated carbon double-bond system are possible throughout the depth of the membrane. [Note that polar carotenoids such as zeaxanthin also act as rivets, strengthening the membrane (40) and they also limit the penetration of oxygen into membranes (65)]. It should also be noted that not all xanthophylls behave the same and small differences in structure alter their behavior, so that, for example, the diols zeaxanthin and lutein orient themselves quite differently in membranes (40). Such factors would, in turn, be expected to affect their antioxidant ability against carotenoids in the lipid and aqueous phases.

β-Carotene has been shown to be effective against *tert*-butyl hydroperoxide–induced lipid peroxidation (66) and DNA damage (67). The mode of action is thought to be via degradation to alkoxyl and peroxyl radicals (1). However, in the presence of H_2O_2 or xanthine/xanthine oxidase [an exogenous source of H_2O_2 and $O_2^{\cdot-}$—both components of cigarette smoke (68) and produced in inflammatory cells in asbestosis (69)] in HT29 adenocarcinoma cells, the ability of β-carotene and lycopene to protect the cells against DNA damage were only seen at low doses ($\sim$1–2 μM; 70) and this protective effect was lost as the dose of carotenoid was increased (<4 μM), so that at the highest doses tested (10 μM) the carotenoid afforded no protection against DNA damage. Relatively high doses of β-carotene also failed to protect against H_2O_2-induced DNA damage in HepG2 cells (67). At high doses of β-carotene, the membranes of HT29 cells became increasingly permeabilized (68), and this was closely correlated with DNA damage, indicating perhaps that the presence of carotenes may increase permeability to aqueous ROS. Interestingly, neither β-carotene nor lycopene exhibits in vitro antioxidant behavior against H_2O_2 and $O_2^{\cdot-}$ at high doses (66). In contrast, zeaxanthin exhibited dose-dependent protection against xanthine/ xanthine oxidase–mediated DNA damage (56). True pro-oxidative effects were not seen in these studies, rather a significant decrease in antioxidant effectiveness. These observations cannot readily be explained unless factors other than the inherent antioxidant properties of these molecules are considered. While carotenoids may have an identical chromophore and very similar electron density profiles (34,35), so that their inherent antioxidant ability is effectively the same, they can behave quite differently once incorporated in a membrane system. It is known not only that these carotenoids influence the properties of membranes into which they are incorporated in a different manner (40) but that their effectiveness against ROS in the aqueous and lipid phases is quite different (34,36; see above). The optimal concentrations of lycopene, lutein, and β-carotene required to protect human fibroblasts against UVB irradiation is very different (44).

At high concentrations or in polar environments, carotenoids exhibit a tendency to aggregate or crystallize out of solution, with different compounds behaving differently depending on their structure, so that some compounds have a greater tendency to aggregate than others (40,41). Cis isomers also have a lower tendency for aggregation compared with their all-trans counterparts (35). Such carotenoid aggregates have been directly observed in membranes, and their presence is thought to have a profound effect on the properties of the membrane itself by leading to an increase in membrane fluidity and permeability, ultimately perhaps, resulting in pro-oxidant-type effects (40). Importantly, the biophysical and electronic properties of aggregates are quite different from that of the monomeric form of the carotenoid in solution (35,40), suggesting differences in their reactivity. There is some preliminary evidence that singlet oxygen quenching by carotenoids may be strongly influenced by their aggregation state (71). For example, in unilamellar dipalmitoylphosphatidylcholine (DPPC) liposomes, zeaxanthin behaves in a very unusual way in that as the concentration of the carotenoid increases its $^1O_2$ quenching properties are progressively lost, possibly due to aggregation of the carotenoid molecules (Fig. 1). This behavior in a model membrane system fits well with the data obtained from some cellular-based studies in which carotenoids have been seen to lose their ability to protect against oxidative damage at high doses (44,67,70).

IV. INTERACTION WITH OTHER DIETARY ANTIOXIDANTS

The potential for the interaction of carotenoids with other antioxidants is discussed in detail in Chapter 3 and only an outline is given here. Truscott (72) first proposed a plausible mechanism for the interaction of vitamins C and E with β-carotene whereby the carotenoid molecule repairs the vitamin E radical [reaction (8)] and the resulting carotenoid cation radical is, in turn, repaired by vitamin C [reactions (9) and (10)]. An additive response has been observed for β-carotene and vitamin E, but a synergistic response was only seen when vitamin C was also present (73). If this model is correct then the reduction in the levels of vitamin C in the plasma of smokers compared with nonsmokers (74) is of significance as the repair of any β-carotene radical cations formed would be impaired. A xanthophyll such as zeaxanthin whose conjugated system spans the membrane (see above) would, in theory, be able to interact much more effectively with both lipid- and water-soluble antioxidants than carotenes such as β-carotene

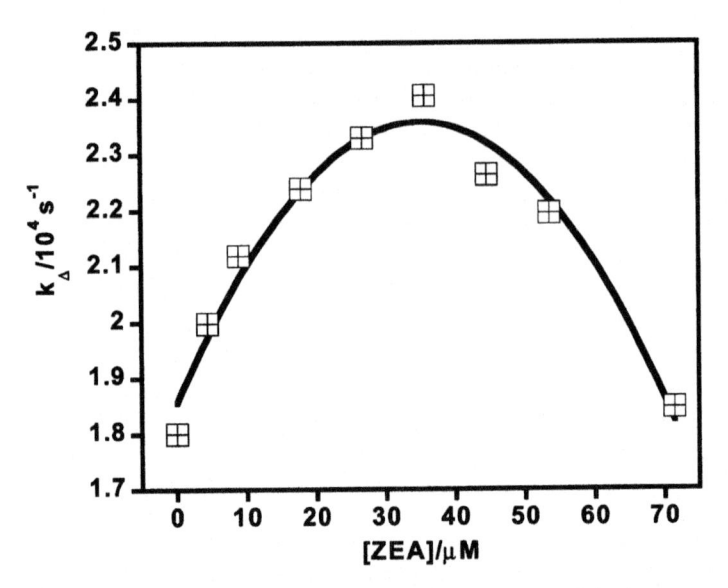

Figure 1 Variation of the rate constant for the decay of singlet oxygen with carotenoid concentration for zeaxanthin in DPPC liposomes (69). At concentrations up to ~45 μM the response is linear with a quenching rate constant of $2.3 \times 10^8 \, M^{-1} \, s^{-1}$. With increasing zeaxanthin concentration the rate progressively decreases and is completely lost at ~70 μM.

and lycopene because the carotene radical cation would first have to migrate from the hydrophobic core to the membrane surface to interact with vitamin C, for example. The relatively long lifetime and polarity of the carotenoid radical cation may permit this (27). Vitamin C has been shown to protect both the carotenoid and vitamin E pools in LDLs from Cu^{2+}-mediated oxidative damage (75). The synergistic protection afforded by carotenoids and other co-antioxidants is dependent on a balance between these components and changes in the concentration of any one of these might disturb this balance, reducing antioxidant effectiveness. An increase in carotenoid content, for example, may result in the formation of carotenoid cation radicals or adducts at a level beyond which the tocopherol/ascorbate pool can effectively repair, resulting in pro-oxidant effects.

$$CAR + TOH^{\bullet +} \longrightarrow TOH + CAR^{\bullet +} \tag{8}$$

$$CAR^{\bullet +} + ASCH_2 \longrightarrow CAR + ASCH^{\bullet} + H^+ \tag{9}$$

$$CAR^{\bullet +} + ASCH^- \longrightarrow CAR + ASCH^{\bullet -} + H^+ \tag{10}$$

Carotenoid–carotenoid interactions have rarely been considered, and the vast majority of studies have focused instead on single compounds in isolation. This belies the natural in vivo state in which a heterogeneous stage of a range of xanthophylls and carotenes coexist. A synergistic response between different carotenoids has been reported (76), with a combination of lutein and lycopene proving to be most effective against 2,2'-azobis(2,4-dimethylvaleronitrile) (AMVN)-induced oxidation in multilamellar liposomes. The potential for electron transfer between different carotenoids [reaction (11)] has been examined (27,37). Lycopene is a strong reducing agent but astaxanthin weak. While lycopene was able to reduce the radical cations of lutein and zeaxanthin, β-carotene could not.

$$CAR1^{\bullet +} + CAR2 \rightarrow CAR1 + CAR2^{\bullet +} \tag{11}$$

V. DO CAROTENOIDS ACT AS ANTIOXIDANTS IN VIVO?

Much of the fundamental information regarding the antioxidant potential of carotenoids with a range of oxidizing species (especially radicals) has been gathered in vitro by challenging individual carotenoids (often simply in organic solvents, simple micelles, or liposomes) with individual ROS or, more rarely, RNS. While these may provide important intrinsic information on the interactions between a carotenoid and an ROS and serve as a guide to potential antioxidant activity, they do not represent the complex in vivo situation. In vivo, the carotenoid content and composition of the vast majority (if not all) tissues are heterogeneous. Physiologically, carotenoids are present in lower concentrations than typically used in vitro (35), and rather than being free in solution they are generally associated with some form of lipoprotein complex or incorporated into biological membranes. All too often, great claims are made with regard to the antioxidant activity of one carotenoid being "x times better" than another (usually β-carotene) purely on the basis of very limited studies (often in one solvent) against one ROS without due consideration for the possible in vivo behavior (e.g., limitations in uptake, differences in tissue and cellular distribution, etc.). Similarly, more antioxidant is often regarded as better. As has been discussed above for both in vitro studies (34,36,44,67,70,71) and indeed in the intervention studies (13–15) this may be a rather naive approach.

Although carotenoid interactions have readily been demonstrated in organic solutions, it is much more difficult to demonstrate such interactions in vivo. Many intervention trials performed using carotenoids depend on an end point, namely, the protection against a given condition or the reduction of a specific biomarker for free radical challenge. The outcomes of such trials will not determine if the effect is simply due to the antioxidant action of the carotenoid being assessed or its synergystic action with other dietary components to diminish oxidant stress. If a reduction in a selected biomarker is sought, then the chosen marker must be unique and its reduction cannot be explained by other means. The source of carotenoids used in such studies is important. Lycopene, for example, can be administered as tomato juice, cooked or raw tomatoes, or tomato oleoresin capsules (Table 3), and while the carotenoid may be present in a very high proportion in these preparations, so can other dietary components such as folate, ascorbate, or polyphenols. These constituents may also act to reduce the selected biomarker making interpretation of data difficult. Other dietary components will also have to be closely monitored and accounted for before an association between carotenoids and antioxidant activity in vivo can be confirmed. One important biomarker for oxidative stress and potentially cancer development is 8-hydroxydeoxyguanosine (8OHdG) (77,78). Several carotenoid studies (Table 3) have used this particular biomarker (in either urine or lymphocytes) to indicate a diminution in oxidative stress. In most cases the introduction of antioxidants (e.g., dietary sources of carotenoids) decreases the amount of 8OHdG present in DNA or urine (86–89), suggesting that the consumption of fruit and vegetables largely results in a significant reduction in markers of oxidative cellular damage to DNA and lipids. However, the interpretation of changes in the levels of markers such as 8OHdG in urine is fraught with difficulties (90), although it is likely to be largely unaffected by diet and the biomarker is also not further metabolized in humans. In particular, 8OHdG excretion rates are not a quantitative index of damage to guanine residues in DNA, and the estimation of 8OHdG in tissues or cells may be of much greater benefit (depending on which tissue is selected and the method of DNA extraction and analysis employed; 90). The actual proof that carotenoids can act as effective antioxidants in vivo has not been presented. Some care must be taken when interpreting results obtained in studies with rodents because in these animals supraphysiological levels of supplementation are required because of poor carotenoid absorption. This may promote pro-oxidant effects if a high-dose supplement is given in situations where there is a preexisting oxidative stress (88,89; see above). The studies that have examined the effect of carotenoids on humans have often suffered from having a limited number of participants, which again makes it difficult to draw conclusions from the results. However, the study of Chen et al. (85) on the effects of lycopene supplementation on oxidative damage in serum and prostate tissue of patients suffering from prostate cancer did have encouraging results. Similarly, decreased consumption of carotenoids, vitamin E, and vitamin C are associated with increased DNA strand breaks, chromosomal breaks, and oxidative base lesions (94).

If studies are to be interpreted correctly, then we must also ensure that any in vitro experiments reflect as far as possible the in vivo state. For example, while human plasma contains mainly the all-*trans* forms of common dietary carotenoids (predominantly reflecting the form in most foods), isomers of a number of

Table 3 Examples of Recent Trials Involving Carotenoid Supplementation Using the Assessment of Specific Biomarkers as an End Point for Oxidative Damage

Carotenoid source	System	Sample size	Marker used	Detection method	Ref.
Fruit and vegetables	Human	28	DNA damage and lipid peroxidation	HPLC ELISA	79
Tomato juice	Human	10	DNA damage	Comet assay	80
Tomato puree	Human	11	Antioxidant capacity	TRAP	81
Tomato ketchup and Lyc-O-Mato	Human	12	Lipid peroxidation and protein oxidation	TBARS and DTNB	82
Tomato products	Human	32	DNA damage	HPLC	83
Lycopene	Hamster	24	Lipid peroxidation	TBARS	84
Paprika and β-carotene	Rat	45	MDA and other metabolites of lipid peroxidation	HPLC	85

carotenoids (e.g., 5-*cis*-lycopene; 93) have been identified. *Cis* isomers may account for a significant proportion of the pool of carotenoid stored in tissues. For example, up to 20% of the carotenoid pools of the human liver, kidneys, adrenals, and testes were composed of 9-*cis*, 13-*cis*, and 15-*cis* isomers of β-carotene (6). The presence of such *cis* isomers raises many questions, particularly, in the context of this chapter, whether they have a physiological role in preventing or possibly even promoting oxidation. The properties, particularly in relation to their antioxidant activity, are poorly understood. It also means that the effect of the environment of the carotenoid (and indeed the ROS) is also taken into account. For example, the interaction of β-carotene with tocopherol radical is greatly affected by the polarity of the solvent used. While TOH$^{\bullet}$ is readily converted to TOH by β-carotene in a nonpolar environment, this radical is deprotonated to TO$^{\bullet}$ in a polar environment and does not react with carotenoids (27).

VI. CONCLUSIONS

The function of dietary carotenoids and of their metabolites in the human body is clearly dependent on a wide range of factors other than the basic chemical properties of these molecules per se. While in vitro studies provide an insight into these properties and into the interactions of carotenoids with ROS and co-antioxidants, it is dangerous to extrapolate the results from such studies too far as the scenario within the body is highly complex. There is no evidence to support the hypothesis that carotenoids may act as pro-oxidants within a biological system (i.e., at physiological relevant pO_2 values). What is more probable is that a number of factors may serve to moderate the antioxidant abilities of carotenoids in vivo. One neglected area of research currently is the potential that carotenoids may have concerning the induction of cell signaling to alter the antioxidant properties of the cell. Future studies that use gene arrays and proteomics may determine if this is another mechanism by which carotenoids may diminish oxidative stress. The proof that carotenoids can act as antioxidants in vivo remains elusive, as indeed it does for a number of other antioxidants.

REFERENCES

1. Halliwell B, Gutteridge JMC. Free Radicals in Biology and Medicine, 3rd ed. Oxford: Oxford University Press, 1999.
2. Pfander H. Key to Carotenoids. Basel: Birkhäuser Verlag, 1987.
3. Paiva SAR, Russell RM. β-Carotene and other carotenoids as antioxidants. J Am Coll Nutr 1999; 18:426–433.

4. Khachik F, Spangler CJ, Smith JC, Canfield LM, Steck A, Pfander H. Identification, quantification, and relative concentrations of carotenoids and their metabolites in human milk and serum. Anal Chem 1997; 69:1873–1881.

5. Khachik F, Pfander H, Traber B. Proposed mechanisms for the formation of synthetic and naturally occurring metabolites of lycopene in tomato products and human serum. J Agric Food Chem 1998; 46:4885–4890.

6. Schweigert FJ. Metabolism of carotenoids in mammals. In: Britton G, Liaaen-Jensen S, Pfander H, eds. Carotenoids, Vol 3, Biosynthesis. Basel: Birkhäuser Verlag, 1998: 249–284.

7. Stahl W, Von Laar J, Martin HD, Emmerich T, Sies H. Stimulation of gap junctional communication: comparison of acyclo-retinoic acid and lycopene. Arch Biochem Biophys 2000; 373:271–274.

8. Handleman GJ, van Kuijk FJ, Chatterjee A, Krinsky NI. Characterization of products formed during the autoxidation of β-carotene. Free Radic Biol Med 1991; 10:427–437.

9. Liebler DC, Kennedy TA. Epoxide products of β-carotene antioxidant reactions. Meth Enzymol 1992; 213:472–479.

10. King TJ, Khachik F, Bortkiewicz H, Fukushima LH, Morioka S, Bertram JS. Metabolites of dietary carotenoids as potential cancer preventive agents. Pure Appl Chem 1997; 69:2135–2140.

11. Ziegler RG, Mayne ST, Swanson CA. Nutrition and lung cancer. Cancer Causes Control 1996; 7:157–177.

12. Peto R, Doll R, Buckley JD, Sporn MB. Can dietary beta-carotene materially reduce human cancer rates? Nature 1981; 290:201–208.

13. Omenn GS, Goodman GE, Thornquist MD, Balmes J, Cullen MR, Glass A, Keogh JP, Meyskens FL, Valanis B, Williams JH, Barnhart S, Hammar S. Effects of a combination of beta-carotene and vitamin A on lung cancer and cardiovascular disease. N Engl J Med 1996; 334:1150–1155.

14. The Alpha-Tocopherol, Beta Carotene Cancer Prevention Study Group. The effects of vitamin E and beta carotene on the incidence of lung cancer and other cancers in male smokers. N Engl J Med 1994; 330:1029–1035.

15. Albanes D, Heinonen OP, Taylor PR, Virtamo J, Edwards BK, Rautalahti M, Hartman AM, Palmgren J, Freedman LS, Haapakoski J, Barrett MJ, Pietinen P, Malila N, Tala E, Liippo K, Salomaa ER, Tangrea JA, Teppo L, Askin FB, Taskinen E, Erozan Y, Greenwald P, Huttunen JK. A-tocopherol and β-carotene supplements and lung cancer incidence in the alpha-tocopherol, beta-carotene cancer prevention study: effects of baseline characteristics and study compliance. J Natl Cancer Inst 1996; 88:1560–1570.

16. Mayne ST, Handelman GJ, Beecher G. β-carotene and lung cancer promotion in heavy smokers—a plausible relationship? J Natl Cancer Inst 1996; 88:1513–1515.

17. Mayne ST. Beta-carotene, carotenoids, and disease prevention in humans. FASEB J 1996; 10:690–701.

18. Wang X-D, Russell RM. Procarcinogenic and anticarcinogenic effects of β-carotene. Nutr Rev 1999; 57:263–272.

19. Conn PF, Schalch W, Truscott TG. The singlet oxygen and β-carotene interaction. J Photochem Photobiol B Biol 1991; 11:41–47.

20. DiMascio P, Kaiser S, Sies H. Lycopene as the most efficient biological carotenoid singlet oxygen quencher. Arch Biochem Biophys 1989; 274:532–538.

21. Burton GW, Ingold KU. β-Carotene: an unusual type of lipid anti-oxidant. Science 1984; 224:569–573.

22. Hill TJ, Land EJ, McGarvey DJ, Schalch W, Tinkler JH, Truscott TG. Interactions between carotenoids and the $CCl_3O_2^{\cdot}$ radical. J Am Chem Soc 1995; 117:8322–8326.

23. Everett SA, Dennis MF, Patel KB, Maddix S, Kundu SC, Willson RL. Scavenging of nitrogen dioxide, thiyl, and sulfonyl free radicals by the nutritional anti-oxidant β-carotene. J Biol Chem 1996; 271:3988–3994.

24. Mortensen A Skibsted LH. Kinetics of parallel electron transfer from β-carotene to phenoxyyl radical and adduct formation between phenoxyl radical and β-carotene. Free Radic Res 1996; 25:515–523.

25. Christensen RL. The electronic states of carotenoids. In: Frank HA, Young AJ, Britton G, Cogdell RJ, eds. The Photochemistry of Carotenoids. Dordrecht: Kluwer Academic, 1999:137–157.

26. Marston G, Truscott TG, Wayne RP. Phosphorescence of beta-carotene. J Chem Soc Faraday Trans 1995; 91:4059–4061.

27. Edge R, Truscott TG. Carotenoid radicals and the interaction of carotenoids with active oxygen species. In: Frank HA, Young AJ, Britton G, Cogdell RJ, eds. The Photochemistry of Carotenoids. Dordrecht: Kluwer Academic, 1999:223–234.

28. Foote CS, Denny RW. Chemistry of singlet oxygen. VIII quenching by β-carotene. J Am Chem Soc 1968; 90:6233–6235.

29. Wilkinson F, Ho WT. Electronic energy transfer from singlet molecular oxygen to carotenoids. Spectrosc Lett 1978; 11:425–436.

30. Baltschun D, Beutner S, Briviba K, Martin H-D, Paust J, Peters M, Röver S, Sies H, Stahl W, Steigel A. Stenhorst F. Liebigs Ann-Recueil 1997; 9:1887–1893.

31. Mathews-Roth MM. Carotenoids in erthyropoeitic protoporphyria and other photosensitivity disease. Ann NY Acad Sci 1993; 691:127–138.

32. Mathews-Roth MM. Carotenoids and photoprotection. Photochem Photobiol 1997; 65S:148–151.

33. Mortensen A, Skibsted LH, Sampson J, Rice-Evans C, Everett SA. Comparative mechanisms and rates of free radical scavenging by carotenoid antioxidants. FEBS Lett 1997; 418:91–94.

34. Woodall AA, Britton G, Jackson MJ. Carotenoids and protection of phospholipids in solution or in liposomes against oxidation by peroxyl radicals: relationship between carotenoid structure and protective ability. Biochim Biophys Acta 1997; 1336:575–586.

35. Britton G. Structure and properties of carotenoids in relation to function. FASEB J 1995; 9:1551–1558.

36. Woodall AA, Lee SW, Weesie RJ, Jackson MJ, Britton G. Oxidation of carotenoids by free radicals: relationship between structure and reactivity. Biochim Biophys Acta 1997; 1336:33–42.

37. Edge R, Land EJ, McGarvey D, Mulroy L, Truscott TG. Relative one-electron reduction of potentials of carotenoids radical cations and the interactions of carotenoids with the vitamin E radical cation. J Am Chem Soc 1998; 120:4087–4090.

38. Rice-Evans CA, Sampson J, Bramley PM, Holloway DE. Why do we expect carotenoids to be antioxidants in vivo? Free Radic Res 1997; 26:381–398.
39. Martin HD, Ruck C, Schmidt M, Sell, S, Beutner S, Mayer B, Walsh R. Chemistry of carotenoid oxidation and free radical reactions. Pure Appl Chem 1999; 71:2253–2262.
40. Gruszecki WI. (1999) Carotenoids in membranes. In: Frank HA, Young AJ, Britton G, Cogdell RJ, eds. The Photochemistry of Carotenoids. Dordrecht: Kluwer Academic, 1999:363–379.
41. Ruban AV, Horton P, Young AJ. Aggregation of higher plant xanthophylls: differences in absorption spectra and in dependency on solvent polarity. J Photobiol Photobiochem B 1993; 21:229–234.
42. Panasenko OM, Sharov VS, Briviba K, Sies H. Interaction of peroxynitrite with carotenoids in human low density lipoproteins. Arch Biochem Biophys 2000; 373:302–305.
43. Palozza P. Prooxidant actions of carotenoids in biological systems. Nutr Rev 1998; 56:257–265.
44. Eichler O, Sies H, Stahl W. Divergent optimum levels of lycopene, β-carotene and lutein protecting against UVB irradiation in human fibroblasts. Photochem Photobiol 2002, 75:503–508.
45. Airley RE, Lancaster J, Raleigh JA, Harris Al, Davidson SE, Hunter RD, West CM, Stratford IJ. GLUT-1 and CAIX as intrinsic markers of hypoxia in carcinoma of the cervix: relationship to pimonidazole binding. Int J Cancer 2003; 104:85–91.
46. Palozza P, Krinsky NI. Astaxanthin and canthaxanthin are potent antioxidants in a membrane model. Arch Biochem Biophys 1992; 297:184–187.
47. El-Tinay AH, Chichester CO. Oxidation of β-carotene. Site of attack. J Org Chem 1970; 35:2290–2293.
48. Kennedy TA, Liebler DC. Peroxyl radical oxidation of beta-carotene: formation of beta-carotene epoxides. Chem Res Toxicol 1991; 4:290–295.
49. Caris-Veyrat C, Amiot M-J, Ramasseul R, Marchon J-C. Mild oxidative cleavage of β,β-carotene by dioxygen induced by a ruthenium porphyrin catalyst: characterization of products and of some possible intermediates. N J Chem 2001; 25: 203–206.
50. Ohtake T, Yokota T, Etoh H, Oshima S, Inakuma T, Terao J. Reaction of lycopene with peroxynitrite. Carotenoid Sci 2002; 5:15–16.
51. Salgo MG, Cueto R, Winston GQ, Pryor WA. Beta-carotene and its oxidation products have different effects on microsome-mediated binding of benzo[a]pyrene to DNA. Free Radic Biol Med 1999; 26:162–173.
52. Koyama Y, Fujii R. Cis-trans carotenoids in photosynthesis: configurations, excited-state properties and physiological functions. In: Frank HA, Young AJ, Britton G, Cogdell RJ, eds. The Photochemistry of Carotenoids. Dordrecht: Kluwer Academic, 1999:161–188.
53. Wang X-D, Liu C, Bronsen RT, Smith DE, Krinsky NI, Russell M. Retinoid signalling and activator protein-1 expression in ferrets given β-carotene supplements and exposed to tobacco smoke. J Natl Cancer Inst 1999; 91:60–66.

54. Baker DL, Krol ES, Jacobsen N, Liebler DC. Reactions of β-carotene with cigarette smoke oxidants. Identification of carotenoid oxidation products and evaluation of the prooxidant/antioxidant effect. Chem Res Toxicol 1999; 12:535–543.

55. Alam SQ, Alam BS. Lipid peroxide, alpha-tocopherol and retinoid levels in plasma and liver of rats fed diets containing beta-carotene and 13-cis-retinoic acid. J Nutr 1983; 113:2608–2614.

56. Young AJ, Lowe G. Antioxidant and prooxidnat properties of carotenoids. Arch Biochem Biophys 2001; 385:20–27.

57. Mortensen A, Skibsted LH. Importance of carotenoid structure in radical-scavenging reactions. J Agric Food Chem 1997; 45:2970–2977.

58. Mortensen A, Skibsted LH. Kinetics of photobleaching of β-carotene in chloroform and formation of transient carotenoid species absorbing in the near infrared. Free Radic Res 1996; 25:355–368.

59. Mortensen A. Mechanisms and kinetics of scavenging of the phenylthiyl radical by carotenoids. A laser flash photolysis study. Asian Chem Lett 2000; 4:135–143.

60. Mortensen A. Scavenging of acetylperoxyl radicals and quenching of triplet diacetyl by beta-carotene: mechanisms and kinetics. J Photochem Photobiol B: Biol 2001; 61:62–67.

61. Mortensen A. Scavenging of benzylperoxyl radicals by carotenoids. Free Radic Res 2002; 36:211–216.

62. Mortensen A, Skibsted LH. Free radical transients in photobleaching of xanthophylls and carotenes. Free Radic Res 1997; 26:549–563.

63. van de Ven M, Kattenberg M, van Ginkel G, Levine YK. Study of the orinetational ordering of carotenoids in lipid bilayers by resonance-Raman spectroscopy. Biophys J 1984; 45:1203–1209.

64. Johansson LB-A, Lindblom G, Wieslander A, Arvidson G. Orientation of β-carotene and retinal in lipid bilayers. FEBS Lett 1981; 128:97–99.

65. Subczynski WK, Markowska E, Sielewiesiuk J. Effect of polar carotenoids on the oxygen diffusion-concentration product in lipid bilayers. Biochim Biophys Acta 1991; 1068:68–72.

66. Palozza P, Luberto C, Ricci P, Sgarlata E, Calviello G, Bartoli GM. Effect of β-carotene and canthaxanthin on tert-butyl hydroperoxide-induced lipid peroxidation in murine normal and tumor thymocytes. Arch Biochem Biophys 1996; 325:145–151.

67. Woods JA, Young AJ, Bilton RF. Measurement of menadione-mediated DNA damage in human lymphocytes using the comet assay. FEBS Lett 1999; 449:255–258.

68. Church DF, Pryor WA. Free-radical chemistry of cigarette smoke and its toxicological implications. Environ Health Perspect 1985; 64:111–126.

69. Rom WN, Bitterman PB, Rennard SI, Cantin A, Crystal RG. Characterization of the lower respiratory-tract inflammation of nonsmoking individuals with interstitial lung disease associated with chronic inhalation of inorganic dusts. Am Rev Respir Dis 1987; 136:1429–1434.

70. Lowe GM, Booth LA, Bilton RF, Young AJ. Lycopene and β-carotene protect against oxidative damage in HT29 cells at low concentrations but rapidly lose this capacity at high doses. Free Radic Res 1999; 30:141–151.

71. Cantrell A, McGarvey DJ, Truscott TG, Rancan F, Böhm F. Singlet oxygen quenching by dietary carotenoids in a model membrane environment. Arch Biochem Biophys 2003; 412:47–54.

72. Truscott TG. β-Carotene and disease: a suggested pro-oxidant and anti-oxidant mechanism and speculations concerning its role in cigarette smoking. J Photochem Photobiol B 1996; 35:233–235.

73. Böhm F, Edge R, McGarvey DJ, Truscott TG. β-Carotene with vitamins E and C offer synergistic cell protection against NO_x. FEBS Lett 1998; 436:387–389.

74. Schectman GM, Byrd JC, Gruchow HW. Am J Public Health 1989; 79:158–162.

75. Jialal J, Grundy SM. Preservation of the endogenous antioxidants in low-density-lipoprotein by ascorbate but not probucol during oxidative modification. J Clin Invest 1991; 87:597–601.

76. Stahl W, Junghans A, de Boer B, Driomina ES, Briviba K, Sies H. Carotenoid mixtures protect multilamellar liposomes against oxidative damage: synergistic effects of lycopene and lutein. FEBS Lett 1998; 427:305–308.

77. Kuchino Y, Mori F, Kasai H, Inoue H, Iwai S, Mirura K, Ohtsuka E, Nishimura S. Misreading of DNA templates containing 8-hydroxydeoxyguanosine at the modified base and at adjacent residues. Nature 1987; 327: 77–79.

78. Cheng KC, Cahill DS, Kasai H, Nishimura S, Loeb LA. 8-Hydroxyguanosine, an abundant form of oxidative DNA damage, causes G...T and A...C substitutions. J Biol Chem 1992; 267:16–172.

79. Thompson HJ, Heimendinger J, Haegele A, Sedlacek SM, Gillette C, O'Neill C, Wolfe P, Conry C. Effect of increased vegetable and fruit consumption on markers of oxidative cellular damage. Carcinogenesis 1999; 20:2261–2266.

80. Riso P, Pinder A, Santangelo A, Porrini M. Does tomato consumption effectively increase the resistance of lymphocyte DNA to oxidative damage? Am J Clin Nutr 1999; 69:712.

81. Pellegrini N, Riso P, Porrini, M. Tomato consumption does not affect the total anti-oxidant capacity of plasma. Nutrition 2000; 16:268–271.

82. Rao Av, Shen H. Effect of low dose lycopene intake on lycopene bioavailability and oxidant stress. Nutr Res 2002; 22:1125–1131.

83. Chen L, Stacewicz-Sapuntzakis M, Duncan C, Sharifa R, Ghosh, van Breemen R, Ashton D, Bowen PE. Oxidative DNA damage in prostate cancer patients consuming tomato based entrees as a whole-food intervention. J Natl Cancer Inst 2001; 93:1872–1879.

84. Bhuvaneswari V, Velmurugen B, Nagini S. Lycopene modulates circulatory anti-oxidants during hamster buccal pouch carcinogenesis. Nutr Res 2001; 21:1447–1453.

85. Seppanen CM, Csallany AS. The effect of paprika carotenoids on in vivo lipid peroxidation measured by urinary excretion of secondary oxidation products. Nutr Res 2002; 22:1055–1065.

86. Baskin CR, Hinchcliff KW, DiSilvestro RA, Reinhart GA, Hayek MG, Chew BP, Burr JR. Effects of dietary antioxidant supplementation on oxidative damage and resistance to oxidative damage during prolonged exercise in sled dogs. Am J Vet Res 2000; 61:886–891.

87. Porrini M, Riso P, Oriani G. Spinach and tomato consumption increases lymphocyte DNA resistance to oxidative stress but this is not related to cell carotenoid concentrations. Eur J Nutr 2002; 41:95–100.

88. Porrini M, Riso P. Lymphocyte lycopene concentration and DNA protection from oxidative damage is increased in women after a short period of tomato consumption. J Nutr 2000; 130:189–192.

89. van den Berg R, van Vliet T, Broekmans WM, Cnubben NH, Vaes WH, Roza L, Haenen GR, Bast A, van den Berg H. A vegetable/fruit concentrate with high antioxidant capacity has no effect on biomarkers of antioxidant status in male smokers. J Nutr 2001; 131:1714–1722.

90. Halliwell B. Effect of diet on cancer development: is oxidative DNA damage a biomarker? Free Radic Biol Med 2002; 32:968–974.

91. Rahman I, MacNee W. Role of oxidants/antioxidants in smoking-induced lung diseases. Free Radic Biol Med 1996; 21:669–681.

92. Leo, MA, Aleynik MK., Lieber CS. β-Carotene beadlets potentiate hepatotoxicity of alcohol. Am J Clin Nutr 1997; 66:1461–1469.

93. Stahl W, Schwarz W, Sundquist AR, Sies H. Cis-trans isomers of lycopene and beta-carotene in human serum and tissues. Arch Biochem Biophys 1992; 294:173–177.

94. French M. Micronutrients and genomic stability: a new paradigm for recommended dietary allowances (RDAs). Food Chem Toxicol 2002; 40:1113–1117.

6

Evidence for Pro-Oxidant Effects of Carotenoids In Vitro and In Vivo: Implications in Health and Disease

Paola Palozza
Catholic University, Rome, Italy

I. INTRODUCTION

Evidence has accumulated from many prospective as well as retrospective epidemiological studies that individuals eating more fruits and vegetables rich in carotenoids (1), or having higher blood concentrations of carotenoids (2), decrease their risk for developing cancer, especially lung cancer. In contrast, the role of carotenoids in the prevention of cancer has been brought into question by the results of several intervention trials. These studies not only failed to detect any protective effect of β-carotene or of a combination of β-carotene and vitamin A on the incidence of diverse cancers, but two of them [the β-Carotene and Retinol Efficacy Trial (CARET; 3) and the Alpha-Tocopherol, Beta-Carotene Cancer Prevention Study (ATBC, 4)] even show that these compounds can increase the incidence of lung cancer. Although these unexpectedly adverse effects have been obtained in populations at risk for lung cancer (smokers, ex-smokers, or asbestos workers) and the supplemented β-carotene has been given at a stage where the cancers were most likely already in the later phase (progression), there is concern that most of the clinical trials giving β-carotene as a supplement have been stopped. A great deal of emphasis has been given to the understanding of the mechanism(s) of action by which carotenoids may modulate physiological functions and influence the progression of chronic diseases, inducing beneficial or adverse health effects. A possible mechanism that can explain the dual role of carotenoid molecules as both beneficial and harmful agents in cancer as well as in other chronic diseases is their ability to modulate intracellular redox status.

Carotenoid molecules may serve as antioxidants (5–7), inhibiting free radical production, or as pro-oxidants (8–10), propagating free radical–induced reactions, depending on their intrinsic properties as well as on the redox potential of the biological environment in which they act. In other words, these compounds may behave as reactants in a continuity of electron-donating and accepting agents commonly found in cells (11). In this context, their antioxidant function may not be inherently good, and their pro-oxidant activity may not necessarily be bad. This review summarizes the available evidence for a pro-oxidant activity of carotenoids in vitro and in vivo. In particular, it focuses on (a) the main factors influencing the pro-oxidant activity of carotenoids, (b) the biological and molecular targets evidencing such an activity, and (c) the possible implications of carotenoid oxidative functions in health and disease.

II. FACTORS INVOLVED IN THE PRO-OXIDANT ACTIVITY OF CAROTENOIDS

Increasing evidence suggests that the antioxidant activity of carotenoids may shift into a pro-oxidant one in biological models, depending on several factors. Some of them have been recently reviewed (8–10) and are summarized in Table 1. As Burton and Ingold suggested (12), carotenoids do not have the structural features commonly associated with chain-breaking antioxidants. The extensive system of conjugated double bonds may impart a pro-oxidant character to the carotenoid molecule and may make it very susceptible to attack by free radical species. It is known that carotenoids may interact with free radicals in three main ways; electron transfer (reaction A), hydrogen abstraction (reaction B), and addition of a radical species (reaction C) (13–15).

$$ROO^{\bullet} + CAR \longrightarrow ROO^{-} + CAR^{\bullet +} \qquad \text{(reaction A)}$$
$$ROO^{\bullet} + CAR \longrightarrow ROOH + CAR^{\bullet} \qquad \text{(reaction B)}$$
$$ROO^{\bullet} + CAR \longrightarrow (ROO\text{-}CAR)^{\bullet} \qquad \text{(reaction C)}$$

Table 1 Factors Involved in the Pro-Oxidant Activity of Carotenoids

A. Intrinsic Factors
  Carotenoid structure
  Carotenoid concentration
  Carotenoid location in cell membranes

B. Extrinsic Factors
  Oxygen tension
  Cell redox status
  Interactions with redox agents (antioxidants/pro-oxidants)

Once produced, the fate of such carotenoid radicals is of interest. The carotenoid radical cation $(CAR^{\cdot+})$ itself is unreactive and decays slowly by second-order kinetics to unknown products, which do not significantly interact with oxygen and which do not continue the chain reaction, as suggested by Truscott (14). However, since such a radical is rather long lived, it could migrate to a site where damaging consequences arise unless a mechanism is available for its removal (14). A recent finding suggests that it can be efficiently repaired by cell antioxidants, such as vitamin C. On the other hand, the carotene radicals $(CAR^{\cdot}$ and $ROO\text{-}CAR^{\cdot})$ may act as pro-oxidants and undergo oxidation, especially under elevated oxygen partial pressures (16). While at low po_2, the $CAR^{\cdot+}$ is mainly formed and carotenoids act as chain-breaking antioxidants, consuming peroxyl radicals (8,17), whereas at high po_2, the carotenoid radicals are hypothesized to react with oxygen to produce carotenoid peroxyl radicals, which are capable of acting as pro-oxidants (12). It has also been suggested that carotenoid oxygenated products may have pro-oxidant activity and may lead to further oxidation of carotenoid molecules (15). Although a number of oxidation products of carotenoids may be produced by the interaction of carotenoids with oxidants (18–21), including tobacco smoke (22,23), their functional significance is under active investigation. The chemical structure of many of these products (i.e., epoxides and apocarotenals) suggests that they would be unstable under oxidative conditions, further contributing to oxidation.

A common finding from in vitro studies is that the pro-oxidant activity of carotenoids is mainly observed when these compounds are used at high concentrations. For instance, it has been demonstrated that in various tumor cells, β-carotene acts as an antioxidant, inhibiting free radical production at low concentrations whereas at high concentrations it acts as a pro-oxidant, increasing such production (24–26). Again, the ability of β-carotene and lycopene in protecting HT29 adenocarcinoma cells from oxidative DNA damage induced by H_2O_2 or xanthine/xanthine oxidase is observed only at low doses (1–2 μM). This protective effect is progressively lost when their doses are increased, so that at the highest concentration tested (10 μM), the carotenoids afford no protection (27). According to these findings, relatively high doses of β-carotene fail to protect HepG2 cells from oxidative DNA damage induced by H_2O_2 (28). How can the concentration affect the redox properties of carotenoids? A high carotenoid concentration might induce a more favorable formation of oxidative carotenoid products and/or a faster rate of carotenoid autoxidation in the presence of free radical species (8). According to this hypothesis, elevated levels of carotenoid oxidative products have been observed in the lung tissues from smoke-exposed ferrets (22). Moreover, it is also possible that a high carotenoid concentration affects cell membrane permeability, increasing the formation of aggregates between carotenoids and other compounds in biological membranes. These aggregates have been found to deeply increase membrane permeability and fluidity, ultimately resulting in prooxidant-type effects (9).

Interestingly, some xanthophylls, such as zeaxanthin, act as antioxidants in protecting cells from oxidative DNA damage, never showing pro-oxidant effects (9). It is possible that cell location as well as orientation of carotenoids within the membrane lipid bilayer may deeply affect carotenoid redox ability. It is well known that while β-carotene and other carotenes, such as lycopene, lie parallel to the membrane face, zeaxanthin and other xanthophylls entirely span the membrane, permitting reactions with the conjugated double-bond system throughout the depth of the membrane (29).

Increasing evidence supports the hypothesis that cell redox status, as well as combinations of antioxidant nutrients, may deeply influence the pro-oxidant character of carotenoids. In recent studies, it has been reported that the pro-oxidant effects of β-carotene are much more pronounced in tumor cells than in normal cells (30) and in undifferentiated then in differentiated leukemic HL-60 cells (25). It is well known that tumor transformation as well as anaplasia deeply impairs the antioxidant status of these cells, rendering them much more susceptible to oxidative stress (31). Moreover, the reduced levels of vitamin C in the plasma of smokers (32) may be a condition of chronic oxidative stress responsible for an enhancement of carotenoid pro-oxidant character. Therefore, the concomitant presence of other antioxidant supplements can be extremely important in limiting carotenoid pro-oxidant effects. According to this hypothesis, numerous studies show that the antioxidant potency of carotenoids is increased by combined addition of other antioxidants (5,6). For instance, it has been demonstrated that β-carotene operates synergistically with α-tocopherol (33) and other antioxidant nutrients (34,35) to provide an effective barrier against oxidation. However, it should be considered that in vivo the synergistic protection afforded by carotenoids and other co-antioxidant nutrients may be dependent on a balance among all these components. An increase in carotenoid concentration may modify the uptake and the subsequent tissue distribution of co-antioxidants, resulting in changes of intracellular redox status, as discussed below.

III. MARKERS OF THE PRO-OXIDANT ACTIVITY OF CAROTENOIDS

One key approach to assess a role for carotenoids as pro-oxidants is the identification of relevant markers of oxidative stress, which can detect potential risks or benefits following carotenoid treatment.

Several markers have been used to assess the pro-oxidant activity of carotenoids in biological systems (Table 2). They include: (a) the increased

Table 2 Markers of the Pro-Oxidant Activity of Carotenoids

---

1. Increased production of bioactive free radical species
2. Changes in cell antioxidant status
   Nonenzymatic antioxidants
      Tocopherols
      Ascorbic acid
      Glutathione
   Enzymatic antioxidants
      Superoxide dismutase
      Catalase
      Glutathione peroxidase
3. Oxidative damage to specific targets
   DNA oxidation
   Lipid oxidation
   Protein oxidation
4. Modulation of redox-sensitive genes
   Genes invoved in cell growth
   Genes involved in detoxification processes
5. Modulation of redox-sensitive transcription factors

---

production of bioactive free radical species; (b) the modulation of cell antioxidant defences; (c) the oxidative damage to specific cell targets, such as DNA, lipids, and proteins; (d) the changes in the expression of redox-sensitive genes and/or genes involved in the maintenance of intracellular redox status; and (e) the modulation of redox-sensitive transcription factors.

A. Increased Production of Bioactive Free Radical Species

In the human body, a range of free radical species are produced, including $^1O_2$, $OH^{\cdot}$, $O_2^{\cdot-}$, and H_2O_2 and many organic products (36). While in the past carotenoids have been exclusively considered for their ability in inhibiting the formation of free radicals (5–7), at the moment they have also been suggested to enhance the formation of these species, under certain conditions. A direct generation of free radical species by β-carotene has been reported in several cultured tumor cells (24,25,37). In these studies, reactive oxygen species (ROS) production is measured by different fluorescent probes, such as dichlorofluorescein diacetate (DCF-DA) and/or dihydrorhodamine (DHR), able to detect ROS produced in whole cytoplasm or mitochondria, respectively. Interestingly, carotenoids may induce enhanced ROS levels at very different concentrations, depending on cell types. Some human colon adenocarcinoma cells (LS-174) show an increase in ROS production at a β-carotene concentration of 2.5 μM (37), whereas others (WiDr) exhibit this effect only at a very high concentration of the carotenoid (50 μM) (24,37). This difference has been related to cell capability in incorporating the carotenoid (38). Moreover, the degree of cell differentiation seems to deeply influence the ability of β-carotene in inducing ROS production. Concerning this, β-carotene is a much more potent inducer of ROS in undifferentiated than in differentiated human leukemic (HL-60) cells (25).

It is still under investigation how carotenoid molecules induce an overproduction of ROS. Several mechanisms have been proposed. These include processes of autoxidation of carotenoid metabolites, alterations in iron levels and in the activity of cytochrome P450 enzymes, and changes in cell antioxidant defenses. In a recent study, it has been also reported that the autoxidation of retinoids leads to the generation of $O_2^{\bullet-}$, as measured by cytochrome c reduction method, in cultured HL-60 and HP100 cells (39). In particular, retinol and retinal, both β-carotene metabolites, show a stronger ability to generate $O_2^{\bullet-}$ than β-carotene itself. This ability is strictly related to the induction of oxidative DNA damage, measured as 8-oxo-dG formation.

Carotenoids have been reported to increase iron levels in animal (40) as well as in human (41) studies. It is well known that iron is able to increase the production of endogenous free radical species through Fenton reactions (42). In addition, it is involved in the transcriptional regulation of antioxidant enzymes (43).

Moreover, it has been demonstrated that β-carotene may act as an endogenous generator of ROS through its ability to induce various P450 isoforms (44).

On the other hand, an increased ROS production by carotenoids may be merely due to an impairment of cell antioxidant status, as described below.

B. Changes in Cell Antioxidant Status

Carotenoids have been reported to affect cell antioxidant status by altering hydrophilic and lipophilic antioxidant absorption and content and by modulating activity and/or gene expression of antioxidant enzymes. Therefore, the measurement of cell antioxidant status may be a necessary and helpful tool in order to reveal pro-oxidant effects by carotenoid molecules in biological systems.

1. Nonenzymatic Antioxidants

Tocopherols.   Several lines of evidence suggest that carotenoids may influence the status of tocopherols both in vitro and in vivo (8). Such a modulation may occur during processes of autoxidation, photo-oxidation and chemically induced oxidation. In particular, it has been demonstrated that α-tocopherol prevents the autoxidation of β-carotene in toluene under 100% oxygen tension at 60°C (19). Moreover, δ-tocopherol enhances the protective effects of β-carotene on $^1O_{2-}$ initiated photo-oxidation of methyl linoleate (45). In addition, γ-tocopherol prevents the pro-oxidant effects of β-carotene in purified triacylglycerol fraction of rapeseed oil exposed to light (46) and the pro-oxidant effects of lutein and lycopene in autoxidized triglycerides (47). Carotenoids have also been reported to increase the loss of α-tocopherol induced by different sources of free radicals in lipid homogeneous solution (48), in isolated membranes (33,49), and in intact cells (50). These studies suggest that tocopherols may be consumed to retard the formation of carotenoid radicals and/or the generation of carotenoid autoxidation products. In accord with this hypothesis, it has been found that photobleached β-carotene in hexane is regenerated by α-tocopherol (51). Interestingly, several studies report that combinations of tocopherol and carotenoids have synergistic positive effects in inhibiting oxidative processes, strongly supporting the hypothesis that tocopherols may limit potential pro-oxidant effects of carotenoids. Recently, it has been reported that a synthetic antioxidant, which combines into a single molecule the chroman head of tocopherols and a fragment of lycopene, consisting of a polyisoprenyl sequence of four conjugated double bonds, provides a higher antioxidant efficiency than α-tocopherol and lycopene, alone or in combination (52), also suggesting the possibility of an oxidative intramolecular cooperation between carotenoids and tocopherols.

Carotenoids have also been reported to interfere with the metabolism of tocopherols in vivo (8). In a recent study, an oral supplementation of canthaxanthin modifies the endogenous concentration of tocopherols in murine tissues (53). The xanthophyll increases α-tocopherol content in spleen and liver and decreases γ-tocopherol content in plasma and several tissues. The mechanism by which such modifications occur is not fully understood. Canthaxanthin and tocopherols may compete for intestinal absorption or for binding with lipoproteins. The possibility that tocopherols and carotenoids may influence one another is suggested by research on ferrets, indicating that α-tocopherol promotes the intestinal absorption of intact β-carotene (54).

Ascorbic Acid. The possibility of oxidative interactions between carotenoids and ascorbic acid is reported by Packer et al., who demonstrate that when ascorbic acid is added to low-density lipoproteins (LDLs), it acts synergistically with β-carotene in protecting LDLs from oxidation and β-carotene from its consumption (55). Ascorbic acid has been also shown to protect both the carotenoid and the tocopherol pools in LDLs from Cu^{2+}-mediated oxidative damage (56). Moreover, in a study of dietary antioxidant (ascorbic acid, α-tocopherol, and β-carotene) supplementation and protection of LDL, the addition of ascorbic acid increases plasma levels of β-carotene (57). A plausible integrated mechanism for the interactions of ascorbic acid and α-tocopherol with β-carotene has been proposed (15). In this model, the carotenoid molecule repairs tocopherol radical (reaction D) and the resulting carotenoid cation radical is, in turn, repaired by ascorbic acid (reactions E and F):

$$CAR + TOH^{\bullet +} \rightarrow TOH + CAR^{\bullet +} \qquad \text{(reaction D)}$$

$$CAR^{\bullet +} + ASCH_2 \rightarrow CAR + ASCH^{\bullet} + H^+ \qquad \text{(reaction E)}$$

$$CAR^{\bullet +} + ASCH^- \rightarrow CAR + ASCH^{\bullet -} + H^+ \qquad \text{(reaction F)}$$

Such a hypothesis has been confirmed in vitro (16). An additive response is observed when β-carotene is added in combination with α-tocopherol, whereas a synergistic response is seen when the carotenoid is added in combination with both α-tocopherol and ascorbic acid.

Glutathione. Recent studies suggest that β-carotene can significantly decrease the content of reduced glutathione (GSH) and to increase that of oxidized glutathione (GSSG) in cultured HL-60 cells (25). Such changes occur at carotenoid concentrations ranging from 10 to 20 μM and are dosedependent. Interestingly, the concomitant presence of α-tocopherol completely prevents the changes in glutathione status induced by the carotenoid in this cell model. In addition, carotenoidrich food extracts are able to reduce plasma glutathione levels in rats treated with aflatoxin B_1 (58).

2. Antioxidant Enzymes

It has been recently reported that carotenoids, including xanthophylls, can substantially modify the activity and/or the expression of enzymatic antioxidants.

In cultured human oral carcinoma cells, β-carotene can reduce the activity of both superoxide dismutase (SOD) and glutathione transferase (59). Interestingly, such a reduction does not occur if the cells are incubated with a combination of β-carotene and α-tocopherol. On the other hand, in vivo dietary supplementation with canthaxanthin has been demonstrated to reduce the activity of glutathione peroxidase (GSH-Px) and to increase that of catalase and MnSOD in murine liver (40). In the same model, the carotenoid can also induce the expression of MnSOD. In addition, carotenoid-rich food extracts can lower blood SOD and catalase in rats treated with aflatoxin B_1 (58). Dietary supplementation of rats with β-carotene modulates the increase of SOD induced by peroxyl radicals produced by a high-fat diet (60). Finally, a decreased erythrocyte SOD activity has been shown in adult women consuming a β-carotene-deficient diet. In the same study, dietary β-carotene repletion increases SOD activity (61).

These results, somewhat controversial, point out that carotenoids may alter the activities of oxygen-protective enzymes and consequently induce cellular oxidative stress. According to this hypothesis, powerful pro-oxidant molecules, such as paraquat, modulate antioxidant enzymes in cultured cells similarly, increasing the activity of SOD and catalase and decreasing that of GSH-Px (62).

Moreover, generators of ROS, such as oxidants, ionizing radiation, cytokines, tumor necrosis factor-α (TNF-α), and lipopolysaccharide have been demonstrated to increase MnSOD activity in different experimental models (43).

It is possible that the dose as well as the concomitant presence of an intracellular oxidative stress may influence the modulating effect of carotenoids on the antioxidant enzymes in vivo. Such a hypothesis is supported by experiments in vitro showing that in chicken embryo fibroblasts β-carotene modulates the activity of SOD, catalase, and GSH-Px in a concentration-dependent manner (63). At a high concentration (10 μM), the carotenoid increases SOD and catalase activities and decreases GSH-Px activity, whereas at a low concentration (0.1 μM) it induces opposite effects. In addition, when a pro-oxidant agent such as paraquat is used in the same cell model, β-carotene prevents the paraquat-induced elevation of catalase and SOD activities and the reduction of GSH-Px at low, but not at high, concentrations (62). It is noteworthy that the modulation of the antioxidant enzymes by carotenoids also varies under different po_2 (62).

C. Oxidative Damage to Specific Targets

1. DNA Oxidation

The potential role of carotenoids in preventing oxidative DNA damage has been recently reviewed and discussed (64). Although some studies have shown that carotenoids are effective in protecting cells from oxidative DNA damage, other studies fail to show it. In particular, the presence of β-carotene increases the susceptibility of HepG2 cells to the DNA-damaging effects of H_2O_2, measured as formation of DNA strand breaks, the most significant DNA lesion produced by peroxides (28). In addition, in the same study, pretreatment with the carotenoid enhances the H_2O_2-induced cytotoxicity as measured by the 3,(4,5-dimethyl-2-thiazolyl)-2,5-diphenyl-2H-tetrazolium bromide (MTT) assay. The failure of β-carotene and lycopene to protect human cells against the DNA-damaging effects of H_2O_2 has been recently demonstrated for HT29 cells (27). Moreover, in two human supplementation trials with β-carotene (65) and with lycopene (66), the concentration of 8-oxo-dG in lymphocyte DNA was not significantly decreased. In addition, human lymphocytes do not acquire resistance to oxidative damage induced by H_2O_2 following consumption of vegetables (67). It has also been shown that whereas β-carotene treatment decreases the number of sister chromatid exchanges induced by H_2O_2 in Chinese hamster ovary (CHO) cells, it significantly increases the number of H_2O_2-induced chromosome aberrations (68). Moreover, an enhancement of the clastogenic effects of bleomycin by β-carotene in CHO cells has also been reported (69). Finally, β-carotene causes concentration-dependent DNA breakdown, although this effect is evidenced only at high po_2 (70). In this case, the protection of DNA from the pro-oxidant effects of β-carotene afforded by α-tocopherol and/or ascorbic acid is limited. A recent study demonstrates that, when oxidized, β-carotene and lycopene lead to oxidative damage to both purified calf thymus DNA and DNA isolated from human Hs68 fibroblasts, as revealed by increases in DNA breakage and 8-OH-dG level (71).

2. Lipid Oxidation

Several studies demonstrate that carotenoids may modulate in vitro and in vivo lipid oxidation. They can alter the formation of both initial (conjugated dienes, hydroperoxide) and terminal [malondialdehyde (MDA), TBARs] products of the lipoperoxidative process. Although a large number of reports demonstrate an inhibitory effect of carotenoids on the formation of lipid oxidative products (5–7), recent observations evidence that they can also enhance such a production, at least under certain circumstances (high po_2, high carotenoid concentration, cell chronic oxidative status) (8). Increases in lipoperoxidation products induced by carotenoids have been reported in both isolated membranes (72) and intact cells (30). Pro-oxidant effects are observed in vitro using β-carotene as well as other carotenoids, such as lycopene. In particular, in human foreskin fibroblasts (Hs68 cells), it has been reported that lycopene may increase TBAR production induced by the lipid-soluble radical generator 2,2′-azobis(2,4-dimethylvaleronitrile) (73). This effect is dosedependent and is not observed when other generators of free radicals, such as the system ferric nitrilotriacetate and the water-soluble 2,2′-azobis(2-amidinopropane)dihydrochloride (AAPH), are used. β-Carotene behaves similarly under the same in vitro oxidative conditions, suggesting that the type of oxidant used may also be an important determinant in the pro-oxidant activity of carotenoids.

Reaven et al. have demonstrated that LDLs isolated from individuals receiving β-carotene supplements are not protected from oxidation (57). In addition, Gaziano et al. also found that β-carotene does not enhance the in vitro resistance of LDLs to copper- or AAPH-induced oxidation (74). Other in vivo studies show that dietary supplementation of β-carotene at high doses enhanced lipid peroxidation in liver, kidney, and brain of CBA mice exposed to methyl mercuric chloride (75). Moreover, a dietary supplement of β-carotene to rats treated with a diet deficient in α-tocopherol and enriched with soybean oil develops a significant increase in MDA production and 15-lipoxygenase in rat testis (76). Again, feeding rats with large amounts of β-carotene increases lipid peroxidation products in liver and plasma (77).

3. Protein Oxidation

It quickly becomes clear that, as compared with DNA and lipid oxidation, the evidence for carotenoids as inducers of protein oxidation in biological systems is very limited. This is mainly due to the fact that the field of protein oxidation is very much in its infancy. On the other hand, it is clear that, since proteins do play a crucial role in many (patho)physiological processes, the area of markers for protein oxidation will grow in years to come. Recently, the effect of β-carotene on protein oxidation has been examined under different oxygen tensions and in the presence of α-tocopherol and ascorbic acid, alone and in combination (78). In this study, human serum albumin is incubated in vitro with AAPH to induce protein oxidation (carbonyl formation). Interestingly, high concentrations of β-carotene produce more protein oxidation in the presence of high pO_2. A mixture of β-carotene, α-tocopherol, and ascorbic acid provides better protective effects on protein oxidation than any single compound. In addition, Andersen and coworkers using Fe^{2+}-mediated oxidation of heme proteins as an early indicator of oxidative stress find that β-carotene exhibits limited protection or a pro-oxidant effect with respect to a pronounced vitamin E antioxidant activity (79).

D. Modulation of Redox-Sensitive Genes

Although the study of the modifications of molecular pathways by carotenoids is in its infancy, it is beginning to reveal that these compounds can bring about a host of changes in the expression of redox-sensitive genes and/or genes involved in the maintenance of cell redox status.

1. Genes Involved in Cell Growth

Increasing evidence shows that β-carotene inhibits tumor cell growth through the involvement of a pro-oxidant mechanism and the modulation of redox-sensitive genes. We recently hypothesized a strict relationship between changes in intracellular redox potential and cell growth by β-carotene in tumor cells (26). The increase in ROS production and/or the levels of oxidized glutathione induced by the carotenoid in human colon adenocarcinoma (24) and leukemia (25) cells are highly coincident with its ability to induce apoptosis and to arrest cell cycle progression. Interestingly, in these cells, the carotenoid is also able to decrease the expression of Bcl-2 (25,38), a protein whose antiapoptotic effects has been at least partially explained by its antioxidant properties (80). In addition, in HL-60 cells, the carotenoid also induces an increased expression of p21WAF-1, which is implicated in the arrest of cell cycle progression at the G_1 phase (25). A recent finding suggests that this protein is regulated by oxidative stress through a mechanism independent of p53 activation (81). The hypothesis of the involvement of a pro-oxidant mechanism in the growthinhibitory effects of β-carotene in these studies is also supported by the finding that α-tocopherol minimizes the effect of the carotenoid on cell growth, apoptosis, and Bcl-2 expression in a dose-dependent manner (25). Moreover, the growthinhibitory effects of the carotenoid in SCC-25 tumor cells are decreased by an oxygen-poor environment in which the pro-oxidant character of the molecule is minimized (82). In addition, β-carotene is able to induce an oxidative stress in tumor oral cells, resulting in the expression of stress proteins, such as the heat-shock protein 70 (hsp 70) and/or hsp90, which are nuclear-binding proteins involved in apoptosis (82,83). Interestingly, both 9-*cis* and all-*trans* β-carotene are able to induce an intracellular accumulation of hsp70 in cervical dysplasia–derived cells and the treated cells showed morphological changes indicative of apoptosis (84). Moreover, β-carotene reduces the expression of mutant p53, which has been associated with the exposure to cigarette smoke (10) and stimulates the expression of TNF-α (85).

2. Genes Involved in Detoxification Processes

Increasing evidence suggests that carotenoids may modulate the expression of detoxification enzymes, involved in oxidative processes. It has been recently found that β-carotene can act as an inducer of several carcinogen-metabolizing enzymes (44,86,87). In the lung of Sprague–Dawley rats, β-carotene is able to induce the following: CYP1A1/2, able to bioactivate aromatic amines, polychlorinated dioxins, and polycyclic aromatic hydrocarbons; CYP3A, able to activate aflatoxins, 1-nitropyrene; CYP2B1, able to activate olefins and halogenated hydrocarbons; and CYP2A, able to activate butadiene, esamethyl phosphoramide, and nitrosamines. In this study, such inductions have been associated with an overgeneration of oxygen-centered radicals (44). In addition, many tobaccosmoke procarcinogens are themselves CYP inducers, and they could act in a synergistic manner with β-carotene or with some of its oxidation products, such as β-apo-8′-carotenal, further contributing to the overall carcinogenic risk (22). Moreover, induction of transformation by benzo[a]pyrene and cigarette-smoke condensate in BALB/c 3T3 cells is markedly enhanced by the presence of β-carotene in either acute or chronic treatment. Such an enhancement has been related to the boosting effect of the carotenoid on the P450 apparatus (87). In addition, β-carotene has been reported to enhance ethanol hepatotoxicity by an induction of CYP2E1 and CYP4A1 in both rodents and nonhuman primates (88). Other carotenoids, such as canthaxanthin and astaxanthin, have been recognized as potent inducers of CYP1A1 and 1A2 in rat liver (89).

Carotenoids have also been suggested to modulate tumor growth by acting as potent inducers of phase II detoxifying enzymes, such as glutathione S-transferase (GST) and quinone reductase (90), as well as of cellular defensive enzymes such as heme-oxygenase-1 (91). In human skin fibroblasts enriched with the carotenoid and exposed to UV light (91), the increase in heme-oxygenase-1 expression by β-carotene is entirely suppressed by vitamin E, but only moderately by vitamin C.

The modulation of these enzymes might occur through an activation of mitogen-activated protein kinase leading to induction of antioxidant/electrophile response element (ARE/EpRE), as suggested for other dietary chemopreventive compounds (92).

E. Modulation of Redox-Sensitive Transcription Factors

Although markers based on transcription factor activation are not considered suitable since their induction tends to be transient and hard to quantify, some indications suggest that carotenoids may modulate the activity of redox-sensitive transcription factors. The nuclear factor κB (NF-κB) pathway is generally thought to be a primary oxidative stress response pathway involved in cell proliferation and apoptosis (93–98). We have recently reported that β-carotene, administrated at concentrations found to induce growthinhibitory and pro-oxidant effects, increases the DNA binding activity of nuclear proteins at the NF-κB site in leukemic as well as in colon adenocarcinoma cells (37). In these cells, the ability of treatments with α-tocopherol or N-acetyl-cysteine to diminish both β-carotene-induced NF-κB DNA binding activity and ROS production further supports the hypothesis that the carotenoid regulates this transcription factor through a pro-oxidant mechanism. It has been recently reported that NF-κB is activated by certain apoptotic stimuli and that some of the NF-κB target genes, such as c-myc, are implicated in apoptosis induction (99). Accordingly, we have recently demonstrated that β-carotene is able to increase the expression of c-myc and that such an increase is directly related to apoptosis induction (37). Interestingly, it has been suggested that β-carotene can also modulate the activation of activator protein-1 (AP-1), which is known to be another redox-sensitive transcription factor involved in the regulation of cell growth (22,100,101).

IV. BENEFITS AND HAZARDS OF CAROTENOIDS
AS PRO-OXIDANT MOLECULES

There is a growing body of literature on the effects of β-carotene and other carotenoids in human chronic diseases, including cardiovascular diseases and cancer. Although epidemiological studies have shown that a high consumption of fruit and vegetables rich in carotenoids is associated with a low risk for chronic diseases (1,2), and numerous in vitro and in vivo experimental studies (102,103) have reported that carotenoids may be beneficial in such diseases, increasing evidence demonstrates more or less detrimental health effects following carotenoid treatment. It has been found that β-carotene acts as an enhancer of cell transforming activity of powerful carcinogens, such as benzo[a]pyrene and cigarettesmoke condensate in BALB/c 3T3 cells in vitro (87). Recently, an enhancement of benzo[a]pyrene-induced mutagenesis in vivo by a lycopene-rich diet was observed in colon and lung from mice, but not in prostate (104). Interestingly, a previous study on dietary supplementation of a lycopene-rich tomato oleoresin demonstrated that lung accumulates this carotenoid to a greater extent than prostate (105). An enhancement of UV-induced skin carcinogenesis by β-carotene has been observed in vivo, as recently reviewed (106,107). An enhancement of lung tumorigenesis by β-carotene has been also observed in ferrets exposed to tobacco smoke (22). β-Carotene-supplemented ferrets exhibit an increased keratinized squamous metaplasia, which can be considered a precancerous lesion and an increased cell proliferation measured as proliferating cell nuclear antigen expression. Interestingly, this effect was only observed using high doses of the carotenoid, while a physiological dose of it does not have potentially detrimental effects in smoke-exposed ferrets and may afford weak protection against lung damage induced by cigarette smoke (108). Moreover, clinical trials not only fail to provide protective effects by β-carotene as a supplement but even result in a significant exacerbation of cancer (3,4). In particular, the ATBC as well as the CARET trials both evidenced that β-carotene-supplemented smokers increase the risk of lung cancer. Although the direct involvement of a pro-oxidant mechanism in the procarcinogenic effects of carotenoids is a matter of debate, these studies highlight several points: (a) Mutagenic or procarcinogenic effects of carotenoid molecules are evidenced mainly at doses that usually exceed the dietary intake. Mayne and colleagues observed that the high dose of β-carotene given as a supplement in clinical trials results in carotenoid levels in the blood (3.0 and 2.1 mg/L in ATBC and CARET, respectively) much higher that those reported for the U.S. population (0.05–0.5 mg/L) (1). This could affect the content and/or the absorption of other dietary nutrients with a better antioxidant profile or favor the formation of β-carotene oxidation products. (b) Procarcinogenic effects of carotenoids are evidenced in tissues, such as lung, in which the oxygen tension is high and therefore able to promote effective pro-oxidant effects of carotenoids. Concerning this, in the human body, the pO_2 is very different among tissues and organs: the lung alveoli have a pO_2 of 100 mm Hg, while the other tissues and venous blood have a pO_2 of 5–15 mm Hg and 40 mm Hg, respectively (36). Therefore, these molecules are expected to be less effective as antioxidants or more effective as pro-oxidants in lung than in other tissues. (c) Either condition, i.e., lack of adequate antioxidant defense (impairment of the antioxidant status) or chronic oxidative stress (UV exposure), results in increased procarcinogenic effects by carotenoid molecules. In this regard, cells from smokers exhibit markedly reduced vitamin C levels, a reflection of severe oxidant exposure (32).

Concomitantly, UV-exposed dermal fibroblasts show an overgeneration of superoxide anions and an enhanced lipid peroxidation, both symptoms of oxidative stress, in the presence of β-carotene (109). (d) The administration of carotenoids with fruit and vegetables instead of carotenoid supplements has never been associated with procarcinogenic effects induced by carotenoids. This can be related to the fact that fruit and vegetables contain, concomitantly, other antioxidant nutrients, which can limit the pro-oxidant effects of carotenoids. Moreover, the use of carotenoids in combination with other nutrients produces more inhibition of carcinogenic processes, such as oral carcinogenesis, than the administration of the single agents (8,10). (e) The CARET trial also evidences an enhancement of lung carcinogenesis in asbestos workers, only 38% of whom were current smokers (3). It is noteworthy that asbestos fibers contain iron, a powerful catalyst for oxidation. Moreover, inflammatory cells recovered by bronchoalveolar lavage from nonsmokers with asbestosis spontaneously release significantly increased amounts of ROS relative to those from normal individuals (110).

On the other hand, it should be considered that the pro-oxidant effects of carotenoids in biological systems are not necessarily bad, but they can also result in beneficial health effects. In accord with this observation, several findings suggest that β-carotene effectively increases intracellular oxidative stress (by increasing ROS production, GSSG content, and/or NF-κBbinding activity) in many tumor cells and this effect is accompanied by antitumor activity: the carotenoid may induce cell cycle arrest and apoptosis and, even, induce the loss of tumor cell viability (26,26,37,38). In addition, the increase of lipid peroxidation products by β-carotene at high po_2 during free radical induced oxidative stress in tumor thymocytes results in cell death (30). Therefore, the development of harmful or beneficial effects by carotenoids may be dependent on the redox potential of carotenoid molecules but also by the cell environment in which these molecules act. A pro-oxidant activity of carotenoids in normal cells may be ineffective because it can be counteracted by the normal endogenous antioxidant defense or may be deleterious because it can alter regulatory functions, damage cell integrity, and/or induce neoplastic transformation. On the other hand, a pro-oxidant activity of carotenoids in already transformed cells may be extremely helpful, because it can block tumor cell growth.

V. CONCLUSIONS

As discussed throughout this chapter 6 increasing evidence shows a role for carotenoids as pro-oxidant agents. These compounds may increase the levels of biochemical and molecular markers of oxidative stress, depending on their intrinsic properties (i.e., structure, concentration, location in cell membranes) as well as on extrinsic factors (i.e., oxygen tension, cell redox status, interactions with other redox agents). Therefore, the possible beneficial or adverse effects of carotenoids as pro-oxidant molecules in health should be considered with an open mind rather than with a preconceived view of their mechanism of action. Nevertheless, numerous gaps still exist in our understanding of the role of carotenoids as pro-oxidants. Many of the results on the pro-oxidant activity of carotenoids have been demonstrated only in vitro. Our knowledge of the influence of carotenoids as pro-oxidants in vivo remains fragmented and incomplete. Moreover, the products of carotenoids directly responsible for their pro-oxidant activity have not been identified yet. Finally, the involvement of the pro-oxidant effects of carotenoids in the carcinogenic process and in the development of chronic diseases need to be clearly elucidated. Improved knowledge of the pro-oxidant role of carotenoids in vitro and in vivo will help in understanding their potential role in health and disease.

REFERENCES

1. Mayne ST. Beta-carotene, carotenoids and disease prevention in humans. FASEB J 1996; 10:690–701.
2. Ziegler RG, Mayne ST, Swanson CA. Nutrition and lung cancer. Cancer Causes Control 1996; 7:157–177.
3. Omenn GS, Goodman GE, Thornquist MD, Balmes J, Cullen MR, Glass A, Keogh JP, Meyskens FL, Valanis B, Williams JH, Barnhart S, Hammar S. Effects of a combination of β-carotene and vitamin A on lung cancer and cardiovascular disease. N Engl J Med 1996; 334:1150–1155.
4. The Alpha-tocopherol, Beta-Carotene Cancer Prevention Study Group. The effect of vitamin E and β-carotene on the incidence of lung cancer and other cancers in male smokers. N Engl J Med 1994; 330:1029–1035.
5. Palozza P, Krinsky NI. Antioxidant effects of carotenoids in vivo and in vitro: an overview. Meth Enzymol 1992; 213:403–420.
6. Krinsky NI. Actions of carotenoids in biological systems. Annu Rev Nutr 1993; 13:561–587.
7. Sies H, Stahl W. Vitamins E and C, β-carotene and other carotenoids as antioxidants. Am J Clin Nutr 1995; 62 (suppl):1315S–1321S.
8. Palozza P. Prooxidant actions of carotenoids in biological systems. Nutr Rev 1998; 56:257–265.
9. Young AJ, Lowe GM. Antioxidant and prooxidant properties of carotenoids. Arch Biochem Biophys 2001; 385:20–27.
10. Schwartz JL. The dual roles of nutrients as antioxidants and prooxidants: their effects on tumor cell growth. J Nutr 1996; 126:1221S–1227S.
11. Olson JA. Benefits and liabilities of vitamin A and carotenoids. J Nutr 1996; 126:1208S–1212S.

12. Burton GW, Ingold KU. β-Carotene: an unusual type of lipid antioxidant. Science 1984; 224:569–573.

13. Britton, G. Structure and properties of carotenoids in relation to functions. FASEB J 1995; 9:1551–1558.

14. Truscott TG. β-Carotene and disease: a suggested prooxidant and antioxidant mechanism and speculations concerning its role in cigarette smoking. J Photochem Photobiol 1996; 35:233–235.

15. Edge R, Truscott TG. Prooxidant and antioxidant reaction mechanisms of carotene and radical interactions with vitamins E and C. Nutr 1997; 13:992–994.

16. Bohm F, Egde R, Land EJ, McGarvey DJ, Schalch W, Truscott TG. Vitamin E and carotenoids: synergetic protection against human cell damage. FEBS Lett 1998; 436:387–389.

17. Mortensen A, Skibsted LH and Truscott TG. The interaction of dietary carotenoids with radical species. Arch Biochem Biophys 2001; 385:13–19.

18. Mayne ST, Handelman GJ, Beecher G. β-Carotene and lung cancer promotion in heavy smokers—a plausible relationship? J Natl Cancer Inst 1996; 88:1513–1515.

19. Handelman GJ, van Kuijk FJGM, Chatterjee A, Krinsky NI. Characterization of products formed during the autooxidation of β-carotene. Free Radic Biol Med 1991; 10:427–437.

20. Liebler DC, McClure TD. Antioxidant reactions of β-carotene: identification of carotenoid-radical adducts. Chem Res Toxicol 1996; 9:8–11.

21. Yamauchi R, Miyake N, Inoue H, Kato K. Products formed by peroxyl radical oxidation of β-carotene. J Agric Food Chem 1993; 41:708–713.

22. Wang XD, Liu C, Bronson RT, Smith DE, Krinsky NI, Russell RM. Retinoid signalling and activator protein-1 expression in ferrets given β-carotene supplements and exposed to tobacco smoke. J Natl Cancer Inst 1999; 91:60–66.

23. Arora A, Willhite CA, Liebler DC. Interactions of β-carotene and cigarette smoke in human bronchial epithelial cells. Carcinogenesis 2001; 22:1173–1178.

24. Palozza P, Calviello G, Serini S, Maggiano N, Lanza P, Ranelletti FO, Bartoli GM. β-Carotene at high concentrations induces apoptosis by enhancing oxy-radical production in human adenocarcinoma cells. Free Radic Biol Med 2001; 30:1000–1007.

25. Palozza P, Serini S, Torsello A, Boninsegna A, Covacci V, Maggiano M, Ranelletti FO, Wolf FI and Calviello G. Regulation of cell cycle progression and apoptosis by β-carotene in undifferentiated and differentiated HL-60 leukemia cells: possible involvement of a redox mechanism. Int J Cancer 2002; 97:593–600.

26. Palozza P, Serini S, Di Nicuolo F and Calviello G. Mitogenic and apoptotic signaling by carotenoids: involvement of a redox mechanism. IUBMB Life 2001; 52:1–5.

27. Lowe GM, Booth LA, Bilton RF, Young AJ. Lycopene and β-carotene protect against oxidative damage in HT29 cells at low concentrations but rapidly lose this capacity at higher doses Free Radic Res 1999; 30:141–151.

28. Woods JA, Young AJ, Bilton RF. Carotene enhances hydrogen peroxide–induced DNA damage in human hepatocellular HepG2 cells. FEBS Lett 1999; 449:255–258.

29. Woodall AA, Britton G, Jackson MJ. Carotenoids and protection of phospholipids in solution or in liposomes against oxidation by peroxyl radicals: relationship between carotenoid structure and protective ability. Biochim Biophys Acta 1997; 1336:575–586.

30. Palozza P, Luberto C, Calviello G, Ricci P, and Bartoli GM. Antioxidant and prooxidant role of β-carotene in murine normal and tumor thymocytes: effects of oxygen partial pressure. Free Radic Biol Med 1997; 22:1065–1073.

31. Shen Q, Chada S, Whiteney C, Newburger PE. Regulation of the human cellular glutathione peroxidase gene during in vitro myeloid and monocytic differentiation. Blood 1994; 84:3902–3908.

32. Lykkesfeldt J, Christen S, Wallock LM, Chang HH, Jacob RA, Ames BN. Ascorbate is depleted by smoking and repleted by moderate supplementation: a study in male smokers and nonsmokers with matched antioxidant intakes. Am J Clin Nutr 2000; 71:530–536.

33. Palozza P and Krinsky NI. β-Carotene and α-tocopherol are synergistic antioxidants. Arch Biochem Biophys 1992; 297:184–187.

34. Leibovitz B, Hu ML, Tappel AL. Dietary supplements of vitamin E, β-carotene, coenzyme Q10 and selenium protect tissues against lipid peroxidation in rat tissue slices. J Nutr 1990; 120:97–104.

35. Chen H, Tappel AL Protection of vitamin E, selenium trolox C, ascorbic acid palmitate, acetylcysteine, coenzyme Q10, β-carotene, canthaxanthin and (+)-catechin against oxidative damage to rat blood and tissues in vivo. Free Radic Biol Med 1995; 5:949–953.

36. Halliwell B and Cross CE. Oxygen derived species: their relation to human diseases and environmental stress. Environ Health Perspect 1994; 102:5–12.

37. Palozza P, Serini S, Torsello A, Di Nicuolo F, Piccioni E, Ubaldi V, Pioli C, Wolf FI, Calviello G. β-Carotene regulates NF-κB DNA-binding activity by a redox mechanism in human leukemia and colon adenocarcinoma cells. J Nutr 2003; 133:381–388.

38. Palozza P, Serini S, Maggiano N, Angelini M, Boninsegna A, Di Nicuolo F, Ranelletti FO, Calviello G. Induction of cell cycle arrest and apoptosis in human colon adenocarcinoma cell lines by β-carotene through down-regulation of cyclin A and Bcl-2 family proteins. Carcinogenesis 2002; 23:11–18.

39. Murata M, Kawanishi S. Oxidative DNA damage by vitamin A and its derivative via superoxide generation. J Biol Chem 2000; 275:2003–2008.

40. Palozza P, Calviello G, De Leo ME, Serini S, Bartoli GM. Canthaxanthin supplementation alters antioxidant enzymes and iron concentration in liver of Balb/c mice. J Nutr 2000; 130:1303–1308.

41. Garcia-Casal MN, Layrisse M, Solano L, Baron MA, Arguello F, Llovera D, Ramirez J, Leets I and Tropper E. Vitamin A and β-carotene can improve nonheme iron absorption from rice, wheat and corn by humans. J Nutr 1998; 128:646–650.

42. Halliwell B, Gutteridge MC. Role of free radicals and catalytic metal ions in human disease: an overview. Meth Enzymol 1990; 186:1–85.
43. De Leo ME, Landriscina M, Palazzotti B, Borrello S, Galeotti T. Iron modulation of LPS-induced manganese superoxide dismutase gene expression in rat tissues. FEBS Lett 1997; 403:131–135.
44. Paolini M, Antelli A, Pozzetti L, Spetlova D, Perocco P, Valgimigli L, Pedulli GF, Cantelli-Forti G. Induction of cytochrome P450 enzymes and overgeneration of oxygen radicals in β-carotene supplemented rats. Carcinogenesis 2001; 22:1483–1495.
45. Terao J, Yamauchi R, Murakami H, Matsushita S. Inhibitory effects of tocopherols and β-carotene on singlet oxygen-initiated photooxidation of methyl linoleate and soybean oil. J Food Proc Preserv 1980; 4:79–93.
46. Haila K, Heinonen M. Action of β-carotene on purified rapeseed oil during light storage. Lebensm Wiss Technol 1994; 27:573–577.
47. Haila KM, Lievonen SM, Heinonen MI. Effects of lutein, lycopene, annatto and γ-tocopherol on autooxidation of triglycerides. J Agric Food Chem 1996; 44:2096–2100.
48. Palozza P, Krinsky NI. The inhibition of radical-initiated peroxidation of microsomal lipids by both α-tocopherol and β-carotene. Free Radic Biol Med 1991; 11:407–414.
49. Palozza P, Moualla S, Krinsky NI. Effects of β-carotene and α-tocopherol on radical-initiated peroxidation of microsomes. Free Radic Biol Med 1992; 13:127–136.
50. Palozza P, Luberto C, Ricci P, Sgarlata E, Calviello G, Bartoli GM. Effect of β-carotene and canthaxanthin on tert-butyl hydroperoxide-induced lipid peroxidation in normal and tumor thymocytes. Arch Biochem Biophys 1996; 325:145–151.
51. Mortensen A, Skibsted LH, Willnow A, Everett, SA. Re-appraisal of the tocopheroxyl radical reaction with β-carotene: evidence for oxidation of vitamin E by the β-carotene radical cation. Free Radic Res 1998; 28:69–80.
52. Palozza P, Piccioni E, Avanzi L, Vertuani S, Calviello G, Manfredini S. Design, synthesis and antioxidant activity of Fe-AOX-6, a novel agent deriving from a molecular combination of the chromanyl and polyisoprenyl moieties. Free Radic Biol Med 2002; 33:1724–1735.
53. Palozza P, Calviello G, Serini S, Moscato P, Bartoli GM. Supplementation with canthaxanthin affects plasma and tissue distribution of α- and γ-tocopherols in mice. J Nutr 1998; 128:1989–1994.
54. Wang XD, Marini RP, Hebuterne X, Fox JG, Krinsky NI, Russell RM. Vitamin E enhances the lymphatic transport of β-carotene and its conversion to vitamin A in the ferret. Gastroenterology 1995; 108:719–726.
55. Packer L. Antioxidant action of carotenoids in vitro and in vivo and protection against oxidation of human low-density lipoproteins. Ann N Y Acad Sci 1993; 691:48–60.
56. Jialal J, Grundy SM. Preservation of the endogenous antioxidants in low-density lipoproteins by ascorbate but not probucol during oxidative modifications. J Clin Invest 1991; 87:597–601.

57. Reaven PD, Ferguson E, Navab M, Pouel FL. Susceptibility of human LDL to oxidative modifications: effects of variations in β-carotene concentration and oxygen tension. Arterioscler Thromb Vasc Biol 1994; 14:1162–1169.

58. He Y, Root MM, Parker RS, Campbell TC. Effects of carotenoid-rich food extracts on the development of preneoplastic lesions in rat liver and on in vivo and in vitro antioxidant status. Nutr Cancer 1997; 27:238–244.

59. Schwartz JL, Tanaka J, Khandekar V. The effectiveness of a mixture of β-carotene, α-tocopherol, glutathione, and ascorbic acid for cancer prevention. Nutr Cancer 1993; 20:145–151.

60. Blakely SR, Slaughter L, Adkins J, Knight EV. Effects of β-carotene and retinyl palmitate on corn oil–induced superoxide dismutase and catalase in rats. J Nutr 1988; 118:152–158.

61. Dixon ZR, Burri BJ, Clifford A, Frankel EN, Schneeman BO, Parks E, Keim NL, Barbieri T, Wu M-M, Fong AKH, Kretsch MJ, Sowell AL, Erdman JW Jr. Effects of a carotene-deficient diet on measures of oxidative susceptibility and superoxide dismutase activity in adult women. Free Radic Biol Med 1994; 17:537–544.

62. Lawlor SM, O'Brien NM. Modulation of paraquat toxicity by β-carotene at low oxygen partial pressure in chicken embryo fibroblasts. Br J Nutr 1997; 77:133–140.

63. Lawlor SM, O'Brien NM. Modulation of oxidative stress by β-carotene in chicken embryo fibroblasts. Br J Nutr 1995; 73:841–850.

64. Collins AR. Carotenoids and genomic stability. Mutat Res 2001; 475:21–28.

65. Lee BM, Lee SK, Kim HS. Inhibition of oxidative DNA damage, 8-OH-dG, and carbonyl contents in smokers treated with antioxidants (vitamin E, vitamin C, β-carotene and red ginseng). Cancer Lett 1998; 132:219–227.

66. Rao AV, Agarwal S. Bioavailability and in vivo antioxidant properties of lycopene from tomato products and their possible role in prevention of cancer. Nutr Cancer 1998; 31:199–203.

67. Pool-Zobel BL, Bub A, Muller H, Wollowski I, Rechkemmer G. Consumption of vegetables reduces genetic damage in humans: first results of a human intervention trial with carotenoid-rich foods. Carcinogenesis 1997; 18:1847–1850.

68. Cozzi R, Ricordy R, Aglitti T, Gatta V, Perticone P, De Salvia R. Ascorbic acid and β-carotene as modulators of oxidative damage. Carcinogenesis 1997; 18:223–228.

69. Salvadori DMF, Ribeiro RR, Natarajan AT. Effects of β-carotene on clastogenic effects of mytomycin C, methyl methanesulphonate and bleomycin in Chinese hamster ovary cells. Mutagenesis 1994; 9:53–57.

70. Zhang P, Omaye ST. DNA strand breakage and oxygen tension: effects of β-carotene, α-tocopherol, and ascorbic acid. Food Chem Toxicol 2001; 39:239–246.

71. Yeh SL, Hu ML. Induction of oxidative DNA damage in human foreskin fibroblast Hs68 cells by oxidized β-carotene and lycopene. Free Radic Res 2001; 35:203–213.

72. Palozza P, Calviello G, Bartoli GM. Prooxidant activity of β-carotene under 100% oxygen pressure in rat liver microsomes. Free Radic Biol Med 1995; 19:887–892.

73. Yeh S, Hu M. Antioxidant and prooxidant effects of lycopene in comparison with β-carotene on oxidant-induced damage in Hs68 cells. J Nutr Biochem 2000; 11:548–554.

74. Gaziano JM, Hatta A, Flyn M, Johnson EJ, Krinsky NI, Ridker PM, Hennekens CH, Frei B. Supplementation with β-carotene in vivo and in vitro does not inhibit low-density lipoprotein oxidation. Atherosclerosis 1995; 112:187–195.

75. Andersen HR, Andersen O. Effects of dietary α-tocopherol and β-carotene on lipid peroxidation induced by methyl mercuric chloride in mice. Pharmacol Toxicol 1993; 73:192–201.

76. Lomnitski L, Bergman M, Schon I, Grossman S. The effect of dietary vitamin E and β-carotene on oxidation processes in rat testis. Biochim Biophys Acta 1991; 1082:101–107.

77. Alam SQ, Alam BS. Lipid peroxide, α-tocopherol, and retinoid levels in plasma and liver of rats fed diets containing β-carotene and 13-cis-retinoic acid. J Nutr 1983; 113:2608–2614.

78. Zhang P, Omaye ST. β-Carotene and protein oxidation: effects of ascorbic acid and α-tocopherol. Toxicology 2000; 146:37–47.

79. Andersen HJ, Chen H, Pellett LJ, Tappel AL. Ferrous-iron-induced oxidation in chicken liver slices as measured by hemichrome formation and thiobarbituric acid-reactive substances: effects of dietary vitamin E and β-carotene. Free Radic Biol Med 1993; 15:37–48.

80. Kane D J, Sarafian TA, Anton R, Hahn H, Gralla EB, Valentine JS, Ord T, Bredesen DE. Bcl-2 inhibition of neural death: decreased generation of reactive oxygen species. Science 1993; 262:1274–1277.

81. Esposito F, Russo L, Russo T, Cimino F. Retinoblastoma protein dephosphorylation is an early event of cellular response to prooxidant conditions. FEBS Lett 2000; 470:211–215.

82. Schwartz JL. In vitro biological methods for determination of carotenoid activity. Meth Enzymol 1993; 214:226–256.

83. Schwartz JL, Singh RP, Teicher B, Wright JE, Trites DH, Shklar G. Induction of a 70 κD protein associated with the selective cytotoxicity of β-carotene in human epidermal carcinoma. Biochem Biophys Res Commun 1990; 169:941–946.

84. Toba T, Shidoji Y, Fujii J, Moriwaki H, Muto Y, Suzuki T, Ohishi N, Yagi K. Growth suppression and induction of heat-shock protein-70 by 9-cis-β-carotene in cervical dysplasia-derived cells. Life Sci 1997; 61:839–845.

85. Abdel-Fatth G, Watzl B, Huang D and Watson RR. β-Carotene in vitro stimulates tumor necrosis factor-α and interleukin-1a secretion by human peripheral blood mononuclear cells. Nutr Res 1993; 13:863–871.

86. Paolini M, Cantelli-Forti G, Perocco P, Pedulli GF, Abdel-Rahman SZ, Legator MS. Co-carcinogenic effect of β-carotene. Nature 1999; 398:760–761.

87. Perocco P, Paolini M, Mazzullo M, Biagi GL, Cantelli-Forti G. β-Carotene as enhancer of cell-transforming activity of powerful carcinogens and cigarette-smoke condensate on Balb/c3T3 cells in vitro. Mutat Res 1999; 440:83–90.

88. Kessova IG, Leo MA, Liebler CS. Effect of β-carotene on hepatic cytochrome P450 in ethanol-fed rats. Alcohol Clin Exp Res 2001; 25:1368–1372.

89. Gradelet S, Le Bon AM, Berges R, Suschetet M. Dietary carotenoids inhibit aflatoxin B1-induced liver preneoplastic foci and DNA damage in the rat: role of the modulation of aflatoxin B1 metabolism. Carcinogenesis 1998; 19:403–411.

90. Sharoni Y, Danilenko M, Walfisch S, Amir H, Nahum A, Ben-Dor A, Hirsch K, Khanin M, Steiner M, Agemy L, Zango G, Levy J. Role of gene-regulation in the anticancer activity of carotenoids. Pure Appl Chem 2002; 74:1469–1477.

91. Obermuller-Jevic UC, Francz PI, Frank J, Flaccus A, Biesalski HK. Enhancement of the UVA-induction of haem oxygenase-1 expression by β-carotene in human skin fibroblasts. FEBS Lett 1999; 460:212–216.

92. Owuor ED, Kong A-N T. Antioxidants and oxidants regulated signal transduction pathways. Biochem Pharmacol 2002; 64:765–770.

93. Schulze-Osthoff K, Los M, Baeuerle PA. Redox signalling by transcription factors NF-κB and AP-1 in the immune system. Biochem Pharmacol 1995; 50:735–741.

94. Sen CH and Packer L. Antioxidant and redox regulation of gene transcription. FASEB J 1996; 10:709–720.

95. Flohé L, Brigelius-Flohé R, Saliou C, Traber MG, Packer L. Redox regulation of NF-kappa;B activation. Free Radic Biol Med 1997; 22:1115–1126.

96. Ginn-Pease ME, Whisler RL. Redox signals and NF-κB activation in T cells. Free Radic Biol Med 1998; 25:346–361.

97. Mercurio F, Manning AM. NF-κB as a primary regulator of the stress response. Oncogene 1999; 18:6163–6171.

98. Bowie A and O'Neill LAJ. Oxidative stress and nuclear factor-κB activation. Biochem Pharmacol 2000; 59:13–23.

99. La Rosa FA, Pierce JW, Sonenshein GE. Differential regulation of the c-myc oncogene promoter by the NF-κB Rel family of transcription factor. Mol Cell Biol 1994; 14:1039–1044.

100. Lotan R. Lung cancer promotion by β-carotene and tobacco smoke: relationship to suppression of retinoic acid receptor-b and increased activator protein-1. J Natl Cancer Inst 1999; 91:7–9.

101. Tibaduiza EC, Fleet JC, Russell RM, Krinsky NI. Excentric cleavage products of β-carotene inhibit estrogen receptor positive and negative breast tumor cell growth in vitro and inhibit activator protein-1-mediated transcriptional activation. Nutr Cancer 2002; 132:1368–1375.

102. Krinsky NI. Effects of carotenoids in cellular and animal systems. Am J Clin Nutr 1991; 53:238S–246S.

103. Gerster H. β-Carotene, vitamin E and vitamin C in different stages of experimental carcinogenesis. Eur J Clin Nutr 1995; 49:155–168.

104. Guttenplan JB, Chen M, Kosinska W, Thompson S, Zhao Z, Cohen LA. Effects of a lycopene-rich diet on spontaneous and benzo(a)pyrene-induced mutagenesis in prostate, colon and lungs of the lacZ mouse. Cancer Lett 2001; 164:1–6.

105. Zhao Z, Khachik F, Richie JP Jr, Cohen LA. Lycopene uptake and tissue disposition in male and female rats. Proc Soc Exp Biol Med 1998; 218:109–114.

106. Black HS. Radical interception by carotenoids and effects on UV carcinogenesis. Nutr Cancer 1998; 31:212–217.

107. Biesalski HK, Obermueller-Jevic UC. UV-light, β-carotene and human skin: beneficial and potentially harmful effects. Arch Biochem Biophys 2001; 389:1–6.

108. Liu C, Wang X-D, Bronson R, Smith DE, Krinsky NI, Russell RM. Effects of physiological versus pharmacological β-carotene supplementation on cell proliferation and histopathological changes in the lungs of cigarette smoke–exposed ferrets. Carcinogenesis 2000; 21:2245–2253.

109. Jones, S, McArdle F, Jack CI, Jackson MJ. Effect of antioxidant supplementation on the adaptive response of human skin fibroblast to UV-induced oxidative stress. Redox Rep 1999; 4:291–299.

110. Rom WN, Bitterman PB, Rennard, SI, Cantin A, Crystal RG. Characterization of the lower respiratory tract inflammation of non-smoking individuals with interstitial lung disease associated with chronic inhalation of inorganic dusts. Am Rev Respir Dis 1987; 136:1429–1434.

7

Carotenoid Orientation: Role in Membrane Stabilization

Wieslaw I. Gruszecki
Maria Curie-Sklodowska University, Lublin, Poland

I. INTRODUCTION

A rod-like molecule of carotenes lacks polar groups and therefore may be expected to be localized in the hydrophobic core of the lipid membrane, owing to the requirement of energy minimization in a system. On the other hand, the terminal groups of polar carotenoids are expected to interact with the polar head group regions of a lipid bilayer via hydrogen bonds. Such a localization of carotenoids, deduced on the basis of their chemical structure, has a strong experimental support from the analysis of a position of light absorption maxima of carotenoid pigments incorporated to lipid membranes (1–4). Specifically, the positions of absorption maxima of carotenoid pigments incorporated to lipid membranes correlate with the polarizability term of the hydrophobic core of the lipid bilayer, representing dielectric properties of the chromophore environment and calculated on the basis of a refractive index. Figure 1 presents such a dependency plotted for lutein, dissolved in a series of organic solvents and incorporated into liposomes formed with dipalmitoylphosphatidylcholine (DPPC). The value of the polarizability term for the hydrophobic core of DPPC correlates very well with the position of the 0-0 transition in the absorption band of lutein incorporated into this membrane system. The rule that polar end groups of xanthophyll pigments have to remain in direct contact with polar groups of lipid molecules, realized in most cases by hydrogen bonding, determines the orientation of carotenoid molecules with respect to the lipid bilayer, as will be discussed below. Both localization and orientation of carotenoid molecules in the membrane are directly responsible for molecular

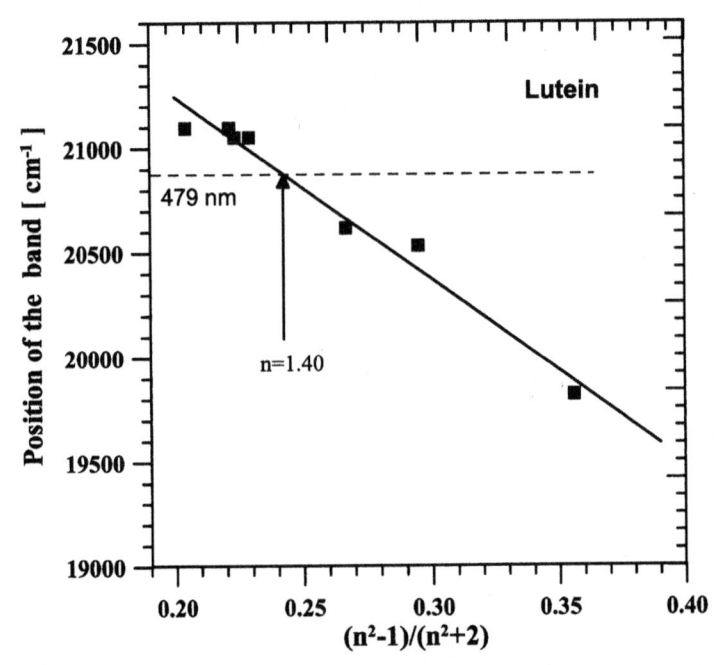

Figure 1 Dependence of the position of the 0-0 vibrational transition in the main electronic absorption band of lutein dissolved in several organic solvents of the refractive index n on the polarizability term. The position of the absorption maximum of lutein embedded to DPPC liposomes [20-879 cm^{-1} (5)] indicated with the dashed line and the value of a polarizability term for the hydrophobic core of DPPC membrane in the L_α phase [0.2424 (6)] indicated by the arrow.

mechanisms of carotenoid–lipid interaction that influence basic physical properties of lipid membranes such as membrane thickness, fluidity, permeability, energy, and cooperativity of phase transitions, etc. Selected aspects of physiologically relevant carotenoid–lipid interactions, directly dependent on carotenoid orientation with respect to the lipid bilayer will also be addressed.

II. ORIENTATION OF CAROTENOIDS IN LIPID MEMBRANES

Figure 2 presents main different patterns of orientation of carotenoid pigments in lipid membranes: not well-defined orientation (as in the case of nonpolar β-carotene), roughly vertical (as in the case of polar zeaxanthin), horizontal (as in the case of *cis*-zeaxanthin), or both horizontal and vertical (as in the case of lutein).

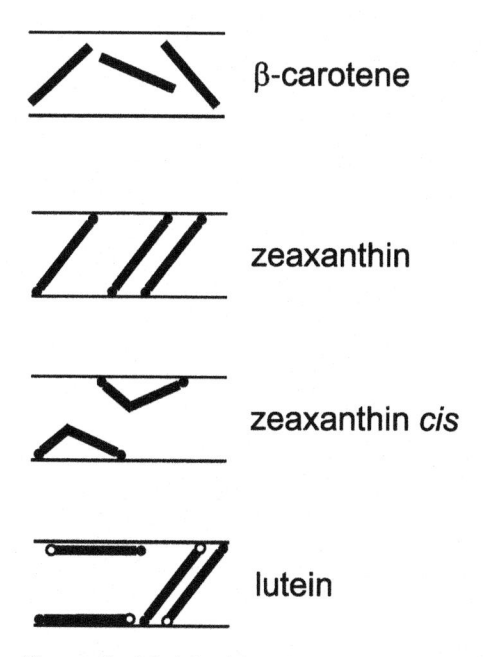

β-carotene

zeaxanthin

zeaxanthin *cis*

lutein

Figure 2 Model of localization and orientation of different in structure carotenoid pigments in the hydrophobic core of lipid membrane. See text for discussion.

Polar groups of xanthophylls are bound to the terminal rings, in almost all physiologically relevant pigments, such as zeaxanthin, lutein, violaxanthin, and astaxanthin. Such localization of polar groups allows the prediction of two essentially different orientation patterns of polar carotenoid pigments in the lipid bilayer: vertical (Fig. 3) and horizontal with respect to the plane of the membrane. The pigment system of C=C bonds has to be located in the hydrophobic core of the membrane in all cases, but polar groups will be anchored in the same head group region or in the opposite polar zones of the bilayer, in the case of horizontal and vertical pigment orientation, respectively. For stereochemical reasons, not all terminally bound polar groups of xanthophylls can remain in contact with the same hydrophobic–hydrophilic interface of the membrane simultaneously. This means that horizontal orientation will be limited to a selected number of polar carotenoids, such as lutein. Lutein and zeaxanthin, the macular pigments, are identical in their chemical composition and very close in structure. Despite that, one essential difference appears that may be responsible for different localization and orientation of these two xanthophyll pigments within a lipid bilayer. Lutein and zeaxanthin contain 11 double bonds but one double bond, in the case of lutein (C_4'-C_5'), is not conjugated to the conjugated double-bond system, in contrast

(A)

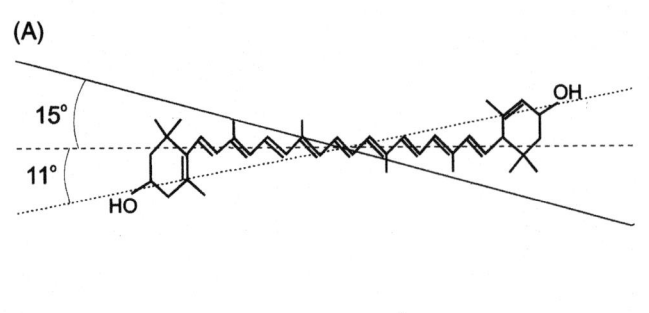

(B)

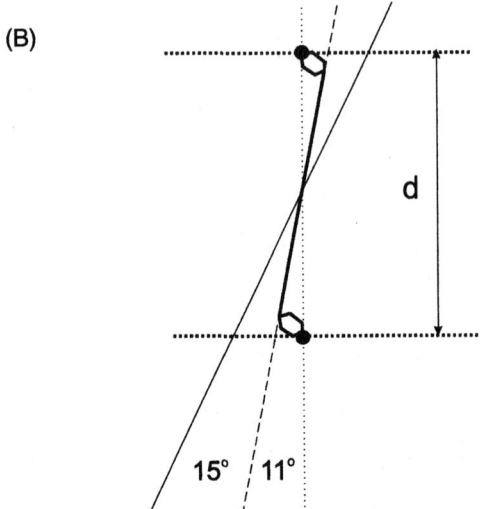

Figure 3 Orientation of the molecular axes of lutein (**A**) and the model of vertical orientation of the pigment incorporated to the lipid membrane (**B**). d is the thickness of the hydrophobic core of the membrane, dotted line the axis connecting opposite hydroxyl groups, dashed line the direction of the chromophore, continuous line the axis of the transition dipole moment tilted by about $15°$ with respect to the linear polyene chromophore (12).

to the terminal double-bond of zeaxanthin (C'_5-C'_6). Such a difference, as may be judged from the spectroscopic point of view, seems to influence stereochemical properties of lutein considerably. Namely, a relative rotational freedom of the entire terminal ring of lutein around the C'_6-C'_7 bond (ε ring) can be predicted, which is unlike in the case of the terminal ring of zeaxanthin. This particular property of lutein is most probably directly responsible for the differences in orientation of lutein and zeaxanthin in model lipid membranes, as determined by means of linear dichroism measurements, carried out in oriented lipid multibilayers composed of several lipid constituents (7,8). Orientation of xanthophyll pigments with terminally located polar groups, such as zeaxanthin (two hydroxyl groups at the C_3 and C_3' positions) can be predicted on the basis of information about the distance between polar groups of the pigment relative to the distance between the opposite polar zones of the lipid bilayer (thickness of the hydrophobic core of the membrane). In several lipid bilayers, the thickness of the hydrophobic core of the membrane [$d = 2.26$ nm in the case of egg yolk phosphatidylcholine (EYPC) and $d = 2.54$ nm in the case of dimyristoylphosphatidylcholine (DMPC)] (7) is less than the distance of hydroxyl groups of C_{40} xanthophyll pigments such as zeaxanthin [$d = 3.2$ nm, (1)] and therefore a tilted orientation of the pigment can be predicted. Such a prediction is in good agreement with experimental linear dichroism data, as can be seen from Table 1. Roughly vertical orientation of the axis connecting the polar groups located at the ends of xanthophyll molecules (Fig. 3) can be predicted in the case of membranes

Table 1 Orientation of Chromophore of Selected Carotenoid Pigments with Respect to the Axis Normal to the Plane of the Lipid Membrane Determined on the Basis of Linear Dichroism Measurements

Carotenoid	Lipid component	Orientation angle (°)	Ref.
β-Carotene	EYPC	55	7
	DOPC	~90	9
	1-Oleoyl-*sn*-glycerol	~90	10
	DMPC	0 and 90	9
Zeaxanthin	EYPC	33	8
	DMPC	25	2
	DPPC	36	8
	DGDG	9	11
	MGDG	17	11
Lutein	EYPC	67	8
	DPPC	57	8
	DHPC	47	8
Violaxanthin	DMPC	22	2
	DGDG	28	11
	MGDG	35	11
Lycopene	EYPC	74	7
Astaxanthin	EYPC	26	7
β-Cryptoxanthin	EYPC	38	7

EYPC, egg yolk phosphatidylcholine; DOPC, dioleoylphosphatidylcholine; DPPC, dipalmitoylphosphatidylcholine; DMPC, dimyristoylphosphatidylcholine; DHPC, dihexadecylphosphatidylcholine; MGDG, monogalactosyldiacylglycerol; DGDG, digalactosyldiacylglycerol.

characterized by a thickness of the hydrophobic core that matches the distance between the polar groups. Such a situation may be expected in the case of thylakoid membranes of chloroplasts ($d = 3$ nm) or the membranes formed with DPPC ($d = 3.2$ nm) (7). The much larger orientation angle values determined in the case of lutein than in the case of zeaxanthin (7,8) may be explained in terms of two pools of the pigment, the first one oriented parallel with respect to the plane of the membrane and the other one oriented the same way or close to that of zeaxanthin. The orientation angles for lutein, with respect to the axis normal to the plane of the membrane, determined as 67° in the case of EYPC or 57° in the case of DPPC correspond to horizontal and roughly vertical pools as 78% and 22% in the case of EYPC or 45% and 55% in the case of DPPC, respectively (8). No distinctly different orientations of lutein and zeaxanthin have been determined in the membranes formed with dihexadecylphosphatidylcholine (DHPC), 47° and 37°, respectively (with the experimental error 4–5°) (8). The fact that DHPC is an analog of DPPC without the keto groups located at the polar–nonpolar interface of the lipid bilayer indicates that the terminal hydroxyl groups of lutein molecules oriented in the plane of the membrane are localized at the interface and interact most probably with the keto groups of lipids.

An essentially different situation, in terms of structural determinants of carotenoid orientation in lipid bilayers, can be expected for membranes containing carotenoid pigments lacking any polar groups that may determine specific pigment localization and orientation. The van der Waals forces between pigment chromophores and alkyl chains of lipid molecules seem to be the sole type of interaction that can potentially influence pigment orientation. Such a situation takes place in membranes containing β-carotene or lycopene. The orientation of lycopene with respect to the axis normal to the plane of the membrane determined as 74° and the orientation of β-carotene determined as 55° in the same system of EYPC membranes (Table 1) are larger or exceptionally close to the magic angle (54.7°), respectively. These results can be interpreted as an indication of roughly horizontal or not well-defined orientations of lycopene and β-carotene, respectively, most probably within the central part of the hydrophobic core of the membrane (Fig. 2). Parallel orientation of β-carotene has also been determined in other experimental systems (Table 1). In some cases, a second possibility of orientation, defined as orthogonal to the parallel one, has been additionally identified for β-carotene (9). This provides a further indication of a complex organization of lipid membranes containing nonpolar carotenoids.

The discussion above refers to the all-*trans* carotenoid pigments, particularly relevant from the physiological point of view. On the other hand, carotenoid pigments in cis conformation are also lipid membrane located and are expected to influence membrane properties at least at a degree comparable to the trans stereoisomers, as can be deduced from the monomolecular layer studies of two-component pigment–lipid systems (Milanowska and Gruszecki, unpublished work). Monomolecular layer technique studies reveals that 9-*cis*- and 13-*cis*-zeaxanthin is oriented in such a way that both hydroxyl groups face the polar–nonpolar interface in the environment of DPPC, at the surface pressure values characteristic of natural biomembranes.

III. EFFECTS OF CAROTENOIDS ON STRUCTURAL AND DYNAMIC PROPERTIES OF LIPID MEMBRANES: BIOLOGICAL CONSEQUENCES

The interaction of membrane-bound carotenoid pigments with both hydrocarbon lipid chains (via van der Waals interactions) and with polar lipid head groups (via hydrogen bonding) determines pigment orientation as discussed above. Furthermore, the interaction influences structural and dynamic properties of the membranes itself. Several techniques have been applied to examine the effect of carotenoid pigments on physical properties of lipid membranes, such as differential scanning calorimetry (DSC) (13–17), ultrasound absorption (18,19), electron spin resonance (ESR) spin label technique (20–26), nuclear magnetic resonance (H^1 NMR, ^{13}C NMR, and P^{31} NMR of lipids) (8,27,28), monomolecular layer technique (4,17,29), X-ray diffractometry (2,11,30–32), fluorescence label technique (16,33), resonance Raman scattering (34), and Fourier transform infrared spectroscopy (35). Theoretical studies have been also carried out, with the application of Monte Carlo simulation of molecular dynamic processes to address this problem (36). The techniques listed above provide information on different aspects of carotenoid–lipid interaction, in particular on dynamics of gauche-trans isomerization of alkyl chains of lipid molecules, that is directly related to membrane fluidity and molecular packing phenomena, both in the head group and hydrocarbon membrane zones, or membrane stability and permeability. As might be expected, the effects of carotenoid pigments on structural and dynamic properties of lipid membranes depend on carotenoid structure (in particular on presence of polar groups). This means that the influence of carotenoids on a membrane is directly related to the molecular localization and orientation of the pigment.

A. Differential Scanning Calorimetry

A calorimetric technique was applied to analyze effect of carotenoid pigments on thermotropic properties of membranes, in particular on a temperature and enthalpy of the phase transition from the ordered to the liquid crystalline phase of lipid bilayers.

In general, the presence of polar carotenoids in the lipid phase decreases enthalpy of the main phase transition of phosphatidylcholines ($P'_\beta \rightarrow L_\alpha$), shifts the transition temperature toward lower values (by about $1°$) and decreases cooperativity of this transition. These effects have been documented in the case of astaxanthin and canthaxanthin in DMPC membranes (15,17), zeaxanthin in DPPC (13,16), lutein in DPPC (37), in DMPC (14), and in lecithin mixtures (16). The effect of β-carotene was found to be much less pronounced and was restricted predominantly to a decrease in the cooperativity of the phase transition (13,14,16,17) which is typical for any additives to the lipid membranes.

B. ESR Spin Labels

The effect of carotenoid pigments on dynamic properties of lipid membranes (directly related to membrane fluidity) was investigated with application of spin labels incorporated into model and natural lipid membranes. The shape of the ESR spectrum of a spin label depends on motional freedom of a free radical segment of a label incorporated into lipid membrane, and therefore spin probes may be applied to follow molecular dynamics phenomena, e.g., associated with phase transitions (20,21). The fact of interaction of paramagnetic molecules of molecular oxygen with the free radical segment of a spin label, manifested in broadening of ESR lines, can be also applied to follow changes in the oxygen diffusion-concentration product in the lipid membrane environment (22). It was found that polar carotenoids decrease cooperativity of the main phase transition of phosphatidylcholines in a concentration-dependent manner. The $P'_\beta \rightarrow L_\alpha$ transition was found to be completely lost at a concentration of 10 mol % of violaxanthin or zeaxanthin (20,21). Polar carotenoids also increase the order parameter of alkyl hydrocarbon chains of membranes formed with unsaturated lipids (in particular in the center of the bilayer) (20), increase the penetration barrier for small molecules and molecular oxygen to the membrane core (22), and increase membrane hydrophobicity (particularly in the center of the bilayer) (23). β-Carotene was found to decrease the penetration barrier for small molecules to the membrane head group region (25,37).

C. H^1 NMR and P^{31} NMR

The molecular dynamics phenomena within lipid membranes, such as very fast gauche–trans isomerization of alkyl chains (correlation time in the order of magnitude of 10^{-9} s), influence the shape of almost all NMR bands associated with lipid molecules involved in formation of membranes. Such a dependency was applied to analyze the effect of carotenoids on dynamic properties of lipid bilayers.

It was found that polar carotenoids broaden spectral lines corresponding to the CH_2 and CH_3 groups of lipid acyl chains (28,37). This effect is due to the restriction of molecular motion of lipids owing to hydrophobic interactions with carotenoids. β-Carotene was demonstrated to increase motional freedom of lipid molecules in the ordered state of the membrane (27). β-Carotene increases also motional freedom of lipids in the head group region (28) and decreases the penetration barrier to the head group region of small charged molecules [praseodymium ions (28)]. From a physiological point of view it is also worth mentioning that polar carotenoids [zeaxanthin (28)] influence mechanical properties of lecithin membranes (reinforcement effect demonstrated in the prolonged sonication during preparation of small unilamellar liposomes).

D. X-Ray Diffractometry

X-ray diffractometry is a technique that, among others, provides the possibility to analyze the thickness of a single bilayer in the experimental system composed of lipid multibilayers. The method is also sensitive to lipid organization in the plane of the membrane and therefore may be applied to analyze the effect of carotenoids on structural properties of lipid bilayers.

Polar carotenoids (in particular lutein) were found to increase the thickness of lipid bilayers. This effect is probably associated, with the molecular mechanism of forcing lipid alkyl chains to adopt extended conformation, owing to the van der Waals interactions with the rigid chromophore (2,11,30,31). Some carotenoids (in particular nonpolar lycopene) were found to disorganize the well-ordered hexagonal molecular packing of lipids [DPPC (32)].

E. Permeability Experiments

Membrane permeability experiments provide direct information on the effect of carotenoid pigments on one of the most important biological function of lipid membranes, namely, providing a barrier for nonspecific transport of ions and small organic molecules. Zeaxanthin incorporated to unilamellar digalactosyldiacylglycerol vesicles at 2 mol % was found to increase significantly the permeability barrier across the lipid membranes for protons (38). Incorporation of polar carotenoids thermozeaxanthins (zeaxanthin glucose esters) to large unilamellar liposomes was found to increase the permeability barrier across the lipid membranes for water-soluble fluorescent dye calcein in the case of membranes formed with EYPC (39). Such a pronounced effect has not been observed in the case of DMPC, DPPC, and DOPC, and the difference was discussed in terms of matching of the thickness of the hydrophobic core of the lipid bilayer with the molecular length and orientation of thermozeaxanthins (39).

The effects of carotenoid pigments on lipid membranes, presented above, clearly demonstrate a crucial role of pigment chemical structure on the extent of an effect and in several cases even on the direction of an effect observed.

Only polar carotenoids have been found to influence essentially membrane properties and stabilize structure of a lipid bilayer. On the contrary, nonpolar carotenoids such as β-carotene and lycopene have been found to destabilize the membranes and reduce the penetration barrier for several classes of molecules to the membrane. These effects coincide with orientation of carotenoid molecules with respect to the membrane: well determined and defined only in the case of xanthophylls. There may be discussion regarding the association of carotenoid orientation with the influence of pigments on the membrane properties. It is rather clear that rigid, rodlike xanthophyll molecules anchored in the opposite polar zones of the membrane restrict molecular motion of lipids, such as rotational diffusion or gauche-trans isomerization of alkyl chains, owing to van der Waals interactions, thus affecting the membrane fluidity and increasing the structural stability. Heterogeneously localized and oriented molecules of nonpolar carotenoids are not involved in that case of membrane stabilization.

ACKNOWLEDGMENTS

The author thanks graduate students Wojtek Grudzinski, Justyna Milanowska, and Monika Herec for help in preparing figures, stimulating discussions, and other means of assistance during preparation of this chapter.

REFERENCES

1. Milon A, Wolff G, Ourisson G, Nakatani Y. Organization of carotenoid-phospholipid bilayer systems. Incorporation of zeaxanthin, astaxanthin, and their C_{50} homologues into dimyristoylphosphatidylcholine vesicles. Helv Chim Acta 1986; 69:12–24.
2. Gruszecki WI, Sielewiesiuk J. Orientation of xanthophylls in phosphatidylcholine multibilayers. Biochim Biophys Acta 1990; 1023:405–412.
3. Andersson PO, Gilbro T, Fergusson L. Absorption spectral shifts of carotenoids related to medium polarizability. Photochem Photobiol 1991; 54:353–360.
4. Sujak A, Gruszecki WI. Organization of mixed monomolecular layers formed with the xanthophyll pigments lutein or zeaxanthin and dipalmitoylphosphatidylcholine at the argon—water interface. J Photochem Photobiol B Biol 2000; 59:42–47.
5. Sujak A, Okulski W, Gruszecki WI. Organization of xanthophyll pigments lutein and zeaxanthin in lipid membranes formed with dipalmitoylphosphatidylcholine. Biochim Biophys Acta 2000; 1509:255–263.
6. Gagos M, Koper R, Gruszecki WI. Spectrophotometric analysis of organization of dipalmitoylphosphatidylcholine bilayers containing the polyene antibiotic amphotericin B. Biochim Biophys Acta 2001; 1511:90–98.

7. Gruszecki WI. Carotenoids in membranes. In: Frank HA, Young AJ, Britton G, Cogdell RJ, eds. The Photochemistry of Carotenoids, Dordrecht: Kluwer Academic, 1999:363–379.

8. Sujak A, Gabrielska J, Grudzinski W, Borc R, Mazurek P, Gruszecki WI. Lutein and zeaxanthin as protectors of lipid membranes against oxidative damage: the structural aspects. Arch Biochem Biophys 1999; 371:301–307.

9. Van de Ven M, Kattenberg M, Van Ginkel G, Levine YK. Study of the orientational ordering of carotenoids in lipid bilayers by resonance Raman spectroscopy. Biophys J 1984; 45:1203–1210.

10. Johansson LB-A, Lindblom G, Wieslander A, Arvidson G. Orientation of β-carotene and retinal in lipid bilayers. FEBS Lett 1981; 128:97–99.

11. Gruszecki WI, Sielewiesiuk J. Galactolipid multibilayers modified with xanthophylls: orientational and diffractometric studies. Biochim Biophys Acta 1991; 1069: 21–26.

12. Shang Q, Dou X, Hudson BS. Off-axis orientation of the electronic transition moment for a linear conjugated polyene. Nature 1991; 352:703–705.

13. Kolev VD, Kafalieva DN. Miscibility of β-carotene and zeaxanthin with dipalmitoylphosphatidylcholine in multilamellar vesicles: a calorimetric and spectroscopic study. Photobiochem Photobiophys 1986; 11:257–267.

14. Castelli F, Caruso S, Giuffrida N. Different effects of two structurally similar carotenoids, lutein and β-carotene, on the thermotropic behaviour of phosphatidylcholine liposomes. Calorimetric evidence of their hindered transport through biomembranes. Thermochim Acta 1999; 327:125–131.

15. Rengel D, Diez-Navajas A, Serna-Rico P, Veiga P, Muga A, Milicua JCG. Exogenously incorporated ketocarotenoids in large unilamellar vesicles. Protective activity against peroxidation. Biochim Biophys Acta 2000; 1463:179–187.

16. Socaciu C, Jessel R, Diehl HA. Competitive carotenoid and cholesterol incorporation into liposomes: effects on membrane phase transition, fluidity, polarity and anisotropy. Chem Phys Lipids 2000; 106:79–88.

17. Shibata A, Kiba Y, Akati N, Fukuzawa K, Terada H. Molecular characteristics of astaxanthin and β-carotene in the phospholipid monolayer and their distributions in the the phospholipid bilayer. Chem Phys Lipids 2001; 113:11–22.

18. Wojtowicz K, Gruszecki WI, Okulski W, Juszkiewicz A, Orzechowski A, Gawda H. Phase transition of zeaxanthin-modified dimyristoylphosphatidylcholine liposomes as monitored by acoustic measurements. Stud Biophys 1991; 140:115–120.

19. Wojtowicz K, Gruszecki WI. Effect of β-carotene, lutein and violaxanthin on structural properties of dipalmitoylphosphatidylcholine liposomes as studied by ultrasound absorption technique. J Biol Phys 1995; 21:73–80.

20. Subczynski WK, Markowska E, Gruszecki WI, Sielewiesiuk J. Effects of polar carotenoids on dimyristoylphosphatidylcholine membranes: a spin-label study. Biochim Biophys Acta 1992; 1105:97–108.

21. Subczynski WK, Markowska E, Sielewiesiuk J. Spin-label studies on phosphatidylcholine-polar carotenoid membranes: effects of alkyl-chain length and unsaturation. Biochim Biophys Acta 1993; 1150:173–181.

22. Subczynski WK, Markowska E, Sielewiesiuk J. Effect of polar carotenoids on the oxygen diffusion-concentration product in lipid bilayers. An EPR spin label study. Biochim Biophys Acta 1991; 1068:68–72.

23. Wisniewska A, Subczynski WK. Effects of polar carotenoids on the shape of the hydrophobic barrier of phospholipid bilayers. Biochim Biophys Acta 1998; 1368:235–246.

24. Yin J-J, Subczynski WK. Effects of lutein and cholesterol on alkyl chain bending in lipid bilayers: a pulse electron spin resonance spin labelling study. Biophys J 1996; 71:832–839.

25. Strzalka K, Gruszecki WI. Effect of β-carotene on structural and dynamic properties of model phosphatidylcholine membranes. I. An EPR spin label study. Biochim Biophys Acta 1994; 1194:138–142.

26. Strzalka K, Gruszecki WI. Modulation of thylakoid membrane fluidity by exogenously added carotenoids. J Biochem Mol Biol Biophys 1997; 1:103–108.

27. Jezowska I, Wolak A, Gruszecki WI, Strzalka K. Effect of β-carotene on structural and dynamic properties of model phosphatidylcholine membranes. II. A ^{31}P-NMR and ^{13}C-NMR study. Biochim Biophys Acta 1994; 1194:143–148.

28. Gabrielska J, Gruszecki WI. Zeaxanthin (dihydroxy-β-carotene) but not β-carotene rigidifies lipid membranes: a ^{1}H NMR study of carotenoid-egg phosphatidylcholine liposomes. Biochim Biophys Acta 1996; 1285:167–174.

29. N'soukpoe-Kossi Ch, Sielewiesiuk J, Leblanc RM, Bone RA, Landrum JT. Linear dichroism and orientational studies of carotenoid Langmuir–Blodgett films. Biochim Biophys Acta 1988; 940:255–265.

30. Gruszecki WI, Smal A, Szymczuk D. The effect of zeaxanthin on the thickness of dimyristoylphosphatidylcholine bilayer: X-ray diffraction study. J Biol Phys 1992; 18:271–280.

31. Sujak A, Mazurek P, Gruszecki WI. Xanthophyll pigments lutein and zeaxanthin in lipid multibilayers formed with dimyristoylphosphatidylcholine. J Photochem Photobiol B Biol 2002; 68:39–44.

32. Suwalsky M, Hidalgo P, Strzalka K, Kostecka-Gugala A. Comparative X-Ray studies on the interaction of carotenoids with a model phosphatidylcholine membranes. Z Naturforsch 2002; 57c:129–134.

33. Socaciu C, Lausch C, Diehl HA. Carotenoids in DPPC vesicles: membrane dynamics. Spectrochim Acta A 1999; 55:2289–2297.

34. Mendelsohn R, Van Holten RW. Zeaxanthin ([3R,3'R]-β,β-carotene-3-3'diol) as a resonance Raman and visible absorption probe of membrane structure. Biophys J 1979; 27:221–236.

35. Varkonyi Z, Masamoto K, Debreczeny M, Zsiros O, Ughy B, Gombos Z, Domonkos I, Farkas T, Wada H, Szalontai B. Low-temperature-induced accumulation of xanthophylls and its structural consequences in the photosynthetic membranes of the cyanobacterium Cylindrospermopsis raciborski: an FTIR spectroscopic study. Proc Natl Acad Sci USA 2002; 99:2410–2415.

36. Okulski W, Sujak A, Gruszecki WI. Dipalmitoylphosphatidylcholine membranes modified with zeaxanthin: numeric study of membrane organization. Biochim Biophys Acta 2000; 1509:216–228.

37. Chaturvedi VK, Kurup CKR. Interaction of lutein with phosphatidylcholine bilayers. Biochim Biophys Acta 1986; 860:286–292.
38. Berglund AH, Nilsson R, Liljenberg C. Permeability of large unilamellar digalactosyldiacylglycerol vesicles for protons and glucose—influence of α-tocopherol, β-carotene, zeaxanthin and cholesterol. Plant Physiol Biochem 1999; 37:179–186.
39. Hara M, Yuan H, Yang Q, Hoshino T, Yokoyama A, Miyake J. Stabilization of liposomal membranes by thermozeaxanthins: carotenoid-glucoside esters. Biochim Biophys Acta 1999; 1461:147–154.

8
Anticancer Activity of Carotenoids: From Human Studies to Cellular Processes and Gene Regulation

Yoav Sharoni, Michael Danilenko and Joseph Levy
Ben-Gurion University of the Negev and Soroka Medical Center of Kupat Holim, Beer-Sheva, Israel

Wilhelm Stahl
Heinrich-Heine Universität, Düsseldorf, Germany

I. INTRODUCTION

Fruits and vegetables have an important role in the prevention of cancer. Carotenoids have been implicated as an important group of phytochemicals that are involved in cancer prevention. However, when reviewing data related to the chemopreventive effects of phytochemicals, one should bear in mind that the use of a single carotenoid or any other micronutrient as a "magic bullet," which had been successful in in vitro and in vivo models, did not prove as favorable in human intervention studies. In contrast, accumulating evidence suggests that a concerted, synergistic action of various micronutrients is more likely to be the basis of the cancer-preventive activity of a diet rich in vegetables and fruit.

The possible mechanisms underlying the anticancer activity of carotenoids will be the focus of this chapter. Carotenoids function as potent antioxidants, and this is clearly a major mechanism of their action. However, accumulating data support other mechanisms as well. In addition, growing evidence indicates that the activity does not always reside in the carotenoid molecule and that metabolites and oxidation products of the carotenoids are the definitive active compounds in certain pathways. We discuss the effects of carotenoids and their derivatives on the basic mechanisms of cell proliferation, growth factor signaling, gap junctional intercellular communication, and detoxification of carcinogens. The existing evidence suggests that carotenoids produce changes in the expression of many proteins participating in these basic processes such as connexins, phase II enzymes, cyclins, cyclin-dependent kinases, and their inhibitors. The changes in protein expression support the hypothesis that the initial effect of carotenoids involves modulation of transcription by certain transcription factors, including ligand-activated nuclear receptors. It is feasible to suggest that carotenoids and their oxidized derivatives interact with a network of transcription systems that are activated by different ligands at low affinity and specificity and that this activation leads to the synergistic inhibition of cell growth.

II. EPIDEMIOLOGICAL EVIDENCE AND HUMAN INTERVENTION STUDIES

Carotenoids have been implicated as important dietary phytonutrients having cancer-preventive activity (1). Interest in carotenoids, especially β-carotene, arose not only because of their antioxidant activity but also because their metabolites, vitamin A and retinoic acid, may be active via other mechanisms, such as induction of cellular differentiation or cell death. β-Carotene has received the most attention because of its provitamin A activity and its prevalence in many foods. However, intervention studies with β-carotene yielded disappointing findings (see below), and thus other carotenoids became the subject of more intensive investigation. Two carotenoids with provitamin A activity, α-carotene and β-cryptoxanthin, are also abundant in foods and contribute substantially to vitamin A intake. Carotenoids without vitamin A activity that are relatively well studied because of their high concentration in serum include lycopene, lutein, and zeaxanthin. Much of the evidence, particularly in terms of cancer prevention, is derived from observational studies of dietary carotenoid intake and thus the findings must be interpreted with caution. In such studies it is not clear if an association between diet and disease is due to the specific carotenoid, other micronutrients present in the specific diet, or the combined effect of several of these active ingredients. Many studies have evaluated the relation between carotenoid intake and cancer. The best evidence for an inverse association exists for lung, colon, breast, and prostate cancer; these data are discussed below.

A. Lung Cancer

Observational studies strongly support an inverse relation between the intake of β-carotene and lung cancer risk. A summary of various epidemiological studies published up to 1995 indicated an inverse relationship for 13 of 14 case-control studies, all of the 5 cohort studies related to dietary β-carotene intake and all of the 7 studies in which the plasma level of the carotenoid was followed (2). Two large cohort studies (3,4) have demonstrated an inverse association with α-carotene intake as well. A recent report combined updated observational data from the Nurses' Health Study and the Health Professional Follow-up Study and found significant risk reduction for lycopene and α-carotene but nonsignificant risk reduction for β-carotene (5). A significant reduction in risk of lung cancer for people consuming a diet high in variety of carotenoids was also observed. In another study, high lycopene intake was associated with lower risk for lung cancer (6). Two large randomized placebo controlled trials, the ATBC study (7) and the CARET study (8), assessed the risk of lung cancer among male smokers or asbestos workers receiving β-carotene supplementation. Both showed statistically significant increases in lung cancer risk among the men who received the supplement. Three other intervention studies did not reveal any beneficial effect of β-carotene supplementation (9–11).

B. Colorectal and Other Digestive Tract Cancers

Several randomized trials have shown no reduction in colorectal cancer risk with β-carotene supplementation (8,10). However, two trials indicated that among regular alcohol users β-carotene supplementation decreases colon cancer risk (12,13). The carotenoid supplementation in alcohol users may be more effective because their serum β-carotene levels appear to be lower than in nonusers (14,15). In another study (16), β-carotene was not effective in preventing colorectal adenoma (a precursor of invasive carcinoma). High lycopene intake was associated with lower risk for gastric cancer (17). In an integrated series of studies in Italy (18), tomato consumption showed a consistent inverse relation with a risk of digestive tract neoplasms. However, these findings were not confirmed by other studies (19,20).

C. Prostate Cancer

The relationship between β-carotene intake and prostate cancer has been examined in observational studies with varied results (21). Intervention trials have revealed either no association of β-carotene supplementation with prostate cancer risk (8,9) or an increase in prostate cancer incidence and mortality (22,23). However, some reduction in prostate cancer risk was evident in these studies in certain subpopulations (15,23). Giovannucci et al. (24,25) reported a reduction in prostate cancer risk among men with high lycopene consumption from tomatoes and tomato products. Additional studies have reported similar findings for tomato products (17,26–28). However, these conclusions were not established in a recent study based on lycopene intake data obtained from food frequency questionnaires (29). Two of three studies in which blood lycopene levels were measured reported an association between higher lycopene levels and reduction of prostate cancer risk (27,28). A third study (30), carried out in Japan, found no association, but its value is limited because of the low lycopene levels in the Japanese population.

Two small-scale, preliminary intervention studies in prostate cancer patients were carried out with natural tomato preparations. In one, Bowen et al. (31) showed that after dietary intervention, serum and prostate lycopene concentrations were increased, and oxidative DNA damage both in leukocytes and in prostate tissue was significantly lower. Furthermore, serum levels of prostate-specific antigen (PSA) decreased after the intervention. In the other study, Kucuk et al. (32) reported that supplementation with tomato extract in men with prostate cancer modulates the grade and volume of prostate intraepithelial neoplasia and tumor, the level of serum PSA, and the level of biomarkers of cell growth and differentiation.

D. Breast Cancer

Observational studies investigating the relationship between carotenoids, mainly β-carotene, and breast cancer have shown varied results. A comprehensive review of the literature published in 1997 (33) reported that the majority of studies did not show reduced breast cancer risk with increased β-carotene consumption. Since that review, four cohort studies have reported no association between the intake of carotenoids and breast cancer risk (34–37). A fifth cohort study found that premenopausal women have a significant reduction in breast cancer risk with an increase in dietary α- and β-carotene, lutein/zeaxanthin, and total vitamin A intake (38). A recent case-control study concluded that increased serum levels of β-carotene, retinol, bilirubin, and total antioxidant status are associated with reductions in breast cancer risk (39). High lycopene intake was associated with lower risk for breast cancer (40,41). Mixed results were obtained in six studies nested within prospective cohorts in which carotenoid serum levels were monitored. Results from the four smaller studies showed no decrease in breast cancer risk with higher serum carotenoid (42–45). In contrast, an inverse relationship for β-cryptoxanthin, lycopene, lutein, and zeaxanthin was found in the two larger studies (46,47).

A comprehensive review of the epidemiological literature on the relation of tomato consumption and cancer risk in general was published by Giovannucci (48). He found that most of the reviewed studies reported inverse associations between tomato intake or blood lycopene level and the risk of various types of cancer. The evidence for a beneficial effect was strongest for cancers of the prostate, lung, and stomach. Data also suggested a beneficial effect for cancers of the pancreas, colon and rectum, esophagus, oral cavity, breast, and cervix. Giovannucci suggests that lycopene may contribute to these beneficial effects of tomato-containing foods but that the anticancer properties could also be explained by interactions among multiple components found in tomatoes.

III. EFFECTS OF CAROTENOIDS ON CANCER IN ANIMAL EXPERIMENTAL MODELS

One of the problems confronting investigators studying the effect of carotenoids in animal models is that rat and mouse, the species most widely utilized for cancer research, poorly absorb dietary carotenoids. In addition, to achieve a clear anticancer effect in short-term experiments, high carotenoid tissue levels are necessary; thus, the animals are fed diets containing large amounts of carotenoids. Therefore, the extrapolation of results to the situation in humans may be even more difficult than anticipated (49). Despite these shortcomings, rodents have been extensively used to evaluate the role of dietary carotenoids in the development of cancer (50–54). Many of these studies have indicated that the formation and growth of various types of tumors are reduced by treatment with different carotenoids.

Lycopene effectively inhibits the growth of glioma cells transplanted in rats (55), development of spontaneous mammary tumors in SHN virgin mice (50,56), and induction of rat mammary tumors by dimethylbenz[a]anthracene (DMBA) (57). Lycopene has also been shown to inhibit the development of aberrant colonic crypt foci induced by N-methylnitrosourea in Sprague–Dawley rats (51), but not the development of preneoplastic aberrant crypt foci induced in mouse by 1,2-dimethylhydrazine (58). β-Carotene, α-carotene, lycopene, and lutein were found to decrease hepatocyte cell injury induced by carbon tetrachloride (59) and to protect against the liver tumor promoter microcystin-LR (60). The incidences and multiplicities of lung adenomas and carcinomas induced by 1,2-dimethylhydrazine in male (but not female) mice were significantly decreased by lycopene treatment (61). Tomato juice containing a combination of lycopene and other antioxidants was observed to exert an inhibitory effect on the development of transitional cell carcinomas in rat urinary bladder initiated with N-butyl-N-(4-hydroxybutyl)nitrosamine (62). Administration of lycopene significantly suppressed the incidence of DMBA-induced hamster buccal pouch tumors (63). An interesting new experimental approach for the prevention of colon cancer was suggested by Arimochi and colleagues in a rat model (64). They found that feeding rats with lycopene-producing *Escherichia coli* strains significantly lowered the number of preneoplastic, azoxymethane-induced, aberrant crypt foci in the colon.

IV. ANTIPROLIFERATIVE EFFECTS OF CAROTENOIDS ON CANCER CELLS

Numerous in vitro studies have been performed to verify the role of carotenoids in cell proliferation and differentiation. In a study on both estrogen receptor–positive (MCF-7) and negative (Hs578T and MDA-MB-231) human breast cancer cells (65), β-carotene significantly inhibited the growth of MCF-7 and Hs578T cells and lycopene inhibited the growth of MCF-7 and MDA-MB-231 cells, whereas cantaxanthin did not affect the proliferation of any of the three cell lines. The same group also studied the effects of synthetic excentric cleavage products of β-carotene in these cells (66). β-Apo-14'-carotenoic acid and β-apo-12'-carotenoic acid significantly inhibited MCF-7 cell growth, whereas only β-apo-14'-carotenoic acid inhibited Hs578T cell growth. None of these treatments inhibited the growth of MDA-MB-231 cells.

Lycopene inhibited proliferation of endometrial (Ishikawa), mammary (MCF-7), leukemic (HL-60), and lung (NCI-H226) human cancer cells with half-maximal inhibitory concentration of $1-2$ μM. β-Carotene was a far less effective inhibitor (67,68). For example, in Ishikawa cells, a 10-fold higher concentration of β-carotene was needed for comparable growth suppression. Lycopene alone was not a potent inhibitor of androgen-independent prostate carcinoma cell proliferation. However, the simultaneous addition of lycopene and α-tocopherol at physiological concentrations resulted in a strong synergistic inhibition of cell growth (69) (see Sec. V for details). The possibility that an oxidation product of lycopene can mediate the inhibitory action of this carotenoid on cell growth is suggested by the following studies. When lycopene was provided as a micellar preparation, which stabilizes the carotenoid and probably prevents formation of oxidation products, it did not inhibit the proliferation of LNCaP human prostate cancer cells (70). By contrast, lycopene solubilized in tetrahydrofuran inhibited growth in LNCaP cells [(71) and authors' unpublished work] and other (71,72) prostate cancer cell lines.

Inhibitory effects of various carotenoids and retinoids on the in vitro growth of rat C-6 glioma cells was reported by Wang (73). The effects of 15 different carotenoids on the viability of three lines of human prostate cancer cells (PC-3, DU-145, and LNCaP) were recently evaluated (71). Prostate cancer cells were cultured in a medium supplemented with carotenoids at 20 μM for 72 h. At this high concentration, several carotenoids, including those present in tomatoes (lycopene, phytoene, phytofluene, ζ-carotene and β-carotene), significantly reduced cell viability due to induction of apoptosis. In another study, phytofluene at 10 μM inhibited HL-60 cell growth (74). The ability of astaxanthin to affect cancer cells in vitro has been addressed in only a few studies. For instance, Kozuki et al. found that 5 μM astaxanthin inhibited the invasion of AH109A rat ascites hepatoma cells (75).

Although carotenoids are not produced by mammalian cells, Nishino succeeded in demonstrating the cancer-preventive activity of phytoene by establishing a mammalian cell clone that produces phytoene (54). This was achieved by introducing the phytoene synthase gene which converts the NIH3T3 cell line to a carotenoid-producing one. This specific genetic manipulation caused the mammalian cells to become resistant to H-ras-induced cell transformation.

The human and animal studies reviewed above suggest a cancer-preventive activity for carotenoids. However, the in vitro effects of carotenoids at the low concentrations that can be achieved in human blood (about 1 μM) have not been studied extensively. At the submicromolar concentrations found in serum of many North Europeans and aging populations, carotenoids exhibit weak, if any, antiproliferative activity on various cancer cells (67). Hence, the preventive effects of carotenoids may be related to the synergistic action of these and other active dietary components.

V. SYNERGISTIC INHIBITION OF CANCER CELL GROWTH BY COMBINATION OF VARIOUS CAROTENOIDS AND OTHER MICRONUTRIENTS

The use of a single plant-derived compound in human prevention studies has not been particularly successful as evidenced from the large intervention studies carried out with β-carotene (7–9,11,16). These results seem to indicate that the beneficial effects of diets rich in vegetables and fruit are not related to the action of a single compound but rather to the concerted action of several micronutrients, which when used alone are active only at high (and sometimes toxic) concentrations. To support this hypothesis, it has to be shown that plant-derived constituents, such as carotenoids, have the ability to act synergistically with other compounds in inhibiting cancer cell growth. We have been studying the anticancer activities of combinations of various micronutrients or their metabolites, including carotenoids (β-carotene, lycopene, phytoene, phytofluene, and astaxanthin), polyphenolic antioxidants (e.g., carnosic acid from rosemary), an organosulfur compound (allicin from garlic), the active metabolite of vitamin D (1,25-dihydroxyvitamin D_3), the metabolite of β-carotene and vitamin A (retinoic acid), and a synthetic derivative of lycopene (*acyclo*-retinoic acid; see Sec. VII.A) in different cancer cell lines. Various combinations of these compounds have resulted in synergistic or additive inhibition of cancer cell growth. For example, a combination of low concentrations of lycopene with 1,25-dihydroxyvitamin D_3 [$1,25(OH)_2D_3$] synergistically suppressed proliferation and induced differentiation in HL-60 leukemic cells (68). Pastori and colleagues have found that the simultaneous addition of lycopene and another vitamin, α-tocopherol, at physiological concentrations resulted in a strong synergistic inhibition of prostate carcinoma cell proliferation (69). This effect was not shared by other antioxidants, such as β-tocopherol, ascorbic acid, and probucol, implying that some natural antioxidant compounds can cooperate with other agents in the antiproliferative action via mechanisms unrelated to their antioxidant properties. Different micronutrients, such as carnosic acid (76,77), α-tocopherol, lipoic acid, β-carotene (78), and curcumin (79), were found to potentiate the effects of $1,25(OH)_2D_3$ on cell growth and differentiation. Furthermore, micronutrients can also cooperate with anticancer drugs. It has been shown that palm oil tocotrienols (80) and indole-3-carbinol found in cabbage, broccoli, and other cruciferous vegetables (81) enhanced the growth-inhibitory effect of the antiestrogen drug tamoxifen in MCF-7 cells.

Some of the above studies have shown that the synergistic suppression of cancer cell growth by combinations of low doses of micronutrients is associated with the augmented inhibition of cell cycle progression (68,76,77,79). Elucidation of the mechanisms underlying the cooperative effects at the level of the cell cycle machinery and other cellular processes may provide a basis for the synergistic inhibition of cancer cell growth by various dietary and pharmacological agents.

VI. CELLULAR AND MOLECULAR MECHANISMS OF CAROTENOID ACTION

As discussed below, carotenoids exert pleiotropic effects on various aspects of cell function that can explain their interference in different stages of cancer development. This chapter focuses on processes that are important for the regulation of cell proliferation, including cell cycle progression, growth factor signaling, and gap junctional intercellular communication. Additional mechanisms have been suggested to underlie the anticancer activity of carotenoids, including antioxidant (this volume, Chapter) and pro-oxidant (this volume, Chapter) effects, antigenotoxic actions (82,83), and immunomodulation (84,85).

A. Regulation of Cell Cycle by Carotenoids

The carotenoid-induced reduction in cancer cell proliferation reported in the in vivo and in vitro studies mentioned above can result from cell death or from inhibition of cell cycle progression or both. Several studies have shown that at high concentrations (20 μM and higher) carotenoids decrease cell viability by inducing apoptosis (71,86). On the other hand, we have demonstrated that the inhibitory effects of low lycopene concentrations (1–4 μM) on the growth of cancer cells are not accompanied by necrotic or apoptotic cell death. This was determined by lactate dehydrogenase release and trypan blue exclusion assays, annexin V binding to plasma membrane, propidium iodide staining of nuclei (68,87), and the proteolytic degradation of poly(ADP-ribose) polymerase (unpublished data). Instead, these antiproliferative effects were accompanied by inhibition of cell cycle progression in the G_0/G_1 phase as measured by flow cytometry (68,87). A similar inhibition of cell cycle progression by α-carotene (88) and fucoxanthin, a carotenoid prepared from brown algae (89), was demonstrated in GOTO human neuroblastoma cells. These data suggest that the inhibitory effects of carotenoids on cancer cell growth at concentrations that can be achieved in human blood are not due to the toxicity of the carotenoids but rather to interference in cell cycle progression. Thus, to understand how carotenoids inhibit cell growth it is important to elucidate their effects on the cell cycle machinery.

Cell cycle transition through a late G_1 checkpoint is governed by a mechanism known as the "pRb pathway" [see (90) for a review]. The central element of this pathway, retinoblastoma protein (pRb), is a tumor suppressor that prevents premature G_1/S transition via interaction with transcription factors of the E2F family. The activity of pRb is regulated by an assembly of cyclins, cyclin-dependent kinases (CDKs) and CDK inhibitors. Phosphorylation of pRb by CDKs results in the release of E2F, which leads to the synthesis of various cell growth–related proteins. CDK activity is modulated in both a positive and a negative manner by cyclins and CDK inhibitors, respectively. It is well documented that growth factors affect the cell cycle apparatus primarily during G_1 phase, and that the main components acting as growth factor sensors are the D-type cyclins (91). Moreover, cyclin D is known as an oncogene and is found to be overexpressed in many breast cancer cell lines as well as in primary tumors (92).

Despite the great body of evidence showing inhibition of the cell cycle by carotenoids, to date few studies have addressed the mode of their effect on the cell cycle machinery. For example, in normal human fibroblasts, β-carotene induced a cell cycle delay in G_1 phase. This delay was associated with an increase in the protein level of the CDK inhibitor $p21^{Cip1/Waf1}$ (p21), an increase in the amount of p21 associated with cdk4, the inhibition of cyclin D_1–associated cdk4 kinase activity, and a decrease in the levels of hyperphosphorylated forms of pRb (93). On the other hand, in prostate cancer cells, β-carotene inhibited growth independently of p21 expression (94). Tibaduiza et al. (66) have found that the inhibition of mammary cancer cell growth by synthetic excentric cleavage products of β-carotene is associated with reduced expression of E2F1 and pRb proteins. In a recent study (95), Nahum et al. demonstrated that cancer cells arrested by serum deprivation in the presence of lycopene are incapable of reentering the cell cycle after serum readdition. This inhibition correlated with a decrease in cyclin D_1 protein levels that resulted in inhibition of cdk4 and cdk2 kinase activity and phosphorylation of pRb. Abundance of p21 was decreased whereas the levels of another CDK inhibitor, $p27^{Kip1}$ (p27), were unchanged. Inhibition of cdk4 was directly related to the lower amount of cyclin D_1–cdk4 complexes while inhibition of cdk2 action was related to a shift of the p27 molecules from cdk4 complexes to cyclin E–cdk2 complexes. Palozza et al. (86,96) demonstrated that β-carotene inhibits the growth of several human colon adenocarcinoma cell lines and promyelocytic leukemia cells by inducing cell cycle arrest in G_2/M phase and apoptosis. These effects were dose and time dependent and strictly related to the ability of cells to accumulate the carotenoid. At inhibitory concentrations, β-carotene lowered the expression of cyclin A, a key regulator of G_2/M progression. Neither p21 nor p27, two cyclin kinase inhibitors, were significantly modified by carotenoid treatment.

Similar to carotenoids, other plant-derived compounds produce diverse effects on the cell cycle machinery. For instance, G_1 phase arrest in human prostate carcinoma and breast carcinoma cells by silymarin, a flavonoid antioxidant isolated from milk thistle, was accompanied by a reduction in CDK activities, mainly due to up-regulation of p21 and p27 (97,98). In breast cancer cells, but not in prostate cancer cells, cyclins D_1 and E decreased as well. Flavone also caused induction of p21 associated with inhibition of pRb phosphorylation in A549 lung adenocarcinoma cells (99). Many other inhibitors of cancer cell growth, such as tamoxifen, pure antiestrogens, retinoids, progestins, transforming growth factor-β and tumor necrosis factor-α have been shown to reduce cyclin D expression (100). Some of these compounds also increase levels of p21 and p27, where as others, such as retinoic acid, decrease cdk2 protein abundance (101). Taken together, these findings demonstrate that various phytochemicals and drugs suppress the cell cycle via different mechanisms. Therefore, synergistic antiproliferative effects of various combinations of low doses of these agents, including carotenoids, can result from their complementary effects on different components of the cell cycle machinery converging at the key regulatory steps, e.g., pRb phosphorylation.

B. Carotenoids and the Insulin-Like Growth Factor System

The identification of risk factors for various types of cancer can lead to appropriate preventive measures. The importance of the sex steroids estradiol and testosterone for the development and progression of breast and prostate cancers, respectively, is well known. Recently, a similar role has been proposed for insulin-like growth factor-I (IGF-I). Chan et al. (102) found a strong positive association between IGF-I levels and prostate cancer risk in participants of the Physicians' Health Study. An equally strong association between the level of this growth factor and breast cancer risk of premenopausal women was also reported in a case control study within the Nurses' Health Study cohort (103) and, more recently, for colorectal cancer (104). Thus, plasma IGF-I levels may be useful for identifying individuals at high risk for some major cancers, similar to the way in which cholesterol levels predict the risk of cardiovascular diseases. As already discussed (Sec. II.C), there is an inverse association between lycopene intake (24) or its blood level (28) and prostate cancer risk. Although it seems justified to make a connection between the reduced risk associated with lycopene and the increased risk associated with IGF-I blood levels, this possibility has only been partially addressed.

Two possible mechanisms can account for the lowering of cancer risk by lycopene. The carotenoid may decrease IGF-I blood level, thereby diminishing the risk associated with its elevation, and/or it can interfere with IGF-I activity in the cancer cell. Studies of the effect of lycopene on IGF-I blood levels are in progress in our clinical center as well as in others. For example, the consumption of cooked tomatoes was substantially and significantly inversely associated with IGF-I levels (105). However, in a small-scale intervention study, no significant effect of tomato oleoresin on IGF-I blood levels was found (32). With respect to the intracellular activity of IGF-I, our findings suggest that cell growth inhibition by lycopene involves interference in the mitogenic pathway of IGF-I. We found that IGF-I-stimulated cell growth was inhibited by lower physiological concentrations of lycopene than those needed for inhibition in unstimulated cells (67,87). These findings suggest that lycopene may affect the IGF signaling pathway.

The IGF system is composed of several components. IGF-I and IGF-II are related peptides and are among the most active growth factors in various types of cancer, including breast cancer (106). The IGF system also includes several IGF-binding proteins (IGFBPs) that exist in secreted and membrane-associated forms and exert mostly a negative effect on IGF action (107,108). The interaction of IGF peptides with the IGF-I receptor results in tyrosine autophosphorylation of the receptor. This, in turn, leads to activation of downstream signaling cascades (109) including tyrosine phosphorylation of the major receptor substrate, insulin receptor substrate-1 (IRS-1), which subsequently leads to activation of transcription systems, such as the activator protein-1 (AP-1) complex. The activation of this transcriptional complex, which includes proteins of the Fos and Jun families, is a middle-term event (1–2 h) in the mitogenic signaling pathway of IGF-I and other growth factors (110). AP-1 activation leads to changes in the expression of many proteins, including those related to the cell cycle machinery, such as cyclin D_1 (Sec. VI.A).

Karas et al. analyzed the effect of lycopene on the IGF-I signaling pathway in mammary cancer cells (87). Lycopene treatment markedly inhibited IGF-I stimulation of both tyrosine phosphorylation of IRS-1 and DNA binding capacity of the AP-1 transcription complex. These effects were not associated with changes in the number or affinity of IGF-I receptors, but rather with an increase in membrane-associated IGFBPs, which may explain the suppression of IGF-I signaling by lycopene. Karas et al. demonstrated (108) that in Ishikawa endometrial cancer cells, membrane-associated IGFBP-3 inhibits IGF-I receptor signaling in an IGF-dependent manner. These results are consistent with our previous findings showing that treatment with different cancer cell growth regulators (e.g., tamoxifen and estradiol) results in modulation of cell surface–associated IGFBPs (111,112).

The reports connecting carotenoids with changes in the IGF-I system suggest that interference in IGF-I signaling may be an essential mechanism for the anticancer activity of carotenoids. In addition, other growth factor systems important in cancer development may be affected by carotenoids. For example, Muto et al. have found that β-carotene-induced growth retardation in cervical dysplasia cell lines is associated with rapid reduction in cell surface binding, as well as internalization of epidermal growth factor (EGF) due to a decrease in EGF receptor levels (113).

C. Carotenoids and Gap Junctional Intercellular Communication

Among the various biological activities of carotenoids, their stimulatory effects on gap junctional intercellular communication (GJIC) have been discussed as one of the possible biochemical mechanisms underlying their cancer-preventive properties (114–117). Although only limited data from in vivo studies are available, a number of cell culture experiments provide evidence for such a mechanism.

Gap junctions are specialized microdomains of the plasma membrane that provide a specific pathway for intercellular signaling and are required for the coordination of cellular functions (118,119). They consist of an array of cell-to-cell channels connecting the cytosol of neighboring cells, which allows small molecules (<1000 Da) to diffuse between coupled cells. A functional unit is formed from two half-channels (connexons), each provided by one of the coupled cells. The half-channel consists of a hexamer of specific proteins that belong to the gene family of connexins. Connexin proteins exhibit four helical transmembrane domains, two extracellular loops, a cytoplasmic loop, and cytoplasmic N- and C-terminal domains (120). In the transmembrane and extracellular domains the sequences are most conserved and the extracellular loop contains three cysteines that are required for channel function. Several subtypes of connexins have been identified, and it has been demonstrated that there are differences in the expression of connexin genes in various tissues. Most cell types express multiple connexin isoforms. Therefore, a spectrum of heteromeric hemichannels and heterotypic gap junctions may be formed that provides the structural basis for the selectivity of signaling via GJIC (119).

GJIC is involved in regulation of growth, transmission of developmental signals, coordination of muscle contraction, and maintenance of metabolic homeostasis. It has been suggested that disturbances in intercellular communication via gap junctions are involved in the regulation of tumor cell growth and differentiation (121,122). Such disturbances may also cause a predisposition for arrhythmias and therefore have a role in the pathogenesis of cardiac diseases (123). Normal cells are contact-inhibited and have functional GJIC, whereas most tumor cells exhibit dysfunctional homologous or heterologous GJIC (121). Typically, cancer cells lack growth control and are not able to terminally differentiate, which has, at least in part, been attributed to disturbed GJIC. Oncogenes like ras, raf, or src down-regulate GJIC, whereas it is up-regulated by tumor suppressor genes (116,117). Furthermore, tumor-promoting compounds such as 12-O-tetradecanoylphorbol-13-acetate or dichlorodiphenyltrichloroethane inhibit GJIC, whereas substances exhibiting antitumor properties, including vitamin D, thyroid hormones, flavonoids retinoids, and carotenoids, stimulate GJIC (116,117,121).

Among the major carotenoids present in human blood and tissues, β-carotene, cryptoxanthine, zeaxanthin, and lutein have been found to be efficient inducers of GJIC. α-Carotene and lycopene are less active compounds (124). In addition, a recent report demonstrated that lycopene enhances GJIC and inhibits proliferation of KB-1 human oral tumor cells (125). Structure–activity relationships reveal that the stimulatory effects of carotenoids on GJIC are not limited to the subgroup of provitamin A compounds (126,127). Carotenoids with substituents at the ionone ring are also active. However, the location and chemical properties of the substituent found in the six-membered ring appears to have little influence on the activity of different carotenoids. Echinenone, canthaxanthin, and 4-hydroxy-β-carotene induce GJIC as does retro-dehydro-β-carotene, a structural analog of β-carotene. Members of the carotenoid family that carry a five-carbon ring system, like dinorcanthaxanthin, have been shown to be less active. The six-carbon ring carotenoid canthaxanthin is about twice as active than its five-membered ring analog. No stimulatory effects were reported for capsorubin or violerythrin (five-ring carotenoids) and methylbixin, which carries a carboxylic acid methyl ester residue at both ends of the conjugated core of the molecule.

The mechanism of up-regulation GJIC in the presence of carotenoids is not yet fully understood. Carotenoids are efficient antioxidants, but at least two studies have demonstrated that the effects of carotenoids on GJIC are independent of their antioxidant activities (126,127). Neither their singlet oxygen–quenching properties nor their inhibitory effects on lipid peroxidation were correlated with the regulatory effects on GJIC.

Known multiple pathways for the regulation of GJIC (128,129) include effects on the transcription rate of connexin genes as well as stabilization of connexin mRNA (130). Connexins may also be modified posttranslationally, and phosphorylation is a common modification of these proteins that affects protein trafficking. GJIC is influenced by the intracellular pH and calcium level and is sensitive to various chemicals or drugs. It has been demonstrated in vitro that carotenoid treatment leads to increased expression of connexin 43, one of the most prominent gap junction proteins (131). The stimulatory effects of various carotenoids have been correlated with their ability to inhibit carcinogen-induced neoplastic transformation. There is some evidence that metabolites and oxidation products of the carotenoids are ultimately the active compounds activating GJIC. It has been suggested that retinoic acid–dependent pathways are involved in the regulation of connexin expression (132). All-*trans* and 13-*cis*-4-oxoretinoic acid were isolated as decomposition products of canthaxanthin and were shown to be active in the cell communication assay (133). Eccentric cleavage products of canthaxanthin (11-apocanthaxanthin-11-oic acid, 13-apocanthaxanthin-13-oic acid, and 14′-apocanthaxanthin-14′-oic acid) are less active than 4-oxoretinoic acid and exhibited no stimulatory effects on GJIC (134). These data suggest that the major biological effects of canthaxanthin on GJIC are related to activities mediated by the products of central cleavage.

Several studies have been published on the metabolites and oxidation products of lycopene. For example, it has been shown that 2,6-cyclolycopene-1,5-diol induces gap junctional communication (135). Another compound, *acyclo*-retinoic acid, the open-chain analog of retinoic acid and a putative metabolite of lycopene, is much less active than retinoic acid and 4-oxoretinoic acid with respect to induction of GJIC and retinoid-related signaling (136). Thus, it was speculated that lycopene affects GJIC independent of the retinoic acid–related pathways.

Most of the studies with carotenoids on GJIC have been performed in cell culture systems. However, α-arotene, β-carotene, and lycopene were also investigated at different dose levels in rats (137). The influence on GJIC in the liver was examined after 5 days of treatment with 0.5, 5, or 50 mg carotenoid/kg body weight. For all of the carotenoids, no effect was found at the level of 0.5 mg carotenoid/kg body weight. Stimulatory effects were observed for all carotenoids after treatment with 5 mg carotenoid/kg body weight. GJIC was lower than the control when the animals were treated with 50 mg carotenoid/kg body weight. Such dose-dependent differences in the biological efficacy of carotenoids should be taken into account when biological activities are discussed.

VII. CAROTENOIDS AND TRANSCRIPTION

As discussed above, carotenoids modulate the basic mechanisms of cell proliferation, growth factor signaling, and GJIC, and produce changes in the expression of many proteins participating in these processes, such as connexins, cyclins, cyclin-dependent kinases, and their inhibitors. Therefore, the question that arises is by what mechanisms do carotenoids affect so many diverse cellular pathways? The changes in the expression of multiple proteins suggest that the initial effect of carotenoids involves modulation of transcription. This may be due to either direct interaction of the carotenoid molecules or their derivatives with transcription factors (e.g., with ligand-activated nuclear receptors) or indirect modification of transcriptional activity (e.g., via changes in status of cellular redox), which affects redox-sensitive transcription systems, such as AP-1, nuclear factor–κB (NF-κB), and antioxidant response element (ARE).

The idea that carotenoid derivatives can activate nuclear receptors is not new, but until recently it was limited to retinoic acid, which is produced from β-carotene and other vitamin A precursors. Emerging evidence now suggests that derivatives of other carotenoids or the carotenoids themselves may also modulate the activity of transcription factors. For example, the synergistic inhibition of cancer cell proliferation by lycopene in combination with $1,25(OH)_2D_3$ or retinoic acid (68) (see Sec. V), the ligands of two members of the nuclear receptor superfamily, suggests that lycopene or one of its derivatives may also interact with members of this family of receptors.

A. Retinoid Receptors

Retinoic acid is the parent compound of ligands known as retinoids. It exerts multiple effects on cell proliferation and differentiation through two classes of nuclear receptors termed retinoic acid receptors (RARs) and retinoid X receptors (RXRs). All-*trans* retinoic acid binds only to RAR, whereas its isomer, 9-*cis*-retinoic acid, binds to both RAR and RXR. Upon DNA binding, RXR/RAR heterodimers regulate gene expression of retinoic acid target genes in a ligand-dependent manner. RXR is also capable of forming heterodimers with other members of the nuclear hormone receptors superfamily, such as the thyroid hormone receptor, the vitamin D receptor, the peroxisome proliferator–activated receptor, and possibly other receptors with unknown ligands designated orphan receptors.

The possibility that a lycopene derivative mediates the inhibitory action of this carotenoid on cell growth is discussed in Section IV. To test the hypothesis that such a derivative acts as a ligand for nuclear receptors and mediates the anticancer activity of lycopene, Ben-Dor et al. (138) analyzed the effect of a hypothetical oxidation product of lycopene, *acyclo*-retinoic acid (136), on cancer cell growth and the transactivation of retinoic acid–regulated reporter gene. *Acyclo*-retinoic acid transactivated a reporter gene containing the retinoic acid response element (RARE) with an approximately 100-fold lower potency than retinoic acid (138). Lycopene exhibited only very modest activity in this system. In contrast to the transactivation data, *acyclo*-retinoic acid, retinoic acid, and lycopene inhibited MCF-7 cell growth and slowed down cell cycle progression from G_1 to S phase with a similar potency. Furthermore, the two retinoids decreased serum-stimulated cyclin D_1 expression. On the other hand, they had dissimilar effects on the level of p21. In the presence of *acyclo*-retinoic acid the level of p21, established during serum stimulation, was comparable to that of control cells, whereas in retinoic acid–treated cells, p21 level was much lower, suggesting that the effects of *acyclo*-retinoic acids are not entirely mediated by the RAR. Moreover, a comparable potency of *acyclo*-retinoic acid and lycopene in inhibition of cell growth suggests that *acyclo*-retinoic acid is unlikely to be the active metabolite of this carotenoid. A similar conclusion was made by Stahl et al. (136) who found that retinoic acid is much more potent than *acyclo*-retinoic acid in transactivation of the retinoic acid–responsive promoter of RAR-β2 and that lycopene and retinoic acid are more active than *acyclo*-retinoic acid in activation of GJIC (Sec. VI). Muto et al. (139) synthesized *acyclo*-retinoic acid and tested its biological activity as part of a series of acyclic retinoids but did not observe transactivation in a RAR or RXR reporter gene system (140). However, they found that other acyclic retinoids, lacking one or two double bonds, caused transactivation of the reporter gene, comparable to that achieved by retinoic acid. One of these acyclic retinoids has recently been shown to inhibit cell cycle progression, which was associated with a reduction in cyclin D_1 level and an increase in the level of p21 (141), similar to the results obtained with *acyclo*-retinoic acid (138). It is interesting to note that the acyclic retinoids described by Muto and colleagues may be potential derivatives of phytoene and phytofluene, two carotenoids present in tomatoes that were found in our laboratory to inhibit the proliferation of various cancer cells (unpublished data).

The anticancer activity of carotenoid derivatives is not necessarily mediated by activation of the retinoid receptors. For example, several cleavage products of β-carotene strongly inhibited AP-1 transcriptional activity (66) (for more detail see chapter by Xiang-Dong Wang). Lycopene was also shown to inhibit AP-1 activation (87). We hypothesize that carotenoids or their oxidized derivatives interact with a network of transcription factors that are activated by different ligands at low affinity and specificity. The activation of several transcription factor systems by different compounds may lead to the synergistic inhibition of cell growth (see Sec. IV). In addition to the retinoid receptors and AP-1, other candidate transcription systems that may participate in this network are the peroxisome proliferator-activated receptors (PPARs) (142–144), the ARE (145,146), the xenobiotic receptor (147,148), NF-κB (149), and unidentified orphan receptors.

B. Peroxisome Proliferator–Activated Receptors

PPARs have a key role in the differentiation of adipocytes, although recently their role in cancer cell growth inhibition and differentiation has also been demonstrated. One of the PPAR subtypes, PPARγ, is expressed at significant levels in human primary and metastatic breast adenocarcinomas (150) and liposarcomas (151). Colon cancer in humans was shown to be associated with loss-of-function mutations in PPARγ (152). Ligand activation of PPARγ in cultured breast cancer cells causes extensive lipid accumulation, changes in breast epithelial gene expression associated with a more differentiated, less malignant state, and a reduction in growth rate and clonogenic capacity of the cells (150). These data suggest that the PPARγ transcription system can induce terminal differentiation of malignant breast epithelial cells and thus may provide a novel therapy for human breast cancer. Human prostate cancer cells were found to express PPARγ at prominent levels while normal prostate tissues demonstrated a very low expression (143). It has recently been shown that PPARγ is expressed in human prostate adenocarcinomas and cell lines derived from these tumors. Activation of this receptor with specific ligands, such as troglitazone, exerts an inhibitory effect on the growth of prostate cancer cell lines (144). In prostate cancer patients with no metastatic disease, troglitazone treatment prevented an increase in PSA level that was evident in the untreated patient group (144). These data suggest that PPARγ may serve as a biological modifier in human prostate cancer and therefore its therapeutic potential in this disease should be investigated further.

The presence of PPARγ receptors in various cancer cells and their activation by fatty acids, prostaglandins and related hydrophobic agents in the micromolar range make these ligand-dependent transcription factors an interesting target for carotenoid derivatives. Takahashi et al. (153) studied the effects of various phytochemicals on activation of human PPARs using a novel reporter gene assay system with coactivator coexpression. This system was activated by the isoprenols farnesol and geranylgeraniol. Moreover, these isoprenols up-regulated the expression of lipid metabolic target genes of PPAR. However, different carotenoids at 100 μM, a concentration hardly achievable in aqueous solutions, did not have any significant effect. We recently compared the relative efficacy of several carotenoids found in tomatoes in transactivation of PPAR response element (PPARRE). Preliminary results indicate that lycopene, phytoene, phytofluene, and β-carotene transactivate PPARRE in MCF-7 cells cotransfected with PPARγ. However, it is not clear whether activation of the PPAR system contributes to the inhibition of cancer cell growth by carotenoids.

C. Antioxidant Response Element

Induction of phase II enzymes, which conjugate reactive electrophiles and act as indirect antioxidants, appears to be an effective means for achieving protection against a variety of carcinogens in animals and humans. Transcriptional control of the expression of these enzymes is mediated, at least in part, through ARE found in the regulatory regions of their genes. The transcription factor Nrf2, which binds to ARE, appears to be essential for the induction of phase II enzymes, such as glutathione S-transferases (GSTs), NAD(P)H:quinone oxidoreductase (NQO1) (154), as well as the thiol-containing reducing factor, thioredoxin (155). Constitutive hepatic and gastric activities of GST and NQO1 were decreased by 50–80% in Nrf2-deficient mice compared with wild-type mice (154). Several studies have shown that antioxidants present in the diet, such as terpenoids, phenolic flavonoids (e.g., green tea polyphenols and epigallocatechin-3-gallate), and isothiocyanates may work as anticancer agents by activating this transcription system (156,157).

Gradelet et al. have shown that some carotenoids are capable of inducing the phase II metabolizing enzymes p-nitrophenol-UDP-glucuronosyltransferase and NQO1 in rats (158). In this study, male rats were fed for 15 days with diets containing different carotenoids, and it was found that canthaxanthin and astaxanthin, but not lutein and lycopene, were active in the induction of these enzymes. In another study, Bhuvaneswari et al. (63) associated the chemopreventive effect of lycopene on the incidence of DMBA-induced hamster buccal pouch tumors with a concomitant rise in the level of GSH, enzymes of the glutathione redox cycle, and glutathione S-transferase in the buccal pouch mucosa. These results suggest that the lycopene-induced increase in the levels of GSH and the phase II enzyme glutathione S-transferase inactivate carcinogens by forming conjugates that are less toxic and readily excreted products. Preliminary results obtained in our laboratory show that in transiently transfected mammary cancer and hepatocarcinoma cells, lycopene transactivates the expression of a reporter gene (luciferase) fused with ARE sequences present in NQO1 and in γ-glutamylcysteine synthetase, the rate-limiting enzyme in glutathione synthesis.

D. Xenobiotic and Other Orphan Nuclear Receptors

Orphan receptors include gene products that are structurally related to nuclear hormone receptors but lack known physiological ligands. The group of orphan nuclear receptors called xenobiotic receptors is part of the defense mechanism against foreign lipophilic chemicals (xenobiotics). This family of receptors includes the steroid and xenobiotic receptor/pregnane X receptor (SXR/PXR), the constitutive androstane receptor (CAR) (147,148), and the aryl hydrocarbon receptor (AhR) (159). These receptors respond to a wide variety of drugs, environmental pollutants, carcinogens, and dietary and endogenous compounds and regulate the expression of cytochrome P450 (CYP) enzymes, conjugating enzymes, and transporters involved in the metabolism and elimination of xenobiotics (148).

Animal studies have shown that in addition to the phase II xenobiotic metabolizing enzymes, as described in Section VII.C, some carotenoids are capable of inducing CYP enzymes, constituents of the phase I detoxification pathway. Canthaxanthin and astaxanthin induced liver CYP1A1 and CYP1A2 in rats, and similar effects were observed with β-apo-8′-carotenal. β-Carotene, lutein, and lycopene were not active (158,160–162). In mice, only canthaxanthin exhibited weak effects whereas the other carotenoids did not stimulate CYP1A1 activity (163). The mechanism underlying CYP enzyme induction by carotenoids is not fully understood, but there is evidence that the AhR-dependent pathway is involved. However, carotenoids did not directly bind to this receptor (164). Of several carotenoids tested in rats (β-carotene, bixin, lycopene, lutein, canthaxanthin, and astaxanthin), only bixin, canthaxanthin, and astaxanthin were capable of inducing the activity of CYP1A1 in liver, lung, and kidney and CYP1A2 in liver and lung (165). In another study, the administration of lycopene to rats at doses ranging from 0.001 to 0.1 g/kg was shown to induce the liver CYP types 1A1/2, 2B1/2, and 3A in a dose-dependent manner (166). The observation that these enzymatic activities were induced at very low lycopene plasma levels led the authors to suggest that modulation of drug-metabolizing enzymes by carotenoids might be relevant to humans (166). Indeed, the activity of CYP1A2 in humans was shown to be correlated with plasma levels of micronutrients (167), and it has been proposed that about one-third of the variation in enzyme activity is related to dietary factors. Plasma lutein levels were negatively associated with CYP1A2 activity whereas lycopene levels were positively correlated with the enzyme activity.

The direct effect of carotenoids on a xenobiotic receptor system was tested in an in vitro transcription system (R. Rühl and F. J. Schweigert, personal communication, 2002). They found that in transiently transfected HepG2 hepatoma cells, β-carotene can transactivate the PXR reporter gene in a manner comparable to that of rifampicin. Furthermore, an up-regulation of CYP3A4 and CYP3A5 was obtained in these cells, pointing to a potential effect of the carotenoid on the metabolism of xenobiotics.

It has become clear that orphan nuclear receptors represent a unique and pivotal resource to uncover new regulatory systems that impact both health and human diseases. The discussion above suggests that at least one group of this receptor family, the xenobiotic receptors, are affected by carotenoids. Thus, it is possible that other, yet unknown, types of orphan receptors are involved in the cellular action of carotenoids.

VIII. CONCLUSION

In studies using cell and animal models, carotenoids have been shown to influence diverse molecular and cellular processes that can form the basis for the beneficial effects of carotenoids on human health and disease prevention. However, despite the promising results it is difficult at the moment to directly relate available experimental data to human pathophysiology. One problem is that many results were obtained in studies using carotenoid levels that are much higher than those achievable in human blood. On the other hand, the presented evidence suggests a synergistic action of low concentrations of various carotenoids and other micronutrients. A growing body of experimental data indicates that this synergy may be based on the ability of different dietary compounds to modulate a network of transcription systems. The concerted action of multiple micronutrients acomplished by activation of transcription and probably by other mechanisms can explain the beneficial effect of diets rich in fruits and vegetables. An important question that is still open is whether the described changes in various cellular pathways are due to direct effects of the carotenoid molecules or are mediated by their derivatives. Although some information on this issue is presented in this chapter, additional studies are needed to identify and characterize these putative active carotenoid derivatives.

ACKNOWLEDGMENTS

Studies from the authors' laboratory were supported in part by the Israel Cancer Association; by the Chief Scientist, Israel Ministry of Health; by the Israel Science Foundation founded by the Israel Academy of Science and Humanities; by the European Community (Project No. FAIR CT 97-3100); by LycoRed Natural Products Industries, Beer-Sheva, Israel and by the S. Daniel Abraham International Center for Health and Nutrition, Ben-Gurion University of the Negev. We thank Dr. Hans-Dieter Martin (Heinrich-Heine-Üniversitat, Düsseldorf), Dr. Colin K.W. Watts (Garvan Institute of Medical Research, Sydney), and Dr. Noa Noy (Cornell University, Ithaca, NY) for fruitful collaboration on various parts of the research.

REFERENCES

1. Van Poppel G. Carotenoids and cancer: an update with emphasis on human intervention studies. Eur J Cancer 1993; 29A:1335–1344.
2. van Poppel G, Goldbohm RA. Epidemiologic evidence for beta-carotene and cancer prevention. Am J Clin Nutr 1995; 62:1393S–1402S.
3. Speizer FE, Colditz GA, Hunter DJ, Rosner B, Hennekens C. Prospective study of smoking, antioxidant intake, and lung cancer in middle-aged women (USA). Cancer Causes Control 1999; 10:475–482.
4. Knekt P, Jarvinen R, Teppo L, Aromaa A, Seppanen R. Role of various carotenoids in lung cancer prevention. J Natl Cancer Inst 1999; 91:182–184.
5. Michaud DS, Feskanich D, Rimm EB, Colditz GA, Speizer FE, Willett WC, Giovannucci E. Intake of specific carotenoids and risk of lung cancer in 2 prospective US cohorts. Am J Clin Nutr 2000; 72:990–997.

6. Garcia Closas R, Agudo A, Gonzalez CA, Riboli E. Intake of specific carotenoids and flavonoids and the risk of lung cancer in women in Barcelona, Spain. Nutr Cancer 1998; 32:154–158.
7. Heinonen OP, Huttunen JK, Albanes D, et al. Effect of vitamin E and beta carotene on the incidence of lung cancer and other cancers in male smokers. New Engl J Med 1994; 330:1029–1035.
8. Omenn GS, Goodman GE, Thornquist MD, et al. Effects of a combination of beta carotene and vitamin A on lung cancer and cardiovascular disease. N Engl J Med 1996; 334:1150–1155.
9. Hennekens CH, Buring JE, Manson JE, et al. Lack of effect of long-term supplementation with beta carotene on the incidence of malignant neoplasms and cardiovascular disease. N Engl J Med 1996; 334:1145–1149.
10. Blot WJ, Li JY, Taylor PR, Guo W, Dawsey S, Wang GQ, Yang CS, Zheng SF, Gail M, Li GY, et al. Nutrition intervention trials in Linxian, China: supplementation with specific vitamin/mineral combinations, cancer incidence, and disease-specific mortality in the general population. J Natl Cancer Inst 1993; 85:1483–1492.
11. Lee IM, Cook NR, Manson JE, Buring JE, Hennekens CH. Beta-carotene supplementation and incidence of cancer and cardiovascular disease: the Women's Health Study. J Natl Cancer Inst 1999; 91:2102–2106.
12. Cook NR, Le IM, Manson JE, Buring JE, Hennekens CH. Effects of beta-carotene supplementation on cancer incidence by baseline characteristics in the Physicians' Health Study (United States). Cancer Causes Control 2000; 11:617–626.
13. Glynn SA, Albanes D, Pietinen P, Brown CC, Rautalahti M, Tangrea JA, Taylor PR, Virtamo J. Alcohol consumption and risk of colorectal cancer in a cohort of Finnish men. Cancer Causes Control 1996; 7:214–223.
14. McLarty JW, Holiday DB, Girard WM, Yanagihara RH, Kummet TD, Greenberg SD. Beta-Carotene, vitamin A, and lung cancer chemoprevention: results of an intermediate endpoint study. Am J Clin Nutr 1995; 62:1431S–1438S.
15. Cook NR, Stampfer MJ, Ma J, Manson JE, Sacks FM, Buring JE, Hennekens CH. Beta-carotene supplementation for patients with low baseline levels and decreased risks of total and prostate carcinoma. Cancer 1999; 86:1783–1792.
16. Greenberg ER, Baron JA, Tosteson TD, et al. Clinical trial of antioxidant vitamins to prevent colorectal adenoma. New Engl J Med 1994; 331:141–147.
17. Tsubono Y, Tsugane S, Gey KF. Plasma antioxidant vitamins and carotenoids in five Japanese populations with varied mortality from gastric cancer. Nutr Cancer 1999; 34:56–61.
18. La Vecchia C. Tomatoes, lycopene intake, and digestive tract and female hormone–related neoplasms. Exp Biol Med (Maywood) 2002; 227:860–863.
19. Terry P, Jain M, Miller AB, Howe GR, Rohan TE. Dietary carotenoid intake and colorectal cancer risk. Nutr Cancer 2002; 42:167–172.
20. Malila N, Virtamo J, Virtanen M, Pietinen P, Albanes D, Teppo L. Dietary and serum alpha-tocopherol, beta-carotene and retinol, and risk for colorectal cancer in male smokers. Eur J Clin Nutr 2002; 56:615–621.
21. Fairfield KM, Fletcher RH. Vitamins for chronic disease prevention in adults: scientific review. JAMA 2002; 287:3116–3126.

22. Albanes D, Heinonen OP, Huttunen JK, Taylor PR, Virtamo J, Edwards BK, Haapakoski J, Rautalahti M, Hartman AM, Palmgren J, et al. Effects of alpha-tocopherol and beta-carotene supplements on cancer incidence in the Alpha-Tocopherol, Beta-Carotene Cancer Prevention Study. Am J Clin Nutr 1995; 62:1427S–1430S.

23. Albanes D, Heinonen OP, Taylor PR, et al. Alpha-Tocopherol and beta-carotene supplements and lung cancer incidence in the Alpha-Tocopherol, Beta-Carotene Cancer Prevention Study: effects of base-line characteristics and study compliance. J Natl Cancer Inst 1996; 88:1560–1570.

24. Giovannucci E, Ascherio A, Rimm EB, Stampfer MJ, Colditz GA, Willett WC. Intake of carotenoids and retinol in relation to risk of prostate cancer. J Natl Cancer Inst 1995; 87:1767–1776.

25. Giovannucci E, Rimm EB, Liu Y, Stampfer MJ, Willett WC. A prospective study of tomato products, lycopene, and prostate cancer risk. J Natl Cancer Inst 2002; 94:391–398.

26. Grant WB. An ecologic study of dietary links to prostate cancer. Altern Med Rev 1999; 4:162–169.

27. Rao AV, Fleshner N, Agarwal S. Serum and tissue lycopene and biomarkers of oxidation in prostate cancer patients: a case-control study. Nutr Cancer 1999; 33:159–164.

28. Gann PH, Ma J, Giovannucci E, Willett W, Sacks FM, Hennekens CH, Stampfer MJ. Lower prostate cancer risk in men with elevated plasma lycopene levels: results of a prospective analysis. Cancer Res 1999; 59: 1225–1230.

29. Cohen JH, Kristal AR, Stanford JL. Fruit and vegetable intakes and prostate cancer risk. J Natl Cancer Inst 2000; 92:61–68.

30. Nomura AM, Stemmermann GN, Lee J, Craft NE. Serum micronutrients and prostate cancer in Japanese Americans in Hawaii. Cancer Epidemiol Biomark Prev 1997; 6:487–491.

31. Chen L, Stacewicz-Sapuntzakis M, Duncan C, Sharifi R, Ghosh L, van Breemen R, Ashton D, Bowen PE. Oxidative DNA damage in prostate cancer patients consuming tomato sauce- based entrees as a whole-food intervention. J Natl Cancer Inst 2001; 93:1872–1879.

32. Kucuk O, Sarkar FH, Sakr W, et al. Phase II randomized clinical trial of lycopene supplementation before radical prostatectomy. Cancer Epidemiol Biomark Prev 2001; 10:861–868.

33. Clavel-Chapelon F, Niravong M, Joseph RR. Diet and breast cancer: review of the epidemiologic literature. Cancer Detect Prev 1997; 21:426–440.

34. Kushi LH, Fee RM, Sellers TA, Zheng W, Folsom AR. Intake of vitamins A, C, and E and postmenopausal breast cancer. The Iowa Women's Health Study. Am J Epidemiol 1996; 144:165–174.

35. Verhoeven DT, Assen N, Goldbohm RA, Dorant E, van 't Veer P, Sturmans F, Hermus RJ, van den Brandt PA. Vitamins C and E, retinol, beta-carotene and dietary fibre in relation to breast cancer risk: a prospective cohort study. Br J Cancer 1997; 75:149–155.

36. Jarvinen R, Knekt P, Seppanen R, Teppo L. Diet and breast cancer risk in a cohort of Finnish women. Cancer Lett 1997; 114:251–253.
37. Michels KB, Holmberg L, Bergkvist L, Ljung H, Bruce A, Wolk A. Dietary antioxidant vitamins, retinol, and breast cancer incidence in a cohort of Swedish women. Int J Cancer 2001; 91:563–567.
38. Zhang S, Hunter DJ, Forman MR, Rosner BA, Speizer FE, Colditz GA, Manson JE, Hankinson SE, Willett WC. Dietary carotenoids and vitamins A, C, and E and risk of breast cancer. J Natl Cancer Inst 1999; 91:547–556.
39. Ching S, Ingram D, Hahnel R, Beilby J, Rossi E. Serum levels of micronutrients, antioxidants and total antioxidant status predict risk of breast cancer in a case control study. J Nutr 2002; 132:303–306.
40. Ronco A, De Stefani E, Boffetta P, Deneo-Pellegrini H, Mendilaharsu M, Leborgne F. Vegetables, fruits, and related nutrients and risk of breast cancer: a case-control study in Uruguay. Nutr Cancer 1999; 35:111–119.
41. Hulten K, Van Kappel AL, Winkvist A, Kaaks R, Hallmans G, Lenner P, Riboli E. Carotenoids, alpha-tocopherols, and retinol in plasma and breast cancer risk in northern Sweden. Cancer Causes Control 2001; 12:529–537.
42. Willett WC, Polk BF, Underwood BA, Stampfer MJ, Pressel S, Rosner B, Taylor JO, Schneider K, Hames CG. Relation of serum vitamins A and E and carotenoids to the risk of cancer. N Engl J Med 1984; 310:430–434.
43. Wald NJ, Boreham J, Hayward JL, Bulbrook RD. Plasma retinol, beta-carotene and vitamin E levels in relation to the future risk of breast cancer. Br J Cancer 1984; 49:321–324.
44. Knekt P, Aromaa A, Maatela J, Aaran RK, Nikkari T, Hakama M, Hakulinen T, Peto R, Teppo L. Serum vitamin A and subsequent risk of cancer: cancer incidence follow-up of the Finnish Mobile Clinic Health Examination Survey. Am J Epidemiol 1990; 132:857–870.
45. Comstock GW, Helzlsouer KJ, Bush TL. Prediagnostic serum levels of carotenoids and vitamin E as related to subsequent cancer in Washington County, Maryland. Am J Clin Nutr 1991; 53:260S–264S.
46. Dorgan JF, Sowell A, Swanson CA, Potischman N, Miller R, Schussler N, Stephenson HE, Jr. Relationships of serum carotenoids, retinol, alpha-tocopherol, and selenium with breast cancer risk: results from a prospective study in Columbia, Missouri (United States). Cancer Causes Control 1998; 9:89–97.
47. Toniolo P, Van Kappel AL, Akhmedkhanov A, Ferrari P, Kato I, Shore RE, Riboli E. Serum carotenoids and breast cancer. Am J Epidemiol 2001; 153:1142–1147.
48. Giovannucci E. Tomatoes, tomato-based products, lycopene, and cancer: review of the epidemiologic literature. J Natl Cancer Inst 1999; 91:317–331.
49. Lee CM, Boileau AC, Boileau TW, Williams AW, Swanson KS, Heintz KA, Erdman JW, Jr. Review of animal models in carotenoid research. J Nutr 1999; 129:2271–2277.
50. Nagasawa H, Mitamura T, Sakamoto S, Yamamoto K. Effect of lycopene on spontanous mammary tumor development in SHN virgin mice. Anticancer Res 1995; 15:1173–1178.

51. Narisawa T, Fukaura Y, Hasebe M, Ito M, Aizawa R, Murakoshi M, Uemura S, Khachik F, Nishino H. Inhibitory effects of natural carotenoids, alpha-carotene, beta-carotene, lycopene and lutein, on colonic aberrant crypt foci formation in rats. Cancer Lett 1996; 107:137–142.

52. Schwartz J, Shklar G. The selective cytotoxic effect of carotenoids and alpha-tocopherol on human cancer cell lines in vitro. J Oral Maxillofac Surg 1992; 50:367–373.

53. Bendich A, Olson JA. Biological actions of carotenoids. FASEB J 1989; 3:1927–1932.

54. Nishino H, Murakosh M, Ii T, et al. Carotenoids in cancer chemoprevention. Cancer Metastasis Rev 2002; 21:257–264.

55. Wang CJ, Chou MY, Lin JK. Inhibition of growth and development of the transplantable C-6 glioma cells inoculated in rats by retinoids and carotenoids. Cancer Lett 1989; 48:135–142.

56. Kobayashi T, Itjima K, Mitamura T, Torilzuka K, Cyong J, Nagasawa H. Effect of lycopene, a carotenoid, on intrathymic T cell differentiation and peripheral CD4/CD8 ratio in a high mammary tumor strain of SHN retired mice. Anticancer Drugs 1996; 7:195–198.

57. Sharoni Y, Giron E, Rise M, Levy J. Effects of lycopene enriched tomato oleoresin on 7,12-dimethyl-benz[a]anthracene-induced rat mammary tumors. Cancer Detect Prevent 1997; 21:118–123.

58. Kim JM, Araki S, Kim DJ, et al. Chemopreventive effects of carotenoids and curcumins on mouse colon carcinogenesis after 1,2-dimethylhydrazine initiation. Carcinogenesis 1998; 19:81–85.

59. Kim H. Carotenoids protect cultured rat hepatocytes from injury caused by carbon tetrachloride. Int J Biochem Cell Biol 1995; 27:1303–1309.

60. Matsushima-Nishiwaki R, Shidoji Y, Nishiwaki S, Yamada T, Moriwaki H, Muto Y. Suppression by carotenoids of microcystin-induced morphological changes in mouse hepatocytes. Lipids 1995; 30:1029–1034.

61. Kim DJ, Takasuka N, Kim JM, Sekine K, Ota T, Asamoto M, Murakoshi M, Nishino H, Nir Z, Tsuda H. Chemoprevention by lycopene of mouse lung neoplasia after combined initiation treatment with DEN, MNU and DMH. Cancer Lett 1997; 120:15–22.

62. Okajima E, Tsutsumi M, Ozono S, Akai H, Denda A, Nishino H, Oshima S, Sakamoto H, Konishi Y. Inhibitory effect of tomato juice on rat urinary bladder carcinogenesis after N-butyl-N-(4-hydroxybutyl)nitrosamine initiation. Jpn J Cancer Res 1998; 89:22–26.

63. Bhuvaneswari V, Velmurugan B, Balasenthil S, Ramachandran CR, Nagini S. Chemopreventive efficacy of lycopene on 7,12-dimethylbenz[a]anthracene-induced hamster buccal pouch carcinogenesis. Fitoterapia 2001; 72:865–874.

64. Arimochi H, Kataoka K, Kuwahara T, Nakayama H, Misawa N, Ohnishi Y. Effects of beta-glucuronidase-deficient and lycopene-producing *Escherichia coli* strains on formation of azoxymethane-induced aberrant crypt foci in the rat colon. Biochem Biophys Res Commun 1999; 262:322–327.

65. Prakash P, Russell RM, Krinsky NI. In vitro inhibition of proliferation of estrogen-dependent and estrogen-independent human breast cancer cells treated with carotenoids or retinoids. J Nutr 2001; 131:1574–1580.

66. Tibaduiza EC, Fleet JC, Russell RM, Krinsky NI. Excentric cleavage products of beta-carotene inhibit estrogen receptor positive and negative breast tumor cell growth in vitro and inhibit activator protein-1-mediated transcriptional activation. J Nutr 2002; 132:1368–1375.

67. Levy J, Bosin E, Feldman B, Giat Y, Miinster A, Danilenko M, Sharoni Y. Lycopene is a more potent inhibitor of human cancer cell proliferation than either α-carotene or β-carotene. Nutr Cancer 1995; 24:257–267.

68. Amir H, Karas M, Giat J, Danilenko M, Levy R, Yermiahu T, Levy J, Sharoni Y. Lycopene and 1,25-dihydroxyvitamin-D_3 cooperate in the inhibition of cell cycle progression and induction of differentiation in HL-60 leukemic cells. Nutr Cancer 1999; 33:105–112.

69. Pastori M, Pfander H, Boscoboinik D, Azzi A. Lycopene in association with alpha-tocopherol inhibits at physiological concentrations proliferation of prostate carcinoma cells. Biochem Biophys Res Commun 1998; 250:582–585.

70. Xu X, Wang Y, Constantinou AI, Stacewicz-Sapuntzakis M, Bowen PE, van Breemen RB. Solubilization and stabilization of carotenoids using micelles: delivery of lycopene to cells in culture. Lipids 1999; 34:1031–1036.

71. Kotake-Nara E, Kushiro M, Zhang H, Sugawara T, Miyashita K, Nagao A. Carotenoids affect proliferation of human prostate cancer cells. J Nutr 2001; 131:3303–3306.

72. Hall AK. Liarozole amplifies retinoid-induced apoptosis in human prostate cancer cells. Anticancer Drugs 1996; 7:312–320.

73. Wang C-J, Lin J-K. Inhibitory effects of carotenoids and retinoids on the in vitro growth of rat C-6 glioma cells. Proc Natl Sci Counc B ROC 1989; 13:176–183.

74. Nara E, Hayashi H, Kotake M, Miyashita K, Nagao A. Acyclic carotenoids and their oxidation mixtures inhibit the growth of HL-60 human promyelocytic leukemia cells. Nutr Cancer 2001; 39:273–283.

75. Kozuki Y, Miura Y, Yagasaki K. Inhibitory effects of carotenoids on the invasion of rat ascites hepatoma cells in culture. Cancer Lett 2000; 151:111–115.

76. Danilenko M, Wang X, Studzinski GP. Carnosic acid and promotion of monocytic differentiation of HL60-G cells initiated by other agents. J Natl Cancer Inst 2001; 93:1224–1233.

77. Steiner M, Priel I, Giat J, Levy J, Sharoni Y, Danilenko M. Carnosic acid inhibits proliferation and augments differentiation of human leukemic cells induced by 1,25-dihydroxyvitamin D_3 and retinoic acid. Nutr Cancer 2001; 41:135–144.

78. Sokoloski JA, Hodnick WF, Mayne ST, Cinquina C, Kim CS, Sartorelli AC. Induction of the differentiation of HL-60 promyelocytic leukemia cells by vitamin E and other antioxidants in combination with low levels of vitamin D-3: possible relationship to NF-kappa B. Leukemia 1997; 11:1546–1553.

79. Liu Y, Chang RL, Cui XX, Newmark HL, Conney AH. Synergistic effects of curcumin on all-trans retinoic acid- and 1α,25-dihydroxyvitamin D_3-induced differentiation in human promyelocytic leukemia HL-60 cells. Oncology Res 1997; 9:19–29.

80. Guthrie N, Gapor A, Chambers AF, Carroll KK. Inhibition of proliferation of estrogen receptor-negative MDA-MB-435 and -positive MCF-7 human breast cancer cells by palm oil tocotrienols and tamoxifen, alone and in combination. J Nutr 1997; 127:544S–548S.

81. Cover CM, Hsieh SJ, Cram EJ, Hong C, Riby JE, Bjeldanes LF, Firestone GL. Indole-3-carbinol and tamoxifen cooperate to arrest the cell cycle of MCF-7 human breast cancer cells. Cancer Res 1999; 59:1244–1251.

82. Halliwell B. Effect of diet on cancer development: is oxidative DNA damage a biomarker? Free Radic Biol Med 2002; 32:968–974.

83. Halliwell B. Why and how should we measure oxidative DNA damage in nutritional studies? How far have we come? Am J Clin Nutr 2000; 72:1082–1087.

84. Hughes DA. Dietary carotenoids and human immune function. Nutrition 2001; 17:823–827.

85. Hughes DA. Effects of carotenoids on human immune function. Proc Nutr Soc 1999; 58:713–718.

86. Palozza P, Serini S, Torsello A, Boninsegna A, Covacci V, Maggiano N, Ranelletti FO, Wolf FI, Calviello G. Regulation of cell cycle progression and apoptosis by beta-carotene in undifferentiated and differentiated HL-60 leukemia cells: possible involvement of a redox mechanism. Int J Cancer 2002; 97:593–600.

87. Karas M, Amir H, Fishman D, Danilenko M, Segal S, Nahum A, Koifmann A, Giat Y, Levy J, Sharoni Y. Lycopene interferes with cell cycle progression and insulin-like growth factor I signaling in mammary cancer cells. Nutr Cancer 2000; 36:101–111.

88. Murakoshi M, Takayasu J, Kimura O, Kohmura E, Nishino H, Okuzumi J, Sakai T, Sugimoto T, Imanishi J, Iwasaki R. Inhibitory effects of β-carotene on proliferation of the human neuroblastoma cell line GOTO. J Natl Cancer Inst 1989; 81:1649–1652.

89. Okuzumi J, Nishino H, Murakoshi M, Iwashima A, Tanaka Y, Yamane T, Fujita Y, Takahashi T. Inhibitory effects of fucoxanthin, a natural carotenoid, on N-myc expression and cell cycle progression in human malignant tumor cells. Cancer Lett 1990; 55:75–81.

90. Bartek J, Bartkova J, Lukas J. The retinoblastoma protein pathway in cell cycle control and cancer. Exp Cell Res 1997; 237:1–6.

91. Sherr CJ. D-type cyclins. Trends Biochem Sci 1995; 20:187–190.

92. Buckley MF, Sweeney KJ, Hamilton JA, Sini RL, Manning DL, Nicholson RI, deFazio A, Watts CK, Musgrove EA, Sutherland RL. Expression and amplification of cyclin genes in human breast cancer. Oncogene 1993; 8:2127–2133.

93. Stivala LA, Savio M, Quarta S, et al. The antiproliferative effect of beta-carotene requires p21waf1/cip1 in normal human fibroblasts. Eur J Biochem 2000; 267:2290–2296.

94. Williams AW, Boileau TW, Zhou JR, Clinton SK, Erdman JW, Jr. Beta-carotene modulates human prostate cancer cell growth and may undergo intracellular metabolism to retinol. J Nutr 2000; 130:728–732.

95. Nahum A, Hirsch K, Danilenko M, Watts CK, Prall OW, Levy J, Sharoni Y. Lycopene inhibition of cell cycle progression in breast and endometrial cancer cells is associated with reduction in cyclin D levels and retention of p27(Kip1) in the cyclin E-cdk2 complexes. Oncogene 2001; 20:3428–3436.

96. Palozza P, Serini S, Maggiano N, Angelini M, Boninsegna A, Di Nicuolo F, Ranelletti FO, Calviello G. Induction of cell cycle arrest and apoptosis in human colon adenocarcinoma cell lines by beta-carotene through down-regulation of cyclin A and Bcl-2 family proteins. Carcinogenesis 2002; 23:11–18.

97. Zi X, Feyes DK, Agarwal R. Anticarcinogenic effect of a flavonoid antioxidant, silymarin, in human breast cancer cells MDA-MB 468: induction of G1 arrest through an increase in Cip1/p21 concomitant with a decrease in kinase activity of cyclin-dependent kinases and associated cyclins. Clin Cancer Res 1998; 4:1055–1064.

98. Zi X, Grasso AW, Kung HJ, Agarwal R. A flavonoid antioxidant, silymarin, inhibits activation of erbB1 signaling and induces cyclin-dependent kinase inhibitors, G1 arrest, and anticarcinogenic effects in human prostate carcinoma DU145 cells. Cancer Res 1998; 58:1920–1929.

99. Bai F, Matsui T, Ohtani Fujita N, Matsukawa Y, Ding Y, Sakai T. Promoter activation and following induction of the p21/WAF1 gene by flavone is involved in G1 phase arrest in A549 lung adenocarcinoma cells. FEBS Lett 1998; 437:61–64.

100. Watts CK, Brady A, Sarcevic B, deFazio A, Musgrove EA, Sutherland RL. Antiestrogen inhibition of cell cycle progression in breast cancer cells in associated with inhibition of cyclin-dependent kinase activity and decreased retinoblastoma protein phosphorylation. Mol Endocrinol 1995; 9:1804–1813.

101. Teixeira C, Pratt MAC. CDK2 is a target for retinoic acid-mediated growth inhibition in MCF-7 human breast cancer cells. Mol Endocrinol 1997; 11:1191–1202.

102. Chan JM, Stampfer MJ, Giovannucci E, Gann PH, Ma J, Wilkinson P, Hannekens CH, Pollak M. Plasma insulin-like growth factor-I and prostate cancer risk: a prospective study. Science 1998; 279:563–566.

103. Hankinson SE, Willett WC, Colditz GA, Hunter DJ, Michaud DS, Deroo B, Rosner B, Speizer FE, Pollak M. Circulating concentrations of insulin-like growth factor I and risk of breast cancer. Lancet 1998; 351:1393–1396.

104. Ma J, Pollak MN, Giovannucci E, Chan JM, Tao Y, Hennekens CH, Stampfer MJ. Prospective study of colorectal cancer risk in men and plasma levels of insulin-like growth factor (IGF)-I and IGF-binding protein-3. J Natl Cancer Inst 1999; 91:620–625.

105. Mucci LA, Tamimi R, Lagiou P, Trichopoulou A, Benetou V, Spanos E, Trichopoulos D. Are dietary influences on the risk of prostate cancer mediated through the insulin-like growth factor system? Br J Urol Int 2001; 87:814–820.

106. LeRoith D, Werner H, Beitner-Johnson D, Roberts Jr. CT. Molecular and cellular aspects of the insulin-like growth factor I receptor. Endocr Rev 1995; 16:143–159.

107. Drop SL, Schuller AG, Lindenbergh KD, Groffen C, Brinkman A, Zwarthoff EC. Structural aspects of the IGFBP family. Growth Regul 1992; 2:69–79.

108. Karas M, Danilenko M, Fishman D, LeRoith D, Levy J, Sharoni Y. Membrane associated IGFBP-3 inhibits insulin-like growth factor-I (IGF-I)-induced IGF-I receptor signaling in Ishikawa endometrial cancer cells. J Biol Chem 1997; 272:16514–16520.

109. Czech MP. Signal transmission by the insulin-like growth factors. Cell 1989; 59:235–238.

110. Angel P, Karin M. The role of Jun, Fos and the AP-1 complex in cell-proliferation and transformation. Biochim Biophys Acta 1991; 1072:129–157.

111. Karas M, Kleinman D, Danilenko M, Roberts CR, Jr, LeRoith D, Levy J, Sharoni Y. Components of the IGF system mediate the opposing effects of tamoxifen on endometrial and breast cancer cell growth. Prog Growth Factor Res 1995; 6: 513–520.

112. Kleinman D, Karas M, Danilenko M, Arbeli A, Roberts Jr. CT, LeRoith D, Levy J, Sharoni Y. Stimulation of endometrial cancer cell growth by tamoxifen is associated with increased IGF-I induced tyrosine phosphorylation and reduction in IGF binding proteins. Endocrinology 1996; 137:1089–1095.

113. Muto Y, Fujii J, Shidoji Y, Moriwaki H, Kawaguchi T, Noda T. Growth retardation in human cervical dysplasia-derived cell lines by beta-carotene through down-regulation of epidermal growth factor receptor. Am J Clin Nutr 1995; 62:1535S–1540S.

114. Hossain MZ, Zhang L-X, Bertram JS. Retinoids and carotenoids upregulate gap-junctional communication: correlation with enhanced growth control and cancer prevention. In: Hall JE, Zampighi GA, Davis RM, eds. Progress in Cell Research, Vol. 3. Amsterdam: Elsevier Science, 1993, pp 301–309.

115. Stahl W, Sies H. The role of carotenoids and retinoids in gap junctional communication. Int J Vitam Nutr Res 1998; 68:354–359.

116. Bertram JS. Carotenoids and gene regulation. Nutr Rev 1999; 57:182–191.

117. Stahl W, Ale-Agha N, Polidori MC. Non-antioxidant properties of carotenoids. Biol Chem 2002; 383:553–558.

118. Goodenough DA, Goliger JA, Paul DL. Connexins, connexons, and intercellular communication. Annu Rev Biochem 1996; 65:475–502.

119. Evans WH, Martin PE. Gap junctions: structure and function (Review). Mol Membr Biol 2002; 19:121–136.

120. Harris AL. Emerging issues of connexin channels: biophysics fills the gap. Q Rev Biophys 2001; 34:325–472.

121. Trosko JE, Chang CC. Mechanism of up-regulated gap junctional intercellular communication during chemoprevention and chemotherapy of cancer. Mutat Res 2001; 480–481:219–229.

122. Omori Y, Zaidan Dagli ML, Yamakage K, Yamasaki H. Involvement of gap junctions in tumor suppression: analysis of genetically-manipulated mice. Mutat Res 2001; 477:191–196.

123. Jongsma HJ, Wilders R. Gap junctions in cardiovascular disease. Circ Res 2000; 86:1193–1197.
124. Zhang L-X, Cooney RV, Bertram J. Carotenoids enhance gap junctional communication and inhibit lipid peroxidation in C3H/10T1/2 cells: relationship to their cancer chemopreventive action. Carcinogenesis 1991; 12:2109–2114.
125. Livny O, Kaplan I, Reifen R, Polak-Charcon S, Madar Z, Schwartz B. Lycopene inhibits proliferation and enhances gap-junction communication of KB-1 human oral tumor cells. J Nutr 2002; 132:3754–3759.
126. Zhang LX, Cooney RV, Bertram JS. Carotenoids up-regulate connexin-43 gene expression independent of their provitamin-A or antioxidant properties. Cancer Res 1992; 52:5707–5712.
127. Stahl W, Nicolai S, Briviba K, Hanusch M, Broszeit G, Peters M, Martin HD, Sies H. Biological activities of natural and synthetic carotenoids: induction of gap junctional communication and singlet oxygen quenching. Carcinogenesis 1997; 18:89–92.
128. Simon AM, Goodenough DA. Diverse functions of vertebrate gap junctions. Trends Cell Biol 1998; 8:477–483.
129. Lampe PD, Lau AF. Regulation of gap junctions by phosphorylation of connexins. Arch Biochem Biophys 2000; 384:205–215.
130. Clairmont A, Sies H. Evidence for a posttranscriptional effect of retinoic acid on connexin43 gene expression via the 3'-untranslated region. FEBS Lett 1997; 419:268–270.
131. Bertram JS, Bortkiewicz H. Dietary carotenoids inhibit neoplastic transformation and modulate gene expression in mouse and human cells. Am J Clin Nutr 1995; 62:1327S–1336S.
132. Acevedo P, Bertram JS. Liarozole potentiates the cancer chemopreventive activity of and the up-regulation of gap junctional communication and connexin43 expression by retinoic acid and beta-carotene in 10T1/2 cells. Carcinogenesis 1995; 16:2215–2222.
133. Hanusch M, Stahl W, Schulz H, Sies H. Induction of gap junction communication by 4-oxo-retinoic acid generated from its precursor canthaxanthin. Arch Biochem Biophys 1995; 317:423–428.
134. Teicher VB, Kucharski N, Martin HD, van der Saag P, Sies H, Stahl W. Biological activities of apo-canthaxanthinoic acids related to gap junctional communication. Arch Biochem Biophys 1999; 365:150–155.
135. Bertram JS, King T, Fukishima L, Khachik F. Enhanced activity of an oxidation product of lycopene found in tomato products and human serum relevant to cancer prevention. In: Sen CK, Sies H, Baeuerle PA, eds. Antioxidant and Redox Regulation of Genes. London: Academic Press, 2000:pp 409–424.
136. Stahl W, von Laar J, Martin HD, Emmerich T, Sies H. Stimulation of gap junctional communication: comparison of acycloretinoic acid and lycopene. Arch Biochem Biophys 2000; 373:271–274.
137. Krutovskikh V, Asamoto M, Takasuka N, Murakoshi M, Nishino H, Tsuda H. Differential dose-dependent effects of alpha-, beta-carotenes and lycopene on gap-junctional intercellular communication in rat liver in vivo. Jpn J Cancer Res 1997; 88:1121–1124.

138. Ben-Dor A, Nahum A, Danilenko M, Giat Y, Stahl W, Martin HD, Emmerich T, Noy N, Levy J, Sharoni Y. Effects of acyclo-retinoic acid and lycopene on activation of the retinoic acid receptor and proliferation of mammary cancer cells. Arch Biochem Biophys 2001; 391:295–302.

139. Muto Y, Moriwaki H, Omori M. In vitro binding affinity of novel synthetic polyprenoids (polyprenoic acids) to cellular retinoid-binding proteins. Gann 1981; 72:974–977.

140. Araki H, Shidoji Y, Yamada Y, Moriwaki H, Muto Y. Retinoid agonist activities of synthetic geranyl geranoic acid derivatives. Biochem Biophys Res Commun 1995; 209:66–72.

141. Suzui M, Masuda M, Lim JT, Albanese C, Pestell RG, Weinstein IB. Growth inhibition of human hepatoma cells by acyclic retinoid is associated with induction of p21(CIP1) and inhibition of expression of cyclin D1. Cancer Res 2002; 62:3997–4006.

142. Butler R, Mitchell SH, Tindall DJ, Young CY. Nonapoptotic cell death associated with S-phase arrest of prostate cancer cells via the peroxisome proliferator-activated receptor gamma ligand, 15-deoxy-delta12,14-prostaglandin J2. Cell Growth Differ 2000; 11:49–61.

143. Kubota T, Koshizuka K, Williamson EA, Asou H, Said JW, Holden S, Miyoshi I, Koeffler HP. Ligand for peroxisome proliferator–activated receptor gamma (troglitazone) has potent antitumor effect against human prostate cancer both in vitro and in vivo. Cancer Res 1998; 58:3344–3352.

144. Mueller E, Smith M, Sarraf P, et al. Effects of ligand activation of peroxisome proliferator–activated receptor gamma in human prostate cancer. Proc Natl Acad Sci U S A 2000; 97:10990–10995.

145. Jaiswal AK. Regulation of genes encoding NAD(P)H:quinone oxidoreductases. Free Radic Biol Med 2000; 29:254–262.

146. Venugopal R, Jaiswal AK. Nrf1 and Nrf2 positively and c-Fos and Fra1 negatively regulate the human antioxidant response element-mediated expression of NAD(P) H:quinone oxidoreductase1 gene. Proc Natl Acad Sci U S A 1996; 93:14960–14965.

147. Xie W, Barwick JL, Simon CM, Pierce AM, Safe S, Blumberg B, Guzelian PS, Evans RM. Reciprocal activation of xenobiotic response genes by nuclear receptors SXR/PXR and CAR. Genes Dev 2000; 14:3014–3023.

148. Xie W, Evans RM. Orphan nuclear receptors: the exotics of xenobiotics. J Biol Chem 2001; 276:37739–37742.

149. Seo JY, Kim H, Seo JT, Kim KH. Oxidative stress induced cytokine production in isolated rat pancreatic acinar cells: effects of small-molecule antioxidants. Pharmacology 2002; 64:63–70.

150. Mueller E, Sarraf P, Tontonoz P, Evans RM, Martin KJ, Zhang M, Fletcher C, Singer S, Spiegelman BM. Terminal differentiation of human breast cancer through PPAR gamma. Mol Cell 1998; 1:465–470.

151. Demetri GD, Fletcher CD, Mueller E, Sarraf P, Naujoks R, Campbell N, Spiegelman BM, Singer S. Induction of solid tumor differentiation by the peroxisome proliferator–activated receptor-gamma ligand troglitazone in patients with liposarcoma. Proc Natl Acad Sci U S A 1999; 96:3951–3956.

152. Sarraf P, Mueller E, Smith WM, Wright HM, Kum JB, Aaltonen LA, de la Chapelle A, Spiegelman BM, Eng C. Loss-of-function mutations in PPAR gamma associated with human colon cancer. Mol Cell 1999; 3:799–804.

153. Takahashi N, Kawada T, Goto T, Yamamoto T, Taimatsu A, Matsui N, Kimura K, Saito M, Hosokawa M, Miyashita K, Fushiki T. Dual action of isoprenols from herbal medicines on both PPARgamma and PPAR-alpha in 3T3-L1 adipocytes and HepG2 hepatocytes. FEBS Lett 2002; 514:315–322.

154. Ramos-Gomez M, Kwak MK, Dolan PM, Itoh K, Yamamoto M, Talalay P, Kensler TW. Sensitivity to carcinogenesis is increased and chemoprotective efficacy of enzyme inducers is lost in nrf2 transcription factor–deficient mice. Proc Natl Acad Sci U S A 2001; 98:3410–3415.

155. Kim YC, Masutani H, Yamaguchi Y, Itoh K, Yamamoto M, Yodoi J. Hemin-induced activation of the thioredoxin gene by Nrf2. A differential regulation of the antioxidant responsive element by a switch of its binding factors. J Biol Chem 2001; 276:18399–18406.

156. Kwak MK, Egner PA, Dolan PM, Ramos-Gomez M, Groopman JD, Itoh K, Yamamoto M, Kensler TW. Role of phase 2 enzyme induction in chemoprotection by dithiolethiones. Mutat Res 2001; 480–481:305–315.

157. Kong AN, Owuor E, Yu R, Hebbar V, Chen C, Hu R, Mandlekar S. Induction of xenobiotic enzymes by the map kinase pathway and the antioxidant or electrophile response element (ARE/EpRE). Drug Metab Rev 2001; 33:255–271.

158. Gradelet S, Astorg P, Leclerc J, Chevalier J, Vernevaut MF, Siess MH. Effects of canthaxanthin, astaxanthin, lycopene and lutein on liver xenobiotic-metabolizing enzymes in the rat. Xenobiotica 1996; 26:49–63.

159. Denison MS, Nagy SR. Activation of the aryl hydrocarbon receptor by structurally diverse exogenous and endogenous chemicals. Annu Rev Pharmacol Toxicol 2003; 43:309–334.

160. Astorg P, Berges R, Suschetet M. Induction of gamma GT- and GST-P positive foci in the liver of rats treated with 2-nitropropane or propane 2-nitronate. Cancer Lett 1994; 79:101–106.

161. Astorg P, Gradelet S, Leclerc J, Canivenc MC, Siess MH. Effects of beta-carotene and canthaxanthin on liver xenobiotic-metabolizing enzymes in the rat. Food Chem Toxicol 1994; 32:735–742.

162. Gradelet S, Leclerc J, Siess MH, Astorg PO. Beta-apo-8′-carotenal, but not beta-carotene, is a strong inducer of liver cytochromes P4501A1 and 1A2 in rat. Xenobiotica 1996; 26:909–919.

163. Astorg P, Gradelet S, Leclerc J, Siess MH. Effects of provitamin A or non-provitamin A carotenoids on liver xenobiotic-metabolizing enzymes in mice. Nutr Cancer 1997; 27:245–249.

164. Gradelet S, Astorg P, Pineau T, Canivenc MC, Siess MH, Leclerc J, Lesca P. Ah receptor–dependent CYP1A induction by two carotenoids, canthaxanthin and beta-apo-8′-carotenal, with no affinity for the TCDD binding site. Biochem Pharmacol 1997; 54:307–315.

165. Jewell C, O'Brien NM. Effect of dietary supplementation with carotenoids on xenobiotic metabolizing enzymes in the liver, lung, kidney and small intestine of the rat. Br J Nutr 1999; 81:235–242.

166. Breinholt V, Lauridsen ST, Daneshvar B, Jakobsen J. Dose–response effects of lycopene on selected drug-metabolizing and antioxidant enzymes in the rat. Cancer Lett 2000; 154:201–210.

167. Le Marchand L, Franke AA, Custer L, Wilkens LR, Cooney RV. Lifestyle and nutritional correlates of cytochrome CYP1A2 activity: inverse associations with plasma lutein and alpha-tocopherol. Pharmacogenetics 1997; 7:11–19.

9

Induction of Cytochrome P450 Enzymes by Carotenoids

Nora O'Brien and Tom O'Connor
University College, Cork, Ireland

I. INTRODUCTION

It is widely acknowledged that diet influences cancer risk in humans. Dietary parameters have been shown to influence the cancer process at many stages, including at the level of xenobiotic (foreign chemical) metabolizing enzymes. The modulatory effects of dietary and other parameters on xenobiotic metabolizing enzyme activities including modulation of the cytochrome P450 enzyme family (phase I metabolism) have been investigated. Modulation of these enzyme activities may influence the activation of potential carcinogens or the detoxification of reactive xenobiotic metabolites. Relatively little has been reported on the effects of carotenoids on the induction of cytochrome P450 enzymes.

II. CYTOCHROME P450 FAMILY OF ENZYMES

Cytochrome P450 enzymes are a large and functionally diverse family of hemothiolate proteins found in all types of organisms from prokaryotes, fungi, plants, arthropods, to mammals, including humans. They catalyze the metabolism of a great variety of lipophilic organic chemicals. Detailed and comprehensive recent reviews of these enzymes have been published (1,2). A special issue of *Archives of Biochemistry and Biophysics* has been published [Volume 409(1), 2003] containing a large number of papers on various aspects of cytochrome P450 enzymes and dedicated to R. W. Estabrook, one of the pioneers of research in this area. P450s are involved in the metabolism of both endogenous and exogenous compounds in humans. They play key roles in the metabolism of xenobiotics including drugs and environmental pollutants; biosynthesis of steroid hormones, vitamin D_3, cholesterol, and bile acids; and eicosanoid metabolism.

A standardized nomenclature system has been established for cytochrome P450 by a Nomenclature Committee (http://drnelson.utmem.edu/Cytochrome-P450.html). The root for all enzymes is CYP. The individual family is then designated by an Arabic numeral and the subfamily by a letter. Individual enzymes within a subfamily are numbered consecutively as they are reported to the Nomenclature Committee. Thus, the first officially named cytochrome P450 was CYP1A1. The completion of the draft sequence of the human genome revealed the presence of approximately 90 (55 functional and 25 pseudogenes) different cytochrome P450 genes (3). The properties of mammalian cytochrome P450s have been summarized (2) as follows:

1. Cytochrome P450 proteins contain approximately 500 amino acids and contain a thiol-ligand for the heme iron.
2. The P450s catalyze the NADPH and oxygen-dependent oxidative transformation of a large number of different chemicals. They are monooxygenases or mixed-function oxygenases.
3. P450s are distributed in almost every human organ with large amounts in the liver.
4. The cellular expression of many P450s is regulated by transcription factors which become activated (induced) by exposure to various chemicals. The ability of a chemical to induce is generally linked to a family of P450s, e.g., polycyclic aromatic hydrocarbons will induce one type of P450 while barbituates will induce a different type of P450.

Cytochrome P450s have a role in the metabolism of drugs and other xenobiotics, some of which may be involved in chemical carcinogenesis. The covalent binding of chemicals to cellular macromolecules (e.g., DNA, RNA, and proteins) is considered to be a key step in the multistage carcinogenesis process. The formation of chemicals with the high electrophilicity necessary to form DNA adducts very often requires metabolism by P450s, e.g., the metabolism by the CYP1A family of benzo[a]pyrene to its diol-epoxide. P450s can also damage macromolecules due to the production of reactive oxygen species as by-products of P450-catalyzed reactions. On the other hand, P450 may also metabolize certain compounds to less reactive metabolites. Many studies have demonstrated that P450 enzymes can be modulated and induced by factors such as smoking and alcohol consumption, prior exposure to drugs and medications, and dietary parameters. The remainder of this chapter will focus on the modulation by carotenoids of P450 enzyme activities.

III. MODULATION BY CAROTENOIDS OF CYTOCHROME P450 ENZYME ACTIVITIES IN ANIMAL STUDIES

The initial studies on this issue involved investigation of the effects of dietary supplements of β-carotene (20, 100, 500 mg/kg diet) on hepatic microsomal drug-metabolizing enzyme activities in mice (4). Supplementation for 14 days resulted in strong diminution of hepatic cytochrome P450 content and biphenyl-4-hydroxylase activity, but unchanged activities of aminopyrine N-demethylase and p-nitroanisol o-demethylase.

Red palm oil (RPO) from *Elaris guineensis* has been reported to be the richest known natural source of β-carotene (5). Tan and Chu (6) reported that the consumption of RPO by rats inhibited cytochrome P450 mediated benzo[a]-pyrene metabolism. They noted the presence of high levels of α- and β-carotene in the RPO. However, in a study of the effects of RPO on both phase I and phase II drug-metabolizing enzymes in rats, no induction of phase I enzyme activity was observed (7). These workers fed a diet containing 10% RPO or control groundnut oil to male Wistar rats for 4 weeks. This level of RPO provided 37 mg β-carotene and 18 mg of other carotenoids (mainly α) per kg diet. Total microsomal cytochrome P450 activity, in addition to microsomal aminopyrine-N-demethylase and microsomal ethoxyresorufin o-deethylase activities, was assessed. RPO resulted in no significant induction of these phase I enzymes compared to control. In contrast, a significant induction of the phase II enzyme glutathione S-transferase (GST) was observed. The authors speculated that the lack of phase I induction in conjunction with the enhancement of GST activity indicated promise for RPO as an inhibitor of carcinogenesis. Further work on the modulatory effects of carotenoids on cytochrome P450 phase I and phase II enzyme activities in animal models was conducted by a research group based in Dijon, France and reported in a series of publications in the 1990s (9,11,12,14,19,20,27,28). These workers noted that many prospective epidemiological studies have suggested a putative cancer prevention role for carotenoids found in fruit and vegetables. Krinsky (8) has also demonstrated the antigenotoxic properties of carotenoids in vivo and in vitro. The antioxidant properties of carotenoids have been commonly cited as a potential explanation for their anticarcinogenic and antigenotoxic effects. However, these effects might also be explained, in part, by modulatory effects on phase I and II enzyme systems. In the French group's initial study (9), the effects of consumption of β-carotene or canthaxanthin (300 mg/kg diet) for 15 days, excess vitamin A (70,000 IU/kg diet), or intraperitoneal injection of β-carotene (7 × 10 mg/kg body weight) on phase I and II liver enzyme activities in male Wistar rats were investigated. Neither β-carotene (fed or injected) nor excess vitamin A resulted in any significant induction of enzyme activity. Similarly, Edes and coworkers (10) showed that β-carotene did not alter hepatic aryl hydrocarbon hydroxylase activity in rats (marker of CYP1A1). However, these workers noted an enhancing effect of β-carotene on the activity of this enzyme in intestinal mucosa. Canthaxanthin, which accumulated in the liver to a much higher extent than ingested or injected β-carotene, proved to be a powerful inducer of liver xenobiotic-metabolizing enzymes (9).

The French research group subsequently expanded their work to investigate the effect of a range of carotenoids on liver xenobiotic-metabolizing enzymes in the rat. Gradelet and coworkers (11) investigated the effects of canthaxanthin, astaxanthin, lycopene, and lutein (up to 300 mg/kg diet of each carotenoid for 15 days) on xenobiotic-metabolizing enzymes in Wistar rats. This study confirmed the group's earlier findings that canthaxanthin (300 mg/kg diet) increased liver content of cytochrome P450 and a substantial increase in ethoxyresorufin o-deethylase (EROD) activity (139-fold) and methoxyresorufin o-demethylase (MROD) activity (26-fold) and decreased nitrosodimethylamine N-demethylase (NDMAD) activity. These enzyme activities are markers for various isozymes of cytochrome P450. Its inducing effect was still detectable at 10 mg/kg diet. Astaxanthin induced the same pattern of enzyme activities but to a lesser extent to canthaxanthin. Lutein had no significant effect and lycopene only decreased NDMAD activity (marker of CYP2E1). The CYP2E1 isozyme is involved in the activation of diethylnitrosamine (DEN), a known liver carcinogen in rats. Interestingly, a subsequent study (12) reported that lycopene (300 mg/kg diet) decreased the initiation of liver preneoplastic foci by diethylnitrosamine in the rat. These workers noted that only carotenoids bearing oxo functions in 4 and 4′ are CYP1A1 and CYP1A2 inducers. Gradelet and coworkers (11) also noted that hydrophobic and planar polyacyclic aromatic molecules such as 2,3,7,8-tetrachlorodibenzo-p-dioxin (TCDD), β-naphthoflavone (β-NF), and 3-methylcholanthrene (3-MC) selectively induce the transcription of the CYP1A1 and CYP1A2 genes through the binding of the molecule to a cytosolic protein known as the Ah receptor. Ligands of the Ah receptor (AhR) must satisfy strict structural requirements, i.e., they are hydrophobic, planar molecules that can fit into a rectangle of 6.8 × 13.7 Å (13). Canthaxanthin and astaxanthin do not satisfy these structural requirements. However, Gradelet and coworkers (11) speculated that both xanthophylls might undergo enzymatic or oxidative cleavage to smaller molecules, one of which might bind to the AhR. A second hypothesis proposed by Gradelet and coworkers (11) was that canthaxanthin and astaxanthin or one of their metabolites could induce CYP1A1 and CYP1A2 via a mechanism not involving the AhR.

Further elegant work by Gradelet and coworkers (14) attempted to enhance understanding of the mechanism of the effect of carotenoids on cytochrome P450 induction and the relationship to the AhR. Canthaxanthin or β-apo-8′-carotenal (300 mg/kg diet for 14 days) were fed to AhR-responsive C57BL/6 mice, AhR-low responsive DBA/2 mice, and AhR gene knockout mice. Liver microsomal cytochrome P450 and associated reductases were measured. The activities of several phase I and II xenobiotic metabolizing enzymes were also measured, in addition to immunoblots of CYP1A. The direct interaction between both carotenoids and cytosolic AhR of C57BL/6 mice was assessed in vitro.

Canthaxanthin induced both EROD (marker of CYP1A1) and MROD (marker of CYP1A2) in the C57BL/6 mice but did not modulate phase II enzyme activities. β-Apo-8′-carotenal induced only MROD activity. No enzyme activities were modified by feeding these carotenoids in either AhR-low responsive DBA/2 mice or in AhR gene knockout mice. Results of the immunoblot analysis correlated well with enzymatic analysis for CYP1A1 and CYP1A2. Neither carotenoid could compete with TCDD for the binding to the AhR in the C57BL/6 mice. However, it is a possibility, that carotenoids may bind to a second binding site on the AhR distinct from the TCDD-binding site. However, the use of the genetically engineered mouse model deficient in the AhR demonstrated that the carotenoids do act through an AhR-dependent signal transduction pathway. The DBA/2 mice have an altered AhR with low binding affinity for polycyclic aromatic hydrocarbons (15). The absence of an effect of dietary canthaxanthin or β-apo-8′-carotenal in the AhR-low responsive DBA/2 mice and in the Ah receptor gene knockout mice, in contrast to their effect in C57BL/6 mice, strongly suggests that cytochrome P450 induction by carotenoids involves the AhR. Furthermore, the fact that canthaxanthin induced both CYP1A1 and CYP1A2 activity in C57BL/6 mice whereas β-apo-8′-carotenal only induced CYP1A2 suggests that the mechanisms of induction of the two isozymes by the two carotenoids are not identical, though both are AhR dependent.

Gradelet and coworkers (14) posed the question as to why some carotenoids (canthaxanthin, astaxanthin, β-apo-8′-carotenal) induce CYP1A1 whereas other carotenoids (β-carotene, lutein, lycopene) do not, even though no obvious structural feature separates the former from the latter. Known metabolites that are potentially formed from canthaxanthin, astaxanthin, or β-apo-8′-carotenal can also be derived from β-carotene, which has no P450 inducing effect.

CYP1A1 and CYP1A2 are involved in the bioactivation of many carcinogens, polycyclic aromatic hydrocarbons, and aromatic amines (16), and high levels of these isozymes have been associated with increased cancer risk (17,18). However, Gradelet and coworkers (11) noted that human intakes of astaxanthin and canthaxanthin are probably less than 1 mg/day and therefore it was unlikely that these xanthophylls could exert an inducing effect in humans, assuming that man's response is similar to the rat's.

Further work by the same group (19) demonstrated that the apocarotenoid β-apo-8′-carotenal is also a strong inducer of CYP1A1 and CYP1A2. The induction profile resembled that produced by canthaxanthin and astaxanthin.

Ethyl β-apo-8'-carotenoate and citraxanthin resulted in similar effects to β-apo-8'-carotenal but of less intensity.

This group (20) has also investigated the effects of carotenoids on mouse liver xenobiotic-metabolizing enzymes. An earlier study described above (4) reported a strong decrease in cytochrome P450 activity in mice fed β-carotene. Astorg and coworkers (20) compared the effects of β-carotene, the three carotenoids that they had previously reported to induce CYP1A in rat liver (canthaxanthin, astaxanthin, and β-apo-8'-carotenal), and the classical CYP1A inducer 3-MC in Swiss mice. In contrast to findings in rat liver, only canthaxanthin showed some significant inducing effect on mouse liver CYP1A–dependent activities with a much weaker intensity than 3-MC. Astaxanthin and β-apo-8'-carotenal showed no inducing effects. These authors noted that the fact that carotenoids have different effects on cytochrome P450 induction in Wistar rats and Swiss mice is not due to a lack of responsivity of Swiss mice to CYP1A inducers, as 3-MC showed approximately the same potency as an inducer in the mice as in rats. In contrast to the findings of Basu and coworkers (4), β-carotene showed no inducing effects on cytochrome P450 in Astorg and coworkers's study (20). No explanation for this discrepancy was apparent. Many studies have reported that β-carotene decreases the potency of several classes of indirect carcinogens such as polycyclic aromatic hydrocarbons (21–24), nitrosamines (22), and cyclophosphamide (25,26). The reported protective effects of β-carotene suggest a decrease in the activation or an increase in the detoxification of the relevant carcinogens. However, this hypothesis is inconsistent with the lack of findings of an effect of β-carotene on cytochrome P450 activities in Astorg and coworkers's report (20). However, these workers noted, the β-carotene is also protective in vivo against genotoxic or cancer-initiating effects induced by direct carcinogens such as methylnitrosourea, which suggests that mechanisms other than the induction of xenobiotic-metabolizing enzymes may be involved.

Dietary carotenoids (canthaxanthin, astaxanthin, β-apo-8'-carotenal) which are inducers of CYP1A have been shown to reduce the carcinogenicity of aflatoxin B_1 (AFB_1) in rat liver by increasing the metabolism of AFB_1 to aflatoxin M_1 (AFM_1), a less genotoxic hydroxylated metabolite formed by CYP1A. β-Carotene did not alter AFB_1 metabolism (27,28). However, dietary β-carotene, as well as canthaxanthin, astaxanthin, and β-apo-8'-carotenal, was very efficient in reducing the number and size of AFB_1-induced preneoplastic glutathione S-transferase positive liver foci. Only canthaxanthin, astaxanthin, and β-apo-8'-carotenal decreased in vivo AFB_1-induced DNA single-strand breaks, the binding of AFB_1 to liver DNA and plasma albumin, and increased in vitro AFB_1 metabolism to AFM_1 (a less toxic metabolite). β-Carotene did not protect hepatic DNA from AFB_1-induced alterations. Thus, the observed protective effect of β-carotene against AFB_1-induced liver preneoplastic foci appears to be mediated by different and unknown mechanisms to the protective effects resulting from the

CYP1A-inducing carotenoids. These workers also demonstrated that dietary lycopene (300 mg/kg diet) or an excess of vitamin A (21,000 RE/kg diet) had protective effects against the AFB_1 induction of liver preneoplastic foci. β-Carotene, which is noted for its antioxidant properties, protected against AFB_1-induced preneoplastic foci whereas lycopene, which is also a good antioxidant, did not. The authors noted that β-carotene is mostly converted to vitamin A in the rat and it possibly protects against AFB_1-induced foci through its provitamin A activity. However, excess dietary vitamin A in their study did not influence the AFB_1 induction of preneoplastic foci.

The ability of dietary carotenoids to modulate xenobiotic-metabolizing enzymes in animal organs other than the liver has received very limited attention. Jewell and O'Brien (29) investigated the effect of 16 day intake of 300 mg/kg diet of β-carotene, bixin, lycopene, lutein, canthaxanthin, or astaxanthin on xenobiotic-metabolizing enzymes in liver, lung, kidney, and small intestine of male Wistar rats. Bixin, canthaxanthin, and astaxanthin significantly induced liver, lung, and kidney EROD (marker of CYP1A1). These three carotenoids also significantly induced MROD (marker of CYP1A2) in liver and lung while only canthaxanthin and astaxanthin significantly induced this activity in kidney. Pentoxyresorufin o-depentylase (marker of CYP2B1/2) and benzyloxyresorufin-o-dearylase (marker of CYP1A1/2, 2B1/2, and 3A) were induced in liver to a lesser degree by canthaxanthin, astaxanthin and bixin. Benzyloxyresorufin o-dearylase in lung was significantly decreased by all carotenoids. None of the marker enzyme activities were detected in the small intestine.

Further work on the ability of β-carotene to induce cytochrome P450 enzymes in organs other than the liver was reported (30). These authors investigated the effects of supplementation with 250 or 500 mg/kg body weight of β-carotene for up to 5 days on liver, kidney, lung, and intestine cytochrome P450 activities in male and female Sprague–Dawley rats. β-Carotene supplementation resulted in induction of a number of cytochrome P450 isozymes in all tissues. The most affected were CYP3A1/2, CYP2E1, CYP1A1/2, and CYP2B1/2 in the liver; CYP3A1/2, CYP2E1 and CYP1A1/2 in the kidney; CYP1A1/2 and CYP3A1/2 in the lung; CYP3A1/2, CYP1A1/2 and CYP2E1 in the intestine. Some sex differences were observed, i.e., males were more responsive to β-carotene in the lung whereas females were more responsive in the kidney. These authors claimed that the recorded induction of cytochrome P450 isozymes is consistent with the cocarcinogenic potential of β-carotene. They noted the possible relevance of this to the risk of lung cancer in heavy smokers, as induction of cytochrome P450 could lead to greater activation of the immense range of procarcinogens in tobacco smoke. Increased bioactivation of pro-carcinogens to final carcinogens could facilitate lung tumorigenesis by saturating DNA repair mechanisms and altering tumor suppressor genes. They further noted the fact that long-term supplementation with β-carotene in two separate intervention trials actually increased the relative risk for lung cancer among heavy smokers. While β-carotene itself may act as an anticarcinogen due to its antioxidant properties, its oxidized products which are particularly high in the lung fluids of smokers may facilitate carcinogenesis (31,32).

Further work in ferrets exposed to cigarette smoke and/or a pharmacological dose of β-carotene demonstrated a three to sixfold induction of CYP1A1 and CYP1A2 but not CYP2E1 and CYP3A1 in lung tissue (33). These authors also speculated that the enhanced lung carcinogenesis seen with pharmacological doses of β-carotene supplementation in cigarette smokers may be due to induction of cytochrome P450 isozymes. Cytochrome P450 enzymes are inducible in human lung and can convert carcinogens present in tobacco smoke into DNA-reactive metabolites (34). Greater cytochrome P450 activity in lung may also increase destruction of retinoic acid, which may suppress carcinogenesis in epithelial tissues such as lung (35). Liu and coworkers (33) demonstrated that low levels of retinoic acid in the lung of ferrets exposed to cigarette smoke and/or pharmacological doses of β-carotene are related to enhanced retinoic acid catabolism by the induced cytochrome P450 isozymes.

A recently published study (36) reported that astaxanthin and canthaxanthin (100 mg/kg diet for 3 weeks) do not induce kidney or liver xenobiotic-metabolizing enzymes in rainbow trout. A range of cytochrome P450 isozyme markers were assessed including ethoxyresorufin o-deethylase, methoxyresorufin o-demethylase, pentoxyresorufin o-dealkylase, and benzoxyresorufin o-dearylase. Their findings are in contrast to the previously documented cytochrome P450–inducing effects of canthaxanthin and astaxanthin in rats and mice.

A detailed study on the dose–response effects of lycopene on liver xenobiotic-metabolizing enzymes in female Wistar rats was conducted by Breinholt and coworkers (37). These authors noted the abundance of lycopene in the human food supply, its strong antioxidant function, its presence at between 21% and 43% of total carotenoids in human plasma and evidence of its cancer preventative effects. Lycopene was administered by gavage at doses of 0.001, 0.005, 0.05, and 0.1 g/kg body weight/day for 2 weeks. In contrast to Gradelet and coworkers (11) where lycopene had no inducting effect on P450 activities in male Wistar rats, benzyloxyresorufin o-dealkylase activity was significantly induced in a dose-dependent fashion at all lycopene doses investigated. Ethoxyresorufin o-dealkylase activity was induced at the two highest lycopene concentrations tested. No induction of pentoxyresorufin o-dealkylase or methoxyresorufin o-dealkylase was observed. Rat plasma lycopene levels ranged from 16 to 67 μM, which is within the lower range of mean human plasma concentrations. Gradelet and coworkers (11) did not determine plasma lycopene concentrations, and it cannot be concluded whether the differences in observed effects of lycopene between the two reports are due to differences in lycopene bioavailability or the use of rat models of different ages and sexes.

IV. CAROTENOIDS AND CYTOCHROME P450 ENZYME ACTIVITIES IN HUMANS

Very limited data have been generated on the induction by carotenoids of cytochrome P450 isozymes in humans. Le Marchand and coworkers (38) examined lifestyle and nutritional correlates of CYP1A2 activity in 43 human subjects with in situ colorectal cancer and 47 healthy population controls. In a stepwise multiple regression analysis, 27% of the overall variation in CYP1A2 activity was explained by seven variables. Plasma lutein accounted for the largest portion (7%) of the variance in CYP1A2 activity and was negatively associated ($p = 0.006$) with activity. The authors suggested that plasma lutein may be a marker of intake of green leafy vegetables which may contain other constituents that inhibit CYP1A2. However, plasma lycopene was positively associated ($p = 0.06$) with CYP1A2 activity. Results were similar for colorectal cancer cases and controls. Almost 73% of the variability in CYP1A2 activity was unaccounted for by any of the correlates examined, which is consistent with the hypothesis that a genetic polymorphism exists that would explain most of the interindividual variation. CYP1A2 is involved in the metabolic activation of various procarcinogens such as aromatic amines and heterocyclic amines through N-oxidation (39). Its activity can be easily measured in humans by monitoring the rate of demethylation of caffeine through analysis of caffeine and its metabolites in urine. These authors noted the desirability of further exploring lifestyle and nutritional correlates of cytochrome P450 activities in humans, preferably with a prospective study design.

Kistler and coworkers (40) recently investigated the capacity of astaxanthin to induce cytochrome P450 genes using human hepatocytes grown in primary cultures as an in vitro model. The human liver samples used for the preparation of the primary hepatocyte cultures were obtained from patients who underwent a partial hepatectomy for the resection of liver metastases of various origins. Their data indicated that astaxanthin induces CYP3A4 and CYP2B6 but not CYP1A1 and CYP1A2, as has been reported in the rat (11,19), when the human hepatocytes were cultured for 96 h in the presence or absence of 3.75 μM astaxanthin. CYP3A4 is the major form of cytochrome P450 in adult human liver.

V. CONCLUSIONS

Limited data exist on the induction of cytochrome P450 isozymes by dietary carotenoids. The poor correlation between findings in rats and mice in relation to factors influencing xenobiotic-metabolizing enzyme activities emphasizes the necessity for a conservative approach in extrapolating findings from rodents to humans. The very few data on induction by carotenoids of cytochrome P450 isozymes in human subjects further point to a conservative approach in interpreting data. Clearly, a need exists for further research, particularly in humans and cultured human cells, to clarify the role and delineate the mechanism(s) of action of dietary carotenoids in the modulation of cytochrome P450 isozyme activities.

REFERENCES

1. Danielson PB. The cytochrome P450 superfamily: biochemistry, evolution and drug metabolism in humans. Curr Drug Metab 2002; 3:561–597.
2. Hasler JA, Estabrook R, Murray M, Pikuleva I, Waterman M, Capdevila J, Holla V, Helvig C, Falck JR, Farrell G, Kaminsky LS, Spivack SD, Boitier E, Beaune P. Human cytochrome P450. Mol Asp Med 1999; 20:1–137.
3. Ingelman-Sundberg M. Polymorphism of cytochrome P450 and xenobiotic toxicity. Toxicology 2002; 181/182:447–452.
4. Basu TK, Temple NJ, No J. Effect of dietary β-carotene on hepatic drug-metabolizing enzymes in mice. Clin Biochem Nutr 1987; 3:95–102.
5. Rukmini C. Carotenes from red palm oil: current status, future prospects. In: Gopalan C, Narsinga B, Seshadri S, eds. Combating Vitamin A Through Dietary Improvement. New Delhi: Nutrition Foundation of India, Special Publication Series 6, 1992; 149–156.
6. Tan B, Chu FL. Effects of palm carotenoids in rat hepatic cytochrome P450–mediated benzo(a)pyrene metabolism. Am J Clin Nut 1991; 53:1071S–1075S.
7. Manorama R, Chinnasamy N, Rukmini C. Effect of red palm oil on some hepatic drug-metabolizing enzymes in rats. Food Chem Toxicol 1993; 31(8): 583–588.
8. Krinsky NA. Effects of carotenoids in cellular and animal systems. Am J Clin Nutr 1991; 53:238S–246S.
9. Astorg P, Gradelet S, Leclerc J, Canivenc MC, Siess, MH. Effects of β-carotene and canthaxanthin on liver xenobiotic-metabolizing enzymes in the rat. Food Chem Toxicol 1994; 32:735–742.
10. Edes TE, Thornton W, Shah J. β-Carotene and aryl hydrocarbon hydroxylase in the rat: an effect of β-carotene independent of vitamin A activity. J Nutr 1989; 119:796–799.
11. Gradelet S, Astorg P, Leclerc J, Chevalier J, Vernevaut MF, Siess MH. Effects of canthaxanthin, astaxanthin, lycopene and lutein on liver xenobiotic-metabolizing enzymes in the rat. Xenobiotica 1996; 26:49–63.
12. Astorg P, Gradelet S, Berges R, Suschetet M. Dietary lycopene decreases the initiation of liver preneoplastic foci by diethylnitrosamine in the rat. Nutr Cancer 1997; 29:60–68.
13. Gillner M, Bergman J, Cambillau C, Fernstrom B, Gustafsson JA. Interactions of indoles with specific binding sites for 2,3,7,8-tetrachloro-p-dioxin in rat liver. Mol Pharmacol 1985; 28:357–363.

14. Gradelet S, Astorg P, Pineau T, Canivenc MC, Siess MH, Leclerc J, Lesca P. Ah receptor–dependent CYP1A induction by two carotenoids, canthaxanthin and β-apo-8′-carotenal, with no affinity for the TCDD binding site. Biochem Pharmacol 1997; 54:307–315.

15. Poland A, Glover E. Genetic expression of aryl hydrocarbon hydroxylase by 2,3,7, 8-tetrachlorodibenzo-p-dioxin: evidence for a receptor mutation in genetically non-responsive mice. Mol Pharmacol 1975; 11:389–398.

16. Guenguerich FP. Metabolic activation of carcinogens. Pharmacol Ther 1992; 54:17–61.

17. Ioannides C, Parke DV. Induction of cytochrome P450 A1 as an indicator of potential chemical carcinogenesis. Drug Metab Rev 1993; 25:485–501.

18. Kawajira K, Nakachi K, Imai K, Watanabe J, Hayashi SI. The CYP1A1 gene and cancer susceptibility. Crit Rev Oncol Hematol 1993; 14:77–87.

19. Gradelet S, Leclerc J, Siess MH, Astorg P. β-Apo-8′-carotenol, but not β-carotene, is a strong inducer of liver cytochromes P450 1A1 and 1A2 in rat. Xenobiotica 1996; 26:909–919.

20. Astorg P, Gradelet S, Leclerc J, Siess MH. Effects of provitamin A or non-provitamin A carotenoids on liver xenobiotic-metabolizing enzymes in mice. Nutr Cancer 1997; 27:245–249.

21. Sorn S, Chatterjee M, Banerjee M. β-Carotene inhibition of 7,12-dimethylbenzan-thracene-induced transformation of murine mammary cells in vitro. Carcinogenesis 1984; 5:937–940.

22. Manoharan K, Banerjee M. β-Carotene reduces sister chromatid exchanges induced by chemical carcinogens in mouse mammary cells in organ culture. Cell Biol Int Rep 1985; 9:783–789.

23. Das SK, Jin TZ, Bandyopadhyay AM, Banerjee M. β-Carotene-mediated inhibitions of a DNA adduct induced by 7,12-dimethylbenz(a)anthracene and 7-hydroxymethyl-12-methylbenz(a)anthracene in mouse mammary gland in vitro. Eur J Cancer 1992; 28A:1124–1129.

24. Lahiri M, Bhide SV. Effect of four plant phenols, β-carotene and α-tocopherol on 3(H)benzo(a)pyrene-DNA interactions in vitro in the presence of rat and mouse postmitochondrial fraction. Cancer Lett 1993; 73:35–39.

25. Mukherjee A, Agarwal K, Aguilar MA, Sharma A. Anticlastogenic activity of β-carotene against cyclophosphamide in mice in vivo. Mutat Res 1991; 263:41–46.

26. Salvadori DMF, Ribeiro LR, Oliveira MDM, Pereira CAB, Becak W. The protective effect of β-carotene on genotoxicity induced by cyclophosphamide. Mutat Res 1992; 265:273–244.

27. Gradelet S, Astorg P, Le Bon AM, Berges R, Suschetet M. Modulation of aflatoxin B1 carcinogenicity, genotoxicity and metabolism in rat liver by dietary carotenoids: evidence for a protective effect of CYP1A inducers. Cancer Lett 1997; 114:221–223.

28. Gradelet S, Le Bon AM, Berges R, Suschetet M, Astorg P. Dietary carotenoids inhibit aflatoxin B1–induced liver preneoplastic foci and DNA damage in the rat: role of the modulation of aflatoxin B1 metabolism. Carcinogenesis 1998; 19:403–411.

29. Jewell C, O'Brien NM. Effect of dietary supplementation with carotenoids on xenobiotic metabolizing enzymes in the liver, lung, kidney and small intestine of the rat. Br J Nutr 1999; 81:235–242.

30. Paolini M, Antelli A, Pozzetti L, Spetlova D, Perocco P, Valgimigli L, Pedulli GF, Cantelli-Forti G. Induction of cytochrome P450 enzymes and over-generation of oxygen radicals in beta-carotene supplemented rats. Carcinogenesis 2001; 22:1483–1495.

31. Salgo MG, Cueto R, Winston GW, Pryor WA. Beta carotene and its oxidation products have different effects on microsome mediated binding of benzo(a)pyrene to DNA. Free Radic Biol Med 1999; 26:162–173.

32. Wang XD, Russell RM. Procarcinogenic and anticarcinogenic effects of beta carotene. Nutr Rev 1999; 57:263–272.

33. Liu C, Russell RM, Wang XD. Exposing ferrets to cigarette smoke and a pharmacological dose of β-carotene supplementation enhance in vitro retinoic acid catabolism in lungs via induction of cytochrome P450 enzymes. J Nutr 2003; 133:173–179.

34. Bartsch H, Nair U, Risch A, Rojas M, Wikman H, Alexandrov K. Genetic polymorphism of CYP genes, alone or in combination, as a risk modifier of tobacco-related cancers. Cancer Epidemiol Biomark Prev 2000; 9:3–28.

35. Lippman SM, Lotan R. Advances in the development of retinoids as chemo-preventative agents. J Nutr 2000; 130:479S–482S.

36. Page GI, Davies SJ. Astaxanthin and canthaxanthin do not induce liver or kidney xenobiotic-metabolizing enzymes in rainbow trout (*Oncorhynchus mykiss* Walbaum). Compar Biochem Physiol, Part C Toxicol Pharmacol 2002; 133:443–451.

37. Breinholt V, Lauridsen ST, Daneshvar B, Jakobsen J. Dose–response effects of lycopene on selected drug-metabolizing and antioxidant enzymes in the rat. Cancer Lett 2000; 154:201–210.

38. Le Marchand L, Franke AA, Custer L, Wilkens LR, Cooney RV. Lifestyle and nutritional correlates of cytochrome CYP1A2 activity: inverse associations with plasma lutein and alpha-tocopherol. Pharmacogenetics 1997; 7:11–19.

39. Guengerich FP, Shimada T. Oxidation of toxic and carcinogenic chemicals by human cytochrome P450 enzymes. Chem Res Toxicol 1991; 4:391–407.

40. Kistler A, Liechti H, Pichard L, Wolz E, Oesterhelt G, Hayes A, Maurel P. Metabolism and CYP-inducer properties of astaxanthin in man and primary human hepatocytes. Arch Toxicol 2002; 75:665–675.

10

Impact of Food Processing on Content and Bioavailability of Carotenoids

Amy C. Boileau
Abbott Laboratories, Columbus, Ohio, U.S.A.

John W. Erdman, Jr.
University of Illinois, Urbana, Illinois, U.S.A.

I. INTRODUCTION

A number of variables determine the carotenoid content of raw whole fruits and vegetables. These include variety (cultivars), maturity at harvest, growing season, indoor versus outdoor growth, growing location, and harvest storage conditions (1–3). When considering the absolute carotenoid content of foods, it is important to keep in perspective the inherent bioavailability differences between carotenoids from fruits versus carotenoids from vegetables, as well as the impact of food processing and cooking on bioavailability. These considerations are important when attempting to reasonably determine individual or population intake of carotenoids from foods.

Carotenoid bioavailability may best be described as a continuum with raw whole-food sources exhibiting the lowest relative bioavailability, mildly processed foods slightly better, and purified sources in oily or water-dispersible preparations having the highest bioavailability (4,5). Results from a number of well-designed studies have led to the conclusion that orange fruits rank above green leafy vegetables on this continuum. Most notably, dePee and colleagues reported that orange fruits (papaya, mango, squash pumpkin) provided twice the vitamin A activity from an equal amount of β-carotene than green-leafy vegetables and carrots provided (6,7). In addition, mean serum response for β-carotene was four times greater for subjects consuming fruits as than vegetables. This superiority may be due to differences between the cellular structures in fruits and vegetables that sequester carotenoids (8). In dark green leafy vegetables, carotenoids are contained in chloroplasts in crystalline form. In orange and yellow fruits, carotenoids are dissolved in oily droplets within the chromoplast structure. The functional result of these differences is that carotenoids dissolved in oily droplets, as they occur in orange and yellow fruits as well as sweet potatoes, are more likely to be solubilized by the digestive milieu during intestinal transit. Carotenoids contained within chloroplasts, in crystalline sheets, or complexed to proteins may not be as accessible to the digestive processes that render these compounds bioavailable. For example carrots, contain α- and β-carotene sequestered in crystalline sheets, surrounded by a number of thickened membranes (9–11). Thermal processing has the potential to improve carotenoid bioavailability by disrupting the matrix of the cellular structures. The extent of this disruption varies depending on the plant type and rigor of the processing applied. Increased extractability of carotenoids following heat treatment offers one fundamental observation to support this conclusion (12,13).

Increased extractability of carotenoids from spinach following blanching and steaming (12,13) has led to the logical assumption that disruption of the food matrix will improve carotenoid bioavailability. If the goal is to maximize carotenoid bioavailability, then disruption must be balanced so that processing severity does not result in excessive degradative loss of carotenoids through heat or oxidation. The type of food, or at least the type of cellular structures containing the carotenoids, in part determins where the optimal balance between maximum bioavailability and minimal nutrient loss will lie. In reality, a processing regimen is dictated by the requirements of food safety and desired organoleptic qualities of the final product. For example, it would not be practical to reduce the temperature or time of retort processing (canning) in order to minimize carotenoid loss. Retort processing is rigorous because canned foods are stored at room temperatures and must remain unspoiled for the duration of shelf life. Blanching of vegetables prior to freezing is also driven by the need to preserve organoleptic characteristics and improve shelf life. However, food storage and preparation methods used by consumers can, in many cases, be selected to maximize nutrient retention.

As consumer awareness of the potential health benefits of carotenoids grows, increasing numbers of food product manufacturers will draw attention to the carotenoid content of their products. For these manufacturers, knowledge of processing effects on carotenoid degradation and isomerization is critical. This knowledge is also equally important to the researchers who study carotenoid and vitamin A intake of individuals and populations. The purpose of the following discussion is to consider the impact of food processing and preparation on carotenoid content of foods in the context of bioavailability. The discussion is focused on β-carotene, lutein, and lycopene because these have been most thoroughly explored by the research community. The tables in this chapter summarize published reports of degradative losses and isomerization of β-carotene, lutein, and lycopene following processing and cooking.

II. β-CAROTENE

β-Carotene is valued because of its unique ability to provide retinol or active vitamin A. For this reason, knowledge of the effects of processing on β-carotene bioavailability is critical for accurate assessment of the provitamin A value of foods for the purpose of food surveys or epidemiological studies. For example, consumption of raw or unprocessed vegetables may provide significantly less bioavailable β-carotene (provitamin A) than consumption of an equal amount of processed vegetable. In addition, food manufacturers may base vitamin A label claims on β-carotene content of the food product. In these cases, it may be useful to consider the use of correction factors to account for β-carotene stability and proportion of cis isomers since they demonstrate less provitamin A value (14,15). A thorough understanding of the effects of processing on carotene bioavailability must include knowledge of degradation and isomer formation during processing and storage.

A. Food Processing

The impact of thermal processing on β-carotene degradation is summarized by process type in Table 1. Experimental commercial-scale deep frying of blanched carrot chips has been shown to result in significant loss of β-carotene (16). In this study, sliced carrots were dehydrated and then rehydrated in boiling water prior to deep frying. The authors further explored the effects of dehydration on carotenoid degradation and found that deep-fried sliced carrots retained approximately 90% of their β-carotene content when the dehydration–rehydration steps were eliminated. Carrots were merely steam blanched for 4 min, cooled under running tap water for 4 min, and soaked in 0.2% metabisulfite solution for 15 min prior to deep frying. When carrot slices were dehydrated in a cabinet dryer to moisture content <10% then rehydrated for 1 min in boiling distilled water, β-carotene retention upon frying was only about 67%, highlighting the detrimental effects of dehydration during processing. This study also included an experimental protocol to determine the optimal antioxidant presoak. In addition to metabisulfite, salt brine, erythorbic acid, and l-cysteine were studied. The results suggested that erythorbic acid was nearly as effective as metabisulfite in preserving carotenoid content.

Table 1 Carotenoid Retention During Commercial Food Processing (% apparent retention, relative to fresh food)

Process	Ref.	Food	β-Carotene (%)	Lycopene (%)	Lutein (%)
Deep frying	16	Carrot chips (sliced), raw	100		
Not dehydrated[a]			91		
Partially dehydrated[a]			79		
Dehydrated and rehydrated at room temperature[a]			68		
Dehydrated and rehydrated in boiling water[a]			67		
Pasteurization	17	Tomato, hot-break extract	114	103	93
Retort sterilization	17	Tomato, paste	97	137	97
Extrusion	22	Starch-based matrix[b]	8		
Spray drying	26	Maltodextrin encapsulate[c]	89		
Drum drying	26	Maltodextrin encapsulate[c]	86		
Freeze-drying	26	Maltodextrin encapsulate[c]	92		
Oven drying 10 h, 65°C	24	Spinach	72		
Sun drying					
10 h	24	Spinach	43		
24 ± 12 h	25	Amaranth leaves[d]	2		

[a]All treatments included a 4-min steam blanch, 4 min cooling under running tap water, followed by a 15-min. soak in 0.2% (w/w) sodium metabisulfite. β-Carotene retention results include total carotene, all-*trans* β-carotene, α-carotene, and *cis*-β-carotene.
[b]Extrudate contained β-carotene, corn starch, and water.
[c]β-Carotene was encapsulated in 25 dextrose equivalent maltodextrin by each of three drying processes. Retention refers to β-carotene retained during first 24 h following drying.
[d]Green leafy vegetable (Amaranthus cruentus).

Table 2 Cis Isomer Formation During Commercial Food Processing and Home Cooking

Process	Ref.	Food	β-Carotene (% cis isomers)	Lycopene (% cis isomers)
Retort	19	Fresh tomato	12.9	
		Canned tomato	31.2	
		Tomato juice	32.7	
	18	Fresh tomato	21.8	4.2
		Tomato juice	78.3	3.6
		Whole tomato, canned	62.0	3.7
		Tomato soup	55.6	4.3
		Tomato sauce	54.1	5.1
		Tomato paste	85.9	4.1
	17	Tomato (fresh)	<1	20.6
		Tomato paste	9.7	25.2
	63	Tomato (fresh)		7.7
		Tomato paste		5.5
	19	Carrot (fresh)	0	
		Carrot, canned	26.8	
		Collards (fresh)	25.0	
		Collards, canned	44.0	
		Spinach (fresh)	11.8	
		Spinach, canned	34.5	
		Peach (fresh)	26.7	
		Peach, canned	40.0	
		Sweet potato (fresh)	0	
		Sweet potato, canned	38.8	
Lye peeling	18	Fresh tomato	21.8	4.2
		Raw, peeled	23.8	5.4
Concentration	18	Tomato (fresh)	21.8	4.2
		Tomato, paste	57.8	5.1
Pasteurization	18	Tomato (fresh)	21.8	4.2
		Tomato, hot-break extract	57.6	6.0
	17	Tomato paste: raw	<1	20.6
		Hot-break extract	3.9	25.5
	63	Tomato (fresh)		7.7
		Tomato sauce (hot break)		6.0
		Tomato sauce (cold break)		6.3
	19	Oranges (fresh)	15.4	
		Orange juice	16.7	
Stewing (high temperature) Temp range: 85°–110°C	53	Spaghetti sauce prepared from canned tomatoes canned tomato spaghetti sauce		16 44–65
Boiling 100°C, 7 min	19	Broccoli (fresh)	29.5	
		Broccoli, boiled	29.8	

A fairly wide range of values has been reported for β-carotene cis isomer content of processed foods (Table 2). Raw whole tomatoes are reported to contain between 1% and 22% cis isomers of β-carotene (17–19). This reported variability is likely due to analytical variation of the high-performance liquid chromatography (HPLC) methods used. Differences in cis-β-carotene content of cultivars may also contribute to reported variability.

Pasteurization of tomatoes during the production of tomato juice, a relatively mild process, does not appear to result in loss of β-carotene and may result in increased extractability (Table 1) (17). While pasteurization of tomatoes during juice production did not appear to result in significant β-carotene degradation, the process has been shown to result in significant conversion of all-trans β-carotene to cis isomers (18). In raw, fresh tomatoes, approximately 22% of β-carotene was present as cis-β-carotene as compared to 58% cis-β-carotene in pasteurized (hot break) tomato juice (Table 2). This was lower than the proportion of cis-β-carotene reported for the same tomatoes processed into juice by retort methods, approximately 78% cis-β-carotene. In the same study, whole canned tomatoes contained 62% cis-β-carotene, tomato soup 56% cis-β-carotene, and tomato sauce 54% cis-β-carotene following retort processing. The retort-processed tomato paste contained the greatest proportion of cis-β-carotene at 86%. The cis versus trans proportions reported for β-carotene are in stark contrast to the cis-lycopene profile of tomatoes reported by these authors (see lycopene section of this chapter).

Retort processing also appears to induce significant changes in the isomer profile of β-carotene in a variety of other foods (19–21). Retort processing of carrots and sweet potatoes resulted in an increase in cis-β-carotene from zero in raw food to 27% cis-β-carotene for carrots and 39% for sweet potatoes (19). In the same study, retort processing was also shown to increase the cis-β-carotene content of collards, spinach, and peaches (Table 2).

Extrusion processing employs high temperature and mechanical pressure in the presence of oxygen. As expected, β-carotene has been shown to be subject to extensive oxidative degradation during this process (22). Extrusion processing of a β-carotene and cornstarch slurry resulted in 92% loss of all-trans β-carotene (22). The degradative products identified in the extrudate were classified into six groups: cis isomers, diepoxides, apocarotenals, a ketone derivative, a dihydroxide derivative; and a monohydroxide diepoxide derivative. It may be possible to mitigate some loss of β-carotene by optimizing extrusion settings such as process temperature, screw speed, moisture content, and residence time for maximal carotenoid stability (23).

Dehydration of foods for long-term storage and shelf stability is likely to have a significant impact on carotenoid content. Temperature, light, and oxygen exposure are variables that determine the destructive potential of various dehydration methods. For example, oven-dried (10 h at 65°C) spinach retained

72% of its raw β-carotene content as opposed to sun-dried spinach (10 h), which retained only 43% (24). When amaranth leaves (green leafy vegetable component of traditional Tanzanian diet) were sun or shade dried for approximately 24 h, only 2–4% of the fresh leaf β-carotene content remained (25). By comparison, freeze-drying methods employ significantly less heat and thus offer the potential to minimize thermal degradation. Freeze-drying of carrots has been reported to prevent significant loss of β-carotene during both processing and shelf storage relative to alternative dehydration methods (11,21).

β-Carotene stability during commercial encapsulation in maltodextrin by different drying methods has also been reported (26). During the first 24-hours following drying, the spray-dried β-carotene and maltodextrin slurry retained 89% of the original β-carotene, the drum dried slurry retained 86%, and the freeze dried slurry retained 92%. Stability beyond the initial 24 h was dependent on the resultant particle size of the dried product and on the proportion of β-carotene present at the surface of the particles.

Oxygen exposure during storage of dehydrated foods is also an important variable. For example, β-carotene retention following shelf storage of dehydrated potato flakes has been shown to be inversely related in a dose-dependent manner to oxygen exposure (27). Consideration should be given to potential sources of oxygen such as head space in finished product packaging and also gas permeability of packaging materials.

B. Food Preparation

Microwave cooking of fresh vegetables is a rapid cooking method that appears to preserve carotenoid content fairly well. Microwave cooking of short duration, 5 min or less at high power, has been shown to preserve 100% of the β-carotene content of fresh broccoli, spinach, and green beans (12). These results were in contrast to earlier publications by this group demonstrating that microwave cooking resulted in small losses of β-carotene, i.e., 5–15% loss following preparation of acorn squash, brussels sprouts, and kale (28,29). Steaming broccoli and spinach for 5 min and 3 min, respectively, also did not result in significant degradative loss of β-carotene. Boiling broccoli for 7 min did not change the isomer profile for β-carotene in this vegetable (19). Collectively, the studies demonstrated that β-carotene is reasonably heat stable and can resist degradative loss during mild to moderate heat exposure.

Simmering amaranth leaves (green leafy vegetable component of traditional Tanzanian diet) for 15–60 min, covered and over medium heat, did not result in loss of β-carotene (25). However, loss of β-carotene from spinach has been reported following blanching (24). While blanching for 5 min resulted in little change, blanching for 15 min resulted in 26% loss of β-carotene from spinach leaves. These results are contrasted with the effects of both stir-frying (open-pan cooking for 30 min) and pressure cooking (10 min) spinach with fat, salt, and spices (24). In these experiments, β-carotene content was not changed.

C. Implications for β-Carotene Bioavailability

The bioavailability of β-carotene is of particular interest owing to its provitamin A properties. Factors such as food matrix, extent of degradation, and isomerization are important in determining the vitamin A value of β-carotene in foods. The current Dietary Reference Intake (DRI) for vitamin A reflects updated scientific knowledge of food matrix effects on bioavailability by suggesting a retinol equivalency ratio of 12 μg of β-carotene from foods to 1 μg retinol versus 2 μg β-carotene from supplemental β-carotene (free of matrix) to 1 μg retinol (30). The dramatic impact of the vegetable matrix itself cannot be ignored. β-Carotene has been reported to be only about 7% bioavailable from green leafy vegetables (7). β-Carotene from raw carrots has been shown to be only about one-forth as bioavailable as purified crystalline β-carotene and juiced carrots only slightly less than half as efficacious as the β-carotene supplement (31). The bioavailability of β-carotene from fruits, where the carotenoid is present in the chromoplast, has been shown to be significantly superior to that of β-carotene from green leafy vegetables (6).

Food processing has the capability to dramatically affect β-carotene bioavailability. At one extreme, physical disruption of the matrix can greatly improve the bioaccessible fraction of carotenoid; at the other extreme, extensive exposure to heat and oxygen can prove detrimental to the content of carotenoids in the food. Physical disruption of the matrix, in its simplest form, occurs when foods are chopped or pureed. This sort of basic processing has been shown to increase the bioavailability of β-carotene (32,33). In one study, food particulate size was significantly inversely associated with serum carotenoid concentration in children (34). Enzymatic liquefaction of spinach, resulting in extensive disruption of the plant matrix, provided a significantly more bioavailable source of β-carotene as compared to whole leaf or minced spinach (35). Although significant, β-carotene was still substantially more bioavailable when provided as a purified carotenoid suspended in vegetable oil. The mean plasma response of subjects who consumed the purified supplement was more than 13-fold greater than the subjects who consumed the liquefied spinach.

In addition to disrupting the matrix, thermal processing of vegetables has the potential to induce appreciable isomerization (see discussion above). The Food and Nutrition Board's DRI report considers *cis*-β-carotene to be half as bioavailable as all-*trans* β-carotene (30). It is well recognized that all-*trans* β-carotene is preferentially absorbed over cis isomers, as assessed by serum and triglyceride response in humans (36–39). This conclusion has been supported by animal models of β-carotene bioavailability (14,15). You et al. have demonstrated that orally administered 9-*cis* β-carotene is isomerized to the all-trans isomer in the gut prior to incorporation into chylomicrons (40). In this study, oral ingestion of $[^{13}C]9$-*cis*-β-carotene by human subjects resulted in the appearance of $[^{13}C]$all-*trans* β-carotene and $[^{13}C]$all-*trans* retinol in plasma. This was the first study to show that β-carotene undergoes isomerization at the level of the gut. However, it is not clear if this finding is physiologically relevant only at very low intraluminal concentrations, thus explaining the observation that all-*trans* β-carotene functionally provides greater vitamin A value.

Extensive isomerization of β-carotene in processed foods may reduce bioavailability. However, for processed vegetables, the positive impact of thermal and mechanical disruption of the matrix on bioavailability may be of greater value. In a cross-over study comparing plasma β-carotene following 4-week periods of feeding either raw vegetables (carrots and spinach) or pureed and retort-processed carrots and spinach, plasma response was increased three-fold following the processed vegetable arm, despite significant β-carotene isomerization (41). The raw vegetable dose was comprised of 94% all-*trans* and 6% *cis*-β-carotene and the processed vegetables provided 76% all-*trans* and 24% *cis*-β-carotene. The daily dose of β-carotene provided by each of these treatments was approximately 9.3 mg. This observation suggests that at this level of daily intake, cis isomerization of β-carotene is not detrimental to β-carotene bioavailability; rather the benefits of thermal processing on the plant matrix outweigh it. A more recent study employing stable isotope technology supports this conclusion. The authors concluded that β-carotene bioavailability from pureed and retort-processed carrots was two times greater than carrots boiled and mashed, despite increased cis isomer content of the more extensively processed carrot puree (42). Additive effects of homogenization on heat treatment have been demonstrated in humans using a factorial study design approach (43). In this approach, β-carotene bioavailability from canned tomatoes was improved following additional homogenization. Additional heat treatment, beyond that provided by the thermal process of canning, did not appear to enhance bioavailability even in samples that were also extensively homogenized.

An interesting approach to maximizing β-carotene bioavailability from processed foods comes from an observation reported in an animal study (44). During intestinal infusion of β-carotene in ferrets, it was noted that α-tocopherol enhanced the lymphatic transport by 4-fold when present at physiological levels and up to 21-fold when present in the infusate at a pharmacological concentration. The addition of optimized antioxidant blends to food ingredients might serve to protect the carotenoid content during processing and also during shelf storage. In addition, antioxidants may improve carotenoid bioavailability during gastrointestinal processing by reducing oxidation of the molecule.

III. LUTEIN

Lutein is primarily present as a fatty acid ester in certain orange fruits and vegetables such as squash and papaya (45). In green leafy vegetables, lutein is present unesterified to fatty acids or as free lutein (45). The impact of this difference on bioavailability and food processing stability is not known. Lutein and its structural isomer, zeaxanthin, have attracted a great deal of attention owing to the plausibility that they function as blue-light filters in protecting the eye (46). Increased epidemiological research has made accurate estimation of dietary lutein intake and absorption increasingly important. A number of food companies have added lutein to products or have focused labeling attention on the inherent content of lutein in their foods. For this reason, knowledge of lutein's stability, isomerization during processing, and bioavailability has become critical.

A. Food Processing

The effects of commercial food processing on lutein stability have been reported only for a small number of applications. In tomatoes, nearly 100% retention of lutein content during the manufacture of tomato puree and paste has been reported (Table 1) (17). Khachik and Beecher have measured lutein in processed foods and have identified a possible dehydration product of lutein that may be produced during the acidic processing conditions during the manufacture of baby food squash (28). Lutein degradation and isomerization has also been noted during retort processing of low-acid canned foods (Abbott Laboratories, personal communication).

The effects of commercial food processing on lutein in foods are not well characterized. Perhaps one reason for this may be that β-carotene and lycopene have historically attracted more health research interest. Analytical limitations have also likely contributed to the lack of literature. Increasing interest in the health impact of lutein will likely result in more published data in the future.

B. Food Preparation

Microwave cooking, for 5 min or less at high power, has been shown to preserve 100% of the lutein content of fresh broccoli, spinach, and green beans (12). While trans and cis isomers of lutein and neoxanthin appeared to be quite stable, this was not the case for all xanthophylls. Violaxanthin and lutein epoxide losses were appreciable even under these mild cooking conditions. Boiling green beans for 1 h did not result in loss of lutein; however, neoxanthin, violaxanthin, and lutein 5,6-epoxide were mostly destroyed (12) (Table 3).

Table 3 Carotenoid Retention During Cooking/Food Preparation
(% Apparent Retention, Relative to Fresh Food)

Cooking method	Ref.	Food	β-Carotene (%)	Lycopene (%)	Lutein (%)
Microwave in water					
6 min	29	Brussels sprouts	85		88
		Kale	86		69
8 min	28	Acorn squash	95		74
Microwave, no water	12	Broccoli	105		116
		Spinach	102		92
		Green beans	113		120
Steaming	12	Broccoli	118		115
		Spinach	111		112
Stewing, medium heat 8 min	12	Tomato	107	112	115
Simmering, covered, med heat	25				
15 min		Amaranth leaves[a]	74		
30 min		Amaranth leaves[a]	83		
60 min		Amaranth leaves[a]	87		
Boiling	12				
9 min		Green beans	115		103
1 h		Green beans	112		107
Blanching					
5 min	24	Spinach	92		
5 min	25	Amaranth leaves[a]	84		
10 min	24	Spinach	83		
15 min		Spinach	74		
Stir-fry, open pan 30 min	24	Spinach	98		
Pressure cooker 10 min	24	Spinach	99		

(continued)

Table 3 Continued

Cooking method	Ref.	Food	β-Carotene (%)	Lycopene (%)	Lutein (%)
Refrigerated storage, in polythene bag 48 h,	24	Spinach	83		
Refrigerated storage, no, bag 48 h	24	Spinach	99		

[a]Green leafy vegetable (*Amaranthus cruentus*).

The overall conclusion of these studies is that lutein, as well as carotenes, are reasonably heat stable during both mild to moderate cooking and may also be stable during more severe cooking procedures, such as boiling.

C. Implications for Lutein Bioavailability

The observation that lutein remains stable during food preparation implies that mild to moderate thermal processing will only improve lutein bioavailability from foods. Independent of thermal processing, the molecular structure of lutein appears to contribute to improved stability and bioavailability, at least relative to β-carotene. Unlike the hydrocarbon structure of β-carotene, lutein contains two hydroxyl groups, one at each end. Increased polarity of lutein relative to a hydrocarbon carotene influences its behavior during digestion and intestinal absorption. For example, when eight subjects were fed Betatene, a source of mixed carotenoids from the alga *Dunaliella salina*, lutein appeared in the chylomicron fraction at a proportion more than 13 times its concentration in Betatene (47). The chylomicron carotenoid content comprised 10.9% lutein and 81.2% β-carotene compared to 0.8% lutein and 93.5% β-carotene in the Betatene supplement. This observation has also been reported in chylomicron lymph samples of ferrets fed a tomato oleoresin source of lycopene (48). The oleoresin was reported to contain 98% lycopene, 2% β-carotene, and <0.1% lutein. The lymph samples obtained following oral ingestion of oleoresin contained only 46% lycopene while β-carotene comprised 9% and 45% of lymph carotenoid was lutein. In humans, lutein has been shown to be significantly more bioavailable than β-carotene from a diet of mixed vegetables (49). Lutein has also been shown to be significantly more bioavailable than β-carotene from spinach (35). These observations demonstrate the important role of polarity when estimating the relative bioavailability of different carotenoids from foods.

Purified lutein for dietary supplements or food ingredients is commercially available in two forms: lutein esters (diesters) or free lutein (unesterified or "free"). A recent study designed to systematically evaluate the bioavailability of lutein from these sources in humans found that lutein esters were slightly more bioavailable at the dose studied, approximately 20 mg for a 70-kg participant (50). In this cross-over study, the two lutein sources were directly administered as a crystalline suspension in gelatin capsules to the subjects. The authors compared their results to that of an earlier study published by Kostic et al. (51). In Kostic's study, the free lutein source was extracted from its crystalline suspension and dissolved in corn oil prior to being fed to human subjects. In their discussion, Bowen et al. (50) noted that lutein dissolved in corn oil appeared to be significantly more bioavailable than free lutein or lutein esters when offered as concentrated crystalline suspensions. These authors suggested that bioavailability of lutein from dietary supplements may be more dependent on the degree of processing or molecular dispersion applied to the lutein source rather than the form of lutein, i.e., free or esterified. By implication, processed foods that contain supplemental lutein may offer a more bioavailable dose of lutein than that of tablet-style supplements. Solubility and stability during processing should also be considered when selecting a commodity for food fortification.

IV. LYCOPENE

Tomatoes provide an abundant source of dietary lycopene, and more than 80% are consumed in the form of processed tomato products (1). The isomer profile of lycopene in foods is different than that observed for β-carotene. Lycopene is present in both fresh and thermally processed foods almost exclusively as all-*trans* lycopene (18,52). During thermal processing, β-carotene undergoes isomerization (see β-carotene section of this chapter) whereas lycopene remains more resistant to isomerization, even during exposure to extreme temperatures. This interesting observation has led to a number of studies testing the stability of lycopene in both food and purified preparations at high temperatures. One inherent difficulty in assessing the impact of processing on lycopene isomerization is that sophisticated separation techniques are required to adequately separate isomers. This difficulty may in part explain the variation in analytical results between studies that have explored this question.

A. Food Processing

During processing for juice, tomatoes typically undergo hot-break procedures for creating a peeled and mashed intermediate. The fruit is then either pasteurized and aseptically packaged or retort processed during canning. In one study, lycopene was not oxidized to an appreciable extent during the processing of fresh tomatoes to both a hot-break extract and retort-sterilized paste (17). In the same study, these processes induced minimal isomerization. The fresh tomatoes were reported to have 20.6% cis-lycopene whereas the processed products contained about 25% cis-lycopene. High-temperature stewing, 85–110°C for up to 1 h, has been shown to result in significant isomerization of lycopene in canned tomatoes (53). A carefully conducted study by Nguyen and Schwartz revealed that standard processing procedures, including lye peeling, hot-break juicing, and retort processing, did not induce isomerization of lycopene (18). In their studies, isomerization was successfully induced when tomatoes were heated, in olive oil, at approximately 200°C for 45 min. These authors also reported that commercially available drum-dried tomato flakes, as well as other processed tomato products, contained cis isomer content consistent with the experimental processed tomatoes products, less than 10% cis-lycopene. Lycopene is clearly quite stable in foods as an all-trans isomer. There is little likelihood that mild to moderate cooking methods applied to tomato products would have an extensive impact on the isomer profile.

B. Food Preparation

Stewing is a typical method used to prepare tomato sauce from fresh or canned tomatoes. In one report, stewing tomatoes over medium heat for 8 min did not change the amount of lycopene present (12). It seems reasonable to assume that extensive cooking time or extensive heat in the presence of oxygen in an open pan would eventually result in degradative losses of lycopene. Oxidation has been identified as a primary factor in degradative losses of lycopene during processing (1). The susceptibility of lycopene to thermal isomerization does not appear to be affected by cultivars, addition of cooking oil, or mechanical disruption of tomato skin during cooking (54). Unlike β-carotene and lutein, where extensive thermal isomerization occurred during tomato cooking, lycopene was stable in its all-trans form.

C. Implications for Lycopene Bioavailability

Thermal processing of tomatoes has been shown to improve lycopene bioavailability (55–57). Lycopene absorption from a single serving of tomato paste, as compared to fresh tomatoes, demonstrated 2.5-fold higher peak serum concentration and 3.8-fold higher total area under the curve (57). Both doses were fed to subjects along with 15 g of corn oil. In a study comparing fresh tomatoes to tomato puree, provision of tomato puree was significantly more effective in raising total plasma lycopene (56). The importance of thermal processing on lycopene bioavailability has also highlighted by the work of Stahl and Sies (58). These authors reported that a single serving of tomato juice (to provide 2.5 μmol/kg body weight or approximately 100 mg of lycopene for an 70-kg subject) did not increase serum lycopene in human subjects. However, when the same dose of tomato juice was heated to 100°C for 1 h with oil, serum lycopene did increase and peaked at 24–48 h. In a factorial study designed to test the interaction of mechanical disruption of the food matrix and thermal processing, it was reported that heat treatment alone was less destructive to the tomato cell wall than extensive homogenization alone (55). As a result, extensive homogenization appeared to be most effective at releasing lycopene from the tomato matrix, as measured by in vitro extractability and postprandial triglyceride-rich lipoprotein lycopene content.

In human plasma, β-carotene is nearly exclusively all-*trans* β-carotene while cis isomers of lycopene makes up at least 50% of the total plasma lycopene (58). The apparent discrepancy between the isomer profile of processed tomato products (mostly all-*trans* lycopene) and the predominance of cis isomers in serum and tissues has lead to speculation regarding the physiological origin of *cis*-lycopene. A number of studies have supported the hypothesis that *cis*-lycopene preferentially accumulates in tissues and serum (52,53,57,59). Data obtained during collection of lymph from ferrets fed tomato oleoresin provided evidence that cis isomers of lycopene are more bioavailable than all-*trans* lycopene (48). While the dose contained more than 90% all-*trans* lycopene, the mesenteric lymph secretions contained more than 75% cis isomers of lycopene. Serum and tissue lycopene was also enriched in cis isomers, representing more than 50% of lycopene present. The bioavailability differences may be due to the extreme hydrophobicity of all-*trans* lycopene and the possibility that *cis*-lycopene may be less likely to aggregate in a crystal structure, rendering it less soluble in the intestinal milieu (60). Thus, lycopene bioavailability appears to be enhanced by thermal and mechanical processing, even when these processes are severe. However, food processing and cooking does not induce appreciable isomerization of lycopene.

V. CONCLUSIONS

Lycopene and β-carotene behave differently during thermal processing of foods. While lycopene remains quite stable in its all-trans form, even during rigorous processing, β-carotene is far more labile to heat. Unlike *cis*-lycopene, cis isomers of β-carotene are not likely to be more bioavailable than the all-trans isomer. Thus, greater care should be taken when processing and cooking foods containing β-carotene. Relative bioavailability of *cis*- versus *trans*-lutein has not yet been explored. Perhaps its polar qualities will supersede any advantage, or disadvantage, observed by the introduction of cis isomers.

Beyond the scope of heat and mechanical disruption, factors such as lipid and antioxidant constituents of processed foods must also be considered. Additional antioxidant ingredients, such as vitamin C and E, seem to provide significant protection from both degradation and isomerization. Carotenoids themselves are recognized for their antioxidant value in foods high in polyunsaturated fatty acids, such as fish (61). The lipid constituent of processed foods may also be of importance to potential bioavailability. For example, lycopene absorption from olive oil has been shown to be more than twice as bioavailable as lycopene suspended in corn oil in rats (62). Many aspects of food composition, processing, storage, and preparation impact carotenoid content and isomer profile. The impact of these effects on bioavailability is quite variable. In order to maximize bioavailability, processing methods could be optimized to maximize carotenoid stability while also providing disruption of the food matrix that sequesters the carotenoids.

REFERENCES

1. Shi J, Le Maguer M. Lycopene in tomatoes: chemical and physical properties affected by food processing. Crit Rev Food Sci Nutr 2000; 40:1–42.
2. Khachik F, Beecher GR, Goli MB. Separation, identification, and quantification of carotenoids in fruits, vegetables and human plasma by high performance liquid chromatography. Pure Appl Chem 1991; 63:71–80.
3. Gross J. Pigments in Vegetables: Chlorophylls and Carotenoids. New York: Van Nostrand Reinhold, 1991: pp 73–254.
4. Yeum KJ, Russell RM. Carotenoid bioavailability and bioconversion. Annu Rev Nutr 2002; 22:483–504.
5. Boileau T, Moore AC, Erdman JW Jr. Carotenoids and vitamin A. In: Papas AM, ed. Antioxidant Status, Diet, Nutrition, and Health. Boca Raton: CRC Press, 1999: 133–158.
6. de Pee S, West CE, Permaesih D, Martuti S, M, Hautvast JG. Orange fruit is more effective than are dark-green, leafy vegetables in increasing serum concentrations of retinol and β-carotene in schoolchildren in Indonesia. Am J Clin Nutr 1998; 68:1058–1067.
7. de Pee S, West CE, Muhilal, Karyadi D, Hautvast J. Lack of improvement in vitamin A status with increased consumption of dark-green leafy vegetables. Lancet 1995; 346:75–81.
8. Castenmiller JJM, West CE. Bioavailability and bioconversion of carotenoids. Annu Rev Nutr 1998; 18:19–38.
9. Zhou JR, Gugger ET, Erdman JW, Jr. Isolation and partial characterization of an 18 kDa carotenoid-protein complex from carrot roots. J Agric Food Chem 1994; 42:2386–2390.

10. Ben-Shaul Y, Treffry T, Klein S. Fine structure studies of carotene body development. J Microsc (Paris) 1968; 7:265–274.

11. Desobry SA, Netto FM, Labuza TP. Preservation of β-carotene from carrots. Crit Rev Food Sci Nutr 1998; 38:381–396.

12. Khachik F, Goli MB, Beecher GR, Holden J, Lusby WR, Tenorio MD, Barrera MR. Effect of food preparation on qualitative and quantitative distribution of major carotenoid constituents of tomatoes and several green vegetables. J Agric Food Chem 1992; 40:390–398.

13. Dietz JM, Sri Kantha S, Erdman JW, Jr. Reversed phase HPLC analysis of α- and β-carotene from selected raw and cooked vegetables. Plant Foods Hum Nutr 1988; 38:333–341.

14. Deming DM, Teixeira SR, Erdman JW, Jr. All-trans β-carotene appears to be more bioavailable than 9-cis or 13-cis β-carotene in gerbils given single oral doses of each isomer. J Nutr 2002; 132:2700–2708.

15. Deming DM, Baker DH, Erdman JW, Jr. The relative vitamin A value of 9-cis β-carotene is less and that of 13-cis β-carotene may be greater than the accepted 50% that of all-trans β-carotene in gerbils. J Nutr 2002; 132:2709–2712.

16. Sulaeman A, Keeler L, Taylor SL, Giraud DW, Driskell JA. Carotenoid content, physicochemical, and sensory qualities of deep-fried carrot chips as affected by dehydration/rehydration, antioxidant, and fermentation. J Agric Food Chem 2001; 49:3253–3261.

17. Abushita AA, Daood HG, Biacs PA. Change in carotenoids and antioxidant vitamins in tomato as a function of varietal and technological factors. J Agric Food Chem 2000; 48:2075–2081.

18. Nguyen ML, Schwartz SJ. Lycopene stability during food processing. Proc Soc Exp Biol Med 1998; 218:101–105.

19. Lessin W, Catigani G, Schwartz SJ. Quantification of cis-trans isomers of provitamin A carotenoids in fresh and processed fruits and vegetables. J Agric Food Chem 1997; 45:3728–3732.

20. Jonsson L. Thermal degradation of carotenes and influence on their physiological functions. Adv Exp Med Biol 1991; 289:75–82.

21. Erdman JW, Jr., Poor CL, Dietz JM. Factors affecting the bioavailability of vitamin A, carotenoids, and vitamin E. Food Technol 1988; 42:214–221.

22. Marty C, Berset C. Degradation products of trans-β-carotene produced during extrusion cooking. J Food Sci 1988; 53:1880–1886.

23. Williams AW, Erdman JW, Jr. Food Processing: Nutrition, Safety, and Quality Balances. In: Shils M, Olson J, Shine M, Ross A, eds. Modern Nutrition in Health and Disease. Baltimore: Williams and Welkins, 1999: 1813–1821.

24. Yadav SK, Sehgal S. Effect of home processing on ascorbic acid and β-carotene content of spinach (*Spinacia oleracia*) and amaranth (*Amaranthus tricolor*) leaves. Plant Foods Hum Nutr 1995; 47:125–131.

25. Mosha TC, Pace RD, Adeyeye S, Laswai HS, Mtebe K. Effect of traditional processing practices on the content of total carotenoid, β-carotene, α-carotene and vitamin A activity of selected Tanzanian vegetables. Plant Foods Hum Nutr 1997; 50: 189–201.

26. Desobry SA, Netto FM, Labuza TP. Comparison of spray-drying, drum-drying and freeze-drying for beta-carotene encapsulation and preservation. J Food Sci 1997; 62:1158–1162.
27. Emenhiser C, Watkins RH, Simunovic N, Solomons N, Bulux J, Barrows J, Schwartz S. Packaging preservation of beta-carotene in sweet potato flakes using flexible film and an oxygen absorber. J Food Qual 1999; 22:63–73.
28. Khachik F, Beecher GR. Separation and identification of carotenoids and carotenol fatty acid esters in some squash products by liquid chromatography.1 Quantification of carotenoids and related esters by HPLC. J Agric Food Chem 1988; 36:929–937.
29. Khachik F, Beecher GR, Whittaker NF. Separation, identification, and quantification of the major carotenoid and cholorphyll constituents in extracts of several green vegetables by liquid chromatography. J Agric Food Chem 1986; 34:603–616.
30. Trumbo P, Yates AA, Schlicker S, Poos M. Dietary reference intakes: vitamin A, vitamin K, arsenic, boron, chromium, copper, iodine, iron, manganese, molybdenum, nickel, silicon, vanadium, and zinc. J Am Diet Assoc 2001; 101:294–301.
31. Torronen R, Lehmusaho M, Hakkinen S, Hanninen O, Mykkanen H. Serum β-carotene response to supplementation with raw carrots, carrot juice or purified β-carotene in healthy non-smoking women. Nutr Res 1996; 16:565–575.
32. Parker RS. Absorption, metabolism, and transport of carotenoids. FASEB J 1996; 10:542–551.
33. Erdman JW, Jr., Bierer TL, Gugger ET. Absorption and transport of carotenoids. Ann N Y Acad Sci 1993; 691:76–85.
34. Patel H, Dunn HG, Tischer B, McBurney AK, Hach E. Carotenemia in mentally retarded children. I. Incidence and etiology. Can Med Assoc J 1973; 108:848–852.
35. Castenmiller JJM, West CE, Linssen JPH, van het Hof KH, Voragen AGJ. The food matrix of spinach is a limiting factor in determining the bioavailability of β-carotene and to a lesser extent of lutein in humans. J Nutr 1999; 129:349–355.
36. Stahl W, Schwarz W, von Laar J, Sies H. All-trans β-carotene preferentially accumulates in human chylomicrons and very low density lipoproteins compared with the 9-cis geometrical isomer. J Nutr 1995; 125:2128–2133.
37. Johnson EJ, Krinsky NI, Russell RM. Serum response of all-trans and 9-cis isomers of β-carotene in humans. J Am Coll Nutr 1996; 15:620–624.
38. Gaziano JM, Johnson EJ, Russell RM, Manson JE, Stampfer MJ, Ridker PM, Frei B, Hennekens CH, Krinsky NI. Discrimination in absorption or transport of β-carotene isomers after oral supplementation with either all-trans- or 9-cis-β-carotene. Am J Clin Nutr 1995; 61:1248–1252.
39. Stahl W, Schwarz W, Sies H. Human serum concentrations of all-trans β- and α-carotene but not 9-cis β-carotene increase upon ingestion of a natural isomer mixture obtained from *Dunaliella salina* (Betatene). J Nutr 1993; 123:847–851.
40. You CS, Parker RS, Goodman KJ, Swanson JE, Corso TN. Evidence of cis-trans isomerization of 9-cis-β-carotene during absorption in humans. Am J Clin Nutr 1996; 64:177–183.
41. Rock CL, Lovalvo JL, Emenhiser C, Ruffin MT, Flatt SW, Schwartz SJ. Bioavailability of β-carotene is lower in raw than in processed carrots and spinach in women. J Nutr 1998; 128:913–916.

42. Edwards AJ, Nguyen CH, You CS, Swanson JE, Emenhiser C, Parker RS. α- and β-carotene from a commercial carrot puree are more bioavailable to humans than from boiled-mashed carrots, as determined using an extrinsic stable isotope reference method. J Nutr 2002; 132:159–167.

43. van het Hof KH, de Boer BC, Tijburg LB, Lucius BR, Zijp I, West CE, Hautvast JG, Weststrate JA. Carotenoid bioavailability in humans from tomatoes processed in different ways determined from the carotenoid response in the triglyceride-rich lipoprotein fraction of plasma after a single consumption and in plasma after four days of consumption. J Nutr 2000; 130:1189–1196.

44. Wang X-D, Marini RP, Hebuterne X, Fox JG, Krinsky NI, Russell RM. Vitamin E enhances the lymphatic transport of β-carotene and its conversion to vitamin A in the ferret. Gastroenterology 1995; 108:719–726.

45. Zaripheh S, Erdman JW, Jr. Factors that influence the bioavailablity of xanthophylls. J Nutr 2002; 132:531S-534S.

46. Junghans A, Sies H, Stahl W. Macular pigments lutein and zeaxanthin as blue light filters studied in liposomes. Arch Biochem Biophys 2001; 391:160–164.

47. Gartner C, Stahl W, Sies H. Preferential increase in chylomicron levels of the xanthophylls lutein and zeaxanthin compared to β-carotene in the human. Int J Vitam Nutr Res 1996; 66:119–125.

48. Boileau AC, Merchan NR, Wasson K, Atkinson CA, Erdman JW, Jr. Cis-lycopene is more bioavailable than trans-lycopene in vitro and in vivo in lymph-cannulated ferrets. J Nutr 1999; 129: 1176–1181.

49. van het Hof KH, Brouwer IA, West CE, Haddeman E, Steegers-Theunissen RP, van Dusseldorp M, Weststrate JA, Eskes TK, Hautvast JG. Bioavailability of lutein from vegetables is 5 times higher than that of β-carotene. Am J Clin Nutr 1999; 70:261–268.

50. Bowen PE, Herbst-Espinosa SM, Hussain EA, Stacewicz-Sapuntzakis M. Esterification does not impair lutein bioavailability in humans. J Nutr 2002; 132:3668–3673.

51. Kostic D, White WS, Olson JA. Intestinal absorption, serum clearance, and interactions between lutein and β-carotene when administered to human adults in separate or combined oral doses. Am J Clin Nutr 1995; 62:604–610.

52. Clinton SK, Emenhiser C, Schwartz SJ, Bostwick DG, Williams AW, Moore BJ, Erdman JW, Jr. Cis-trans lycopene isomers, carotenoids, and retinol in the human prostate. Cancer Epidemiol Biomark Prev 1996; 5:823–833.

53. Schierle J, Bretzel W. Content and isomeric ratio of lycopene in food and human blood plasma. Food Chem 1997; 59:459–465.

54. Nguyen M, Francis D, Schwartz S. Thermal isomerization susceptibility of carotenoids in different tomato varieties. J Sci Food Agric 2001; 81:910–917.

55. van het Hof KH, de Boer BC, Tijburg LBM, Lucius BRHM, Zijp I, West CE, Hautvast JGAJ, Westrate JA. Carotenoid bioavailability in humans from tomatoes processed in different ways determined from the carotenoid response in the triglyceride-rich lipoprotein fraction of plasma after a single consumption and in plasma after four days of consumption. J Nutr 2000; 130:1196–2000.

56. Porrini M, Riso P, Testolin G. Absorption of lycopene from single or daily portions of raw and processed tomato. Br J Nutr 1998; 80:353–361.

57. Gartner C, Stahl W, Sies H. Lycopene is more bioavailable from tomato paste than from fresh tomatoes. Am J Clin Nutr 1997; 66:116–122.

58. Stahl W, Sies H. Uptake of lycopene and its geometrical isomers is greater from heat-processed than from unprocessed tomato juice in humans. J Nutr 1992; 122:2161–2166.

59. Yeum KJ, Booth SL, Sadowski JA, Liu C, Tang G, Krinsky NI, Russell RM. Human plasma carotenoid response to the ingestion of controlled diets high in fruits and vegetables. Am J Clin Nutr 1996; 64:594–602.

60. Britton G. Structure and properties of carotenoids in relation to function. FASEB J 1995; 9:1551–1558.

61. Eriksson CE, Na A. Antioxidant agents in raw materials and processed foods. Biochem Soc Symp 1995; 61:221–234.

62. Clark RM, Yao L, Furr HC. A comparison of lycopene and astaxanthin absorption from corn oil and olive oil emulsions. Lipids 2000; 35:803–806.

63. Re R, Bramley PM, Rice-Evans C. Effects of food processing on flavonoids and lycopene status in a Mediterranean tomato variety. Free Radic Res 2002; 36:803–810.

11
Transport, Uptake, and Target Tissue Storage of Carotenoids

Harold C. Furr
Craft Technologies, Inc., Wilson, North Carolina, U.S.A.

Richard M. Clark
University of Connecticut, Storrs, Connecticut, U.S.A.

I. INTRODUCTION

This chapter focuses on metabolism of carotenoids in humans. However, research from animal models also cited is because of the many gaps in our knowledge of human carotenoid metabolism. Some previous reviews on this topic include those of Goodwin (1), Davies (2), Olson (3), van Vliet (4), Erdman et al. (5), Parker (6,7), Furr and Clark (8), Castenmiller and West (9), van den Berg (10), Lee et al. (11), Parker et al. (12), Krinsky and Russell (13), and Khachik et al. (14).

The pathway for carotenoids from foods (or carotenoids in intestinal contents) to carotenoids in plasma and other tissues consists of many steps. Our understanding of carotenoid metabolism is complicated by the fact that examination of each individual step is difficult; most of the observations to date are of carotenoids at the beginning and ending stages (carotenoid content in foods and carotenoid content in plasma), but not of the intermediate steps. In addition, human studies suffer from substantial inter- and intraindividual variability, as pointed out by Dimitrov et al. (15,16) and confirmed by numerous subsequent studies.

As discussed elsewhere in this volume, the carotenoids may be classified as carotenes (hydrocarbon compounds, such as β-carotene, α-carotene, and lycopene) and xanthophylls (oxygen-containing carotenoids, such as lutein, zeaxanthin, β-cryptoxanthin, astaxanthin, and canthaxanthin). Hydroxycarotenoids (cryptoxanthins, lutein, zeaxanthin, astaxanthin) in plant food sources are often present as esters with long-chain fatty acids, but are invariably hydrolyzed in the intestinal lumen so that only the free carotenoids are taken up by enterocytes (as discussed in Chapter 12). The differences in polarity among carotenoids (astaxanthin > lutein ~ zeaxanthin > β-cryptoxanthin > α-carotene ~ β-carotene > lycopene) (17) are highly correlated with — and we presume are partially responsible for — differences in their metabolism.

A. Assessing Bioavailability of Carotenoids

Plasma concentrations of carotenoids are determined not only by rate of intake but also by rates of uptake from plasma into tissues and reflux from tissues to plasma. Individual carotenoids differ in plasma transport, uptake (and presumably release) by tissues, and undoubtedly in rates of catabolism and loss. Relative bioavailability of a specific carotenoid from different dietary sources can be estimated, but comparison of bioavailabilities of different carotenoids is problematic. And as pointed out by van den Berg et al. (18), absolute absorption cannot be calculated from area under the concentration curve (AUC) in plasma because the kinetics of absorption, transfer from plasma to tissues, and reflux from tissues to plasma are not known. Thus, attempting to assess bioavailability of carotenoids solely from plasma concentrations is risky!

B. Species Differences in Selective Accumulation of Carotenoids; Animal Models

It has become clear that there are species differences in the types of carotenoids found in tissues. Human plasma and other tissues, for example, contain lutein, zeaxanthin, α- and β-cryptoxanthin, α- and β-carotene, and lycopene in greatest quantities. Bovine plasma contains almost exclusively β-carotene (despite the presence of large amounts of lutein in the diet) (19). The iguana (*Iguana iguana*), on the other hand, seems to selectively take up xanthophylls (20). These differences may be due to (a) diet, (b) selectivity in intestinal absorption, (c) discrimination in plasma transport, (d) selectivity in tissue uptake from plasma, and (e) differences in metabolism in tissues. Even within a zoological family there can be substantial differences among species in plasma carotenoid concentrations, as shown by Crissey et al. for 12 members of the Felidae (21) and for 9 primate species (22).

    In general, mammals are categorized as either white-fat or yellow-fat animals: the carotenoid content and color of adipose tissue in yellow-fat animals is due to their ability to absorb and transport and store carotenoids reasonably well, whereas white-fat animals lack this ability at some point. Humans and other primates, cattle, ferrets, gerbils, and chickens are yellow-fat animals; pigs, rats, and mice have white-fat. Lee et al. have provided a useful review of the use of animal models in studying carotenoid metabolism (11).

Although the rat is generally considered a poor absorber of carotenoids, non-provitamin A carotenoids are absorbed in a dose-dependent manner, and it has been used in many studies of carotenoid metabolism. For example, van Vliet et al. showed that feeding high levels of β-carotene or canthaxanthin (0.2% of diet) resulted in accumulation of the dietary carotenoid not only in plasma but also in liver, lung, and mammae (23).

Ferrets, a species known to absorb carotenoids, can accumulate lycopene in tissues, with liver > intestine > stomach ~ prostate (and not detectable in testes) (24,25). Rats fed lycopene at the same amount per kg body weight accumulated greater concentrations of lycopene in tissues than do ferrets, but with the same order of relative concentration (25). In contrast, rats normally do not have detectable β-carotene in liver when fed at the same concentrations at which ferrets do accumulate β-carotene in liver (25). Lack of accumulation of β-carotene in rat is perhaps due to greater β-carotene cleavage activity in the rat.

C. Cleavage of Provitamin A Carotenoids

Provitamin A carotenoids (β-carotene, α-carotene, β-cryptoxanthin) are cleaved in intestinal cells (and in other tissues) by oxygenase enzymes to form retinoids as well as apocarotenoids and aporetinoids. This cleavage can be central (between the 15- and 15′carbons in the center of the polyene chain, producing retinoids as symmetrical products), or excentric (releasing asymmetrical products, i.e., apocarotenoids and aporetinoids). The mechanisms of these cleavage enzymes and the relative importance of these two pathways are discussed in detail elsewhere in this volume. Apocarotenoids are seldom detected in animal tissues but have been identified in some experiments (26); they have been used as analogs for study of carotenoid metabolism and show the same patterns of rise and fall in plasma concentrations as do other carotenoids (27,28). For our purposes in this chapter, it is important to note that cleavage is relatively inefficient in humans; significant quantities of provitamin A carotenoids escape cleavage and are released into the circulation for uptake by other tissues. This is in contrast to rodents, for example, where provitamin A carotenoids are efficiently cleaved to vitamin A, with little release of intact carotenoid into the blood unless massive doses are fed. This difference in cleavage efficiency among different species exacerbates the problem of finding appropriate animal models to help elucidate human carotenoid metabolism.

II. PLASMA TRANSPORT OF CAROTENOIDS

A. Overview of Lipoprotein Metabolism

Transport of hydrophobic constituents follows this scenario: Freshly absorbed lipophilic components from the diet are packaged primarily into chylomicrons, and small amounts of very-low-density lipoproteins (VLDLA) in the intestines. The intestinal lipoproteins are released into the lymph, and pass from the lymph into the general circulation (but thus are circulated through the entire body instead of passing via the portal circulation, which transfers nutrients from the intestines directly to the liver). Although triglycerides are removed from the intestinal lipoproteins during their circulation through the body (after hydrolysis of triglycerides by lipases), other components of intestinal lipoproteins are taken up by the liver. Endogenous lipids are released from liver as VLDL, which are transformed into intermediate-density lipoproteins (IDLs) and thence into low-density lipoproteins (LDLs) as components are removed during their circulation. High-density lipoproteins (HDLs) are formed by release from extrahepatic tissues and by exchange of components among lipoproteins in circulation. Chylomicrons are cleared rapidly from plasma (half-life on the order of minutes); VLDLs and IDLs have somewhat longer half-lives (cleared from circulation within hours); LDLs circulate for 2 or 3 days; and HDLs have half-lives of approximately 5–6 days.

The general structure of a lipoprotein (whether chylomicron, VLDL, LDL, or HDL) is of a nonpolar core (composed primarily of triglycerides and cholesteryl esters) surrounded by an amphipathic layer of phospholipids and apoproteins. Specific apoproteins originate in different tissues and can give an indication of the tissue of origin of the lipoprotein; however, there is considerable exchange of apoproteins among lipoproteins during circulation in plasma. The apoproteins are also responsible for interaction with lipoprotein receptors on tissues and hence uptake of lipoprotein components by tissues. It is assumed that carotenes (the most lipophilic carotenoids) are transported in the inner hydrophobic core of lipoproteins and that xanthophylls are incorporated in the outer, more hydrophilic phospholipid layer, with some hydrogen bonding between solvent water and the hydroxyl (or keto) functions of the xanthophylls; this presumption is by analogy with the lipoprotein transport of α-tocopherol, and there is supporting evidence from studies of xanthophylls in lipid bilayers (29–33). Borel et al. (34) found that β-carotene was more soluble than zeaxanthin in bulk triglyceride solution; in lipid droplets composed of a triglyceride core with a phospholipid outer coating (a model for lipoprotein structure), the solubility of zeaxanthin increased markedly with increasing phospholipid content whereas that of β-carotene increased only slightly.

It should be remembered that the conventional classification of lipoproteins by density (chylomicrons, VLDLs, IDLs, LDLs, and HDLs) is not definitive, especially when one considers that enterocytes are not only the source of chylomicrons, but that they also release VLDL and small amounts of HDL. This may be an important point when attempting to study kinetics of carotenoid plasma transport on lipoprotein fractions.

B. Carotenoid Packaging into Chylomicrons in the Intestine

It might be hoped that understanding the absorption and transport of other lipid-soluble nutrients could give insight into transport of carotenoids. Vitamin A also is delivered from the intestines to the liver in chylomicrons, as retinyl esters. However, at this point the similarity to carotenoid transport ends: in the liver the retinyl esters are hydrolyzed to retinol, and retinol is released from liver for delivery to other tissues on a specific carrier protein (retinol-binding protein). Vitamin E is perhaps a better model because there is no specific carrier protein for vitamin E in plasma; it is transported nonspecifically by lipoproteins, as are carotenoids. However, there is a protein in liver (α-tocopherol transfer protein) which discriminates in favor of α-tocopherol in the transfer of vitamin E compounds to nascent lipoproteins there; thus, although all forms of vitamin E are equally well absorbed in the intestines and transported via chylomicrons to the liver, it is α-tocopherol that is almost exclusively packaged into other lipoproteins for release into plasma and uptake by extrahepatic tissues.

The mechanism by which carotenoids are taken up by the enterocyte is unknown. Equally puzzling is how carotenoids are controlled once they enter the cell. Rao et al. isolated and partially characterized a cellular carotenoid-binding protein from ferret liver (35,36). In contrast, others have reported finding no cytosolic carotenoid-binding proteins (37,38). There are no reports of a carotenoid-binding protein in the enterocyte.

Within the enterocyte several proteins are known to bind lipophilic compounds. There are two fatty acid-binding proteins (LFABP and IFABP), acyl-CoA-binding proteins, sterol-binding proteins, and other proteins that control trafficking of lipophilic compounds within the enterocyte (39). The poor solubility of carotenoids in aqueous solutions suggests the need for some protein intracellular transporter of carotenoids. It is very possible, but not yet demonstrated, that one or more of these known binding proteins, or perhaps specific carotenoid-binding proteins yet to be discovered, are used for intracellular transfer of carotenoids. We call to the reader's attention the existence of sterol-binding proteins in human intestinal tissue, members of the ATP-binding cassette (ABC) family that can discriminate between phytosterols and cholesterol (40), and we raise the possibility of similar carotenoid-binding proteins, which may impart some specificity to intestinal carotenoid absorption.

The intestine synthesizes VLDLs and chylomicrons for transport of dietary lipids including carotenoids into the lymph. The assembly of the intestinal lipoproteins is not fully understood. Two models have been proposed. The first model is based on work by Tso and colleagues suggesting the existence of two independent pathways for VLDL synthesis and chylomicron synthesis (41). The VLDL pathway constantly functions even with low-fat diets. The chylomicron pathway becomes very active when dietary lipid is provided. With this model, one could envision a preferential incorporation of certain carotenoids in VLDLs and others in chylomicrons based on their structure. A more recent model is one of sequential assembly of lipoproteins (42). This involves the synthesis of a primordial lipoprotein containing primarily apoprotein B (apoB) and phospholipid. An independent synthesis of triglyceride-rich droplets within the enterocyte provides the hydrophobic domain for fat-soluble vitamins and carotenoids, and its size varies with dietary lipid load. The final step in synthesis involves fusion of the primordial lipoprotein with the lipid droplet. The production of VLDLs or chylomicrons depends on the size of the triglyceride-rich droplet. With this second model there would be no discrimination between carotenoids for incorporation into VLDLs or chylomicrons.

The bulk of chylomicron triglycerides and a substantial fraction of chylomicron cholesterol are taken up by extrahepatic tissues. By analogy, it is possible that carotenoids could be taken up from chylomicrons by extrahepatic tissues as they circulate through the body before reaching the liver. It should be noted that retinyl esters (which have polarity similar to that of carotenes) are situated in the inner lipid core of the chylomicron particle, are not hydrolyzed before reaching the liver, and so are taken up almost exclusively by liver cells. Therefore, it is tempting to speculate that the relatively polar xanthophylls, which are believed to be located in the outer layer of the chylomicron lipoprotein particle, may be taken up from chylomicrons by extrahepatic tissues but that the very nonpolar carotenes, which are buried in the inner lipid core, remain in the chylomicron remnants and are taken up almost entirely by the liver. To our knowledge this possibility has not been investigated experimentally.

C. Lipoprotein Transport of Carotenoids in Plasma

As early as 1936, Willstaedt and Lindquist identified the predominant carotenoids (lutein, zeaxanthin, lycopene, and β-carotene, as well as several unidentified carotenoids, most likely β-cryptoxanthin) in human serum and liver (43), but they did not provide dietary intake data on their subjects. The carotenoids that have been identified in human plasma samples are listed in Table 1.

A number of experiments have delineated the time-course of carotenoid concentrations on specific lipoprotein classes after an oral dose of carotenoid; the findings are consistently similar to the early observations of Cornwell et al. (44) (Fig. 1): an early peak in carotenoid content in chylomicrons followed quickly by a peak in VLDLs, with slower accumulation in LDLs and HDLs. Maximal concentrations of β-carotene associated with LDL in human plasma are much higher than those of β-carotene associated with HDL (see discussion below), but the rates of appearance and disappearance are the same in those two lipoprotein classes. Very similar kinetics have been observed for canthaxanthin in human

Table 1   Carotenoids Identified in Human Plasma

Carotenoids provided by diet (identified in foodstuffs)	Carotenoids presumably arising from metabolism rather than from diet (not identified in foodstuffs)
α-Carotene	3'-Hydroxy-ε,ε-caroten-3-one
β-Carotene	3-Hydroxy-ε,ε-caroten-3'-one
γ-Carotene	3-Hydroxy-β,ε-caroten-3'-one
Lycopene	ε,ε-Caroten-3,3'-dione
Neurosporene	3-Hydroxy-3',4'-didehydro-β,γ-carotene
ζ-Carotene	3-Hydroxy-2',3'-didehydro-β,ε-carotene
(7,8,7',8'-tetrahydrolycopene)	
Phytofluene	3'-Epilutein
Phytoene	2,6-Cyclolycopene-1,5-diol
α-Cryptoxanthin	Anhydrolutein
β-Cryptoxanthin	
Lutein	
Zeaxanthin	

Source: Modified from Ref. 14.

plasma after oral dosing (45). The time-course of the appearance and disappearance of squalene (46), another nonpolar lipid, is similar to that observed for carotenoids.

It is well documented that there is exchange of cholesterol esters among lipoproteins, mediated by the cholesterol ester exchange protein (CETP) and lecithin-cholesterol acyltransferase (LCAT). The fact that carotenoids disappear at equal rates from both LDL and HDL suggests that there is interchange of carotenoids between those two lipoprotein fractions also; Borel et al. predicted that dihydroxyxanthophylls (e.g., lutein and zeaxanthin) would exchange between lipoproteins faster than monohydroxyxanthophylls (e.g., β-cryptoxanthin) because of their localization in the outer shell of lipoproteins, and that carotenes (e.g., β-carotene, α-carotene, lycopene) would exchange very slowly because they are localized in the inner core (34). However, Cornwell et al. (44) argued against any such exchange, and Romanchik et al. (47) found no evidence for net exchange of carotenoids between lipoproteins. Tyssandier et al. (48) found bidirectional exchange of carotenoids between VLDL and HDL of trout, and bidirectional transfer of lutein between VLDL and HDL of human plasma, but not exchange of other carotenoids between these two lipoprotein classes; transfer to and from LDL was not reported. [Tyssandier et al. also found that carotenoid transfer between lipoprotein classes, both trout and human, was reduced in the presence of inhibitors of cholesteryl ester transfer protein and of LCAT (48).] In our opinion, the question of transfer of carotenoids between lipoproteins remains

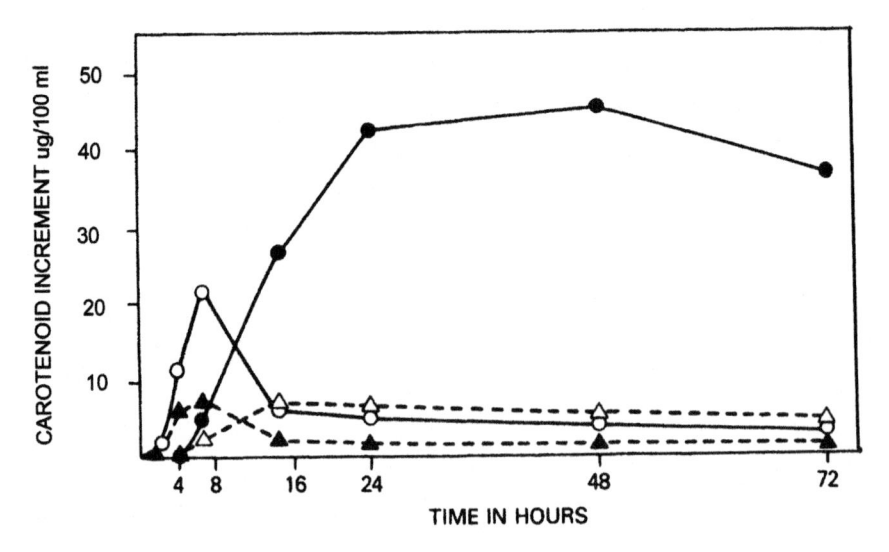

Figure 1 Average lipoprotein increments (over baseline plasma β-carotene concentrations) in plasma lipoprotein fractions for three normal subjects: chylomicrons (▲), VLDL (○), LDL (●), HDL (△) (44).

unresolved, as well as the possible importance of this mechanism in carotenoid transport and tissue uptake. An alternate explanation for the parallel disappearance of carotenoids from LDL and HDL is that exchange of carotenoids occurs not directly between lipoproteins but indirectly via tissue uptake from LDL and subsequent release of carotenoids into HDL.

Krinsky et al. first studied the distribution of carotenoids among lipoproteins and determined the distribution of xanthophylls versus carotenes between high-density lipoproteins and low-density lipoproteins (49). These studies were extended by Cornwell et al. (44) and by Bjornson et al. (50). Kaplan et al. found preferential uptake of specific carotenoids by isolated lipoprotein fractions in vitro (239). The consistent conclusion from these experiments is that carotenoids are not distributed equally among plasma lipoproteins: carotenes (lycopene, α-carotene, β-carotene) are found predominantly in LDLs in humans (approximately two-thirds of total carotene), with much smaller amounts in HDLs; dihydroxyxanthophylls (lutein and zeaxanthin) are found in higher amounts in HDLs than in LDLs; and the monohydroxyxanthophyll β-cryptoxanthin has an intermediate distribution (see Table 2 for an example of such results). The distribution shows an obvious relationship to the polarity of the carotenoids, i.e., less polar carotenoids are associated predominantly with LDL and more polar carotenoids are associated predominantly with HDL. Romanchik et al. pointed out that the distribution of hydrocarbon carotenes among lipoproteins is similar to that of total cholesterol, but

Table 2 Distribution of Carotenoids Among Human Plasma Lipoproteins

A. Concentrations of Carotenoids in Plasma Lipoproteins in Healthy Older Women (μM)

Lipoprotein	Lutein + zeaxanthin	Lycopene	β-Carotene
VLDL	0.06	0.10	0.06
LDL	0.26	0.63	0.34
HDL	0.25	0.16	0.07

Source: Adapted from Ref. 70.

B. Percentage Distribution of Carotenoids Among Human Lipoproteins (22 Male Subjects)

	Total carotenoids	Lutein + zeaxanthin	β-Cryptoxanthin	Lycopene	α-Carotene	β-Carotene	Cholesterol
VLDL	14	16	19	10	16	11	6
LDL	55	31	42	73	58	67	65
HDL	31	53	39	17	26	22	29

Source: Adapted from Ref. 232.

that distribution of xanthophylls (and α-tocopherol) is similar to that of phospholipids (47). As one measure of surface to core volumes, VLDL has a ratio of phospholipid to neutral lipid (triglycerides plus cholesteryl esters) of 0.3 : 1, LDL a ratio of 0.5 : 1, and HDL a ratio of 1.4 : 1 (34). It has been suggested that the nonpolar carotenes are "buried" in the nonpolar core (composed predominantly of triglycerides and cholesteryl esters) of the larger LDL particles and that xanthophylls are associated with the more polar phospholipid outer layer of lipoproteins (34). Such a model is consistent with the distribution of carotenoids in phospholipid bilayer model systems (29,31,32,51). Dialysis or gel filtration of LDL results in little or no loss of carotenoids (when recoveries are expressed per unit cholesterol), indicating that carotenoids are tightly associated with the lipoprotein (52). Lin et al. used resonance Raman spectroscopy to study the localization of lycopene and β-carotene in LDL, and concluded that at least some if not all of the carotenes are actually present close to the surface of the LDL (their study did not exclude the possibility of carotenes being in the inner core also); they suggest that lycopene is closer to the apoB-100 protein than is β-carotene and raise the possibility that this difference in proximity to apoB-100 may control differences in tissue uptake of carotenes (53). Parker suggested that the actual content of β-carotene per unit core lipid (triglyceride plus cholesterol) may be greater in HDL than in LDL. He also noted that although the total surface area of LDL in human plasma is approximately twice that of HDL, the content of lutein plus zeaxanthin is greater in HDL than in LDL (7). Thus, the partitioning into HDL needs further explanation.

In human umbilical cord blood, a greater fraction of β-carotene is transported on HDL than on LDL, but this is also true of cholesterol transport; the ratio of LDL β-carotene to HDL β-carotene increases from children to adults (54), apparently in concert with increasing LDL cholesterol concentrations.

The total amount of carotenoids in plasma is low: Romanchik et al. (47) estimated from their samples that each VLDL particle contained about four molecules of carotenoids (total), each LDL contained about one carotenoid molecule, and that only 25 of 1000 HDL particles contains a molecule of carotenoid (Table 3). The endogenous carotenoid composition of human LDL samples (nmol/mg protein) in 13 U.S. subjects (55) was: lutein, 0.08 $\pm$ 0.06; β-cryptoxanthin, 0.08 $\pm$ 0.05; lycopene 1.61 $\pm$ 2.39; β-carotene 0.37 $\pm$ 0.34; contrasted with α-tocopherol, 5.62 $\pm$ 2.87.

Although there is always concern that carotenoids added to lipoproteins in vitro may not incorporate physiologically, it is of interest that lutein added (in tetrahydrofuran solution) to human plasma incorporates preferentially into HDL, lycopene incorporates into LDL, and β-carotene incorporates into VLDL and LDL (56). This is consistent with the general distribution of carotenoids among human lipoproteins.

Reference ranges reported for plasma (or serum) carotenoids are given in Table 4. Although considerable differences exist from one nationality to another (not surprisingly, considering the differences in diet), in general it can be noted

Table 3 Molar Ratios of Carotenoids and Other Lipid Components in Human Plasma Lipoproteins (mol/mol Lipoprotein)[a]

	Lutein + zeaxanthin	β-Cryptoxanthin	Lycopene	β-Carotene	α-Tocopherol	Triglyceride	Unesterified cholesterol	Esterified cholesterol	Phospholipid
VLDL	0.68	0.36	2.12	0.52	145	11500	3539	3600	4545
LDL	0.05	0.09	0.72	0.23	12	298	475	1310	653
HDL	0.005	0.004	0.011	0.005	0.71	9.5	13	32	51

Source: Adapted from Ref. 47.
[a]Six subjects.

Table 4 Median or Mean Carotenoid Concentrations in Serum or Plasma in Different Populations[a]

Country	Ref.		Lutein Male	Female	Zeaxanthin Male	Female	β-Cryptoxanthin Male	Female	Lycopene Male	Female	α-Carotene Male	Female	β-Carotene Male	Female
Japan (618 M, 1196 F; 7–86 y)	233	Mean	35.2 (0.62)	39.2 (0.69)			19.9 (0.36)	33.1 (0.60)	20.4 (0.38)	26.8 (0.50)	6.4 (0.12)	9.6 (0.18)	18.8 (0.35)	34.3 (0.64)
Malaysia (58 M, 42 F; 17–78 y)	234	Median	31.8 (0.56)	31.8 (0.56)			29.3 (0.53)	28.2 (0.51)	16.6 (0.31)	21.4 (0.40)	7.5 (0.14)	8.6 (0.16)	21.4 (0.40)	27.9 (0.52)
Spain (210 M, 240 F; 5–79 y)	235	Median	10.8 (0.19)	10.2 (0.18)	3.4 (0.06)	19.9 (0.35)	15.5 (0.28)	21.5 (0.39)	18.9 (0.35)	19.3 (0.36)	2.7 (0.05)	3.2 (0.06)	11.8 (0.22)	15.0 (0.28)
UK (England) (944 /M, 938 F; adults)	236	Median	16.5 (0.29)	16.5 (0.29)			7.2 (0.13)	8.8 (0.16)	13.4 (0.25)	13.4 (0.25)	3.2 (0.06)	3.8 (0.07)	12.9 (0.24)	17.2 (0.32)
UK (Scotland) (100 M; 50–59 y)	237	Mean	27.3 (0.48)				5.5 (0.10)		27.9 (0.52)		5.4 (0.1)		28.9 (0.54)	
US	238	Mean	17.6	19.3			8.3	9.9	20.9	18.8	2.7	3.8	16.6	23.6

			C1	C2	C3	C4	C5	C6	C7	C8	C9	C10	C11	C12
(55 M, 55 F; 49–69 y)			(0.31)	(0.34)			(0.15)	(0.18)	(0.39)	(0.35)	(0.05)	(0.07)	(0.31)	(0.44)
US (121 M, 186 F; 45–65 y)	66	Mean	15.9 (0.28)	15.3 (0.27)	4.0 (0.07)	3.4 (0.06)			44.0 (0.82)	40.7 (0.76)	5.9 (0.11)	6.4 (0.12)	24.7 (0.46)	31.1 (0.58)
United States	103													
smokers		Mean	17.5 (0.31)	16.9 (0.30)			6.9 (0.12)	6.5 (0.12)	25.7 (0.48)	23.5 (0.44)	2.7 (0.05)	3.2 (0.06)	11 (0.21)	14.2 (0.26)
		Median	15.5 (0.27)	15.2 (0.27)			5.3 (0.10)	5.1 (0.09)	23.9 (0.45)	21.5 (0.40)	1.3 (0.02)	1.9 (0.04)	8.3 (0.15)	10.4 (0.19)
Nonsmokers		Mean	21.8 (0.38)	21.6 (0.38)			10 (0.18)	10.1 (0.18)	27.4 (0.51)	23.8 (0.44)	4.5 (0.08)	5.6 (0.10)	17.7 (0.33)	21.9 (0.41)
		Median	19 (0.33)	18.8 (0.33)			7.8 (0.14)	7.7 (0.14)	25.6 (0.48)	22.2 (0.41)	3.2 (0.06)	3.9 (0.07)	12.8 (0.24)	16.6 (0.31)
United States (137 M, 193 F; 18–45+)	239	Mean							33.9 (0.63)	35.7 (0.67)	4.5 (0.08)	7.4 (0.14)	18.5 (0.35)	31.8 (0.59)

Source: Adapted in part from Ref. 235.
[a](Values are given in μg/dL, and in μM in parentheses).

that (a) lycopene and β-carotene are present in highest concentrations; (b) lutein is present in higher concentrations than is zeaxanthin; and (c) females have higher concentrations than do males.

As another example of species differences, HDL are the predominant lipoprotein class in cattle and transport most of the β-carotene (57). Calves fed a ration of haylage/hay/straw (dietary intake of carotenoid not given) showed approximately twice as much β-carotene in HDL as in LDL, and approximately two-thirds as much in VLDL as in LDL (58).

Because carotenoids are transported by lipoproteins, and because lipoprotein concentrations themselves can be affected by a variety of factors, it has been suggested that plasma carotenoid concentrations should be expressed in terms of plasma lipids as a form of standardization. It has been found in fact that concentrations of carotenoids correlated well with HDL cholesterol, less well with LDL cholesterol, and not at all with VLDL (59); lycopene and lutein plus zeaxanthin correlated with plasma lipids better than did other carotenoids.

1. Interactions Among Carotenoids

In principle, it would seem that there is a possibility for competition among carotenoids for absorption and transport because they follow the same pathways. A variety of studies in humans and animal models suggest that some, but not all, carotenoids interfere with plasma appearance and deposition in tissues of other carotenoids; this subject has been recently reviewed by van den Berg (10). Kelley and Day reported as early as 1950 that high doses of lutein inhibited tissue storage of β-carotene (60). White et al. found that β-carotene inhibited the appearance of canthaxanthin but that canthaxanthin had no effect on apparent absorption and transport of β-carotene (61); β-carotene inhibited the appearance of lutein but the effect of lutein on β-carotene was not consistent among subjects (62). Van den Berg and van Vliet reported that lutein, but not lycopene, reduced β-carotene appearance in chylomicrons after oral dosing (63), but Tyssandier et al. found competition between lutein, lycopene, and β-carotene for incorporation into chylomicrons (64). High and Day reported that lycopene increased utilization of β-carotene for tissue deposition of vitamin A in rats (65). It is not clear if interference among carotenoids also occurs at the level of intestinal micelle formation and absorption, or incorporation into other lipoproteins, uptake into other tissues, or possibly enhanced rates of catabolism and loss (10).

2. Relationship of Plasma Carotenoid Concentration to Dietary Intake and Supplementation

Many studies have examined the relationship between dietary intake (as assessed by food frequency questionnaires, 24-hour recalls, or other instruments) and plasma concentrations of carotenoids. In general, it is found that plasma concentrations are correlated with dietary intake, but rather weakly, e.g., correlation coefficients ranging between 0.26 and 0.58 (66–68). The problem is, of course, complicated by the fact that it is difficult to assess dietary intake accurately; different instruments for assessing dietary intake do not correlate perfectly (67). Another great body of studies has assessed the impact of dietary supplementation with carotenoids on increasing plasma carotenoid concentrations; again, it is clear that plasma concentrations can be increased by use of supplements, but the effect is subject to considerable individual variation (69). Dietary supplementation with large amounts of β-carotene (90 mg/day for 3 weeks) results in enrichment of β-carotene in all plasma lipoprotein fractions, but the relative distribution of β-carotene was not changed (70). All this suggests that additional factors, such as those listed below, are involved in determining plasma carotenoid concentrations (71).

3. Seasonal Variations

Not surprisingly, it has been possible to demonstrate seasonal variation of serum β-carotene concentrations (68); in a Finnish male population, serum concentrations were highest in October–November and lowest in April–June, in correlation with seasonal variations in dietary carotenoid intake (72). In the same study, serum α-tocopherol concentrations did not show a seasonal variation. These and other observations lead to the reasonable conclusion that cultural differences in food availability, food choices, and consumption will affect plasma carotenoid concentrations.

4. Effect of Age on Plasma Carotenoid Concentrations

In a series of animal studies conducted by Hollander and colleagues, an increased capacity to absorb lipid-soluble nutrients, such as cholesterol, vitamins A, D, and E, was observed in aging rats (73–76). This improved absorption may be due to increased intestinal permeability and thinning of the unstirred water layer adjacent to the brush border (74). These physiological changes in the rat would influence absorption of all lipid-soluble dietary components, including carotenoids. It is not known if these changes observed in the rat occur in aging humans. There are limited data suggesting improved absorption of certain carotenoids by humans with age.

Winklhofer-Roob et al. (77) found consistent age-related increases in plasma cholesterol, lycopene, and β-carotene, but not α-carotene in a Swiss population aged 0.4–39 years. (They did not find seasonal influences on plasma carotenoid concentrations in this population.) Concentrations of lycopene and β-carotene, but not α-carotene, were correlated with plasma cholesterol concentrations. It would have been even more useful to have data on additional carotenoids and wider age spread. Kolb et al. found that concentrations of β-carotene (and vitamin A) increased with age in liver and testes of cattle (78), which is strongly suggesting of age-related accumulation of carotenoids in tissues.

Maiani et al. found that elderly women ($n = 10$, mean age 71 years) displayed higher serum responses (area under the time curve, AUC) for both β-carotene and retinyl esters after a large (15-mg) oral dose of β-carotene than did young women ($n = 17$, mean age 28 years) (79). Baseline concentrations of carotenoids were slightly higher in the elderly than in the young subjects. However, baseline cholesterol and baseline triglyceride concentrations were also higher in the elderly cohort, and the serum triglyceride AUC was also higher in the elderly cohort, suggesting that overall utilization of lipid-soluble nutrients increased.

5. Effect of Sunlight Exposure on Plasma Carotenoid Concentrations

It has been observed that serum β-carotene concentrations are decreased by exposure to sunlight (80). In another study, both plasma and cutaneous β-carotene concentrations were depressed on exposure to intense sunlight (81).

6. Effect of Menstrual Cycle on Serum Lipoprotein Carotenoid Distributions

Forman et al. studied fluctuations in total plasma carotenoid concentrations across the female menstrual cycle (82) and the changes in carotenoids in individual lipoprotein fractions (83). When adjusted for serum cholesterol concentrations, plasma concentrations of individual carotenoids varied independently during the cycle: β-carotene concentrations peaked at menses, lycopene and phytofluene concentrations peaked at midluteal phase, and lutein/zeaxanthin concentrations peaked during the last three phases of the menstrual cycle (82). Calculation of percentage distributions among lipoprotein fractions from the data of Forman et al. (83) does not show a marked shift in lipoprotein distributions across the menstrual cycle.

7. Effect of Body Composition on Plasma Concentrations of Carotenoids

Because of the lipid solubility of carotenoids, it is reasonable to hypothesize relationships of carotenoid content to body composition. Ringer et al. (84), Fuller et al. (85), Rock and Swendseid (86), and Zhu et al. (87) observed inverse correlations between body mass index (BMI) and plasma carotenoid concentrations. Zhu et al. further showed that plasma concentrations of β-carotene are inversely related to both fat mass (FM) and to fat-free mass (FFM), but that plasma concentrations of total carotenoids were inversely related only to FFM, not to FM.

Because increases in plasma concentration of β-carotene during a period of supplementation were negatively correlated with FFM but not with FM, Zhu et al. suggested that nonadipose tissue may have a more active role than adipose tissue in uptake of β-carotene from plasma. As one indication of mobilization of carotenoids from tissues back into plasma, it was found that decline in plasma carotenoid concentrations after cessation of β-carotene supplementation was also inversely related to BMI and FFM but not to FM. It is not surprising that nonadipose body tissue might be an important reservoir of total body carotenoids because it constitutes a large fraction of total body mass. [As points of reference, the mean FM was 31.0 kg, FFM was 59.0 kg, and BMI was 28.7 kg/m^2 in the study group; mean age 65.6 years (87).] These differences in rates of apparent uptake of carotenoids by adipose versus nonadipose tissue might be due, at least in part, to differences in lipoprotein receptors between these tissue types, as suggested by Parker (6).

Elevated plasma concentrations of carotenoids are generally associated with anorexia nervosa (54,86,88–98) [with the exception of one report (99), which also did not find the elevated lipoprotein levels characteristically associated with anorexia nervosa]. It has been reported that both plasma carotenoids (measured spectrophotometrically) and LDL cholesterol concentrations were elevated in cases of anorexia nervosa, but that they were not correlated (100) (perhaps because total carotenoids, not individual carotenoids, were measured). It might be illuminating to correlate these findings with the alterations in lipoprotein profiles associated with anorexia nervosa, but we have not been able to do so, in part because of differences among studies in criteria for defining anorexia nervosa.

8. Effect of Ethnicity

Serum concentrations of carotenoids in U.S. children and adolescents (data from the NHANES III study) were compiled by Ford et al. (101). Age and BMI were inversely related to serum concentrations of all carotenoids except lycopene. Statistically significant differences in serum concentrations were found between African-American, Mexican-American, and white European-American subjects, presumably due to dietary differences. Similarly, in adults sampled by the NHANES III study, Mexican-American adults tended to have higher plasma concentrations of α-carotene, β-cryptoxanthin, and lutein/zeaxanthin; African-Americans had high lutein/zeaxanthin but low α-carotene and β-cryptoxanthin; and those of European ancestry had high lycopene but low lutein/zeaxanthin and β-cryptoxanthin concentrations (102). At this time we assume that these differences are due to ethnic determinants of dietary intake more than to ethnic differences in carotenoid metabolism.

9. Effect of Tobacco Smoking on Plasma Carotenoid Levels

The effects of tobacco smoking on carotenoid metabolism are addressed elsewhere in this volume. In human studies, it has been found that smokers have lower plasma concentrations of lutein/zeaxanthin, β-cryptoxanthin, α-carotene, and β-carotene [data from the 1988–1994 NHANES study (103)]. It has been generally assumed that this reflects higher oxidative stress in smokers than in nonsmokers. However, interpretation of this observation is complicated by the concurrent observation that smokers tend to have lower dietary intake of carotenoids.

10. Other Factors Affecting Plasma Carotenoid Concentrations

Multivariate analysis found that statistically significant correlations of total serum carotenoid concentration in 85 elderly patients included serum cholesterol ($\beta = 0.38$), total serum proteins ($\beta = -0.35$), gender ($\beta = 0.34$, higher concentrations in women), carotene intake ($\beta = 0.28$), and midarm circumference ($\beta = 0.20$); these variables accounted for 46% of the variance in serum carotenoid concentrations (104).

Brady et al. found that the association between alcohol intake and reduced plasma concentrations of carotenoids was similar to the association between dietary intake and plasma concentration, suggesting a lifestyle effect rather than an effect of ethanol per se (105). It has been noted that infection with the coccidum *Eimeria acervulina* results in impaired absorption and plasma concentrations of canthaxanthin by chickens and loss of tissue carotenoids (106). To our knowledge, similar effects have not been studied in humans, but might be expected to reduce carotenoid absorption in our species as well.

There is one report of a patient suffering from a brain tumor who developed and maintained very high plasma concentrations of β-carotene while on a carotenoid-free diet, as concentrations of other carotenoids declined to barely detectable levels (107). The etiology of this condition is unknown.

11. Time-Course of Plasma Carotenoid Concentrations After Oral Intake

Observed peak concentrations of carotenoids in plasma occur at 6–24 hours after an oral dose in humans. Similar results have been noted using radioactive β-carotene in monkeys (108). This is slower than the time of appearance of cholesterol or triglycerides after a fatty meal, typically at 4–6 h (passage of ingesta through the ileum takes no longer than 6 h total), and at first sight raises several questions. What explains such a delay? An additional problem is raised (sometimes) by the presence of a second peak in plasma carotenoid concentration, which seems to accompany a later meal.

A reasonable explanation is provided by a model such as this: (a) The carotenoid from the diet is absorbed into enterocytes at the same time and rate as dietary triglycerides and cholesterol. (b) The dietary carotenoid is packaged into chylomicrons and released into the lymph, again in concert with freshly absorbed trigylcerides and cholesteryl esters. (c) After rapid circulation through the body, chylomicron remnants (with their carotenoid contents) are taken up by the liver. Plasma transit and clearance of chylomicrons is a rapid process, with half-lives of chylomicrons estimated to be 2.5–11.5 min (18). (d) Carotenoids are repackaged in liver into VLDL and released into plasma. Carotenoids are then taken up from VLDL and LDL to a limited extent by extrahepatic tissues. (e) Carotenoids efflux from tissues into HDL. (f) Carotenoids are taken up by liver from LDL and HDL, with potential repetition of the release and transport process. Support for point (c) is provided by observations by van Vliet et al. (109), van het Hof (110), and O'Neill and Thurnham (111) on transport of carotenoids in the triglyceride-rich (i.e., chylomicron and VLDL) fractions of plasma after a carotenoid-rich meal. Furthermore, the half-life of a carotenoid in plasma is approximately the same as the half-life of LDL measured in different experiments. This hypothesis is consistent with the delayed and prolonged elevation of plasma carotenoid concentrations after a large oral dose.

O'Neill and Thurnham (111) noted that lutein concentrations in the triglyceride-rich fraction (chylomicrons plus VLDL) peaked earlier (about 2 h postprandially) than did β-carotene and lycopene concentrations in this fraction (about 4–6 h after an oral dose in humans). [Similar observations were made by Bierer et al. (112) in total serum in calves, but the comparison is clouded by the very different lipoprotein composition and metabolism in calves than in humans (113).] Whether this difference between xanthophyll and carotene peak concentrations in triglyceride-rich lipoproteins kinetics represents more rapid intestinal absorption (and release) or more rapid clearance from plasma has not been investigated further.

A different problem is presented by a second peak in chylomicron carotenoid concentrations which sometimes accompanies a low-carotenoid meal following a carotenoid-rich meal (114). van den Berg et al. suggest that this is due to release of carotenoids from liver on VLDL and LDL (18). We suggest, however, that this is due to sequestration of absorbed carotenoids in enterocytes, with release prompted by the availability of a later dose of lipid; a very similar phenomenon has been observed with absorption of fatty acids (115). The time-course for the (relatively) very polar carotenoid astaxanthin showed two peaks in the triglyceride-rich lipoprotein fraction (at about 7 and 16 h) in three male human subjects (116), coinciding with peak plasma triglyceride concentrations. There was considerable variability, but most of the carotenoid was present in the triglyceride-rich fraction (chylomicrons plus VLDLs) at all time points (36–64% of total plasma astaxanthin), with the remainder approximately equally distributed between LDLs and HDL. [Because this was a kinetic (single-dose) study, not a long-term feeding study, equilibrium distribution of astaxanthin among lipoproteins was not determined.]

Plasma concentrations of carotenoids depend not only on input from diet (i.e., via the intestines) but also on rates of uptake into and efflux from other tissues. Considering the difficulty of direct measurement of human tissue uptake and release, another approach is kinetic modeling of carotenoid transfer (117). However, because of the lack of suitably labeled carotenoids, very few studies of carotenoids kinetics have been reported to date. To distinguish the oral carotenoid "tracer" dose from carotenoids already present in diet and tissues, von Reinersdorff (45) and Zeng et al. (28) used carotenoids that are not present normally in human tissues. The AUC varied considerably from one carotenoid to another, and was also dependent on dose. "Mean sojourn time" [MST, defined as the mean distribution of times that tracer molecules spend in the system from time of first entry until the time of irreversible exit from plasma (118)] was quite similar for three carotenoids that undergo little or no known catabolism in humans: MST was 144 ± 23 h for 4,4'-dimethoxy β-carotene and 209 ± 71 h for ethyl β-apo-8'-carotenoate (100 μmol oral doses) (28), and 192 ± 13 h (133 μmol oral dose) or 192 ± 19 h (265 μmol dose) for canthaxanthin (L. Yao and H. C. Furr, unpublished analysis of data of von Reinersdorff). Zeng et al. did not study distribution of carotenoids on plasma lipoproteins; von Reinersdorff separated lipoprotein classes, and MST of 194 ± 17 h for LDL-canthaxanthin and 208 ± 26 h for HDL canthaxanthin have been calculated from those data (L. Yao and H. C. Furr, unpublished observations), i.e., the same as MST for whole plasma. The terminal slopes of the concentration-time curves were the same for LDL canthaxanthin, HDL canthaxanthin, and whole-plasma canthaxathin (45), suggesting exchange among lipoprotein classes (direct or indirect; see discussion above). Depletion of serum carotenoids was followed in a long-term depletion study in young women by Burri et al. (119); the estimated half-lives were lycopene, 26 days; β-carotene, 37 days; zeaxanthin, 38 days; β-cryptoxanthin, 39 days; α-carotene, 45 days; lutein, 76 days. It is not known why the half-lives differ so much, unless there are substantial differences in tissue uptake, release, and catabolism. The rate of disappearance of plasma carotenoids in that depletion study seems slower than the rate of turnover of human lipoproteins, suggesting that plasma carotenoids concentrations are maintained by exchange with other tissues.

The stochastic kinetic modeling summarized above gives some hints about carotenoid metabolism, but cannot give estimates of rates of tissue uptake and release of carotenoids. Thorough understanding of such a multiple-pool model of carotenoid metabolism requires compartmental modeling techniques. The only compartmental modeling of carotenoid metabolism reported to date is that of Novotny et al. (120,121). The use of increasingly sophisticated methods for study of stable-isotope-labeled carotenoids should lead to more refined compartmental models of carotenoid metabolism (122–124). This is an area that deserves further investigation.

12. And Now for an Exception

Structurally, the apocarotenoid bixin (and its metabolite norbixin) is a dicarboxylic acid carotenoid of only 30 carbons; one of the carboxyl groups of bixin is methylated, whereas the analog norbixin has both carboxyl groups free and ionizable at physiological pH. These compounds are of more than academic interest because bixin is used as a food colorant (it is the major colorant in annatto). After a single oral dose of 16 mg of bixin, maximal concentrations in human plasma were seen at 2–4 h, and maximal concentrations of the metabolite norbixin were seen at 4 h (a broad peak with appreciable concentrations over the period 2–6 h); complete plasma clearance (to below levels of detection) occurred by 8 h for bixin and 24 h for norbixin (125). It was not determined whether the plasma bixin and norbixin were associated with lipoproteins. We suggest that this uniquely polar carotenoid, which possesses appreciable water solubility, is released from enterocytes into the portal circulation instead of into lymph chylomicrons and that it does not appreciably associate with lipoproteins in contrast to the metabolism of other carotenoids.

III. UPTAKE AND RELEASE OF CAROTENOIDS BY EXTRAHEPATIC TISSUES

A. Tissue Distribution

Although there are now many published data on human plasma carotenoid concentrations, the information available on other tissues is limited. The older studies used nonspecific spectrophotometric methods, which do not provide information on carotenoid profiles but often expressed total carotenoid as β-carotene. Almost no studies provide dietary information, so it is difficult to correlate dietary intake and tissue concentrations in more than qualitative terms. A limited number of human tissues have been analyzed for carotenoid content: liver (126–130), kidney (127,128,130), adipose tissue (126–128,131), adrenal glands (127,128), pancreas (126,127), breast tissue (6), lung (127,130), prostate (132–134), muscle (127), spleen (127), testes (127), thyroid (127), and skin (135).

There are definite differences in carotenoid profiles in different tissues. For example, the macula of the primate eye has relatively high concentrations of the xanthophylls lutein and zeaxanthin and in fact displays a marked spatial distribution. Certain other tissues, such as the prostate of the male primate seem to accumulate lycopene. Human milk concentrations of lutein and zeaxanthin are several times higher than those of β-carotene, in contrast to their concentrations in maternal plasma. These tissue differences are discussed in more detail below. Some typical human tissue carotenoid concentrations are presented in Table 5.

There is extreme paucity of information on mechanisms of uptake of carotenoids from plasma lipoproteins by tissues. Martin et al. studied uptake of carotenoids by HepG2 cells in culture and reported that uptake of β-carotene from LDL was similar to that from HDL (136); Kirkiles et al. found that BeWo human choriocarcinoma cells can take up canthaxanthin from human LDL and HDL (137). It has been suggested that lipoprotein receptors such as the LDL receptor may be involved in carotenoid uptake (and release?) (131), but this has not been confirmed experimentally. It is known that subcelllar structures such as the caveolae and their associated lipid transport proteins (such as caveolin and sterol carrier protein-2) are involved in cellular uptake and release of cholesterol, cholesterol esters, and fatty acids (138). Thus, it seems reasonable that these structures and similar proteins are involved in tissue uptake and release of carotenoids, but this mechanism has not been investigated.

It should be remembered that data such as those in Table 5 are based on a small number of samples and that these values are undoubtedly dependent on long-term dietary intake.

Table 5 Carotenoid Concentrations in Human Tissues (Average Concentrations, ng/g)

Carotenoid	Liver	Lung	Breast	Cervix	Prostate	Colon	Skin
α-Carotene	67	47	128	24	50	128	8
β-Carotene	470	226	356	125	163	256	26
γ-Carotene	nd	nd	nd	nd	48	nd	20
Lycopene	352	300	234	95	374	534	69
ζ-Carotene	150	25	734	57	187	134	13
Phytofluene	261	195	416	106	201	116	15
Phytoene	168	1275	69	nd	45	70	65
α-Cryptoxanthin	127	31	23	4	32	21	nd
β-Cryptoxanthin	363	121	37	24	146	35	nd
Lutein	1701	212	90	24	128	452	26
Zeaxanthin	591	90	14	nd	35	32	6
2,6-Cyclolycopene-1,5-diols	576	20	42	nd	7	19	7
3'-Hydroxy-ε,ε-caroten-3-one	527	22	15	nd	nd	12	nd
3-Hydroxy-β,ε-3'-one	319	24	32	nd	nd	17	nd
ε,ε-Caroten-3,3'-dione	314	nd	52	nd	nd	15	nd
3'-Epilutein	96	11	10	nd	nd	27	nd

Adapted from Ref. 14.
Source: nd, not detected.

1. Liver

There are marked differences in the capacity of different organs to take up carotenoids and release them back to the bloodstream. It has been suggested that organs with the greatest number of LDL receptors have the greatest uptake of lipoproteins and generally have the greatest concentrations of carotenoids (131). These organs include the liver, adrenal glands, and testes.

Regardless of the species studied, the liver has been reported to have a high capacity to accumulate carotenoids (130). Schmitz et al. measured liver concentrations of major carotenoids in samples from 20 humans of various ages (130); plasma concentrations were not measured, but the ratio of each carotenoid to total liver carotenoid content was quite similar to that of typical plasma concentrations, over a range of total liver carotenoid content from 2.5 to 77.1 nmol/g tissue. Others report that accumulation of individual carotenoids in the liver varies greatly with the type of carotenoid: Jewell and O'Brien (139) fed six different types of carotenoids to rats for 16 days, and the order of accumulation of carotenoids in the liver was canthaxanthin > lutein > bixin > lycopene > β-carotene > astaxanthin. The relatively poor accumulation of astaxanthin compared to the other carotenoids is difficult to explain but has been observed in several other rat feeding studies (Table 6) (140–142). Canthaxanthin deposition in the liver was consistently greater than that of the other carotenoids (139–142). It appears that large doses of canthaxanthin can be consumed without toxic effects. Tang et al. (143) provided pharmacological levels of canthaxanthin for 24 months via gavage to ferrets. Liver canthaxanthin was at its greatest level at 12 months and did not increase during the second year of the study. One possible explanation for the lack of a further increase in liver canthaxanthin was that the large amounts of dietary canthaxanthin initially consumed reduce the

Table 6 Liver Accumulation of Carotenoids in Rats Supplemented with a Variety of Carotenoids (Each Carotenoid Fed at 300 mg/kg Diet in Individual Feeding Studies)

Carotenoid reference	(nmol/g) (139)	(μg/g) (140)[a]	(nmol/g) (141)[a]	(μg/g) (142)[a]
Control	0.0 ± 0.0	0.0 ± 0.0	0.0 ± 0.0	0.0 ± 0.0
β-Carotene	76.6 ± 4.7	1.9 ± 0.5	—	9.2 ± 1.4
Lycopene	145.0 ± 6.0	16.3 ± 1.9	80.2 ± 12.5	15.8 ± 3.0
Lutein	547.7 ± 13.6	—	—	—
Canthaxanthin	1200.0 ± 14.9	26.2 ± 4.7	397.0 ± 83.0	20.0 ± 4.4
Astaxanthin	57.1 ± 6.6	0.25 ± 0.06	3.7 ± 2.1	0.10 ± 0.03

[a]Same diet.

subsequent accumulation of the carotenoid (144); it may be that the liver had become saturated with canthaxanthin.

In human autopsy samples, lycopene concentrations in liver were higher than those in kidney or lung, ranging between 0.2 and 20.7 nmol/g tissue (130) (lycopene concentrations in kidney ranged between 0.1 and 2.4 nmol/g, and in lung between <0.1 and 4.2 nmol/g).

There is relatively little information on the tissue turnover rates of different carotenoids. The kinetic characteristics of β-carotene uptake and depletion of several organs in rats fed semipurified diets for 21 weeks were reported (145); among the organs studied, the liver accumulated the greatest amount of β-carotene per unit weight and had the fastest turnover rate ($t_{1/2} = 9$ days). Carotenoid cleavage activity (conversion of β-carotene to vitamin A) has been demonstrated in human liver (146) and may be partially responsible for the disappearance of provitamin A carotenoids. An additional possible fate of liver carotenoids is their removal from the body by excretion in the bile; Leo et al. (147) reported that all the major carotenoids in human serum (β-carotene, α-carotene, lycopene, cryptoxanthin, and lutein/zeaxanthin) undergo biliary excretion.

2. Testes and Ovaries

All the major carotenoids in blood accumulate in human testes and ovaries (148). In populations that consume tomato products the testes accumulate very high concentrations of lycopene whereas the accumulation in the ovaries is moderate (148). In humans the adrenal gland and testes have similar high capacities for accumulation of lycopene, but in the rat the adrenal has a much greater capacity than the testes (149). Compared to the liver and other tissues in the rat, the testes accumulate only small amounts of lycopene in response to lycopene supplementation (25,144). The rat ovary accumulated canthaxanthin and lycopene to a greater degree than did the testes (144). In rats supplemented with β-carotene the ovary accumulated high levels of β-carotene and was still accumulating β-carotene after 21 weeks of supplementation (145).

It is well known that the yellow color of avian egg yolks is due to carotenoids, and commercial poultry feeds contain carotenoids to achieve appropriate coloration (150). During avian embryogenesis, the concentration of yolk carotenoids (which are predominantly lutein) decreases and liver content increases (151).

3. Prostate Gland

Epidemiological studies suggested that consumption of tomato products is associated with reduced risk of prostate cancer in men. It was soon shown that there is also an association between intake of tomato products and increased levels of lycopene in human prostate (132,152), and this has been confirmed in other studies. The intake-dependent accumulation of lycopene in prostate in the rat has also been demonstrated (149). The percentage of lycopene present as cis isomers is greater in human prostate than in serum and higher in serum than in food products (132,134,153), suggesting either isomerization or preferential retention of *cis* isomers in tissues.

4. Adrenal Glands

Based on analysis of various tissues obtained from human autopsies, the adrenal was reported to have the highest concentration of carotenoids (128). All the major carotenoids in serum were present with lycopene observed in the highest concentration. Stahl et al. (148) also reported large concentrations of lycopene in adrenal tissue. In a rat study involving feeding of varying levels of lycopene, the adrenal was the tissue that accumulated the highest concentration of lycopene (149). In another study, in which β-carotene was fed to rats, the adrenal gland accumulated a large amount of β-carotene and had not reached saturation after 21 weeks of feeding (145). The release of β-carotene from the adrenal was much slower than from liver (145). In a study with ferrets fed canthaxanthin, the adrenal accumulated moderate amounts of canthaxanthin but less than the liver, lungs, and small intestine (143).

5. Lung

Several studies have reported accumulation of a wide range of carotenoids in the lungs. Levels of carotenoids in human lung tissue are correlated with their serum levels (154). In a long-term feeding study with rats, Shapiro et al. (145) observed that, compared to the liver, the lungs accumulate β-carotene more slowly and have a slower turnover rate ($t_{1/2} = 16$ days versus 9 days). Pollack et al. (155) fed gerbils a test meal and measured tissue changes in β-carotene in response to the meal: liver β-carotene levels increased after the meal whereas lung concentrations did not change significantly. This response is consistent with the slower accumulation of β-carotene by the lungs reported by Shapiro et al. (145). It should be noted that the accumulation of carotenoid from a test meal may be influenced by previous consumption of the carotenoid. Mathews-Roth et al. (144) observed that prior feeding of canthaxanthin to rats almost completely prevented subsequent accumulation of labeled canthaxanthin in the lung, i.e., it seems that the tissue was saturated.

The type of carotenoid influences its deposition into the lung. Jewell and O'Brien (139) observed in rats fed equal amounts of individual carotenoids that the accumulation of carotenoid in lung tissue was similar to the pattern observed in the liver. The order of accumulation (nmol/g) was canthaxanthin (582.9) > bixin (84.6) > lutein (57.7) > lycopene (15.9) > astaxanthin (12.8) >

β-carotene (3.6). There is no obvious correlation of these tissue levels with polarity or with carotenoid solubility in organic solvents.

6. Spleen

Several studies have identified the spleen as one of the more active accumulators of carotenoids. In some instances the spleen accumulates more carotenoids than does the liver. Rats fed a diet of 0.2% canthaxanthin for 66 weeks accumulated 175 μg/g canthaxanthin in the spleen and 14.1 μg/g in the liver (156). Mongolian gerbils fed a standard rodent diet had 34 pmol/g β-carotene in the liver and 312 pmol/g in the spleen (155). Park et al. (157) fed BALB/c mice a 0.4% carotenoid diet for 14 days and observed that the accumulation of β-carotene, lutein, and astaxanthin in the spleen reflected changes observed in the plasma. β-Carotene deposition in the spleen was the least and astaxanthin accumulation the greatest.

7. Adipose Tissue

Adipose tissue appears to accumulate all carotenoids but not as quickly as other organs in the body. It has been suggested that adipose tissue levels of carotenoid can be used to assess long-term body carotenoid status (158). In humans the carotenoids found in the serum are also found in measurable quantities in the adipose tissue (128). Of the major carotenoids, lycopene and zeaxanthin/lutein were observed in the greatest amounts in one study (128), whereas β-carotene and lycopene were found to predominate in another (131). β-Carotene concentrations in adipose tissue were found to correlate with plasma β-carotene concentrations ($r = 0.56$), although this study did not find a correlation of plasma or adipose β-carotene concentrations with baseline dietary intake (159); adipose β-carotene concentrations did respond to supplementation with 30 mg daily. In a human study involving feeding of foods rich in lutein, adipose tissue lutein concentrations changed in response to diet though not as quickly as other tissues measured (160). Interestingly, the percent body fat was not correlated with accumulation of lutein in adipose tissue. Lycopene concentration in adipose is correlated with the long-term dietary levels in the rat (149). Pharmacological doses of canthaxanthin provided to ferrets for 2 years resulted in increases in adipose canthaxanthin at 12 months but no further increase during the second year (143). No change in β-carotene content of adipose tissue after a single test meal was observed in Mongolian gerbils (155).

　　　In a study in Costa Rica, human plasma and adipose tissue carotenoid concentrations were compared with dietary intake (161). The relative concentrations of carotenoids in plasma were more similar to dietary intake than were concentrations in adipose tissue (Table 7).

Table 7 Correlations Between Dietary Intake (as Determined by Dietary Interview and Food Frequency Questionnaire) and Adipose Tissue Concentrations of Carotenoids

Factor	α-Carotene	β-Carotene	β-Cryptoxanthin	Lutein + zeaxanthin	Lycopene
Plasma, women	0.26	0.13	0.55	0.22	0.19
Plasma, men	0.24	0.22	0.44	0.20	0.35
Adipose, women	0.25	0.29	0.44	0.17	0.14
Adipose, men	0.04	0.07	0.23	0.06	0.26

Source: Adapted from Ref. 161.

8. Skin

It has long been known that prolonged high dietary intakes of carotenoids can result in their accumulation in skin (carotenodermia) (162). The condition has been reported as being common in Cameroon, an area where consumption of red palm oil is high (163), and can be induced by consumption of 30 mg purified β-carotene daily (164). One case of hypercarotenemia and carotenodermia was reported in an infant who had been fed proprietary baby food with a high carrot content (165). Increased concentrations of carotenoids in skin after feeding β-carotene or mixed carotenoids can be measured by reflection spectroscopy, a technique used measure total carotenoid content but not individual carotenoids (166). Prince and Frisoli quantitated this accumulation and found a lag of up to 2 weeks between increase in plasma concentration and increase in skin (167), implying a slow transfer from lipoproteins to the dermal layer. It is also noteworthy that the absorption spectrum of β-carotene was shifted approximately 40 nm to higher wavelengths, suggesting that the carotenoid in skin was in a very nonpolar environment. In poultry, it is found that xanthophylls are more effective than carotenes in enhancing skin pigmentation (168). Xanthophyll esters (esters of lutein, zeaxanthin, anhydrolutein, α-cryptoxanthin, and β-cryptoxanthin) have been detected in very low concentrations (pmol/g) in human skin (169); it is not known if they are absorbed and transported intact or esterified in situ.

It has been shown that cells accessible to sampling, such as those of buccal mucosa (135) and urogenital tract (170), increase β-carotene content with increasing dietary intake. It was suggested that exfoliated cells from these sites might be useful in assessing tissue carotenoid levels (170).

9. Atherosclerotic Plaque

β-Carotene can accumulate in atherosclerotic plaque (of New Zealand white rabbits) (171). This has been used to advantage in experimental visualization and laser ablation of aortic plaque (171–173).

10. Pineal Gland and Brain

It has long been known that the pineal gland contains retinoids and rhodopsin analogs, and that it seems to be involved in light perception. Shi et al. found that bovine pineal gland contains β-carotene but not measurable quantities of other carotenoids (174). Of course, bovine plasma would provide predominantly β-carotene to all its tissues. Human brain contains low but detectable amounts of the carotenoids found in human plasma (175).

11. Lutein and Zeaxanthin in the Eye

The important role of lutein and zeaxanthin in macular pigment is discussed in Chapter 22. Nearly all ocular structures contain predominantly lutein, zeaxanthin (and their E/Z isomers), as well as lesser amounts of the metabolites 3'-epilutein (3R,3'S,6'R-lutein) and 3-hydroxy-β,ε-caroten-3'-one, and details of tissue distribution are given by Bernstein et al. (176). Small amounts of mono-hydroxycarotenoids and carotenes were also present in some structures of the eye. Correlations of macular pigment density with serum lutein, serum zeaxanthin, and adipose lutein concentrations were found in men but not in women (177). Some, but not all, human subjects respond to increased dietary lutein and zeaxanthin with increased serum and macular pigment xanthophyll concentrations (178).

Khachik et al. (179) have argued for a series of oxidation-reduction and double-bond isomerization reactions to create the characteristic metabolites found in ocular tissues. Both lutein and zeaxanthin have the greatest concentration at the center of the fovea, but zeaxanthin concentrations decrease more rapidly than lutein at increasing distances from the center (180–183) this is unexplained. *meso*-Zeaxanthin is apparently formed by metabolism of lutein in the eye, since it is not found in diet (181). It has been suggested that the class of proteins known as tubulins may be xanthophyll-binding proteins in primate retina (184–186).

Only trace amounts of other carotenoids are found in retinal tissue (187), so it is surprising that canthaxanthin accumulates in the retina after chronic high dosing (188,189). Canthaxathin is a xanthophyll, but it is less polar than the dihydroxycarotenoids lutein and zeaxanthin because it is a diketocarotenoid; study of its accumulation in retina may yield clues to xanthophyll accumulation there.

B. Subcellular Distribution of Carotenoids

While the incorporation of carotenoids into membranes is essential for many of their proposed activities in cells, there is little information available on the subcellular distribution of carotenoids. β-Carotene has been found in all subcellular fractions examined, e.g., nuclear, mitochondrial, microsomal, and cytosolic fractions, in bovine corpus luteum (190), in livers of chicks (191), and in livers of rats given prolonged high dietary doses of β-carotene (192). It is not known if other carotenoids have similar intracellular distribution. After supplementation with high doses (50 or 100 mg/day for 30 days), β-carotene could be measured in neutrophils and lymphocytes of dog plasma; within cells, concentrations in cytosol $>$ mitochondria $\sim$ microsomes $>$ nuclei (193). The incorporation of carotenoids into subcellular membranes most likely depends on the structure of the carotenoid and type of membrane. Lancrajan et al. studied the incorporation of β-carotene, lutein, and canthaxanthin into plasma, mitochondria, and microsomal membranes in vitro (37). They concluded that membrane fluidity is a major determinant of carotenoid uptake: nonpolar β-carotene is preferentially incorporated into the more fluid membranes (i.e., mitochondria and microsomes) while the polar carotenoids, lutein and canthaxanthin, are incorporated into the less fluid plasma membranes (37). The orientation of carotenoids in membranes also appears to depend on carotenoid structure. Socaciu et al. reported efficient incorporation of β-carotene, lycopene, lutein, zeaxanthin, canthaxanthin, and astaxanthin into pig liver microsomes (194). The xanthophylls and β-carotene span the membrane, while the very nonpolar carotenoid, lycopene, is located preferentially in the lipid core of the membrane (194).

C. Biotransformations of Carotenoids in Animal Tissues

1. Examples of Carotenoid Biotransformations

Solely on the basis of structural considerations, the types of metabolism to be expected of carotenoids include cleavage (both polyene chain and ionone ring) and chain shortening, hydroxylation/oxidation, and dehydration (of xanthophylls) (195). Cleavage of the polyene chain, either symmetrical or asymmetrical, is well known; opening of ionone rings has not been reported. Esterification of xanthophylls might be expected (by analogy with retinol and cholesterol) but has not been definitively proven to occur.

Cleavage of provitamin A carotenoids such as β-carotene is discussed in detail elsewhere in this volume. In the current context, it should be remembered that retinoic acid (as well as retinal) can be produced by cleavage of β-carotene in some tissues (196).

Khachik et al. have proposed that metabolism of lycopene in human tissues might involve formation of epoxides, specifically at the 1,2- and 5,6 double bonds, with subsequent rearrangement of the strained three-carbon epoxide rings to five-membered rings (197). To what extent these are enzymatically catalyzed reactions within human tissues and to what extent they occur nonenzymatically during processing of tomato products is not yet clear.

Anhydrolutein, a dehydration product of lutein, has been found in human plasma (198). Subsequently the structural configuration of the major anhydrolutein product in human plasma was identified as (3R,6'R)-3-hydroxy-3',4'-didehydro-β,γ-carotene, with lower concentrations of (3R,6'R)-3-hydroxy-2',3'-didehydro-β,γ-carotene (199). To date these compounds have been detected in few foodstuffs (200,201); thus it is assumed that the amounts found in human plasma are due to transformation from dietary lutein, perhaps catalyzed in the acid milieu of the stomach (199). Savithry et al. found that anhydrolutein is converted to 3-dehydroretinol (vitamin A_2) in rat intestines (202). Vitamin A_2 is found in human tissues also, but its source in humans has not been determined; we suggest that it may arise from this process as well as preformed from diet.

Evidence for biotransformation of carotenoids in humans is mostly indirect at best. This is in large part because of lack of appropriate labeled compounds. However, there is evidence of biotransformation in other species, in particular, in birds. McGraw et al. have demonstrated that cardinals (*Cardinalis cardinalis*) are capable of transforming dietary yellow carotenoids to red carotenoids for plumage coloration (203), and also suggested that the zebra finch (*Taeniopygia guttata*) is capable of transforming dietary lutein to anhydrolutein (204). As in the cardinal, the American goldfinch (*Carduelis tristis*) also shows gender-specific biotransformation of carotenoids (205). Selective distribution of carotenoids among different tissues and organs has been shown in avian species. In the free-living gull (*Larus fucus*), liver contained the highest carotenoid concentrations, and β-carotene was the most prominent carotenoid in liver; in all other tissues studied, lutein was the predominant carotenoid, with zeaxanthin, canthaxanthin, β-cryptoxanthin, echinenone, and β-carotene present in lesser concentrations (206). Surai et al. found that β-carotene was the predominant carotenoid in the egg yolks of common moorhen (*Gallinula chloropus*), American coot (*Fulica americana*), and lesser black-backed gull (*Larus fuscus*), in contrast to the domestic chicken (*Gallus domesticus*) in whose yolk xanthophylls are predominant (207). In the newly hatched gull, proportions of lutein and zeaxanthin were high in heart and muscle (but low in liver) when compared to the yolk; proportions of canthaxanthin, echinenone, and β-carotene were lower in heart and muscle than in yolk. In the newly hatched coot and moorhen, the liver was relatively enriched in β-cryptoxanthin and β-carotene (as well as echinenone in the moorhen) compared to the egg yolks. Plumage coloration in wild house finches (*Carpodacus mexicanus*) is related to dietary carotenoid intake (208). Red coloration of male barn swallows (*Hirundo rustica*) correlated with plasma concentrations of lutein (209).

Khachik et al. (179) studied carotenoid concentrations in the eyes of several species and identified nondietary carotenoids; they concluded that biotransformations of xanthophylls involve oxidation–reduction reactions and double-bond isomerizations. Similar carotenoid profiles were found in humans, frogs (179), and quail (187), suggesting the presence of similar biotransformation pathways.

Esters of xanthophylls are generally not detectable in human tissues [except when vary large quantities are fed (169)]. This suggests that intact esters are not absorbed at usual dietary intake levels, and that either (a) they must be hydrolyzed in the intestinal lumen or (b) they are generally not available for absorption. A variety of evidence indicates that xanthophyll esters are bioavailable and that they are hydrolyzed by esterases in the intestinal lumen. However, some animals, such as the lobster, can accumulate appreciable quantities (as much as 80% of total carotenoids) of xanthophyll esters (210), and lutein esters have been detected in tissues of the chicken (211).

Tyckowski and Hamilton found that canthaxanthin is reduced to an alcohol in chickens (212), but similar metabolism has not yet been described in humans.

Enzymatic cleavage of carotenoids is discussed elsewhere in this volume. Although the quantitatively greater pathway is that of central cleavage, there is evidence for excentric cleavage to retinoids and apocarotenoids in animal and human tissues [reviewed in (213)]. After rats had been fed β-apo-8'-carotenal, shorter chain apocarotenoic acids could be identified in their intestinal mucosa (214); it is not yet known whether this is due to activity of a carotenoid cleavage enzyme, or to β oxidation of the polyene chain, as is seen with chain shortening of α-tocopherol (215,216).

2. cis/trans Isomerization In Vivo

Lycopene and Phytoene Isomers. Sakamoto et al. [cited in (217)] found some evidence of *trans*-to-*cis* isomerization of lycopene in vivo. It has been shown that cis isomers of lycopene are better absorbed than the all-*trans* isomer (24,148), and it has been suggested that this is because *cis*-lycopene isomers are more soluble in organic solvents and thus more soluble in bile acid micelles (24); it may be that the *cis* isomers of lycopene are more soluble (more readily incorporated) in chylomicrons than the all-*trans* form. In marked contrast, the ratio of 9-*cis*-phytoene to all-*trans* phytoene was much lower in liver, spleen, and kidney than in the diet in rats fed phytoene, while the isomer ratio in plasma and adrenals was similar to that of the ratio in diet (218). Again, this difference may reflect differences in efficiency of uptake of the isomers by tissues or differences in rates of catabolism.

β-Carotene Isomers. After an oral dose containing both all-*trans* and 9-*cis*-β-carotene, human subjects showed a much higher concentration of the all-*trans* isomer than of 9-*cis* in chylomicrons and the VLDL fractions of plasma (62,219). Consistent with this observation, Erdman et al. (220) showed that all-*trans* β-carotene is absorbed much better than is 9-*cis*-β-carotene into intestinal mucosal cells by ferrets. However, 9-*cis*-β-carotene could be detected in liver, kidneys, and adrenals of the ferrets, even when they were fed only the all-*trans* isomer, and ratios of 9-*cis*/all-*trans* β-carotene were higher in adrenals and kidneys than in livers. This is a particularly striking finding because only all-*trans* β-carotene, not the 9-*cis* isomer, was detectable in serum. Hence, either (a) 9-*cis*-β-carotene is taken up by tissues more efficiently than is the all-trans isomer, and/or (b) all-*trans* β-carotene is recycled to plasma or is catabolized more rapidly than is the 9-*cis* isomer, and/or (c) there is appreciable isomerization of all-*trans* β-carotene to its 9-*cis* isomer in tissues.

3. Other Factors Affecting Tissue Uptake and Metabolism of Carotenoids

Boileau et al. (149) found that accumulation of lycopene in livers of castrated male rats was significantly greater than in noncastrated animals (and concentrations of lycopene in liver were greater than in adrenal, kidney, lung, adipose tissue, prostate, or testes of intact animals). There was also a trend (but not statistically significant) toward greater deposition of lycopene in adrenals of castrated animals, but not in kidney, lung, or adipose tissue. The *cis*/*trans* isomer ratio increased with increasing dietary lycopene. It is possible that these effects are due to androgen effects on lipoprotein metabolism and/or on hepatic lycopene metabolism, but details are not clear.

D. Carotenoids in Milk

Colostrum, the first milk secreted after giving birth, has a distinct yellow color that decreases during the first week of lactation. The yellow color is due to carotenoids associated with milk fat. It has been suggested that a large portion of the carotenoids in colostrum may come from carotenoids stored in adipose tissue of the breast (221).

Breast milk carotenoids serve many functions for the developing neonate. The provitamin A carotenoids, β-carotene, β-cryptoxanthin, and α-carotene, collectively provide 50% of the breast milk carotenoid during early lactation and are potentially an important source of vitamin A for the infant (222). The carotenoids devoid of vitamin A activity and the metabolites of carotenoids may be equally important. There are many trophic components in human milk that contribute to digestive tract development. Breast milk carotenoids may join this list of components by influencing developing gut immunity and cellular communication (223). Much current interest in lutein and zeaxanthin is centered on their role in potentially preventing or slowing the development of age-related macular degeneration. In the neonate these carotenoids have an equally important protective role for the retinal pigment epithelium of the newborn's eye (224).

The breast-fed infant's source of lutein and zeaxanthin is the mother's milk. While carotenoid concentrations are known to decrease as lactation progresses, the decline in lutein is not as great as that in the other carotenoids (225). Lutein represented approximately 25% of the total carotenoids in milk at 4 days postpartum and 50% at 32 days postpartum. This maintenance of lutein in milk may be due to an increased flow from the blood as there is a significant postpartum decline in plasma lutein concentrations (225).

Thirty-four carotenoids, including 13 geometrical isomers and 8 metabolites, have been identified in human milk and are identical to those observed in serum (223). The major carotenoids in human milk are lutein, zeaxanthin, β-cryptoxanthin, lycopene, α- and β-carotene (222,223,226–228). Although carotenoids in milk are derived from the serum, their concentrations in milk are several fold less than in the serum (222,223). Furthermore, there is discrimination in transfer of carotenoids for incorporation into milk (Table 8): the efficiency of transfer is directly related to the relative polarity of the carotenoid (229).

Not surprisingly, milk carotenoid concentrations show some correlation with dietary intake (226). A number of studies have shown that human breast milk concentrations of β-carotene can be increased by dietary supplementation (230). When healthy lactating mothers were supplemented with 30 mg β-carotene daily, β-carotene concentrations increased both in serum and in breast milk (231); the rise in concentrations in breast milk seemed to lag slightly behind the rise in serum, but the reductions in concentrations after cessation of supplementation were parallel.

Carotenoid content in milk varies greatly but to a large degree is correlated with the amount of lipid in the milk. In a study of variability of major carotenoids in milk, some carotenoids were seen to vary as much as fourfold within a single day (227). This makes sampling of breast milk a challenge and explains some of the differences in breast milk carotenoid concentrations reported in the literature. Kim et al. found only weak correlations between estimated dietary intake of individual carotenoids and human milk carotenoid concentrations (but plasma caroteneoid concentrations were not provided) (226). Patton et al. claimed that mean carotenoid concentration in colostrum of multiparous human mothers was greater than that of primiparous mothers (and observed a similar phenomenon in lactating cattle), although dietary information was not provided (221). They also found that concentrations of carotenoids in breast milk decreased with time after delivery (221).

IV. SUMMARY

This chapter has summarized some of the observations on accumulation and metabolism of carotenoids in plasma and other tissues. At this point, it is difficult

Table 8   Carotenoid Content in Humans
A. Carotenoid Content of Human Breast Milk and Correlation with
Dietary Intake (Mean ± Standard Deviation)

Factor	Lutein	Lycopene	α-Carotene	β-Carotene
Milk concentration (μg/100 g) ($n = 54$)	11.5 ± 3.4	3.8 ± 2.1	3.2 ± 0.9	4.6 ± 1.6
Estimated dietary intake (μg/d) ($n = 42$)	3106 ± 2611	389 ± 213	651 ± 393	3247 ± 2093
Correlation between dietary intake and milk concentration	+0.2487	+0.0279	+0.5216 ($p < 0.01$)	+0.4174 ($p < 0.01$)

Source: Adapted from Ref. 226.

B. Carotenoid Concentrations in Human Milk and Serum (3 Subjects,
More than 1 Month Postparturition)

Carotenoid	Mean serum concentration (μg/dL)	Mean breast milk concentration (μg/dL)	Ratiomilk/serum
Lutein	16.5	2.6	0.16
Zeaxanthin	2.1	0.4	0.21
Epilutein	1.2	0.2	0.13
Anhydrolutein	2.0	0.3	0.16
α-Cryptoxanthin	3.4	0.4	0.11
β-Cryptoxanthin	12.8	1.8	0.14
α-Carotene	6.4	0.4	0.06
β-Carotene	19.7	1.3	0.06
Phytofluene	9.4	0.9	0.1
Phytoene	2.4	0.1	0.05
Lycopene	36.4	1.1	0.03

Source: Adapted from Ref. 223.

to elucidate the factors that control uptake and retention of specific carotenoids. This is an aspect of carotenoid metabolism that deserves much more experimental attention because of the roles of carotenoids as antioxidants and as precursors of retinoids, and perhaps as modulators of gene expression in their own right.

ACKNOWLEDGMENT

Preparation of this review was supported in part by a USDA Competitive Research Grant USDA NRI 2002-35200-12312 (RMC).

REFERENCES

1. Goodwin TW. Mammals. In: Goodwin TW, ed. The Biochemistry of the Carotenoids, Vol. 25 Animals. New York: Chapman and Hall, 1984:173–195.
2. Davies BH. Carotenoid metabolism as a preparation for function. Pure Appl Chem 1991; 63:131–140.
3. Olson JA. 1992 Atwater lecture. The irresistible fascination of carotenoids and vitamin A. Am J Clin Nutr 1993; 57:833–839.
4. Van Vliet T. Absorption of beta-carotene and other carotenoids in humans and animal models. Eur J Clin Nutr 1996; 50(suppl 3):S32–S37.
5. Erdman JW Jr, Bierer TL, Gugger ET. Absorption and transport of carotenoids. Ann NY Acad Sci 1993; 691:76–85.
6. Parker RS. Carotenoids in human blood and tissues. J Nutr 1989; 119:101–104.
7. Parker RS. Absorption, metabolism, and transport of carotenoids. FASEB J 1996; 10:542–551.
8. Furr HC, Clark RM. Intestinal absorption and tissue distribution of carotenoids. J Nutr Biochem 1997; 8:364–377.
9. Castenmiller JJ, West CE. Bioavailability and bioconversion of carotenoids. Annu Rev Nutr 1998; 18:19–38.
10. van den Berg H. Carotenoid interactions. Nutr Rev 1999; 57:1–10.
11. Lee CM, Boileau AC, Boileau TW, Williams AW, Swanson KS, Heintz KA, Erdman JW Jr. Review of animal models in carotenoid research. J Nutr 1999; 129:2271–2277.
12. Parker RS, Swanson JE, You CS, Edwards AJ, Huang T. Bioavailability of carotenoids in human subjects. Proc Nutr Soc 1999; 58:155–162.
13. Krinsky N, Russell RM. Regarding the conversion of beta-carotene to vitamin A. Nutr Rev 2001; 59:309.
14. Khachik F, Carvalho L, Bernstein PS, Muir GJ, Zhao DY, Katz NB. Chemistry, distribution, and metabolism of tomato carotenoids and their impact on human health. Exp Biol Med (Maywood) 2002; 227:845–851.
15. Dimitrov NV, Boone CW, Hay MB, Whetter P, Pins M, Kelloff GJ, Malone W. Plasma beta-carotene levels—kinetic patterns during administration of various doses of beta-carotene. Nutr Growth Cancer 1987; 3:227–238.
16. Dimitrov NV, Meyer C, Ullrey DE, Chenoweth W, Michelakis A, Malone W, Boone C, Fink G. Bioavailability of beta-carotene in humans. Am J Clin Nutr 1988; 48:298–304.
17. Cooper DA, Webb DR, Peters JC. Evaluation of the potential for olestra to affect the availability of dietary phytochemicals. J Nutr 1997; 127:1699S–1709S.

18. van den Berg H, Faulks R, Fernando Granado H, Hirschberg J, Olmedilla B, Sandmann G, Southon S, Stahl W. The potential for the improvement of carotenoid levels in foods and the likely systemic effects. J Sci Food Agric 2000; 80:880–912.

19. Hidiroglou N, McDowell LR, Boning A. Liquid chromatographic determination of carotenes in cattle serum and liver. Int J Vitam Nutr Res 1986; 56:339–344.

20. Raila J, Schuhmacher A, Gropp J, Schweigert FJ. Selective absorption of carotenoids in the common green iguana (*Iguana iguana*). Comp Biochem Physiol A Mol Integr Physiol 2002; 132:513–518.

21. Crissey SD, Ange KD, Jacobsen KL, Slifka KA, Bowen PE, Stacewicz-Sapuntzakis M, Langman CB, Sadler W, Kahn S, Ward A. Serum concentrations of lipids, vitamin D metabolites, retinol, retinyl esters, tocopherols and selected carotenoids in twelve captive wild felid species at four zoos. J Nutr 2003; 133:160–166.

22. Crissey SD, Barr JE, Slifka KA, Bowen PE, Stacewicz-Sapuntzakis M, Langman C, Ward A, Ange K. Serum concentrations of lipids, vitamins A and E, vitamin D metabolites, and carotenoids in nine primate species at four zoos. Zoo Biology 1999; 18:551–564.

23. Van Vliet T, Van Schaik F, Van Schoonhoven J, Schrijver J. Determination of several retinoids, carotenoids and E vitamers by high-performance liquid chromatography. Application to plasma and tissues of rats fed a diet rich in either beta-carotene or canthaxanthin. J Chromatogr 1991; 553:179–186.

24. Boileau AC, Merchen NR, Wasson K, Atkinson CA, Erdman JW Jr. cis-Lycopene is more bioavailable than trans-lycopene in vitro and in vivo in lymph-cannulated ferrets. J Nutr 1999; 129:1176–1181.

25. Ferreira AL, Yeum KJ, Liu C, Smith D, Krinsky NI, Wang XD, Russell RM. Tissue distribution of lycopene in ferrets and rats after lycopene supplementation. J Nutr 2000; 130:1256–1260.

26. Singh H, Mallia AK, Cama HR. Chemistry and metabolism of beta-apocarotenals and their epoxides. Biochem Soc Symp 1972; 219–232.

27. Zeng S, Furr HC, Olson JA. Metabolism of carotenoid analogs in humans. Am J Clin Nutr 1992; 56:433–439.

28. Zeng S, Furr HC, Olson JA. Human metabolism of carotenoid analogs and apocarotenoids. Methods Enzymol 1993; 214:137–147.

29. Sujak A, Mazurek P, Gruszecki WI. Xanthophyll pigments lutein and zeaxanthin in lipid multibilayers formed with dimyristoylphosphatidylcholine. J Photochem Photobiol B 2002; 68:39–44.

30. Gruszecki WI, Grudzinski W, Banaszek-Glos A, Matula M, Kernen P, Krupa Z, Sielewiesiuk J. Xanthophyll pigments in light-harvesting complex II in monomolecular layers: localisation, energy transfer and orientation. Biochim Biophys Acta 1999; 1412:173–183.

31. Gruszecki WI, Sujak A, Strzalka K, Radunz A, Schmid GH. Organisation of xanthophyll-lipid membranes studied by means of specific pigment antisera, spectrophotometry and monomolecular layer technique lutein versus zeaxanthin. Z Naturforsch [C] 1999; 54:517–525.

32. Gabrielska J, Gruszecki WI. Zeaxanthin (dihydroxy-beta-carotene) but not beta-carotene rigidifies lipid membranes: A H-1-NMR study of carotenoid-egg phosphatidylcholine liposomes. Biochim Biophys Acta Biomembranes 1996; 1285:167–174.

33. Gruszecki WI, Sielewiesiuk J. Orientation of xanthophylls in phosphatidylcholine multibilayers. Biochim Biophys Acta 1990; 1023:405–412.

34. Borel P, Grolier P, Armand M, Partier A, Lafont H, Lairon D, Azais-Braesco V. Carotenoids in biological emulsions: solubility, surface-to-core distribution, and release from lipid droplets. J Lipid Res 1996; 37:250–261.

35. Rao MN, Ghosh P, Lakshman MR. Purification and partial characterization of a cellular carotenoid- binding protein from ferret liver. J Biol Chem 1997; 272:24455–24460.

36. Lakshman MR, Rao MN. Purification and characterization of cellular carotenoid-binding protein from mammalian liver. Meth Enzymol 1999; 299:441–456.

37. Lancrajan I, Diehl HA, Socaciu C, Engelke M, Zorn-Kruppa M. Carotenoid incorporation into natural membranes from artificial carriers: liposomes and beta-cyclodextrins. Chem Phys Lipids 2001; 112:1–10.

38. Gugger ET, Erdman JW Jr. Intracellular beta-carotene transport in bovine liver and intestine is not mediated by cytosolic proteins. J Nutr 1996; 126:1470–1474.

39. Storch J. The role of fatty acid binding proteins in enterocyte fatty acid transport. In: Mansbach CM, Tso P, Kuksis A, eds. Intestinal Lipid Metabolism. New York: Kluwer Academic/Plenum Press, 2001:153–170.

40. Berge KE, Tian H, Graf GA, Yu L, Grishin NV, Schultz J, Kwiterovich P, Shan B, Barnes R, Hobbs HH. Accumulation of dietary cholesterol in sitosterolemia caused by mutations in adjacent ABC transporters. Science 2000; 290:1771–1775.

41. Tso P, Drake DS, Black DD, Sabesin SM. Evidence for separate pathways of chylomicron and very low-density lipoprotein assembly and transport by rat small intestine. Am J Physiol 1984; 247:G599–G610.

42. Hussain MM. A proposed model for the assembly of chylomicrons. Atherosclerosis 2000; 148:1–15.

43. Willstaedt H, Lindqvist T. Uber die carotenoide des serums und der leber beim menschen. I. (About the carotenoids of serum and liver in humans). Hoppe Seylers Z Physiol Chem 1936; 240:10–18.

44. Cornwell DG, Kruger FA, Robinson HB. Studies on the absorption of beta-carotene and the distribution of total carotenoid in human serum lipoproteins after oral administration. J Lipid Res 1962; 3:65–70.

45. von Reinersdorff D. Biokinetische Untersuchungen zur Resorption von Canthaxanthin (Biochemical studies on the absorption of canthaxanthin). Giessen, Germany: Wissenschaftlicher Fachverlag, 1990.

46. Gylling H, Relas H, Miettinen TA. Postprandial vitamin A and squalene clearances and cholesterol synthesis off and on lovastatin treatment in type III hyperlipoproteinemia. Atherosclerosis 1995; 115:17–26.

47. Romanchik JE, Morel DW, Harrison EH. Distributions of carotenoids and alpha-tocopherol among lipoproteins do not change when human plasma is incubated in vitro. J Nutr 1995; 125:2610–2617.

48. Tyssandier V, Choubert G, Grolier P, Borel P. Carotenoids, mostly the xanthophylls, exchange between plasma lipoproteins. Int J Vitam Nutr Res 2002; 72:300–308.

49. Krinsky NI, Cornwell DG, Oncley JI. The transport of vitamin A and carotenoids in human plasma. Arch Biochem Biophys 1958; 73:233–246.

50. Bjornson LK, Kayden HJ, Miller E, Moshell AN. The transport of alpha-tocopherol and beta-carotene in human blood. J Lipid Res 1976; 17:343–352.

51. Jezowska I, Wolak A, Gruszecki WI, Strzalka K. Effect of beta-carotene on structural and dynamic properties of model phosphatidylcholine membranes. II. A ^{31}P-NMR and ^{13}C-NMR study. Biochim Biophys Acta 1994; 1194:143–148.

52. Chopra M, Fitzsimons P, Hopkins M, Thurnham DI. Dialysis and gel filtration of isolated low density lipoproteins do not cause a significant loss of low density lipoprotein tocopherol and carotenoid concentration. Lipids 2001; 36:205–209.

53. Lin S, Quaroni L, White WS, Cotton T, Chumanov G. Localization of carotenoids in plasma low-density lipoproteins studied by surface-enhanced resonance Raman spectroscopy. Biopolymers 2000; 57:249–256.

54. Manago M, Tamai H, Ogihara T, Mino M. Distribution of circulating beta-carotene in human plasma lipoproteins. J Nutr Sci Vitaminol (Tokyo) 1992; 38:405–414.

55. Dugas TR, Morel DW, Harrison EH. Impact of LDL carotenoid and alpha;-tocopherol content on LDL oxidation by endothelial cells in culture. J Lipid Res 1998; 39:999–1007.

56. Romanchik JE, Harrison EH, Morel DW. Addition of lutein, lycopene or beta-carotene to LDL or serum in vitro: effects on carotenoid distribution, LDL composition, and LDL oxidation. J Nutr Biochem 1997; 8:681–688.

57. Schweigert FJ, Rambeck WA, Zucker H. Transport of beta-carotene by the serum lipoproteins in cattle. J Anim Physiol Anim Nutr 1987; 57:162–167.

58. Chew BP, Wong TS, Michal JJ. Uptake of orally administered beta-carotene by blood plasma, leukocytes, and lipoproteins in calves. J Anim Sci 1993; 71:730–739.

59. Gross M, Yu X, Hannan P, Prouty C, Jacobs DR Jr. Lipid standardization of serum fat-soluble antioxidant concentrations: the YALTA study. Am J Clin Nutr 2003; 77:458–466.

60. Kelley B, Day HG. Effect of xanthophyll on the utilization of carotene and vitamin A by the rat. J Nutr 1950; 40:159–168.

61. White WS, Stacewicz-Sapuntzakis M, Erdman JW Jr, Bowen PE. Pharmacokinetics of beta-carotene and canthaxanthin after ingestion of individual and combined doses by human subjects. J Am Coll Nutr 1994; 13:665–671.

62. Gaziano JM, Johnson EJ, Russell RM, Manson JE, Stampfer MJ, Ridker PM, Frei B, Hennekens CH, Krinsky NI. Discrimination in absorption or transport of beta-carotene isomers after oral supplementation with either all-trans- or 9-cis-beta-carotene. Am J Clin Nutr 1995; 61:1248–1252.

63. van den Berg H, Van Vliet T. Effect of simultaneous, single oral doses of beta-carotene with lutein or lycopene on the beta-carotene and retinyl ester responses in the triacylglycerol-rich lipoprotein fraction of men. Am J Clin Nutr 1998; 68:82–89.

64. Tyssandier V, Cardinault N, Caris-Veyrat C, Amiot MJ, Grolier P, Bouteloup C, Azais-Braesco V, Borel P. Vegetable-borne lutein, lycopene, and beta-carotene compete for incorporation into chylomicrons, with no adverse effect on the medium-term (3-wk) plasma status of carotenoids in humans. Am J Clin Nutr 2002; 75:526–534.

65. High EG, Day HG. Fate of lycopene in the rat and its effects on the utilization of carotene and vitamin A. J Nutr 1952; 48:369–376.

66. Ascherio A, Stampfer MJ, Colditz GA, Rimm EB, Litin L, Willett WC. Correlations of vitamin A and E intakes with the plasma concentrations of carotenoids and tocopherols among American men and women. J Nutr 1992; 122:1792–1801.

67. Yong LC, Forman MR, Beecher GR, Graubard BI, Campbell WS, Reichman ME, Taylor PR, Lanza E, Holden JM, Judd JT. Relationship between dietary intake and plasma concentrations of carotenoids in premenopausal women: application of the USDA-NCI carotenoid food-composition database. Am J Clin Nutr 1994; 60:223–230.

68. Scott KJ, Thurnham DI, Hart DJ, Bingham SA, Day K. The correlation between the intake of lutein, lycopene and beta-carotene from vegetables and fruits, and blood plasma concentrations in a group of women aged 50–65 years in the UK. Br J Nutr 1996; 75:409–418.

69. Brown ED, Micozzi MS, Craft NE, Bieri JG, Beecher G, Edwards BK, Rose A, Taylor PR, Smith JC Jr. Plasma carotenoids in normal men after a single ingestion of vegetables or purified beta-carotene. Am J Clin Nutr 1989; 49:1258–1265.

70. Ribaya-Mercado JD, Ordovas JM, Russell RM. Effect of beta-carotene supplementation on the concentrations and distribution of carotenoids, vitamin E, vitamin A, and cholesterol in plasma lipoprotein and non-lipoprotein fractions in healthy older women. J Am Coll Nutr 1995; 14:614–620.

71. Rock CL, Thornquist MD, Kristal AR, Patterson RE, Cooper DA, Neuhouser ML, Neumark-Sztainer D, Cheskin LJ. Demographic, dietary and lifestyle factors differentially explain variability in serum carotenoids and fat-soluble vitamins: baseline results from the sentinel site of the olestra post-marketing surveillance study. J Nutr 1999; 129:855–864.

72. Rautalahti M, Albanes D, Haukka J, Roos E, Gref CG, Virtamo J. Seasonal variation of serum concentrations of beta-carotene and alpha-tocopherol. Am J Clin Nutr 1993; 57:551–556.

73. Hollander D, Morgan D. Aging: its influence on vitamin A intestinal absorption in vivo by the rat. Exp Gerontol 1979; 14:301–305.

74. Hollander D, Tarnawski H. Influence of aging on vitamin D absorption and unstirred water layer dimensions in the rat. J Lab Clin Med 1984; 103:462–469.

75. Hollander D, Dadufalza V. Lymphatic and portal absorption of vitamin E in aging rats. Dig Dis Sci 1989; 34:768–772.

76. Hollander D, Dadufalza V. Influence of aging on vitamin A transport into the lymphatic circulation. Exp Gerontol 1990; 25:61–65.

77. Winklhofer-Roob BM, van't Hof MA, Shmerling DH. Reference values for plasma concentrations of vitamin E and A and carotenoids in a swiss population from infancy to adulthood, adjusted for seasonal influences. Clin Chem 1997; 43:146–153.

78. Kolb E, Dittrich H, Dobeleit G, Schmalfuss R, Siebert P, Stauber E, Wahren M. [The content of beta-carotene, vitamin A and ascorbic acid in different tissues of bulls, short-scrotum bulls and oxen of different body weights]. Berl Munch Tierarztl Wochenschr 1991; 104:423–427.

79. Maiani G, Mobarhan S, Ceccanti M, Ranaldi L, Gettner S, Bowen P, Friedman H, De Lorenzo A, Ferro-Luzzi A. Beta-carotene serum response in young and elderly females. Eur J Clin Nutr 1989; 43:749–761.

80. Roe DA. Photodegradation of carotenoids in human subjects. Fed Proc 1987; 46:1886–1889.

81. Biesalski HK, Hemmes C, Hopfenmuller W, Schmid C, Gollnick HP. Effects of controlled exposure of sunlight on plasma and skin levels of beta-carotene. Free Radic Res 1996; 24:215–224.

82. Forman MR, Beecher GR, Muesing R, Lanza E, Olson B, Campbell WS, McAdam P, Raymond E, Schulman JD, Graubard BI. The fluctuation of plasma carotenoid concentrations by phase of the menstrual cycle: a controlled diet study. Am J Clin Nutr 1996; 64:559–565.

83. Forman MR, Johnson EJ, Lanza E, Graubard BI, Beecher GR, Muesing R. Effect of menstrual cycle phase on the concentration of individual carotenoids in lipoproteins of premenopausal women: a controlled dietary study. Am J Clin Nutr 1998; 67:81–87.

84. Ringer TV, DeLoof MJ, Winterrowd GE, Francom SF, Gaylor SK, Ryan JA, Sanders ME, Hughes GS. Beta-carotene's effects on serum lipoproteins and immunologic indices in humans. Am J Clin Nutr 1991; 53:688–694.

85. Fuller CJ, Faulkner H, Bendich A, Parker RS, Roe DA. Effect of beta-carotene supplementation on photosuppression of delayed-type hypersensitivity in normal young men. Am J Clin Nutr 1992; 56:684–690.

86. Rock CL, Swendseid ME. Plasma carotenoid levels in anorexia nervosa and in obese patients. Meth Enzymol 1993; 214:116–123.

87. Zhu YI, Hsieh WC, Parker RS, Herraiz LA, Haas JD, Swanson JE, Roe DA. Evidence of a role for fat-free body mass in modulation of plasma carotenoid concentrations in older men: studies with hydrodensitometry. J Nutr 1997; 127:321–326.

88. Crisp AH, Stonehill E. Hypercarotenaemia as a symptom of weight phobia. Postgrad Med J 1967; 43:721–725.

89. Pops MA, Schwabe AD. Hypercarotenemia in anorexia nervosa. JAMA 1968; 205:533–534.

90. Robboy MS, Sato AS, Schwabe AD. The hypercarotenemia in anorexia nervosa: a comparison of vitamin A and carotene levels in various forms of menstrual dysfunction and cachexia. Am J Clin Nutr 1974; 27:362–367.

91. Frumar AM, Meldrum DR, Judd HL. Hypercarotenemia in hypothalamic amenorrhea. Fertil Steril 1979; 32:261–264.

92. Bhanji S, Mattingly D. Anorexia nervosa: some observations on "dieters" and "vomiters," cholesterol and carotene. Br J Psychiatry 1981; 139:238–241.

93. Kemmann E, Pasquale SA, Skaf R. Amenorrhea associated with carotenemia. JAMA 1983; 249:926–929.

94. Curran-Celentano J, Erdman JW Jr, Nelson RA, Grater SJ. Alterations in vitamin A and thyroid hormone status in anorexia nervosa and associated disorders. Am J Clin Nutr 1985; 42:1183–1191.

95. Thibault L, Roberge AG. The nutritional status of subjects with anorexia nervosa. Int J Vitam Nutr Res 1987; 57:447–452.

96. Sherman P, Leslie K, Goldberg E, Rybczynski J, St. Louis P. Hypercarotenemia and transaminitis in female adolescents with eating disorders: a prospective, controlled study. J Adolesc Health 1994; 15:205–209.

97. Rock CL, Vasantharajan S. Vitamin status of eating disorder patients: relationship to clinical indices and effect of treatment. Int J Eat Disord 1995; 18:257–262.

98. Rock CL, Gorenflo DW, Drewnowski A, Demitrack MA. Nutritional characteristics, eating pathology, and hormonal status in young women. Am J Clin Nutr 1996; 64:566–571.

99. Mehler PS, Lezotte D, Eckel R. Lipid levels in anorexia nervosa. Int J Eat Disord 1998; 24:217–221.

100. Boland B, Beguin C, Zech F, Desager JP, Lambert M. Serum beta-carotene in anorexia nervosa patients: a case-control study. Int J Eat Disord 2001; 30:299–305.

101. Ford ES, Gillespie C, Ballew C, Sowell A, Mannino DM. Serum carotenoid concentrations in US children and adolescents. Am J Clin Nutr 2002; 76:818–827.

102. Ford ES. Variations in serum carotenoid concentrations among United States adults by ethnicity and sex. Ethn Dis 2000; 10:208–217.

103. Wei W, Kim Y, Boudreau N. Association of smoking with serum and dietary levels of antioxidants in adults: NHANES III, 1988–1994. Am J Public Health 2001; 91:258–264.

104. Kergoat MJ, Leclerc BS, PetitClerc C, Imbach A. Determinants of total serum carotene concentrations in institutionalized elderly. J Am Geriatr Soc 1988; 36:430–436.

105. Brady WE, Mares-Perlman JA, Bowen P, Stacewicz-Sapuntzakis M. Human serum carotenoid concentrations are related to physiologic and lifestyle factors. J Nutr 1996; 126:129–137.

106. Tyczkowski JK, Hamilton PB, Ruff MD. Altered metabolism of carotenoids during pale-bird syndrome in chickens infected with *Eimeria acervulina*. Poult Sci 1991; 70:2074–2081.

107. Olmedilla B, Granado F, Blanco I. Hyper-beta-carotenemia unrelated to diet: a case of brain tumor. Int J Vitam Nutr Res 1995; 65:21–23.

108. Krinsky NI, Mathews-Roth MM, Welankiwar S, Sehgal PK, Lausen NC, Russett M. The metabolism of [^{14}C]beta-carotene and the presence of other carotenoids in rats and monkeys. J Nutr 1990; 120:81–87.

109. Van Vliet T, Schreurs WH, van den Berg H. Intestinal beta-carotene absorption and cleavage in men: response of beta-carotene and retinyl esters in the triglyceride-rich lipoprotein fraction after a single oral dose of beta-carotene. Am J Clin Nutr 1995; 62:110–116.

110. van het Hof KH, de Boer BC, Tijburg LB, Lucius BR, Zijp I, West CE, Hautvast JG, Weststrate JA. Carotenoid bioavailability in humans from tomatoes processed in different ways determined from the carotenoid response in the triglyceride-rich lipoprotein fraction of plasma after a single consumption and in plasma after four days of consumption. J Nutr 2000; 130:1189–1196.

111. O'Neill ME, Thurnham DI. Intestinal absorption of beta-carotene, lycopene and lutein in men and women following a standard meal: response curves in the triacylglycerol-rich lipoprotein fraction. Br J Nutr 1998; 79:149–159.

112. Bierer TL, Merchen NR, Erdman JW Jr. Comparative absorption and transport of five common carotenoids in preruminant calves. J Nutr 1995; 125:1569–1577.

113. Jenkins KJ, Griffith G, Kramer JK. Plasma lipoproteins in neonatal, preruminant, and weaned calf. J Dairy Sci 1988; 71:3003–3012.

114. Borel P, Tyssandier V, Mekki N, Grolier P, Rochette Y, Alexandre-Gouabau MC, Lairon D, Azais-Braesco V. Chylomicron beta-carotene and retinyl palmitate responses are dramatically diminished when men ingest beta-carotene with medium-chain rather than long-chain triglycerides. J Nutr 1998; 128:1361–1367.

115. Fielding BA, Callow J, Owen RM, Samra JS, Matthews DR, Frayn KN. Postprandial lipemia: the origin of an early peak studied by specific dietary fatty acid intake during sequential meals. Am J Clin Nutr 1996; 63:36–41.

116. Osterlie M, Bjerkeng B, Liaaen-Jensen S. Plasma appearance and distribution of astaxanthin E/Z and R/S isomers in plasma lipoproteins of men after single dose administration of astaxanthin. J Nutr Biochem 2000; 11:482–490.

117. van Lieshout M, West CE, van Breemen RB. Isotopic tracer techniques for studying the bioavailability and bioefficacy of dietary carotenoids, particularly beta-carotene, in humans: a review. Am J Clin Nutr 2003; 77:12–28.

118. Green MH, Green JB. The application of compartmental analysis to research in nutrition. Ann Rev Nutr 1990; 10:41–61.

119. Burri BJ, Neidlinger TR, Clifford AJ. Serum carotenoid depletion follows first-order kinetics in healthy adult women fed naturally low carotenoid diets. J Nutr 2001; 131:2096–2100.

120. Novotny JA, Dueker SR, Zech LA, Clifford AJ. Compartmental analysis of the dynamics of beta-carotene metabolism in an adult volunteer. J Lipid Res 1995; 36:1825–1838.

121. Novotny JA, Zech LA, Furr HC, Dueker SR, Clifford AJ. Mathematical modeling in nutrition: constructing a physiologic compartmental model of the dynamics of beta-carotene metabolism. Adv Food Nutr Res 1996; 40:25–54.

122. Lin Y, Dueker SR, Burri BJ, Neidlinger TR, Clifford AJ. Variability of the conversion of beta-carotene to vitamin A in women measured by using a double-tracer study design. Am J Clin Nutr 2000; 71:1545–1554.

123. Yao L, Liang Y, Trahanovsky WS, Serfass RE, White WS. Use of a 13C tracer to quantify the plasma appearance of a physiological dose of lutein in humans. Lipids 2000; 35:339–348.

124. Hickenbottom SJ, Follett JR, Lin Y, Dueker SR, Burri BJ, Neidlinger TR, Clifford AJ. Variability in conversion of beta-carotene to vitamin A in men as measured by using a double-tracer study design. Am J Clin Nutr 2002; 75:900–907.

125. Levy LW, Regalado E, Navarrete S, Watkins RH. Bixin and norbixin in human plasma: determination and study of the absorption of a single dose of Annatto food color. Analyst 1997; 122:977–980.
126. Dagadu JM. Distribution of carotene and vitamin A in liver, pancreas and body fat of Ghanaians. Br J Nutr 1967; 21:453–456.
127. Raica N, Scott J, Lowry L, Sauberlich HE. Vitamin A concentration in human tissues collected from five areas in the United States. Am J Clin Nutr 1972; 25:291–296.
128. Kaplan LA, Lau JM, Stein EA. Carotenoid composition, concentrations, and relationships in various human organs. Clin Physiol Biochem 1990; 8:1–10.
129. Tanumihardjo SA, Furr HC, Amedee-Manesme O, Olson JA. Retinyl ester (vitamin A ester) and carotenoid composition in human liver. Int J Vitam Nutr Res 1990; 60:307–313.
130. Schmitz HH, Poor CL, Wellman RB, Erdman JW. Concentrations of selected carotenoids and vitamin A in human liver, kidney and lung tissue. J Nutr 1991; 121:1613–1621.
131. Parker RS. Carotenoid and tocopherol composition of human adipose tissue. Am J Clin Nutr 1988; 47:33–36.
132. Clinton SK, Emenhiser C, Schwartz SJ, Bostwick DG, Williams AW, Moore BJ, Erdman JW Jr. Cis-trans lycopene isomers, carotenoids, and retinol in the human prostate. Cancer Epidemiol Biomark Prev 1996; 5:823–833.
133. Freeman VL, Meydani M, Yong S, Pyle J, Wan Y, Arvizu-Durazo R, Liao Y. Prostatic levels of tocopherols, carotenoids, and retinol in relation to plasma levels and self-reported usual dietary intake. Am J Epidemiol 2000; 151:109–118.
134. van Breemen RB, Xu X, Viana MA, Chen L, Stacewicz-Sapuntzakis M, Duncan C, Bowen PE, Sharifi R. Liquid chromatography–mass spectrometry of cis- and all-trans-lycopene in human serum and prostate tissue after dietary supplementation with tomato sauce. J Agric Food Chem 2002; 50:2214–2219.
135. Peng YM, Peng YS, Lin Y, Moon T, Roe DJ, Ritenbaugh C. Concentrations and plasma–tissue–diet relationships of carotenoids, retinoids, and tocopherols in humans. Nutr Cancer 1995; 23:233–246.
136. Martin KR, Loo G, Failla ML. Human lipoproteins as a vehicle for the delivery of beta-carotene and alpha-tocopherol to HepG2 cells. Proc Soc Exp Biol Med 1997; 214:367–373.
137. Kirkiles NC, Rubin LP, Furr HC. Uptake of canthaxanthin by human placental choriocarcinoma (BeWo) cells from human plasma lipoproteins. FASEB J 1996; 10:A239.
138. Schroeder F, Gallegos AM, Atshaves BP, Storey SM, McIntosh AL, Petrescu AD, Huang H, Starodub O, Chao H, Yang H, Frolov A, Kier AB. Recent advances in membrane microdomains: rafts, caveolae, and intracellular cholesterol trafficking. Exp Biol Med (Maywood) 2001; 226:873–890.
139. Jewell C, O'Brien NM. Effect of dietary supplementation with carotenoids on xenobiotic metabolizing enzymes in the liver, lung, kidney and small intestine of the rat. Br J Nutr 1999; 81:235–242.

140. Astorg P, Gradelet S, Berges R, Suschetet M. Dietary lycopene decreases the initiation of liver preneoplastic foci by diethylnitrosamine in the rat. Nutr Cancer 1997; 29:60–68.

141. Gradelet S, Astorg P, Leclerc J, Chevalier J, Vernevaut MF, Siess MH. Effects of canthaxanthin, astaxanthin, lycopene and lutein on liver xenobiotic-metabolizing enzymes in the rat. Xenobiotica 1996; 26:49–63.

142. Gradelet S, Le Bon AM, Berges R, Suschetet M, Astorg P. Dietary carotenoids inhibit aflatoxin B1-induced liver preneoplastic foci and DNA damage in the rat: role of the modulation of aflatoxin B1 metabolism. Carcinogenesis 1998; 19:403–411.

143. Tang G, Blanco MC, Fox JG, Russell RM. Supplementing ferrets with canthaxanthin affects the tissue distributions of canthaxanthin, other carotenoids, vitamin A and vitamin E. J Nutr 1995; 125:1945–1951.

144. Mathews-Roth MM, Welankiwar S, Sehgal PK, Lausen NC, Russett M, Krinsky NI. Distribution of [^{14}C]canthaxanthin and [^{14}C]lycopene in rats and monkeys. J Nutr 1990; 120:1205–1213.

145. Shapiro SS, Mott DJ, Machlin LJ. Kinetic characteristics of beta-carotene uptake and depletion in rat tissue. J Nutr 1984; 114:1924–1933.

146. During A, Smith MK, Piper JB, Smith JC. beta-carotene 15,15′-dioxygenase activity in human tissues and cells: evidence of an iron dependency. J Nutr Biochem 2001; 12:640–647.

147. Leo MA, Ahmed S, Aleynik SI, Siegel JH, Kasmin F, Lieber CS. Carotenoids and tocopherols in various hepatobiliary conditions. J Hepatol 1995; 23:550–556.

148. Stahl W, Schwarz W, Sundquist AR, Sies H. cis-trans Isomers of lycopene and beta-carotene in human serum and tissues. Arch Biochem Biophys 1992; 294:173–177.

149. Boileau TW, Clinton SK, Erdman JW Jr. Tissue lycopene concentrations and isomer patterns are affected by androgen status and dietary lycopene concentration in male F344 rats. J Nutr 2000; 130:1613–1618.

150. Marusich WL, Bauernfeind JC. Oxycarotenoids in poultry feed. In: Bauernfeind JC, ed. Carotenoids as Colorants and Vitamin A Precursors. New York: Academic Press, 1981:320–462.

151. Surai PF, Noble RC, Speake BK. Tissue-specific differences in antioxidant distribution and susceptibility to lipid peroxidation during development of the chick embryo. Biochim Biophys Acta 1996; 1304:1–10.

152. Stahl W, Sies H. Lycopene: a biologically important carotenoid for humans? Arch Biochem Biophys 1996; 336:1–9.

153. Bowen P, Chen L, Stacewicz-Sapuntzakis M, Duncan C, Sharifi R, Ghosh L, Kim HS, Christov-Tzelkov K, van Breemen R. Tomato sauce supplementation and prostate cancer: lycopene accumulation and modulation of biomarkers of carcinogenesis. Exp Biol Med (Maywood) 2002; 227:886–893.

154. Redlich CA, Grauer JN, van Bennekum AM, Clever SL, Ponn RB, Blaner WS. Characterization of carotenoid, vitamin A, and alpha-tocopheral levels in human lung tissue and pulmonary macrophages. Am J Respir Crit Care Med 1996; 154:1436–1443.

155. Pollack J, Campbell JM, Potter SM, Erdman JW Jr. Mongolian gerbils (*Meriones unguiculatus*) absorb beta-carotene intact from a test meal. J Nutr 1994; 124:869–873.

156. Bendich A, Shapiro SS. Effect of beta-carotene and canthaxanthin on the immune responses of the rat. J Nutr 1986; 116:2254–2262.

157. Park JS, Chew BP, Wong TS, Zhang JX, Magnuson NS. Dietary lutein but not astaxanthin or beta-carotene increases pim-1 gene expression in murine lymphocytes. Nutr Cancer 1999; 33:206–212.

158. Wallstrom P, Wirfalt E, Lahmann PH, Gullberg B, Janzon L, Berglund G. Serum concentrations of beta-carotene and alpha-tocopherol are associated with diet, smoking, and general and central adiposity. Am J Clin Nutr 2001; 73:777–785.

159. Kardinaal AF, Van 't Veer P, Brants HA, van den Berg H, Van Schoonhoven J, Hermus RJ. Relations between antioxidant vitamins in adipose tissue, plasma, and diet. Am J Epidemiol 1995; 141:440–450.

160. Johnson EJ, Hammond BR, Yeum KJ, Qin J, Wang XD, Castaneda C, Snodderly DM, Russell RM. Relation among serum and tissue concentrations of lutein and zeaxanthin and macular pigment density. Am J Clin Nutr 2000; 71:1555–1562.

161. El-Sohemy A, Baylin A, Kabagambe E, Ascherio A, Spiegelman D, Campos H. Individual carotenoid concentrations in adipose tissue and plasma as biomarkers of dietary intake. Am J Clin Nutr 2002; 76:172–179.

162. Mathews-Roth MM. Carotenoids in medical applications. In: Bauernfeind JC, ed. Carotenoids as Colorants and Vitamin A Precursors. New York: Academic Press, 1981:755–785.

163. Le François P. Carotenodermia. Am J Clin Nutr 1989; 49:1330–1331.

164. Micozzi MS, Brown ED, Taylor PR, Wolfe E. Carotenodermia in men with elevated carotenoid intake from foods and beta-carotene supplements. Am J Clin Nutr 1988; 48:1061–1064.

165. Stirling HF, Laing SC, Barr DG. Hypercarotenaemia and vitamin A overdosage from proprietary baby food. Lancet 1986; 1:1089.

166. Heinrich U, Gartner C, Wiebusch M, Eichler O, Sies H, Tronnier H, Stahl W. Supplementation with beta-carotene or a similar amount of mixed carotenoids protects humans from UV-induced erythema. J Nutr 2003; 133:98–101.

167. Prince MR, Frisoli JK. Beta-carotene accumulation in serum and skin. Am J Clin Nutr 1993; 57:175–181.

168. Hencken H. Chemical and physiological behavior of feed carotenoids and their effects on pigmentation. Poult Sci 1992; 71:711–717.

169. Wingerath T, Sies H, Stahl W. Xanthophyll esters in human skin. Arch Biochem Biophys 1998; 355:271–274.

170. Cameron LM, Rosin MP, Stich HF. Use of exfoliated cells to study tissue-specific levels of beta-carotene in humans. Cancer Lett 1989; 45:203–207.

171. Mitchell DC, Prince MR, Frisoli JK, Smith RE, Wood RF. Beta carotene uptake into atherosclerotic plaque: enhanced staining and preferential ablation with the pulsed dye laser. Lasers Surg Med 1993; 13:149–157.

172. LaMuraglia GM, Mathews-Roth MM, Parrish JA, Abbott WM, Brewster DC, McAuliffe DJ, Prince MR. Enhancing the carotenoid content of atherosclerotic plaque: implications for laser therapy. J Vasc Surg 1989; 9:563–567.

173. Ye B, Abela GS. Beta-carotene enhances plaque detection by fluorescence attenuation in an atherosclerotic rabbit model. Lasers Surg Med 1993; 13:393–404.

174. Shi HL, Furr HC, Olson JA. Retinoids and carotenoids in bovine pineal gland. Brain Res Bull 1991; 26:235–239.

175. Craft N, Garnett K, Hedlye-Whyte ET, Fitch K, Haitema T, Dorey CK. Carotenoids, tocopherols, and vitamin A in human brain. FASEB J 1998; 12:A967 (Abstract).

176. Bernstein PS, Khachik F, Carvalho LS, Muir GJ, Zhao DY, Katz NB. Identification and quantitation of carotenoids and their metabolites in the tissues of the human eye. Exp Eye Res 2001; 72:215–223.

177. Broekmans WM, Berendschot TT, Klopping-Ketelaars IA, de Vries AJ, Goldbohm RA, Tijburg LB, Kardinaal AF, van Poppel G. Macular pigment density in relation to serum and adipose tissue concentrations of lutein and serum concentrations of zeaxanthin. Am J Clin Nutr 2002; 76:595–603.

178. Hammond BR Jr, Johnson EJ, Russell RM, Krinsky NI, Yeum KJ, Edwards RB, Snodderly DM. Dietary modification of human macular pigment density. Invest Ophthalmol Vis Sci 1997; 38:1795–1801.

179. Khachik F, de Moura FF, Zhao DY, Aebischer CP, Bernstein PS. Transformations of selected carotenoids in plasma, liver, and ocular tissues of humans and in nonprimate animal models. Invest Ophthalmol Vis Sci 2002; 43:3383–3392.

180. Snodderly DM, Handelman GJ, Adler AJ. Distribution of individual macular pigment carotenoids in central retina of macaque and squirrel monkeys. Invest Ophthalmol Vis Sci 1991; 32:268–279.

181. Bone RA, Landrum JT, Friedes LM, Gomez CM, Kilburn MD, Menendez E, Vidal I, Wang W. Distribution of lutein and zeaxanthin stereoisomers in the human retina. Exp Eye Res 1997; 64:211–218.

182. Landrum JT, Bone RA, Moore LL, Gomez CM. Analysis of zeaxanthin distribution within individual human retinas. Meth Enzymol 1999; 299:457–467.

183. Rapp LM, Maple SS, Choi JH. Lutein and zeaxanthin concentrations in rod outer segment membranes from perifoveal and peripheral human retina. Invest Ophthalmol Vis Sci 2000; 41:1200–1209.

184. Kimler VA, Taylor JD. Ultrastructural immunogold localization of some organelle-transport relevant proteins in wholemounted permeabilized nonextracted goldfish xanthophores. Pigment Cell Res 1995; 8:75–82.

185. Crabtree DV, Ojima I, Geng X, Adler AJ. Tubulins in the primate retina: evidence that xanthophylls may be endogenous ligands for the paclitaxel-binding site. Bioorg Med Chem 2001; 9:1967–1976.

186. Yemelyanov AY, Katz NB, Bernstein PS. Ligand-binding characterization of xanthophyll carotenoids to solubilized membrane proteins derived from human retina. Exp Eye Res 2001; 72:381–392.

187. Toyoda Y, Thomson LR, Langner A, Craft NE, Garnett KM, Nichols CR, Cheng KM, Dorey CK. Effect of dietary zeaxanthin on tissue distribution of zeaxanthin and lutein in quail. Invest Ophthalmol Vis Sci 2002; 43:1210–1221.

188. Daicker B, Schiedt K, Adnet JJ, Bermond P. Canthaxanthin retinopathy. An investigation by light and electron microscopy and physicochemical analysis. Graefes Arch Clin Exp Ophthalmol 1987; 225:189–197.

189. Goralczyk R, Barker FM, Buser S, Liechti H, Bausch J. Dose dependency of canthaxanthin crystals in monkey retina and spatial distribution of its metabolites. Invest Ophthalmol Vis Sci 2000; 41:1513–1522.

190. O'Fallon JV, Chew BP. The subcellular distribution of beta-carotene in bovine corpus luteum. Proc Soc Exp Biol Med 1984; 177:406–411.

191. Mayne ST, Parker RS. Subcellular distribution of dietary beta-carotene in chick liver. Lipids 1986; 21:164–169.

192. Bianchi-Santamaria A, Stefanelli C, Cembran M, Gobbi M, Peschiera N, Vannini V, Santamaria L. Hepatic subcellular storage of beta-carotene in rats following diet supplementation. Int J Vitam Nutr Res 1999; 69:3–7.

193. Chew BP, Park JS, Weng BC, Wong TS, Hayek MG, Reinhart GA. Dietary beta-carotene is taken up by blood plasma and leukocytes in dogs. J Nutr 2000; 130:1788–1791.

194. Socaciu C, Jessel R, Diehl HA. Carotenoid incorporation into microsomes: yields, stability and membrane dynamics. Spectrochim Acta A Mol Biomol Spectrosc 2000; 56:2799–2809.

195. Davies BH. Carotenoid metabolism in animals: a biochemist's view. Pure Appl Chem 1985; 57:679–684.

196. Napoli JL, Race KR. Biogenesis of retinoic acid from beta-carotene. Differences between the metabolism of beta-carotene and retinol. J Biol Chem 1988; 263:17372–17377.

197. Khachik F, Pfander H, Traber B. Proposed mechanisms for the formation of the synthetic and naturally occurring metabolites of lycopene in tomato products and human serum. J Agric Food Chem 1998; 46:4885–4890.

198. Khachik F, Beecher GR, Goli MB, Lusby WR, Smith JC Jr. Separation and identification of carotenoids and their oxidation products in the extracts of human plasma. Anal Chem 1992; 64:2111–2122.

199. Khachik F, Englert G, Beecher GR, Smith JC Jr. Isolation, structural elucidation, and partial synthesis of lutein dehydration products in extracts from human plasma. J Chromatogr B Biomed Appl 1995; 670:219–233.

200. Khachik F, Beecher GR. Separation and identification of carotenoids and carotenol fatty acid esters in some squash products by liquid chromatography. 1. Quantification of carotenoids and related esters by HPLC. J Agric Food Chem 1988; 36:929–937.

201. Khachik F, Beecher GR, Lusby WR. Separation and identification of carotenoids and carotenol fatty acid esters in some squash products by liquid chromatography. 2. Isolation and characterization of carotenoids and related esters. J Agric Food Chem 1988; 36:938–946.

202. Savithry KN, Mallia AK, Cama HR. Metabolism and biological activity of anhydrolutein (3'-hydroxy-3,4-dehydro-beta-carotene) in rat. Indian J Biochem Biophys 1972; 9:325–327.

203. McGraw KJ, Hill GE, Stradi R, Parker RS. The influence of carotenoid acquisition and utilization on the maintenance of species-typical plumage pigmentation in male American goldfinches (*Carduelis tristis*) and northern cardinals (*Cardinalis cardinalis*). Physiol Biochem Zool 2001; 74:843–852.

204. McGraw KJ, Adkins-Regan E, Parker RS. Anhydrolutein in the zebra finch: a new, metabolically derived carotenoid in birds. Comp Biochem Physiol B Biochem Mol Biol 2002; 132:811–818.

205. McGraw KJ, Hill GE, Stradi R, Parker RS. The effect of dietary carotenoid access on sexual dichromatism and plumage pigment composition in the American goldfinch. Comp Biochem Physiol B Biochem Mol Biol 2002; 131:261–269.

206. Surai PF, Royle NJ, Sparks NH. Fatty acid, carotenoid and vitamin A composition of tissues of free living gulls. Comp Biochem Physiol A Mol Integr Physiol 2000; 126:387–396.

207. Surai PF, Speake BK, Wood NA, Blount JD, Bortolotti GR, Sparks NH. Carotenoid discrimination by the avian embryo: a lesson from wild birds. Comp Biochem Physiol B Biochem Mol Biol 2001; 128:743–750.

208. Hill GE, Inouye CY, Montgomerie R. Dietary carotenoids predict plumage coloration in wild house finches. Proc R Soc Lond B Biol Sci 2002; 269:1119–1124.

209. Saino N, Stradi R, Ninni P, Pini E, Moller AP. Carotenoid plasma concentration, immune profile, and plumage ornamentation of male barn swallows (*Hirundo rustica*). Am Nat 1999; 154:441–448.

210. Coral-Hinostroza GN, Bjerkeng B. Astaxanthin from the red crab langostilla (*Pleuroncodes planipes*): optical R/S isomers and fatty acid moieties of astaxanthin esters. Comp Biochem Physiol B Biochem Mol Biol 2002; 133:437–444.

211. Tyczkowski JK, Hamilton PB. Lutein as a model dihydroxycarotenoid for the study of pigmentation in chickens. Poult Sci 1986; 65:1141–1145.

212. Tyczkowski JK, Hamilton PB. Canthaxanthin as a model for the study of utilization of oxycarotenoids by chickens. Poult Sci 1986; 65:1350–1356.

213. Wang XD, Krinsky NI. The bioconversion of beta-carotene into retinoids. Subcell Biochem 1998; 30:159–180.

214. Sharma RV, Mathur SN, Dmitrovskii AA, Das RC, Ganguly J. Studies on the metabolism of beta-carotene and apo-beta-carotenoids in rats and chickens. Biochim Biophys Acta 1977; 486:183–194.

215. Birringer M, Pfluger P, Kluth D, Landes N, Brigelius-Flohe R. Identities and differences in the metabolism of tocotrienols and tocopherols in HepG2 cells. J Nutr 2002; 132:3113–3118.

216. Pope SA, Burtin GE, Clayton PT, Madge DJ, Muller DP. New synthesis of $(+/-)$-alpha-CMBHC and its confirmation as a metabolite of alpha-tocopherol (vitamin E). Bioorg Med Chem 2001; 9:1337–1343.

217. Shi J, Le Maguer M. Lycopene in tomatoes: chemical and physical properties affected by food processing. Crit Rev Food Sci Nutr 2000; 40:1–42.

218. Werman MJ, Mokady S, Ben-Amotz A. Bioavailability of the isomer mixture of phytoene and phytofluene-rich alga *Dunaliella bardawil* in rat plasma and tissues. J Nutr Biochem 2002; 13:585–591.

219. Stahl W, Schwarz W, von Laar J, Sies H. All-trans beta-carotene preferentially accumulates in human chylomicrons and very low density lipoproteins compared with the 9-cis geometrical isomer. J Nutr 1995; 125:2128–2133.

220. Erdman JW Jr, Thatcher AJ, Hofmann NE, Lederman JD, Block SS, Lee CM, Mokady S. All-trans beta-carotene is absorbed preferentially to 9-cis beta-carotene, but the latter accumulates in the tissues of domestic ferrets (*Mustela putorius puro*). J Nutr 1998; 128:2009–2013.

221. Patton S, Canfield LM, Huston GE, Ferris AM, Jensen RG. Carotenoids of human colostrum. Lipids 1990; 25:159–165.

222. Canfield LM, Giuliano AR, Neilson EM, Yap HH, Graver EJ, Cui HA, Blashill BM. Beta-carotene in breast milk and serum is increased after a single beta-carotene dose. Am J Clin Nutr 1997; 66:52–61.

223. Khachik F, Spangler CJ, Smith JC Jr, Canfield LM, Steck A, Pfander H. Identification, quantification, and relative concentrations of carotenoids and their metabolites in human milk and serum. Anal Chem 1997; 69:1873–1881.

224. Jewell VC, Northrop-Clewes CA, Tubman R, Thurnham DI. Nutritional factors and visual function in premature infants. Proc Nutr Soc 2001; 60:171–178.

225. Gossage CP, Deyhim M, Yamini S, Douglass LW, Moser-Veillon PB. Carotenoid composition of human milk during the first month postpartum and the response to beta-carotene supplementation. Am J Clin Nutr 2002; 76:193–197.

226. Kim Y, English C, Reich P, Gerber LE, Simpson KL. Vitamin A and carotenoids of human milk. J Agric Food Chem 1990; 38:1930–1933.

227. Giuliano AR, Neilson EM, Yap HH, Baier M, Canfield LM. Quantitation of and inter/intraindividual variability in major carotenoids of mature human milk. J Nutr Biochem 1994; 5:551–556.

228. Schweigert FJ, Hurtienne A, Bathe K. Improved extraction procedure for carotenoids from human milk. Int J Vitam Nutr Res 2000; 70:79–83.

229. Li Y, Craft NE, Handelman GJ, Nommsen-Rivers LA, McCrory MA, Dewey KG. Associations between serum and breast milk carotenoids, vitamins A and E. FASEB J 1999; 13:A240 (Abstract).

230. Johnson EJ, Qin J, Krinsky NI, Russell RM. Beta-carotene isomers in human serum, breast milk and buccal mucosa cells after continuous oral doses of all-trans and 9-cis beta-carotene. J Nutr 1997; 127:1993–1999.

231. Canfield LM, Giuliano AR, Neilson EM, Blashil BM, Graver EJ, Yap HH. Kinetics of the response of milk and serum beta-carotene to daily beta- carotene supplementation in healthy, lactating women. Am J Clin Nutr 1998; 67:276–283.

232. Clevidence BA, Bieri JG. Association of carotenoids with human plasma lipoproteins. Meth Enzymol 1993; 214:33–46.

233. Morinobu T, Tamai H, Tanabe T, Murata T, Manago M, Mino M, Hirahara F. Plasma alpha-tocopherol, beta-carotene, and retinol levels in the institutionalized elderly individuals and in young adults. Int J Vitam Nutr Res 1994; 64:104–108.

234. Tee ES, Lim CL, Chong YH. Carotenoid profile and retinol content in human serum—simultaneous determination by high-pressure liquid chromatography (HPLC). Int J Food Sci Nut 1994; 45:147–157.
235. Olmedilla B, Granado F, Gil-Martinez E, Blanco I, Rojas-Hidalgo E. Reference values for retinol, tocopherol, and main carotenoids in serum of control and insulin-dependent diabetic Spanish subjects. Clin Chem 1997; 43:1066–1071.
236. Thurnham DI, Flora PS. Do higher vitamin A requirements in men explain the difference between the sexes in plasma provitamin A carotenoids and retinol? Proc Nutr Soc 1988; 47:181A (Abstract).
237. Ross MA, Crosley LK, Brown KM, Duthie SJ, Collins AC, Arthur JR, Duthie GG. Plasma concentrations of carotenoids and antioxidant vitamins in Scottish males: influences of smoking. Eur J Clin Nutr 1995; 49:861–865.
238. Stacewicz-Sapuntzakis M, Bowen PE, Kikendall JW, Burgess M. Simultaneous determination of serum retinol and various carotenoids: their distribution in middle-aged men and women. J Micronutr Anal 1987; 3:27–45.
239. Kaplan LA, Stein EA, Kaplan JM. Specificity of in vitro loading of lipoproteins with carotenoids [abstr]. Clin Chem 1987; 33:935–936.

12

Bioequivalence of Provitamin A Carotenoids

Guangwen Tang and Robert M. Russell
Tufts University, Boston, Massachusetts, U.S.A.

I. INTRODUCTION

In 1930, Moore discovered that β-carotene (β-C) could be converted in vivo to vitamin A (1). Since then, the vitamin A value of dietary β-C and other provitamin A carotene products, in addition to their other biological activities, have been investigated. It is now known that the bioequivalence of provitamin A carotenoids in humans varies greatly, probably as a result of environmental and genetic factors.

Vitamin A is an essential vitamin for the promotion of general growth, maintenance of visual function, cellular differentiation, immune function, and embryonic development (2). Recent reports from developing countries have demonstrated that vitamin A also plays an important role in the prevention of morbidity and mortality from infectious diseases (3,4). In developing countries, provitamin A carotenes in vegetables and fruits may provide >70% of daily vitamin A intake (5). Thus, food-based interventions to increase the availability of provitamin A rich foods have been suggested as a realistic and sustainable option to overcome vitamin A deficiency globally (2). However, the efficacy of carotenoid-rich foods in the prevention of vitamin A deficiency has been questioned in several recent studies (6,7).

In contrast to developing countries, in Western societies provitamin A carotenoids derived from plants provide <30% of daily vitamin A intake (8). However, interest in studying the vitamin A value of dietary carotenoids in developed countries has arisen due to epidemiological data that show that diets rich in carotenoid-containing foods correlate with a reduced risk of certain types of chronic diseases such as cancer (aerodigestive, primarily) (9), cardiovascular disease (10), age-related macular degeneration (11,12), and cataract (13,14). The possible disease-preventing activities of β-C and other provitamin A carotenoids may be ascribed to their conversion into retinoids as well as to their antioxidant activity as intact molecules (15). However, the results of several human intervention studies indicate that high-dose supplementation with β-C, either alone (16) or with vitamin E (16) or vitamin A (17), do not decrease the risk of cancer or cardiovascular disease, and might even be harmful to smokers or former asbestos workers in terms of causing more lung cancers. Thus, it appears that carotenoids and β-C may be health promoting when taken at physiological levels in foods but may have adverse properties when given in high doses and under highly oxidative conditions.

As is well known, after an oral dose of β-C, intact β-C as well as one of its metabolites, retinol, can be found in the circulation as seen below:

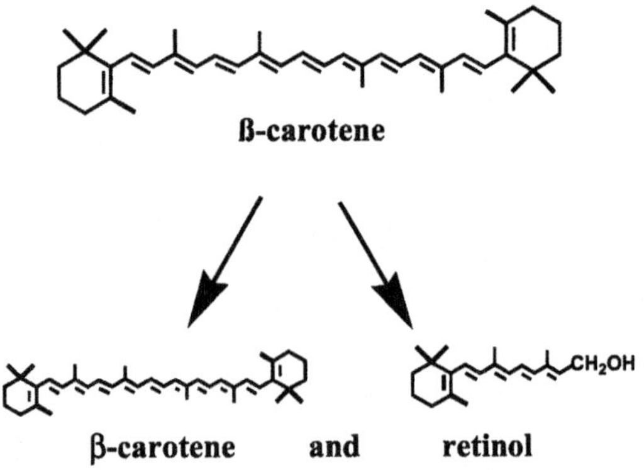

ß-carotene

β-carotene   and   retinol

β-C conversion to vitamin A in humans takes place in the intestine, liver, and possibly other tissues (18). The amount of a given oral dose of β-C to the amount of vitamin A derived from the β-C dose is defined as the β-C to vitamin A conversion factor. In theory, if all the β-C converted to retinol, the conversion factor will be 0.94 : 1 (1 mol of β-C = 536 g to 2 mol of retinol = 572 g) by weight or 1 : 2 by mole. Two pathways have been proposed for the conversion of β-C to vitamin A in mammals: the central cleavage pathway (19,20) is the major pathway that postulates the formation of 2 mol of retinaldehyde from a single β-C molecule by cleaving the 15,15′ double bond; whereas the excentric pathway is the minor pathway that postulates a single mole of retinaldehyde formed by a stepwise oxidation of β-C beginning at any of the double bonds of the polyene chain (18,21,22). A recent study confirmed that both central and random (excentric) cleavage of β-C take place in the postmitochondrial fraction of rat intestine, but that the pathway used depends on the presence or absence of other antioxidants, such as α-tocopherol (23).

Recently, the enzyme β-carotene 15, 15'-oxgenase that cleaves β-carotene to retinal has been identified in chicken intestinal mucosa and subsequently sequenced and expressed in two different cell lines (24). In addition, the existence an excentric cleavage enzyme of β-C has been reported in the mouse (25). Both central and random (excentric) cleavage enzymes of β-C can be found together in small intestine and liver (18). The existence of at least two different β-C oxygenases makes the estimation of bioequivalence of β-C quite complex.

II. EARLY STUDIES ON BIOEQUIVALENCE OF DIETARY SYNTHETIC β-CAROTENE TO VITAMIN A IN HUMANS

Several studies (26,27) on bioequivalence used a depletion–repletion method to determine the β-C equivalence (conversion factor) to vitamin A. Hume and Krebs (26) reported a depletion study conducted on 16 healthy subjects between the ages of 19 and 34 years (7 additional subjects served as positive controls). The investigation used both a blood concentration of retinol below 0.35 μmol/L (<10 μg/dL) and deterioration in dark adaptation to define "unmistakably deficient" subjects. After 12 months of depletion, only three of the subjects were vitamin A deficient. Of the three subjects with "unmistakable" signs of vitamin A deficiency, two were given β-C and one was given preformed vitamin A (as supplements). The results showed that daily doses of 1500 μg of β-C or 390 μg of retinol were sufficient to treat vitamin A deficiency in these subjects. Therefore, from this human study, the β-C to vitamin A conversion factor was 3.8 : 1 by weight.

In 1974, Sauberlich et al. (27) reported another extensive and well controlled vitamin A depletion–repletion study in human subjects. They recruited 8 healthy male subjects between 31 and 43 years of age. These volunteers were depleted in vitamin A over 359–771 days. Depletion was based on a plasma retinol level below 0.3 μmol/L (<10 μg/dL) and clinical signs of vitamin A deficiency (dark adaptation impairment, abnormal electroretinogram, or follicular hyperkeratosis). The investigators repleted 5 subjects with vitamin A and 3 subjects with β-C, and found that daily doses of 600 μg retinol or 1200 μg of β-C were required to cure vitamin A deficiency. In this study, the β-C to vitamin A equivalence was therefore 2 : 1 by weight.

These studies used depletion–repletion approaches. Whether a 3.8- or 2-μg equivalence of supplementary β-C to 1 μg of retinol is applicable in vitamin A–sufficient individuals cannot be determined from these studies, since all subjects had been made deficient in vitamin A.

On the basis of these earlier investigations using synthetic β-C in humans and vitamin A–depleted subjects and the lack of any specific data on food carotene bioavailability or bioconversion, the availability of β-C from the diet has been taken as one-third of the provitamin A carotenoids ingested, with a maximal conversion of absorbed β-C of 50% on a weight basis (28). Since other provitamin A carotenoids (α-C, cryptoxanthin, etc.) have only half the molecular structure that is identical to the all-*trans* β-C molecule, they are thought to exhibit approximately half of the vitamin A activity of β-C (28). Therefore, the retinol equivalence of carotenoids in food was (until recently) generally assumed and accepted as follows (29): 6 μg of all-*trans* β-C or 12 μg of other provitamin A carotenoids is equivalent to 1 μg of retinol (6:1 or 12:1). Since one retinol equivalent (RE) is equal to 1 μg of retinol, 1 RE is equal to 6 μg of β-C or 12 μg of other provitamin A carotenoids (30,31). Using these assumptions, the National Health and Nutrition Examination Survey (NHANES) of 1970–1980 in the United States showed that the median adult dietary intake of vitamin A was 624 RE with $\sim$25% coming from carotenoids and $\sim$75% coming from preformed vitamin A sources, as calculated from food composition tables (29). However, whether the β-C conversion factor of 6:1 can be used in vitamin A–sufficient population or accurately reflects β-C conversion from foods requires further investigation.

The National Academy of Science (USA) recently revised the dietary β-C:retinol equivalency ratio from 6:1 to 12:1 (μg:μg) for the following reasons: (a) a recent study demonstrated the relative absorption of β-C from food versus β-C in oil to be 14% [or, approximately 1/6 (not 33% as previously thought)]; (b) considering that the metabolism of β-C after absorption of the molecule is the same (when from food or from oil) and the maximal conversion of β-C in oil is 2:1 (2 μg of β-C in oil yields 1 μg of retinol), the retinol equivalency ratio from the food is therefore (6 × 2):1 or 12:1. So as not to confuse the old nomenclature of 1 RE = 1 μg retinol = 6 μg of dietary β-C, the Academy coined the term RAE (retinol activity equivalent; 1 RAE = 1 μg retinol = 12 μg of dietary β-C). Since the vitamin A activity of β-cryptoxanthin and α-C is one half that of β-C, 1 RAE = 24 μg dietary provitamin A carotenoids other than β-C. The Academy recognized that these conversion ratios might change as more data become available (32).

III. LESS BIOEQUIVALENCE OF PLANT PROVITAMIN A CAROTENOIDS

Recent studies have reported that dietary provitamin A carotenoids have much less biopotency to provide vitamin A nutrition than previously was accepted.

de Pee et al. (33) reported changes of serum retinol levels in vitamin A–deficient ($\sim$0.7 μmol/L) anemic school children aged 7–11 years, who were fed one of four supplements (1 RE = 1 μg of retinol; therefore, REs were calculated by dividing the amount of all-*trans* β-C by 6 and of other provitamin A carotenoids by 12): (a) 556 RE/day from retinol rich foods, $n = 48$; (b) 509 RE/day from fruits, $n = 49$; (c) 684 RE/day from vegetables, $n = 45$; and (d) 44 RE/day from low-retinol and low-carotene foods, $n = 46$. The authors assessed the changes in serum retinol in the groups eating these foods for 9 weeks (6 days/week) to determine a relative conversion efficiency of β-C from vegetables or fruits versus the from vitamin A rich food (egg, chicken liver, fortified margarine, and fortified chocolate milk). That is, they compared the increase in serum retinol concentrations after consumption of fruit (509 RE/day, serum retinol increased 0.12 μmol/L) and vegetables (684 RE/day, serum retinol increased 0.07 μmol/L) with that in the group consuming foods rich in preformed vitamin A (556 RE/day, serum retinol increased 0.23 μmol/L). From this they calculated that the relative mean conversion factor of vegetable β-C to retinol was 26:1 and of orange fruit β-C to retinol was 12:1 (33).

However, changes of serum retinol would not be a sensitive indicator of vitamin A status. Instead of measuring the serum retinol changes, we have used isotope dilution techniques to measure changes of total body stores of vitamin A in children with marginal to normal vitamin A status, who participated in a food-based intervention using either green–yellow vegetables or light-colored vegetables during the winter months (34). In this study we found that the serum carotenoid concentrations of children fed green–yellow vegetables increased, whereas the serum concentration of vitamin A did not change. In contrast, the isotope dilution tests carried out before and after the vegetable intervention showed that while the body stores of vitamin A [calculated by using modified Baush-Rietz equation (35)] were stable in the group fed green–yellow vegetables, the body stores of vitamin A became decreased in the group fed light-colored vegetables. As compared to the children fed light-colored vegetables, 205.8 mg of calculated β-C from green–yellow vegetables fed over a 10-week period prevented the loss of 7.7 mg vitamin A from body stores. Thus, from this study, we calculated that the vegetable β-C to retinol equivalence was 26.7 μg β-C to 1 μg retinol. This conversion factor is very similar to that reported by de Pee et al. for vegetable carotenoids (33).

Another study (on one subject) also reported (36) that the mass equivalency of carrot β-C to vitamin A was 13:1 (without considering the contribution of 5.2 μmol α-C to vitamin A). If the contribution of α-C were to be considered, the ratio could be higher than 13:1, i.e., 16:1 (assuming that α-C has half of the β-C activity).

IV. FACTORS ON THE BIOEQUIVALENCE OF DIETARY PROVITAMIN A CAROTENOIDS

Until now, the vitamin A value of a food has been calculated based on the amount of specific preformed vitamin A and provitamin A carotenoids contained in that food. Many factors affect the bioavailability and bioconversion of carotenoids to vitamin A, as summarized by the acronym SLAMENGHI (*s*pecies of carotenoids, molecular *l*inkage, *a*mount of carotenoids consumed in a meal, *m*atrix of the carotenoids associated, *e*ffectors of absorption, *n*utritional status, *g*enetic factors, *h*ost-related factors, *i*nteractions) (37). However, the major factors that affect the bioavailability of food carotenoids and the bioconversion of food carotenoids to vitamin A in humans are likely food matrices and the fat content of a meal.

A. Food Matrix

The absorption and conversion of carotenoids from various food matrices can be investigated utilizing plant food material in which the carotenoids have been endogenously or intrinsically labeled with a low-abundance stable isotope.

Plant carotenoids can be intrinsically labeled through the addition of a hydrogen-stable isotope presented to the plant's roots in the form of heavy water, ^2H_2O. Plants can be easily grown hydroponically (38) on a nutrient solution composed of a fixed ^2H_2O atom percentage. Figure 1 demonstrates the isotope profiles of β-C from spinach (top graph) and carrot (bottom graph) grown hydroponically with 25 atom % ^2H_2O and analyzed by liquid chromatograph/atmospheric pressure chemical ionization-mass spectrometry (LC/APCI-MS). In deuterated β-C molecules from these vegetables, the highest abundance peak is 547 (molecular mass 536 + H + 10).

Spinach and carrots were harvested 32 and 60 days, respectively, after initiation of hydroponic growth. The spinach leaves (or sliced carrots) were steamed in thin layers (2–3 leaves) for 10 min. The cooked spinach leaves (or sliced carrots) were immersed in cold water (1 L water per 200 g vegetable) for 2 min. The labeled spinach or carrots were then drained, pureed, sealed in a plastic container, and stored at $-70°C$ until used for the analysis of contents and for human consumption experiments.

Four adult men (average age 56 years) took two different plant foods (spinach, carrot) 3 months apart. β-C in spinach may be in the form of chromoproteins (39) located in chloroplasts, whereas carrot is a root vegetable, and β-C in carrot is in the form of carotene crystals in chromoplasts (40). The 3-month interval was required to avoid a possible interference between the doses, and the doses were given in random order. A fasting blood sample (10 mL, time = 0 h) was drawn on day 0. Then a liquid formula breakfast was given (35% energy from fat). In the middle of this meal, the subject took either an oral dose of pureed spinach (300 g, thawed), or pureed carrot (100 g, thawed). On day 7, the volunteer repeated the procedures described for day 0 of the study, except that he received a 3.0-mg $^2H_8$ retinyl acetate capsule together with a liquid formula meal. No vitamin supplements or large amounts of β-C or vitamin A in the diet were permitted during this period. These procedures were repeated on day 90 using the other vegetable. The serum samples were analyzed by using GC/electron

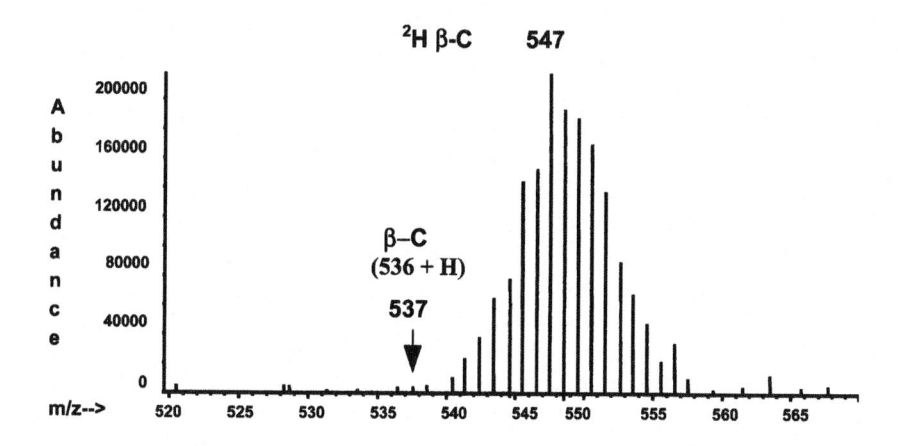

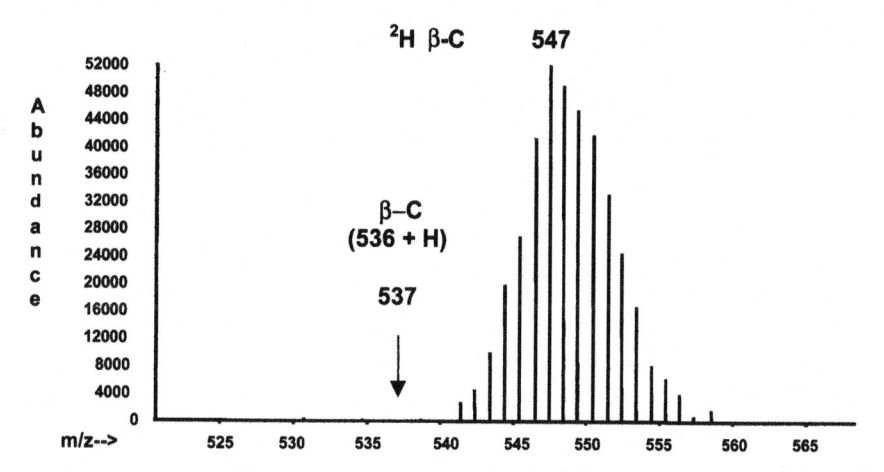

Figure 1 Isotope profiles of β-C from spinach (*top*) and carrot (*bottom*) grown hydroponically with 25 atom% ^2H_2O.

capture negative chemical ionization-MS (41) to determine the enrichment of labeled retinol in the circulation formed from the labeled vegetables. Because there is a distribution of several isotopomers of the β-C molecule, we included the enrichment of each isotopomer in our calculation. By doing this, we found that conversion of food carotenoids to vitamin A could be accurately evaluated.

The 300 g of labeled spinach and 100 g of labeled carrots contained $\sim$11 mg calculated β-C, and it was assumed that α-C and *cis*-β-C have half the activity of all-*trans* β-C. The results from this labeled vegetable study on 4 subjects showed that the retinol equivalence of spinach β-C was 29 μg spinach β-C to 1 μg retinol, and the retinol equivalence of carrot β-C dose was 19 μg carrot β-C to 1 μg retinol.

Since both spinach and carrots were pureed and were given with an equal amount of fat, this study provides evidence that provitamin A carotenoids from different foods have different conversion factors, and thus have different bioequivalence to vitamin A.

A recent bioengineered golden rice introduced β-C to rice endosperm (42). Rice endosperm contains starch and protein, and cooked rice is easy to digest. The bioavailability and bioconversion of golden rice β-C are probably different from spinach β-C and carrot β-C due to the more simple rice endosperm matrix in which it is contained. The question "what is the vitamin A equivalence of golden rice β-C?" has not yet been answered.

B. Fat Content of a Meal

The effects of fat content of a meal on the bioavailability of β-C have been investigated (43). It has been generally accepted that a higher fat content in the diet facilitates the formation of intestinal micelles needed for vitamin A and carotene absorption. A recent publication (44) reported dietary fat effects on the conversion of β-C to vitamin A by assessing the accumulation of β-C and vitamin A (derived from the β-C doses) in tissues (liver, kidney, and adrenal tissue) of Mongolian gerbils that were given a β-C-deficient diet for 1 week and followed by one of eight isocaloric, semipurified diets supplemented with carrot powder [1 μg β-C and 0.5 μg α-C/kJ diet] for 2 weeks ($n = 12$/group). The authors observed that increasing dietary fat from 10% to 30% of total energy resulted in higher vitamin A tissue levels and lower β-C stores in the liver, suggesting that consumption of high-fat diets enhances conversion of β-C to vitamin A.

V. OTHER FACTORS

A. Vitamin A Status

The vitamin A activity of provitamin A carotenoids may be affected by vitamin A status. It has been found that the activity of intestinal β-C cleavage enzyme in vitamin A-sufficient rats is 50% of that in vitamin A-deficient rats (45). This was also observed in human in vivo studies. For example, it was reported (46) that after the intervention with 40 g amaranth, children aged 2–6 years with initial serum retinol <25 μg/dL increased their serum retinol by 12.6 μg/dL while those with initial serum retinol >25 μg/dL increased their serum retinol only by 6.2 μg/dL. These observations were further confirmed by a recent report (47) that children with inadequate vitamin A status (<25 μg/dL) showed the greatest response in increasing serum vitamin A concentration, where $<$ as the children with serum retinol >25 μg/dL showed very little or no response in serum retinol concentration. However, as mentioned earlier, the change in serum retinol concentration before and after an intervention is not a good indicator for judging vitamin A status because in subjects with normal vitamin A status the vitamin A formed may contribute to increased body (liver) stores of vitamin A—but not to the serum retinol concentration.

B. Isomers of Carotenoids

In plants, provitamin A carotenoids are not only in all-trans form but also in other isomeric forms. The bioequivalence of other isomers of provitamin A carotenes have been defined as possessing 50% of the activity of all-*trans* β-C. This is based on structures, since in theory, 1 mol of all-*trans* β-C may cleave to 2 mol of all-*trans* retinol, whereas the other isomers of β-C can only cleave to yield 1 mol of all-*trans* retinol. However, structural differences may also result in differences in absorption efficiencies by the intestine, and this has not been rigorously researched. A recent paper (48) reported a study in gerbils wherein the relative vitamin A bioequivalence of 9-*cis*-β-C was less (38%) and 13-*cis*-β-C (62%) was more than the defined value of 50% of all-*trans* β-C.

C. Dose Levels on the Bioequivalence of Provitamin A Carotenoids

From our early study (49), it was reported that the $^2H_4$ retinol formed from 6 mg of $^2H_8$β-C (11.2 μmol) in oil was calculated to be equivalent to 1.6 mg of retinol (i.e., 3.8 : 1). However, the $^2H_4$ retinol formed from 126 mg of $^2H_8$β-C (235 μmol) in oil was only equivalent to 2.3 mg of retinol (i.e., 55 : 1). These results demonstrate that there is an inverse dose-dependent efficiency of bioconversion of β-C to retinol. The variation of the bioequivalence of all-*trans* β-C ranged between 2.4 : 1 and 20.2 : 1 with an average figure of 9 : 1 by weight (50) when using 6 mg of all-*trans* β-C in oil dose. Lower doses of isotopically labeled β-C have not yet been studied extensively (51,52). Another report used 16.3 mg of all-*trans* β-C in oil dose, and showed a conversion factor of all-*trans* β-C in oil as 16 to 1 by weight (53).

From these results, it is clear that bioavailability of β-C as vitamin A is dose dependent. This implies that the conversion capability of β-C to vitamin A is under physiological regulation.

D. Influence of Other Micronutrients and Antioxidants

A reduction of the plasma β-C response by simultaneously administered lutein has been reported by Kostic et al. (54). Whether this reduction also interferes the cleavage of β-C to provide retinol requires study. A recent report using the postprandial chylomicron method to evaluate the effect of other carotenoids on the absorption and cleavage of β-C demonstrated that lutein, but not lycopene, reduced β-C absorption but that neither carotenoid affected the formation of retinyl palmitate (55).

E. Protein Malnutrition

The β-C 15,15'-oxygenase cleavage enzyme and excentric oxygenase enzymes have been found mainly in intestine and liver. It is possible that populations with protein malnutrition will have diminished capability to convert β-C to vitamin A. This hypothesis is corroborated in a recent report of a study conducted in rats (56).

F. Intraluminal Infections

It is common that populations at heightened risk of vitamin A deficiency have a high prevalence of parasitic infestation and have a high intake of plant foods. Until now, data on whether parasitic infection affects vitamin A nutrition have been somewhat conflicting (43). The level or severity of ascaris/hookworm infections needed to affect the absorption of vitamin A and/or bioconversion of dietary provitamin A carotenoids to vitamin A remains to be studied.

G. Macronutrient Factors

A recent publication (44) reported that type of dietary fiber, in addition to dietary fat, affects conversion of β-C to vitamin A. By assessing the accumulation of β-C and vitamin A (derived from the β-C doses) in tissues (liver, kidney, and adrenal tissue) of Mongolian gerbils that were given β-C deficient diet for 1 week, investigators found that consumption of citrus pectin resulted in lower hepatic vitamin A stores and higher hepatic β-C stores compared with all other groups, suggesting less conversion of β-C to vitamin A. In contrast, consumption of oat gum resulted in higher vitamin A and lower β-C stores in liver than those of citrus pectin-fed gerbils. Furthermore, the level of dietary fat consumed with soluble fiber had no interactive effects on hepatic vitamin A, β-C, or α-C stores. These results demonstrate that β-C absorption is independently affected by type of soluble fiber and suggest that these dietary components modulate the conversion of β-C to vitamin A.

H. Food Preparation

Food preparation practices have some effect on the bioavailability of carotenoids as vitamin A, since carotenoid bioavailability depends on the type and extent of food processing as well (57). To study the effect of variously processed spinach products on serum carotenoid concentrations, subjects received, over a 3-week period, a control diet ($n = 10$) or a control diet supplemented with carotenoids or one of three spinach products ($n = 12$ per group): whole-leaf spinach with an almost intact food matrix, minced spinach with the matrix partially disrupted, and liquefied spinach. It was found that serum total β-C responses differed significantly between the whole-leaf and liquefied spinach groups, and between the minced and liquefied spinach groups. The relative bioavailability as compared to bioavailability of the carotenoid supplement for whole-leaf, minced, and liquefied spinach for β-C was 5.1%, 6.4%, and 9.3%, respectively. The investigators concluded that disruption of the matrix (cell wall structure) enhanced the bioavailability of β-C from whole-leaf and minced spinach. However, the effect of the food preparation on the conversion of β-C to retinol was not observed in this population due to the insensitivity of the serum retinol measurement (57).

I. Genetic Factors

Using an isotope reference method, a recent study conducted in the east central region of China found that 4 of 15 adult subjects showed abnormal poor conversion of β-C to vitamin A, although their absorptions of β-C and vitamin A were normal (personal communication with Drs. Shi-an Yin and Zhixu Wang). These four subjects were healthy and without any biomedical abnormality. We speculate that this may due to polymorphism of the 15,15'-oxygenase gene in this population. Another study on the genetic profile of these subjects may provide important information about possible genetic factors on the conversion of provitamin A carotenoids to vitamin A.

VI. BIOEQUIVALENCE OF β-C TO RETINOIC ACID

β-C can be converted to retinoic acid via an excentric cleavage pathway in ferret intestine (58,59) and in human intestinal mucosa (60). The concentration of all-*trans* retinoic acid in the serum of rabbits fed β-C was found to be higher than those fed no β-C (61). Retinoic acid plays an important role in the prevention and therapy of cancers through its control of gene expression (62); thus, factors that affect the formation of retinoic acid from dietary β-C warrant further investigation.

VII. CONCLUSION

The present reported values for bioequivalence of provitamin A carotenoids to vitamin A varies from 2 μg β-C to 1 μg retinol (synthetic pure β-C in oil) to 27 μg β-C to 1 retinol (vegetable β-C). Factors affecting β-C conversion to vitamin A are dietary factors including food matrix (e.g., vegetables, fruits) and dietary fat and fiber content (macronutrient), host nutritional status (vitamin A status and protein nutrition status), and host intestinal health (parasitic infection and other infections). Provitamin A carotenoids (mainly β-C) can provide vitamin A nutrition for humans, but the efficiency of production of vitamin A from dietary carotene is quite a bit less than previously thought.

ACKNOWLEDGMENT

This work was supported by grants from the U.S. Department of Agriculture, Agricultural Research Service under Cooperative Agreement Numbers 1950-51000-047-SQR and 99-35200-7564. The contents of this publication do not necessarily reflect the views or policies of the U.S. Department of Agriculture, nor does mention of trade names, commercial products, or organizations imply endorsement by the U.S. Government.

REFERENCES

1. Moore T. Vitamin A and carotene. VI. The conversion of carotene to vitamin A in vivo. Biochem J 1930; 24:696–702.
2. Underwood BA, Arthur P. The contribution of vitamin A to public health. FASEB J 1996; 10:1040–1048.
3. Underwood BA. Overcoming micronutrient deficiencies in developing countries: is there a role for agriculture. Food Nutr Bull 2000; 21(4):356–360.
4. The current situation of VAD in progress in controlling vitamin A deficiency. Micronutrient Initiative/UNICEF/Tulane University, 1998. p. 3.
5. Ge K, Zhai F, Ye H. The dietary and nutritional status of Chinese populations in 1990s. Acta Nutr Sinica 1995; 123–134.
6. de Pee S, West C, Muhila K, Hautvast G. Lack of improvement in vitamin A status with increased consumption of dark green leafy vegetables. Lancet 1995; 346(July 8):75–81.
7. Bulux J, Serrano JD, Giuliano A, Perez R, Lopez CY, Rivera C, Solomons NW, Canfield LM. Plasma response of children to short-term chronic β-carotene supplementation. Am J Clin Nutr 1994; 59:1369–1375.
8. Olson J. Recommended dietary intakes (RDI) of vitamin A in humans. Am J Clin Nutr 1987; 45:704–716.

9. van Poppel G, Goldbohm R. Epidemiologic evidence for β-carotene and cancer prevention. Am J Clin Nutr 1995; 62:1393S–1402S.

10. Gaziano J, Hennekens CH. The role of beta-carotene in the prevention of cardiovascular disease. Ann NY Acad Sci 1993; 691:148–155.

11. Goldberg J, Flowerdew G, Smith E, Brody J, Tso M. Factors associated with age-related macular degeneration. Am J Epidemiol 1988; 128:700–710.

12. Seddon JM, Ajani UA, Sperduto RD, Hiller R, Blair N, Burton TC, Farber MD, Gragoudas ES, Haller J, Miller DT, et al. Dietary carotenoids, vitamins A, C, and E, and advanced age-related macular degeneration. Eye Disease Case-Control Study Group. JAMA 1994; 272(18):1413–1420.

13. Hankinson SE, Stampfer MJ, Seddon JM, Colditz GA, Rosner B, Speizer FE, Willett WC. Nutrient intake and cataract extraction in women: a prospective study. BMJ 1992; 305:335–339.

14. Jacques PF, Chylack LT, McGandy RB, Hartz SC. Antioxidant status in persons with and without senile cataract. Arch Ophthalmol 1988; 106:337–340.

15. Hennekens CH, Buring UE, Peto R. Antioxidant vitamins—benefits not yet proved. N Engl J Med 1994; 330:1080–1081.

16. The α-Tocopherol, β-Carotene Cancer Prevention Study Group. The effect of vitamin E and beta-carotene on the incidence of lung cancer and other cancers in male smokers. N Engl J Med 1994; 330:1029–1035.

17. Omenn G, Goodman G, Thongquist M, et al. Effects of a combination of β-carotene and vitamin A on lung cancer and cardiovascular disease. N Engl J Med 1996; 334:1150–1155.

18. Wang X-D, Tang G, Fox JG, Krinsky NI, Russell RM. Enzymatic conversion of β-carotene into β-apo-carotenals and retinoids by human, monkey, ferret, and rat tissues. Arch Biochem Biophys 1991; 258:8–16.

19. Olson JA, Hayaishi O. The enzymatic cleavage of β-carotene into vitamin A by soluble enzymes of rat liver and intestine. Proc Natl Acad Sci USA 1965; 54:1364–1370.

20. Goodman DS, Huang HS, Shiratori T. Mechanism of the biosynthesis of vitamin A from β-carotene. J Biol Chem 1966; 241:1929–1932.

21. Glover J, Redfearn ER. The mechanism of the transformation of β-carotene into vitamin A in vivo. Biochem J 1954; 58:15–16.

22. Krinsky NI, Wang X-D, Tang G, Russell R. Mechanism of carotenoid cleavage to retinoids. Carotenoids in human health. Ann NY Acad Sci 1993; 691:167–176.

23. Yeum K-J, Ferreira ALA, Smith D, Krinsky NI, Russell RM. The effect of α-tocopherol on the oxidative cleavage of β-carotene. Free Radic Biol Med 2000; 29(2):105–114.

24. von Lintig J, Vogt K. Filling the gap in vitamin A research. J Biol Chem 2000; 275(16):11915–11920.

25. Kiefer C, Hessel S, Lampert JM, Vogt K, Lederer MO, Breithaupt DE, von Lintig J. Identification and characterization of a mammalian enzyme catalyzing the asymmetric oxidative cleavage of provitamin A. J Biol Chem 2001; 276(17):14110–14116.

26. Hume EM, Krebs HA. Vitamin A requirement of human adults. An experimental study of vitamin A deprivation in man. Medical Research Council Special Report Series No. 264. London: His Majesty's Stationary Office, 1949.

27. Sauberlich HE, Hodges RE, Wallace DL, et al. Vitamin A metabolism and requirements in the human studied with the use of labeled retinol. Vitam Horm 1974; 32:251–275.

28. Bauernfeind JC. Carotenoid vitamin A precursors and analogs in foods and feeds. J Agric Food Chem 1972; 20(3):456–473.

29. Olson J. Recommended dietary intakes (RDI) of vitamin A in humans. Am J Clin Nutr 1987; 45:704–716.

30. Food and Agriculture Organization/World Health Organization. Requirement of vitamin A, thiamine, riboflavin, and niacin. Report of a joint Food and Agriculture Organization/World Health Organization Experts Committee. FAO Nutrition Meeting Report Series No. 41. WHO Technical Report Series No. 362. World Health Organization, Geneva, 1967.

31. National Research Council. Recommended Dietary Allowances, 9th revised ed. Report of the Committee on Dietary Allowance, Food and Nutrition Board, Division of Biological Sciences, Assembly of Life Sciences. National Academy of Sciences, Washington, DC, 1980.

32. Dietary reference intakes for vitamin A, vitamin K, arsenic, boron, chromium, copper, iodine, iron, manganese, molybdenum, nickel, silicon, vanadium, and zinc. A Report of the Panel on Micronutrients, Subcommittees on Upper Reference Levels of Nutrients and of Interpretation and Use of Dietary Reference Intakes, and the Standing Committee on the Scientific Evaluation of Dietary Reference Intakes. Food and Nutrition Board, Institute of Medicine, National Academy Press, Washington, DC, 2002.

33. de Pee S, West CE, Permaesih D, Martuti S, Muhila K, Hautvast G. Orange fruit is more effective than are dark-green, leafy vegetables in increasing serum concentrations of retinol and β-carotene in school children in Indonesia. Am J Clin Nutr 1998; 68:1058–1067.

34. Tang G, Gu X, Xu Q, Zhao X, Qin J, Fjeld C, Dolnikowski GG, Russell RM, Yin S. Green and yellow vegetables can maintain vitamin A nutrition of Chinese children. Am J Clin Nutr 1999; 70:1069–1076.

35. Furr HC, Amedee-Manesme O, Clifford AJ, Bergen HR, Jones AD, Anderson LD, Olson JA. Vitamin A concentrations in liver determined by isotope dilution assay with tetradeuterated vitamin A and by biopsy in generally healthy adult humans. Am J Clin Nutr 1989; 49:713–716.

36. Parker RS, Swanson JE, You C-S, Edwards AJ, Huang T. Bioavailability of carotenoids in human subjects. Proc Nutr Soc 1999; 58:1–8.

37. West CE, Castenmiller JJ. Quantification of the "SLAMENGHI" factors for carotenoid bioavailability and bioconversion. Int J Vitam Nutr Res 1998; 68(6):371–377.

38. Grusak M. Intrinsic stable isotope labeling of plants for nutritional investigations in humans. J Nutr Biochem 1997; 8:164–171.

39. McEvoy F, Lynn W. Chloroplast membrane proteins. II. Solubilization of the lipophilic components. J Biol Chem 1973; 248:4568–4573.

40. Goodwin T. The Biochemistry of the Carotenoids. London: Chapman and Hall, 1980.

41. Tang G, Qin J, Dolnikowski GG. Deuterium enrichment of retinol in humans determined by gas chromatography electron capture negative chemical ionization mass spectrometry. J Nutr Biochem 1998; 9:408–414.

42. Ye X, Al-Babili S, Kloti A, Zhang J, Lucca P, Beyer P, Potrykus I. Engineering the provitamin A (β-carotene) biosynthetic pathway into (carotenoid-free) rice endosperm. Science 2000; 287:303–305.

43. Jalal F, Nesheim MC, Agus Z, Sanjur D, JP H. Serum retinol concentrations in children are affected by food sources of β-carotene, fat intake, and anthelminthic drug treatment. Am J Clin Nutr 1998; 68(3):623–629.

44. Deming DM, Boileau AC, Lee CM, Erdman JW Jr. Amount of dietary fat and type of soluble fiber independently modulate postabsorptive conversion of β-carotene to vitamin A in mongolian gerbils. J Nutr 2000; 130:2789–2796.

45. Villard L, Bates C. Carotene dioxygenase [EC1.13.11.21] activity in rat intestine: effects of vitamin A deficiency and pregnancy. Br J Nutr 1986; 56:115–122.

46. Lala VR, Reddy V. Absorption of β-carotene from green leafy vegetables in under nourished children. Am J Clin Nutr 1970; 23:110–113.

47. Bulux J, de Serrano JQ, Perez R, Rivera C, Solomons NW. The plasma β-carotene response to a single meal of carrots in Guatemalan schoolchildren. Am J Clin Nutr 1998; 49:173–179.

48. Deming DM, Baker DH, Erdman JW Jr. The relative vitamin A value of 9-cis β-carotene is less and that of 13-cis β-carotene may be greater than the accepted 50% that of all-trans β-carotene in gerbils. J Nutr 2002; 132:2709–2712.

49. Tang G, Qin J, Dolnikowski GG, Russell RM. Vitamin A equivalence of β-carotene in a woman as determined by a stable isotope reference method. Eur J Nutr 2000; 39:7–11.

50. Tang G, Qin J, Dolnikowski, Russell RM. Short-term (intestinal) and long-term (post intestinal) conversion of β-carotene to retinol in adults using a stable isotope reference method. Am J Clin Nutr 2003; 78:259–266.

51. Parker BS, Swanson JE, Marmor B, Goodman KJ, Spielman AB, Brenna JT, Viereck SM, Canfield WK. Study of β-carotene metabolism in humans using ^{13}C-β-carotene and high precision isotope ratio mass spectrometry. Ann NY Acad Sci 1993; 691:86–95.

52. van Lieshout M, West CE, Muhilal, Permaesih D, Wang Y, Xu X, van Breemen RB, Creemers AFL, Verhoeven MA, Lugtenburg J. Bioefficacy of β-carotene dissolved in oil studied in children in Indonesia. Am J Clin Nutr 2001; 73:949–958.

53. Hickenbottom SJ, Lemke SL, Dueker SR, Lin Y, Follett JR, Carkeet C, Buchholz BA, Vogel JS, Clifford AJ. Dual isotope test for assessing β-carotene cleavage to vitamin A in humans. Eur J Nutr 2002; 41:141–147.

54. Kostic D, White WS, Olson JA. Intestinal absorption, serum clearance, and interactions between lutein and β-carotene when administered to human adults in separate or combined oral doses. Am J Clin Nutr 1995; 62:604–610.

55. Van den Berg H, van Vliet T. Effect of simultaneous, single oral doses of β-carotene with lutein or lycopene on the β-carotene and retinyl ester responses in the triacylglycerol-rich lipoprotein fraction of men. Am J Clin Nutr 1998; 68:82–89.

56. Parvin SG, Sivakumar B. Nutrition status affects intestinal carotene cleavage activity and carotene conversion to vitamin A in rats. J Nutr 2000; 130:573–577.

57. Castenmiller JJ, West CE, Linssen JP, Van het Hof KH, Voragen AG. The food matrix of spinach is a limiting factor in determining the bioavailability of β-carotene and to a lesser extent of lutein in humans. J Nutr 1999; 129:349–355.

58. Wang XD, Russell RM, Marini RP, Tang G, Dolnikowski GG, Fox GJ, Krinsky NI. Intestinal perfusion of β-carotene in the ferret raises retinoic acid level in portal blood. Biochim Biophys Acta 1993; 1167:159–194.

59. Hebuterne X, Wang XD, Smith DEH, Tang G, Russell RM. In vivo biosynthesis of retinoic acid from β-carotene involves an excentric cleavage pathway in ferret. J Lipid Res 1996; 37:482–492.

60. Wang X-D, Krinsky NI, Tang G, Russell RM. Retinoic acid can be produced from excentric cleavage of β-carotene in human intestinal mucosa. Arch Biochem Biophys 1992; 293(2):298–304.

61. Folman Y, Russell RM, Tang G, Wolf G. Rabbit fed β-carotene have higher serum levels of all-trans retinoic acid than those receiving no β-carotene. Br J Nutr 1989; 62:195–201.

62. Chambon P. A decade of molecular biology of retinoic acid receptors. FASEB J 1996; 10:940–954.

13
Bioconversion of Provitamin A Carotenoids

Arun B. Barua
Iowa State University, Ames, Iowa, U.S.A.

I. PROVITAMIN A CAROTENOIDS

Although the association of vitamin A potency with yellow color in foods was known in the early 1900s, the exact relationship between the yellow color and vitamin A was not known until Moore (1) demonstrated that the yellow-colored orally fed carotene was converted to colorless vitamin A in rats. Elucidation of the chemical structures of β-carotene and vitamin A by Karrer and his coworkers (2) confirmed the relationship.

There are more than 600 carotenoids in nature. However, less than 10% of them can serve as provitamin A. Preformed vitamin A is found in animals only and is derived exclusively from the provitamin A carotenoids, which in turn are not synthesized by animals. Therefore, provitamin A carotenoids are the major source of vitamin A for a large proportion of the world's population. Certainly, β-carotene is a potent provitamin A as well as the major provitamin A carotenoid in many vegetables and fruits consumed by humans. In general, any carotenoid with one unsubstituted β-ionone ring attached to a polyene chain containing at least five conjugated double bonds as shown in Figure 1 may serve as a provitamin A. Like the provitamin A carotenoids, several other carotenoids, i.e., lutein, zeaxanthin, and lycopene, are absorbed very well by humans from dietary fruits and vegetables but are not converted to vitamin A.

The source and biological activity of some of the provitamin A carotenoids are listed in Table 1. The chemical structures of the most common provitamin A carotenoids are shown in Figure 2.

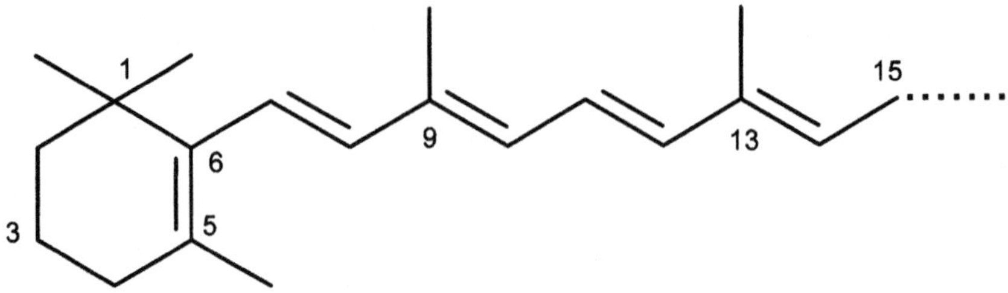

Figure 1   Structural requirement for any carotenoid to show vitamin A activity.

II. BIOAVAILABILITY OF CAROTENOIDS

After ingestion, carotenoids must be released from the food matrix and incorporated into mixed micelles before they can be absorbed and cleaved to vitamin A. Bioavailability is defined as the fraction of an ingested carotenoid that is available for normal physiological functions including storage (4). After a carotenoid becomes bioavailable, part or all of it is converted to vitamin A (bioconversion). The bioavailability and bioconversion of carotenoids are governed by many factors. The factors that may affect bioavailability have been discussed in excellent reviews (4–8). Various techniques, including isotopic tracer technique, can be used for studying the bioavailability and bioefficacy of dietary carotenoids. A review has appeared on the bioavailability of β-carotene in humans (9). The term SLAMENGHI (*s*pecies of carotenoids, molecular *l*inkage, *a*mount of carotenoids consumed in a meal, *m*atrix in which the carotenoid is incorporated, *e*ffectors of absorption and bioconversion, *n*utrient status of the host, *g*enetic factors, *h*ost-related factors, and mathematical *i*nteractions) was coined by Dee Pee and West (10) to describe the factors that can affect the bioavailability and bioconversion of carotenoids. These factors are briefly mentioned below.

A. Species of Carotenoids

Carotenoids can exist in many isomeric forms. The all-*trans* form is usually the most abundant and biologically active form. The all-trans form of β-carotene is the major isomer in circulation in humans. However, cis isomers of β-carotene are present in substantial amounts in processed foods and thus can be an important source of dietary β-carotene (11). The provitamin A activity is usually markedly reduced by isomerization to a cis form at one or more double bonds. The possible number of cis isomers of any carotenoid is very high, the theoretically possible number of cis isomers for β-carotene being 272. However, only 12 are observed out of the 20 unhindered isomers expected. The ease of

Table 1   Provitamin A Carotenoids

Name	Biological activity	Source
β-Apo-2'-carotenal	Active	Citrus fruit
β-Apo-8'-carotenal	36–72	Citrus fruit, green plants, alfalfa meal
β-Apo-10'-carotenal	76–78	Citrus fruit, green plants, alfalfa meal
β-Apo-12'-carotenal	44–72	Alfalfa meal
β-Apo-8'-carotenoic acid	78	Corn, animal tissue
β-Apo-10'-carotenoic acid	Active	Egg yolks
β-Apo-12'-carotenoic acid	Active	Egg yolks
β-Apo-8'-carotenoic acid ethyl ester	Active	—
β-Carotene	100	Green vegetables, carrots, sweet potatoes, squash, paprika, orange, cranberries, grapes, all colored fruits, yellow corn, eggs, milk, etc.
9-*cis*-β-Carotene	38	Processed foods
13-*cis*-β-Carotene	53	Processed foods
15-*cis*-β-Carotene	30–50	Processed foods, green vegetables
α-Carotene	50–54	Accompanies β-carotene (listed above), palm oil
9-*cis*-α-Carotene	13	—
9,13-Di-*cis*-α-carotene	16	—
γ-Carotene	42–50	Carrots, sweet potatoes, corn, tomatoes, some fruits (apricots, water melons), palm oil
β-Carotene 5',6'-monoepoxide	21	Plants, potatoes, red peppers, mangoes
α-Carotene 5,6-monoepoxide	25	Plants, flowers, bleached paprika
β-Carotene 5',8'-monofuranoxide (mutatochrome, citroxanthin)	50	Orange peel, red peppers, tomatoes, sweet potatoes, cranberries, bleached paprika
Citranaxanthin	44	Citrus fruits
β-Cryptoxanthin	50–60	Yellow corn, green peppers, persimmons, papayas, citrus fruits, prunes, apples, apricots, peaches, strawberries, cranberries, paprika, eggs, poultry

(*continued*)

Table 1 *Continued*

Name	Biological activity	Source
α-Cryptoxanthin	Active	Accompanies β-cryptoxanthin
Cryptoxanthin monoepoxide (3-hydroxy-β-carotene 5,6-monoepoxide)	Active	Potato, orange, prune, flowers
3,4-Dehydro-β-carotene	75	Microorganisms
2,2'-Dimethyl-β-carotene	Active	
5,6-Dihydroxy-β-carotene	Active	—
3,4-Diketo-β-carotene	Active	Algae
Echinenone/aphanin/myxoxanthin (4-keto-β-carotene)	44–54	Algae, sea urchins, brine shrimp, crustaceans
3-Keto-β-carotene	Active	Algae
3-Hydroxy-4-keto-β-carotene (hydroxyechinenone)	Active	Algae, bacteria, flowers
4-Hydroxy-β-carotene (isocryptoxanthin)	48	Brine shrimp
β-Semicarotenone	Active	—
Torularhodin	~50	Red yeast, plants, microorganisms, fungus
Torulene (3',4'-Dehydro-γ-carotene)	Active	Red yeast
β-Zeacarotene (7',8'-Dihydro-γ-carotene)	20–40	Corn, tomatoes, yeast, cherries

Source: Adapted from Refs. 1 and 3.

formation of cis–trans equilibrium mixtures under exposure to light, heat, and acids makes it difficult to determine the exact information of the isomers occurring in the native state. Very little is known about the bioavailability of the cis isomers. The effect of food processing and the interaction of carotenoids during the absorption process have been presented in Chapter 12. In general, β-carotene is more bioavailable than 9-*cis* or 13-*cis*-β-carotene (11). The most likely reasons for a cis isomer being less active than the trans isomer are reduced interaction with the cleavage enzyme due to the molecular arrangement or less bioavailability than the trans isomer.

B. Molecular Linkage

Although most carotenoids, hydrocarbon carotenoids in particular, occur unbound to other compounds in fruits and vegetables, hydroxycarotenoids can

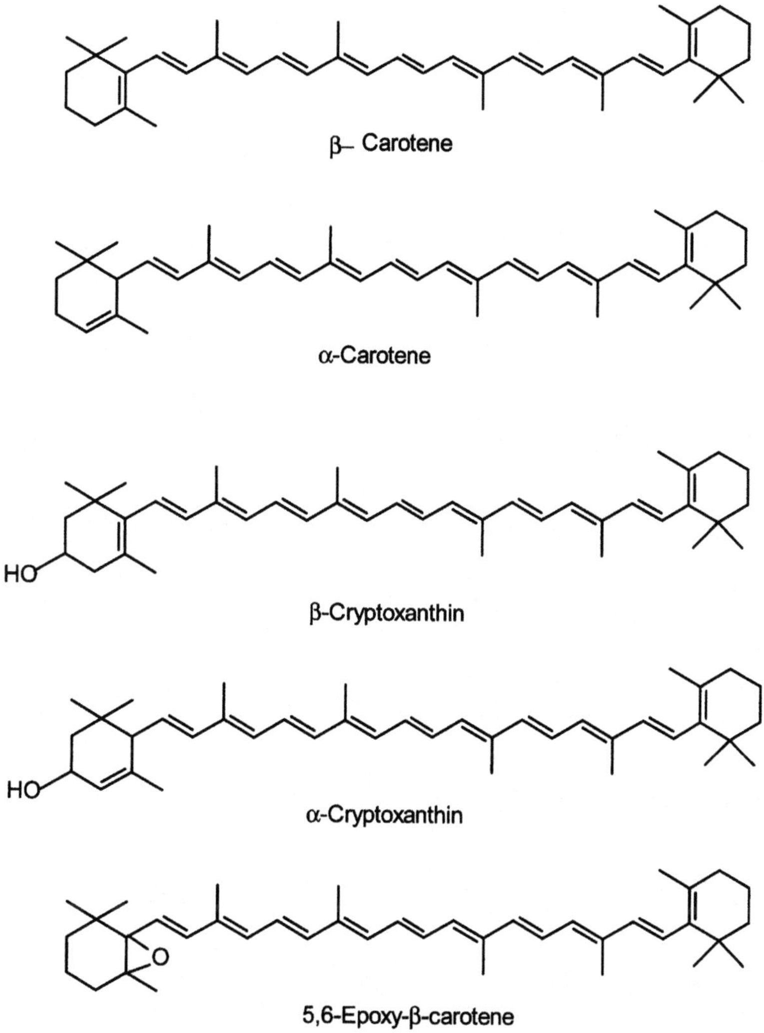

β– Carotene

α-Carotene

β-Cryptoxanthin

α-Cryptoxanthin

5,6-Epoxy-β-carotene

Figure 2 Chemical structures of some of the most common provitamin A carotenoids.

be present as esters bound to fatty acids. For example, cryptoxanthin, a monohydroxy provitamin A carotenoid, is usually present as esters in fruits and vegetables (3). In general, esters are not bioavailable and must be hydrolyzed to become bioavailable (12). The bioavailability can also depend on the amount of carotenoid present in the food. It is reported that β-carotene is more bioavailable when given several times in small doses than when given once as a large

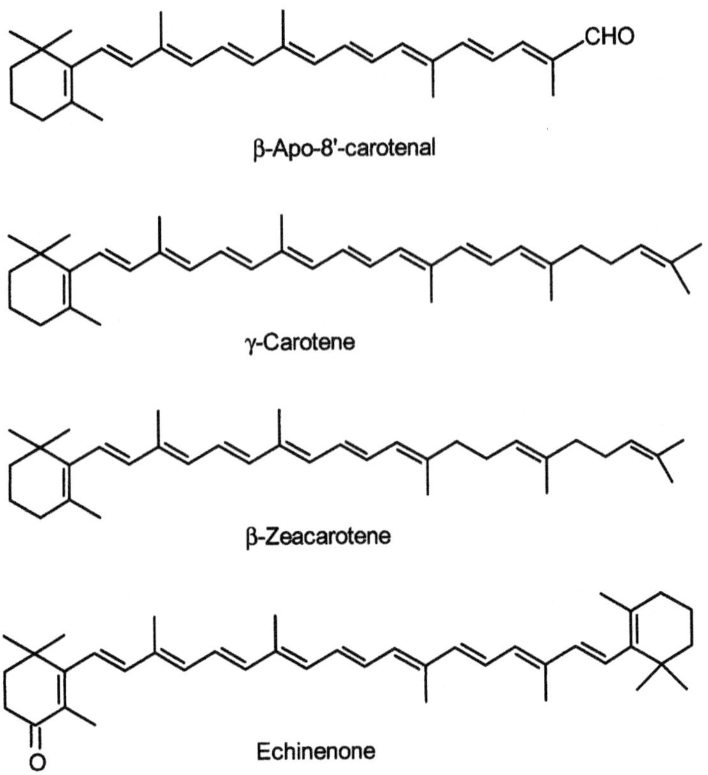

β-Apo-8'-carotenal

γ-Carotene

β-Zeacarotene

Echinenone

Figure 2 Continued.

dose (13). Bioavailability of the carotenes (hydrocarbon carotenoids) such as β-carotene and α-carotene is relatively lower than that of the carotenols (hydroxycarotenoids) such as lutein (14) and zeaxanthin. Xanthophylls and carotenes associate differently with micelles (12). This may be why the absorption of β-carotene from vegetables is much lower than that of lutein.

C. Matrix

Dietary carotenoids exist as true solutions in oil (as in red palm oil) or as parts of matrices within the vegetable or fruit. The matrix may be very complex and may not be fully disrupted during food preparation and during its passage through the intestine. Several investigators had shown that the absorption of β-carotene depends on the food matrix (15,16). The absorption of β-carotene from oil or aqueous dispersion is much higher than from vegetables. The bioavailability of

β-carotene from stir-fried vegetables, carrots, and spinach was found to be 7%, 18–26%, and 7%, respectively (4).

D. Effectors

The bioavailability of carotenoids can be effected by the presence of other nutrients. Moreover, carotenoids may interfere with each other's absorption (12). The presence of protein in the diet can stabilize fat emulsions and enhance micelle formation and carotenoid uptake (4). There can be an interaction of carotenoids with fat and fiber in the food. It has been shown that the presence of fat in the diet can enhance absorption (17). On the other hand, the presence of fiber such as pectin, guar, and alginate can reduce the absorption of carotenoids by as much as 43% (18,19). Gastric pH can have a role in the absorption of carotenoids (20).

E. Nutritional Status

The effect of nutritional status on the absorption of carotenoids is not clearly known (8), although studies had indicated that absorption might be affected by the amount of vitamin A present in the food or by the vitamin A status (4,21,22). It has been shown that a greater β-carotene cleavage activity was present in vitamin A-deficient rats, and a lower activity in protein-deficient rats (22).

F. Genetic Factors

The carotenoid levels in people of different races show different plasma carotenoid profiles (4). It is not clearly known whether such a difference is a genetic difference or due to the diet.

G. Host-Related Factors

Differences in sex and age may explain many of the differences observed in the serum response to ingestion of dietary carotenoids (4). Infection by malaria parasites (23) or intestinal parasites (24) can have an effect on absorption. Deworming before dosing with β-carotene resulted in increased serum retinol in children (24).

H. Mathematical Interactions

This refers to the difference in effect observed when two factors have a shared role compared with the product of the effects observed separately (4). No data are yet available for such an interaction.

I. Responders and Nonresponders

Following a dose of β-carotene, some human subjects respond with a marked increase in the β-carotene concentration in plasma. These subjects are considered as responders. However, some subjects, called nonresponders, show little or no increase in the plasma concentration of β-carotene. Although the cause of such difference is not known with certainty, it is possible that the absorbed carotene is rapidly converted to vitamin A, or that the absorption of β-carotene is extremely slow, or that absorbed β-carotene is cleared from plasma very rapidly (12,25).

III. SITE OF CONVERSION OF PROVITAMIN A CAROTENOIDS TO VITAMIN A

A. Small Intestine

Moore (1) found that vitamin A formed from orally fed carotene was deposited in the liver. This pointed the liver as the likely site of conversion of carotene to vitamin A. In vitro experiments using liver homogenates to study the conversion of β-carotene to vitamin A gave conflicting results (1). That the intestinal wall can be the site of conversion came almost by accident. Sexton et al. (26) found that when a single dose or repeated doses of β-carotene were administered by intraperitoneal or intravenous injection to vitamin A-deficient rats, the growth response and times of survival were much less than when the same doses were given orally. Surprisingly, the livers of the rats that died contained considerable amounts of β-carotene. If β-carotene was converted in the liver, why did the rats die? Sexton et al. (26) suggested that the site of conversion was probably not the liver but more likely the intestinal wall. Following this report, three groups of investigators almost simultaneously demonstrated that the small intestine was the site of conversion of carotenoids to vitamin A (27–29). Morton and his colleagues (30) demonstrated that retinal was also reduced to retinol in the small intestine. Retinol formed this way is immediately esterified to retinyl esters (31,32). Further support that the small intestine is the primary site of conversion of β-carotene to vitamin A was provided by Olson (33) who showed the formation of radioactive retinal, retinol, and other products by injecting ^{14}C-β-carotene in aqueous Tween intraperitoneally into the intestinal loop of rats.

B. Other Sites: Extraintestinal Cleavage

Following parenteral, intravenous, or intramuscular administration, the conversion of β-carotene to vitamin A was noted in animals whose intestines were removed prior to dosing (34,35). Bieri and Pollard (36) showed that the liver was the main site of conversion of β-carotene to vitamin A when β-carotene was administered by intravenous injection. The discrepancy between this finding and the Sexton et al. finding (26) cannot be explained. Treatment of β-carotene with liver homogenates resulted in the formation of retinal and retinol (31) demonstrating extraintestinal cleavage of β-carotene. The formation of retinoic acid and retinol by incubation of liver, lung, kidney, and testes homogenates has been reported (37). A study of the distribution of carotene 15,15'-dioxygenase activity on various rat organs showed that the intestine had the highest activity followed by liver, brain, lung, and kidney (38). These results are in accord with other reports that the conversion of carotene to vitamin A was much less by extraintestinal tissues than by small intestinal mucosa (1). Wang et al. (39) showed β-carotene cleavage activity in liver, kidney, and fat tissues of rats, ferrets, monkeys, and human adipose tissue as well. A recent study demonstrated that besides the small intestine, many other tissues express relatively high levels of the enzyme β,β-carotene 15,15'-dioxygenase, leading to the conclusion that an additional vitamin A supply can be achieved by tissue-specific cleavage of β-carotene (40). By performing reverse-phase polymerase chain reaction (RT-PCR), it has been demonstrated that the expression of carotene 15,15'-dioxygenase mRNA was highest in testes, followed by liver and kidney, and lowest in small intestine (41). In situ hybridization studies showed that the carotene cleavage enzyme was expressed in maternal tissue surrounding the rat embryo (41). Thus, it is now clear that the small intestine is the most common site of conversion of β-carotene to vitamin A, but the liver, testes, and many other tissues may serve as alternative sites.

IV. PATHWAYS OF CONVERSION

Two pathways, i.e., central cleavage and excentric cleavage, for the conversion of provitamin A carotenoids to vitamin A are known. The carotene molecule can undergo fission at the central 15,15' double bond by "central cleavage" to produce theoretically two molecules of vitamin A. Alternatively, the carotene molecule can undergo progressive fission from one end of the polyene chain by "excentric cleavage" to produce a number of β-apocarotenoids of different chain length, ultimately giving rise to one molecule of vitamin A.

A. Central Cleavage Mechanism

If β-carotene is cleaved by the central cleavage pathway, 2 mol of retinal should be formed from 1 mol of β-carotene (Fig. 3) whereas only 1 mol of retinal should be formed from 1 mol of α-carotene or γ-carotene. The finding that α-carotene and γ-carotene possess only half the biological activity of β-carotene supported the central cleavage pathway. However, many factors, such as the relatively slow

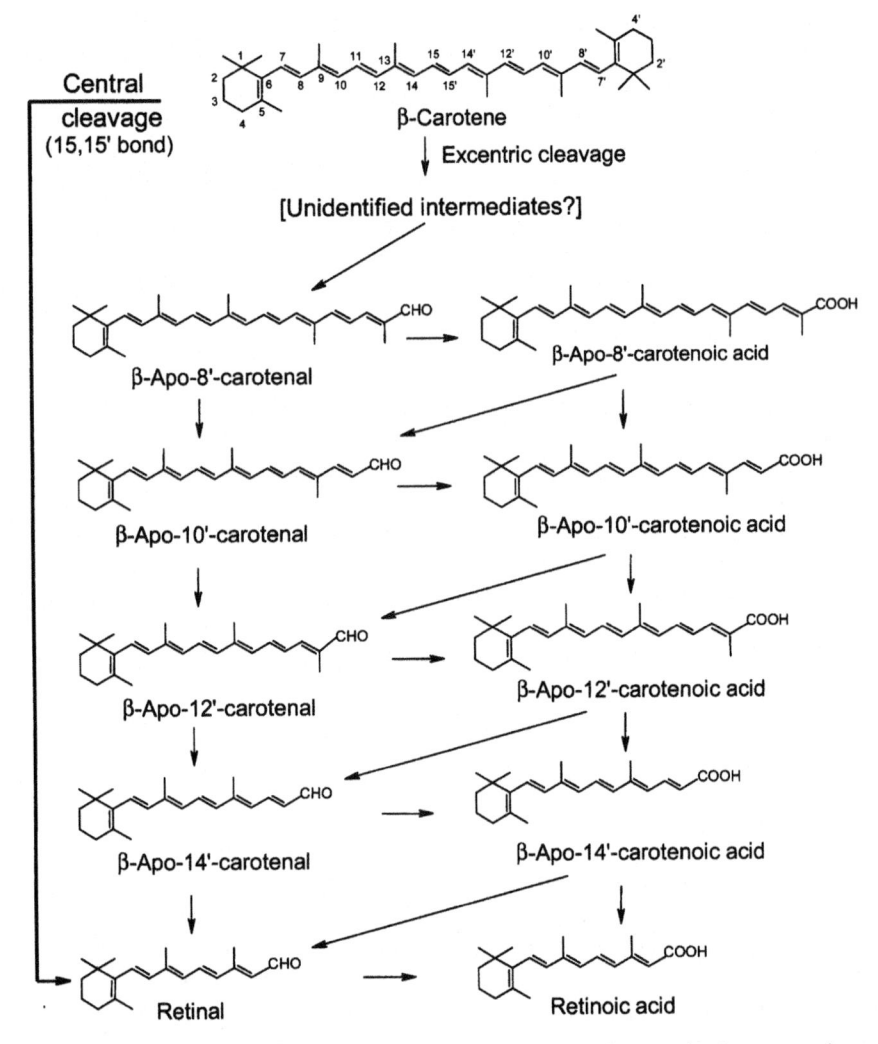

Figure 3 Central cleavage pathway (primary pathway) and excentric cleavage pathway involved in the conversion of provitamin A carotenoids to vitamin A.

conversion of carotene to vitamin A, rapid chemical oxidation of β-carotene during incubation studies, lack of resolving power of metabolites, and low sensitivity of detection, made it difficult to resolve the exact pathway of conversion of β-carotene to vitamin A (12).

The enzyme β,β-carotene 15,15′-dioxygenase (the details of which are discussed in Chapters 17 and 18) involved in the cleavage of β-carotene to vitamin A was first isolated in the mid-1960s (31,42,43). By use of this enzyme it was demonstrated that ^{14}C-β-carotene was cleaved solely to ^{14}C-retinal, pointing to central cleavage of β-carotene. These investigators found that the ratio of the moles of retinal formed to the moles of β-carotene consumed was 1.1–1.5. Any value greater than 1 would favor the central cleavage pathway, whereas any value lower than 1 would favor the excentric cleavage pathway. Support for the central cleavage pathway came from several other studies (44–52) where retinal was shown to be the only cleavage product of β-carotene. In one study, the formation of small amounts of retinol and retinoic acid in addition to retinal as the major product (87%) was reported (53). Using whole intestinal homogenates, Devery and Milborrow (54) found a molar ratio of 1.72 : 1 for retinal/β-carotene. Nagao et al. (50) used pig intestinal enzyme and found a molar ratio of 1.88 : 1 for retinal/β-carotene. After correction for efficiency of extraction, the value was raised to 2.07, a value the same as the theoretical value of 2 : 1 for retinal/β-carotene if cleavage occurs by the central cleavage pathway. The cleavage of many other provitamin A carotenoids, including α-carotene, β-apocarotenals, and 5,6- and 5,8-monoepoxides of β-carotene and of α-carotene, by 15,15'-dioxygenase to retinal has been reported (44,45,55,56). However, the rate of cleavage is considerably lower than that of β-carotene (56). The intestinal absorption of 5,6- and 5,8-monoepoxides of β-carotene in humans has been demonstrated (57).

In an in vivo study, a single oral dose of β-carotene in oil was given to rats of normal vitamin A status. Analysis of carotenoids and retinoids 1 and 3 h after the dose showed that only retinoids were detected as the primary cleavage products of β-carotene in the small intestinal mucosa, liver, kidney, and serum (58). Because only retinoids and no apocarotenoids were detected in the small intestinal mucosa, serum, and other tissues, it was concluded that β-carotene was converted primarily by the central cleavage pathway (58,59). In another in vivo study, ^{3}H-β-carotene was administered to rats of normal and marginal vitamin A status. Analysis of the entire gastrointestinal tract, liver, kidney, and other tissues of these rats showed the presence of ^{3}H-retinoids as the only cleavage products (60). No apocarotenoids or other radioactive metabolites were detected.

Goodman et al. (61) dosed lymph-cannulated rats with a mixture of uniformly labeled ^{14}C-β-carotene and β-carotene labeled at the central 15,15' double bond with tritium. They found that during cleavage of β-carotene the H atoms attached to the central carbon atoms were not lost. Vartapetyan et al. (62) showed that [18]O_2 from molecular oxygen, and not from water, was incorporated into the liver retinyl esters when vitamin A-deficient rats were fed β-carotene. A dioxygenase reaction mechanism and need for a cofactor containing iron was suggested for this conversion (43,45,63,64).

The successful cloning and sequencing of β-carotene 15,15'-dioxygenase activity from chicken, as well from *Drosophila melanogaster*, has been reported (65,66). Details about this enzyme are described in Chapter 17.

Recently, it has been demonstrated that the enzymatic cleavage of the central 15,15' double bond in β-carotene takes place by a monooxygenase-type mechanism. By use of a chicken intestinal β-carotene 15,15'-oxygenase preparation and isomerically pure α-carotene as substrate, it was shown that both $^{17}O_2$ and $H_2{}^{18}O$ were incorporated into the two retinal products (67). Therefore, the enzyme was renamed β-carotene 15,15'-monooxygenase. The isolation of the enzyme from several human tissues and its characterization has been reported (68). These workers also report the role of the enzyme in peripheral vitamin A synthesis from plasma-borne provitamin A carotenoids.

B. Excentric Cleavage Mechanism

An earlier finding that on a weight-by-weight basis β-carotene was half as active as vitamin A in promoting growth led investigators to hypothesize that the cleavage of β-carotene occurred by excentric cleavage. Glover (34) showed that β-carotene administered orally in arachis oil containing an appropriate amount of vitamin E for production of vitamin A was metabolized to small fragments that entered the metabolic pool. He was able to isolate small amounts of β-apo-12'-carotenal, β-apo-12'-carotenol, and β-apo-12'-carotenoic acid ester after feeding rats with ^{14}C-β-carotene. This implied oxidative attack at more than one position in the chain (Fig. 3). β-Apo-12'-carotenal showed excellent biological activity but resulted in a low yield of vitamin A (34). However, while favoring asymmetrical cleavage, Glover found that the amounts of radiolabeled carbon dioxide produced by the metabolism of ^{14}C-β-carotene and ^{14}C-retinol in rats were the same, indicating that asymmetrical cleavage was not a major pathway. Glover concluded that although terminal oxidation of β-carotene could yield vitamin A, β-oxidation of the larger fragment was not the method by which it was degraded to vitamin A. Sharma et al. (69) isolated 8'-, 10'-, and 12'-β-apocarotenals along with much larger amounts of retinal from the intestine of chickens fed β-carotene. The corresponding β-apocarotenoic acids were also isolated and identified. Based on these findings, a pathway of conversion of β-carotene to vitamin A similar to the one shown in Figure 3 was proposed (69,70). Although a distinction between central cleavage and excentric cleavage could not be made, it was shown that the β-apocarotenals could serve as substrates for an enzyme isolated from the intestines of guinea pigs and rabbits (44,45,55). Hansen and Maret (71) followed the procedure of Goodman and Olson (43) for the preparation of the carotene cleavage enzyme, but they failed to demonstrate the cleavage of β-carotene to retinal by incubation with this enzyme preparation. However, they showed that small amounts of β-apocarotenoids were formed chemically in presence of oxygen under normal incubation conditions even in the absence of the enzyme preparation. Wang et al. (39) incubated β-carotene with intestinal mucosal homogenates of human, monkey, ferret, and rat, and showed the formation of β-apo-12'-, β-apo-10'-, and β-apo-8'-carotenal, in addition to retinal and retinoic acid. In a subsequent paper, these investigators showed the formation of two additional products, β-apo-13-carotenone and β-apo-14'-carotenal, thereby demonstrating the sequential excentric cleavage of β-carotene (72). Because retinal was obtained as a relatively minor product in these studies, the investigators concluded that sequential asymmetrical cleavage was a major pathway for the conversion of β-carotene to vitamin A. In the presence of the retinal oxidase inhibitor citral, formation of retinoic acid as a product from both β-carotene and β-apo-8'-carotenal was demonstrated, thereby supporting cleavage of β-carotene by an excentric pathway and β-oxidation (39,73–75). Furthermore, it was shown that citral completely inhibited the conversion of added retinal to retinoic acid in human intestinal mucosa homogenates, without affecting the conversion of β-carotene to retinoic acid. It is possible that the reported very high growth-promoting activity of β-apo-12'-carotenal by Glover (34) was due to retinoic acid formed from β-apo-12'-carotenal by the β-oxidation pathway.

In an in vivo study, vitamin A-deficient rats were orally fed a single dose of β-carotene in oil, and when the small intestinal mucosa was analyzed 1 h after the dose, small amounts of several β-apocarotenals were present (58). However, mucosa of rats killed 3 h after the dose did not show any β-apocarotenals.

It has been reported that the pathway of conversion might depend on the presence or absence of antioxidants such as α-tocopherol (76). When α-tocopherol was present, retinal was the predominant cleavage product favoring the central cleavage pathway. On the other hand, when α-tocopherol was absent, both retinal and β-apocarotenals, indicative of excentric cleavage, were produced. A mammalian enzyme capable of cleaving the 9',10' double bond of β-carotene to produce β-apo-10'-carotenal has been described (77). Dmitrovskii et al. (78) reported the presence of an enzyme capable of cleaving β-apo-8'-carotenol to β-apo-14'-carotenal. When β-carotene was incubated with an intestinal postnuclear homogenate from cytochrome P450-induced rats, traces of 8'-, 10'-, and 12'-apocarotenals were identified (79).

These findings show that the conversion of provitamin A carotenoids to vitamin A can also take place by excentric cleavage mechanism.

C. Other Pathways

The breakdown of carotenoids by free radicals produced by enzymes such as lipoxygenase is known (8). The formation of random cleavage products of β-carotene by lipoxygenase in the presence of linoleic acid or by linoleic acid hydroperoxide has been reported (80). Oxidative cleavage of β-carotene by oxygen was induced by a ruthenium catalyst leading to the formation of several apocarotenals, indicating involvement of free radicals (81).

V. CONCLUSIONS

Carotenoids are not only colorful and attractive to the human eye, but are also beneficial to human health. From more than 600 carotenoids that occur in nature, only a few carotenoids can serve as the source of vitamin A, an essential micronutrient required for growth, development, vision, and immunity. The bioavailability and bioconversion of provitamin A carotenoids depend on a number of factors. Following absorption, provitamin A carotenoids are cleaved primarily by central cleavage of the 15,15′ double bond by an enzyme called carotene 15,15′-monooxygenase. The cleavage of provitamin A carotenoids by excentric cleavage of other double bonds to produce retinoids via β-apocarotenoids is also well documented. The major site of conversion of carotenoids to vitamin A is the small intestine, but the conversion may take place in the liver and many other tissues.

ACKNOWLEDGMENTS

The writing of this chapter, as well as some of the studies on which it was based, was supported by grants from USDA-NRICGP 00-035200-9074 and NIH-DK 39733. Twenty years of fruitful association with the late James Allen Olson in pursuing research in carotenoids and vitamin A is gratefully acknowledged.

REFERENCES

1. Moore T. Vitamin A. Amsterdam: Elsevier, 1957.
2. Karrer P, Jucker E. Carotenoids. Amsterdam: Elsevier, 1950.
3. Bauernfeind JC, Adams CR, Marusich WL. Carotenes and other vitamin A precursors in animal feed. In: Bauernfeind JC, ed. Carotenoids as Colorants and Vitamin A Precursors. New York: Academic Press, 1981:563–743.
4. Castenmiller JJ, West CE. Bioavailability and bioconversion of carotenoids. Annu Rev Nutr 1998; 18:19–38.
5. Erdman JW Jr, Bierer TL, Gugger ET. Absorption and transport of carotenoids. Ann N Y Acad Sci 1993; 691:76–85.
6. Parker RS, Swanson JE, You CS, Edwards AJ, Huang T. Bioavailability of carotenoids in human subjects. Proc Nutr Soc 1999; 58:155–162.
7. van Vliet T. Absorption of β-carotene and other carotenoids in humans and animal models. Eur J Clin Nutr 1996; 50(Suppl 3):S32–S37.
8. Yeum K, Russell RM. Carotenoid bioavailability and bioconversion. Annu Rev Nutr 2002; 22:483–504.
9. van Lieshout M, West CE, van Breemen, RB. Isotopic tracer technique for studying the bioavailability and bioefficacy of dietary carotenoids, particularly β-carotene, in humans: a review. Am J Clin Nutr 2003; 77:12–28.

10. De Pee S, West CE. Dietary carotenoids and their role in combating vitamin A deficiency: a review of the literature. Eur J Clin Nutr 1996; 50(Suppl 3):S38–S53.
11. Deming DM, Teixeira SR, Erdman JW Jr. All-trans β-carotene appears to be more bioavailable than 9-cis or 13-cis β-carotene in gerbils given single doses of each isomer. J Nutr 2002; 132:2700–2708.
12. Olson JA. Carotenoids. In: Shils ME, Olson JA, Shike M, Ross AC. ed. Modern Nutrition in Health and Disease. Baltimore: Williams & Wilkins, 1999:525–541.
13. Prince MR, Frisoli JK. β-Carotene accumulation in serum and skin. Am J Clin Nutr 1993; 175–181.
14. Kostic D, White WS, Olson JA. Intestinal absorption, serum clearance, and interactions between lutein and β-carotene when administered to human adults in separate or combined oral doses. Am J Clin Nutr 1995; 62:604–610.
15. Castenmiller JJ, West CE, Linssen JP, van het Hof KH, Voragen AG. The food matrix of spinach is a limiting factor in determining the bioavailability of β-carotene and to a lesser extent of lutein in humans. J Nutr 1999; 129:349–355.
16. van het Hof KH, Tijburg LB, Pietrzik K, Weststrate JA. Influence of feeding different vegetables on plasma levels of carotenoids, folate and vitamin C. Effect of disruption of the vegetable matrix. Br J Nutr 1999; 82:203–212.
17. Dimitrov NV, Meyer C, Ullrey DE, Chenoweth W, Michaelakis A, Malone W, Boone C, Fink G. Bioavailability of β-carotene in humans. Am J Clin Nutr 1988; 48:298–304.
18. Rock CL, Swendseid ME. Plasma β-carotene response in humans after meals supplemented with dietary pectin. Am J Clin Nutr 1992; 55:96–99.
19. Riedl J, Linseisen J, Hoffmann J, Wolfram G. Some dietary fibers reduce the absorption of carotenoids in women. J Nutr 1999; 129:2170–2176.
20. Tang G, Serfaty-Lacrosniere C, Camilo ME, Russell RM. Gastric acidity influences the blood response to a β-carotene dose in humans. Am J Clin Nutr 1996; 64:622–626.
21. van Vliet T, Fentener van Vlissingen M, van Schaik F, van den Berg H. β-Carotene absorption and cleavage in rats is affected by the vitamin A concentration of the diet. J Nutr 1996; 126:499–508.
22. Parvin SG, Sivakumar B. Nutritional status affects intestinal carotene cleavage activity and carotene conversion to vitamin A in rats. J Nutr 2000; 130:573–577.
23. Das BS, Thurnham DI, Das DB. Plasma α-tocopherol, retinol and carotenoids in children with falciparum malaria. Am J Clin Nutr 1996; 64:94–100.
24. Dee Pee S, West CE, Muhilal, Karyadi D, Hautvast JGAJ. Lack of improvement in vitamin A status with increased consumption of dark-green leafy vegetables. Lancet 1995; 346:75–81.
25. Furr HC, Clark RM. Intestinal absorption and tissue distribution of carotenoids. J Nutr Biochem 1997; 8:364–377.
26. Sexton EL, Mehl JW, Deuel HJ Jr. Studies on carotenoid metabolism. VI. The relative provitamin A activity of carotene when introduced orally and parenterally in the rat. J Nutr 1946; 31:299–320.
27. Mattson FH, Mehl JW, Deuel HJ Jr. Studies on carotenoid metabolism. VII. The site of conversion of carotene to vitamin A in the rat. Arch Biochem 1947; 15:65–73.

28. Glover J, Goodwin TW, Morton RA. Studies in vitamin A. VIII. Conversion of
     β-carotene to vitamin A in the intestine of the rat. Biochem J 1948; 43:512–518.
29. Thompson SY, Ganguly J, Kon SK. The conversion of β-carotene to vitamin A in the
     intestine. Br J Nutr 1949; 3:50–78.
30. Glover J, Goodwin TW, Morton RA. Studies in vitamin A. IV. Conversion in vivo of
     vitamin A aldehyde (retinene$_1$). Biochem J 1948; 43:109–112.
31. Olson JA, Hayaishi O. The enzymatic cleavage of β-carotene into vitamin A by soluble
     enzymes of rat liver and intestine. Proc Natl Acad Sci U S A 1965: 54:1364–1370.
32. Blomhoff R, Green MH, Norum RR. Vitamin A: physiological and biochemical
     processing. Annu Rev Nutr 1992; 12:37–57.
33. Olson JA. The conversion of radioactive β-carotene into vitamin A by the rat
     intestine in vivo. J Biol Chem 1961; 236:349–356.
34. Glover J. The conversion of β-carotene to vitamin A. In: Harris RS, Ingle DJ, eds.
     Vitamins and Hormones. Vol. 18. New York: Academic Press, 1960:371–386.
35. Ganguly J, Sastry PS. Mechanism of conversion of β-carotene into vitamin A:
     central cleavage versus random cleavage. Wld Rev Nutr Diet. 1985; 45:198–220.
36. Bieri JG, Pollard CJ. Studies on the site of conversion of β-carotene injected
     intravenously into rats. Br J Nutr 1954; 8:32–35.
37. Napoli JL, Race KR. Biogenesis of retinoic acid from β-carotene. Differences between
     the metabolism of β-carotene and retinal. J Biol Chem 1988; 263:17372–17377.
38. During A, Nagao A, Hoshino C, Terao J. Assay of β-carotene 15,15′-dioxygenase
     activity by reverse-phase high pressure liquid chromatography. Anal Biochem 1996;
     241:199–205.
39. Wang X, Tang G, Fox JG, Krinsky NI, Russell, RM. Enzymatic conversion of
     β-carotene into β-apo-carotenals and retinoids by human, monkey, ferret, and rat
     tissues. Arch Biochem Biophys 1991; 285:8–16.
40. Wyss A, Wirtz GM, Woggon W, Brugger R, Wyss M, Friedlein A, Riss G,
     Bachmann H, Hunziker W. Expression pattern and localization of β,β-carotene
     15,15′-dioxygenase in different tissues. Biochem J 2001; 354:521–529.
41. Paik J, During A, Harrison EH, Mendelsohn CL, Lai K, Blaner WS. Expression and
     characterization of a murine enzyme able to cleave β-carotene. J Biol Chem 2001;
     276:32160–32168.
42. Goodman DS, Huang HS. Biosynthesis of vitamin A with rat intestinal enzymes.
     Science 1965; 149:879–880.
43. Goodman DS, Olson JA. The conversion of all-trans β-carotene to retinal. Meth
     Enzymol 1969; 15:462–475.
44. Lakshmanan MR, Pope JL, Olson JA. The specificity of a partially purified
     carotenoid cleavage enzyme of rabbit intestine. Biochem Biophys Acta 1968;
     33:347–352.
45. Lakshmanan MR, Chansang H, Olson JA. Purification and properties of carotene
     15,15′-dioxygenase of rabbit intestine. J Lipid Res 1972; 13:477–482.
46. Lakshman MR, Mychkovsky I, Attlesey M. Enzymatic conversion of all-trans
     β-carotene by cytosolic enzyme from rabbit and rat intestinal mucosa. Proc Natl
     Acad Sci U S A 1989; 86:9124–9128.

47. van Vliet T, Schaik FV, Berg HVD, Schreurs WHP. Effect of vitamin A and β-carotene intake on dioxygenase activity in rat intestine. Ann N Y Acad Sci 1993; 691:220–222.
48. Nagao A, Olson JA. Enzymatic formation of 9-cis, 13-cis, and all-trans retinals from isomers of β-carotene. FASEB J 1994; 8:968–973.
49. Lakshman MR, Okoh C. Enzymatic conversion of all-trans β-carotene to retinal. Meth Enzymol 1993; 214:256–269.
50. Nagao A, During A, Hoshino C, Terao J, Olson JA. Stoichiometric conversion of all-trans β-carotene to retinal by pig intestinal extract. Arch Biochem Biophys 1996; 328:57–63.
51. During A, Nagao A, Hoshino C, Terao J. Assay of β-carotene 15,15′-dioxygenase activity by reverse-phase high pressure liquid chromatography. Anal Biochem 1996; 241:199–205.
52. Duszka C, Groiler P, Azim EM, Alexandre-Gouabau MC, Borel P, Azais-Braesco V. Rat intestinal β-carotene dioxygenase activity is located primarily in the cytosol of mature jejunal enterocytes. J Nutr 1996; 126:2550–2556.
53. Crain FD, Lotspeich FJ, Krause RF. Biosynthesis of retinoic acid by intestinal enzyme of the rat. J Lipid Res 1967; 8:249–254.
54. Devery J, Milborrow BV. β-Carotene-15,15′-dioxygenase (EC 1.13.11.21) isolation reaction mechanism and an improved assay procedure. Br J Nutr 1994; 72:397–414.
55. Singh H, Cama HR. Enzymatic cleavage of carotenoids. Biochim Biophys Acta. 1974; 370:49–61.
56. Olson JA. Formation and function of vitamin A. In: Porter JW, Spurgeon DL, eds. Biosynthesis of Isoprenoid Compounds. New York: John Wiley and Sons, 1983:371–412.
57. Barua A. Intestinal absorption of epoxy-β-carotenes by humans. Biochem J 1999; 339:359–362.
58. Barua AB, Olson JA. β-Carotene is converted primarily to retinoids in rats in vivo. J Nutr 2000; 130:1996–2001.
59. Wolf G. The enzymatic cleavage of β-carotene: end of a controversy. Nutr Rev 2001; 59:116–118.
60. Goswami BC, Ivanoff K, Barua AB. Absorption and conversion of 11,12-^{3}H-β-carotene to vitamin A in Sprague–Dawley rats of different vitamin A status. J Nutr 2003; 133:148–153.
61. Goodman DS, Huang HS, Shiratori T. Mechanism of the biosynthesis of vitamin A from β-carotene. J Biol Chem 1966; 241:1929–1932.
62. Vartapetyan BB, Dmitrovskii AA, Alkhazov DG, Lemberg IK, Girshin AB, Gusinskii GM, Starikova NA, Erofeeva NN, Bogdanova IP. A new approach to the study of the mechanism of biosynthesis of vitamin A from carotene by activation of oxygen O^{18} as a result of nuclear reaction O^{18} (α,nγ) Ne^{21} by means of α-particles accelerated in a cyclotron. Biokhimia 1966; 31:881–886.
63. Goodman DS, Blomstrand R, Werner B, Huang HS, Shiratori T. The intestinal absorption and metabolism of vitamin A and β-carotene in man. J Clin Invest 1966; 45:1615–1623.
64. Fidge NH, Goodman DS. Vitamin A and carotenoids. The enzymic conversion of β-carotene into retinal in hog intestinal mucosa. Biochem J 1969; 114:689–694.

65. Von Lintig J, Vogt K. Filling the gap in vitamin A research: molecular identification of an enzyme cleaving β-carotene to retinal. J Biol Chem 2000; 275:11915–11920.

66. Wyss A, Wirtz G, Woggon W, Brugger R, Wyss M, Friedlein A, Bachmann H, Hunziker W. Cloning and expression of β,β-carotene 15,15′-dioxygenase. Biochem Biophy Res Commun 2000; 271:334–336.

67. Leuenberger MG, Engeloch-Jarret C, Woggon W. The reaction mechanism of the enzyme-catalyzed central cleavage of beta-carotene to retinal. Angew Chem Int Ed Engl 2001; 40:2614–2617.

68. Lindqvist A, Andersson S. Biochemical properties of purified recombinant human β-carotene 15,15′-monooxygenase. J Biol Chem 2002; 277:23942–23948.

69. Sharma RV, Mathur SN, Dimitrovskii AA, Das RC, Ganguly J. Studies on the metabolism of β-carotene and apo-β-carotenoids in rats and chickens. Biochim Biophys Acta 1977; 486:183–194.

70. Ganguly J, Sastry PS. Mechanism of conversion of β-carotene into vitamin A: central cleavage versus random cleavage. Wld Rev Nutr Diet 1985; 45:198–220.

71. Hansen S, Maret W. Retinal is not formed in vitro by enzymatic central cleavage of β-carotene. Biochemistry 1988; 27:200–206.

72. Tang G, Wang X, Krinsky NI, Russell RM. Characterization of β-apo-13-carotenone and β-apo-14′-carotenal as enzymatic products of the excentric cleavage of β-carotene. Biochemistry 1991; 30:9829–9834.

73. Wang X, Russell RM, Liu C, Stickel F, Smith DE, Krinsky NL. β-Oxidation in rabbit liver in vitro and in the perfused ferret liver contributes to retinoic acid biosynthesis from β-apocarotenoic acid. J Biol Chem 1996; 271:26490–26498.

74. Krinsky, NI, Wang X, Tang G, Russell RT. Mechanism of carotenoid cleavage to retinoids. Ann NY Acad Sci 1993; 691:167–176.

75. Wang X, Krinsky NI, Tang G, Russell RM. Retinoic acid can be produced from excentric cleavage of β-carotene in human intestinal mucosa. Arch Biochem Biophys 1992; 293:293–304.

76. Yeum KJ, dos Anjos Ferreira AL, Smith D, Krinsky NI, Russell RM. The effect of α-tocopherol on the oxidative cleavage of β-carotene. Free Radic Biol Med 2000; 29:105–114.

77. Keifer C, Hessel S, Lampert JM, Vogt K, Lederer MO, Breithaupt DE, von Lintig J. Identification and characterization of a mammalian enzyme catalyzing the assymetric oxidative cleavage of provitamin A. J Biol Chem 2001; 276:14110–14116.

78. Dmitrovskii AA, Gessler NN, Gomboeva SB, Ershov Yu V, Bykhovsky V. Enzymatic oxidation of β-apo-8′-carotenol to β-apo-14′-carotenal by an enzyme different from β-carotene 15,15′-dioxygenase. Biochemistry (Moscow) 1997; 62:787–792.

79. Bachmann H, Desbarats A, Pattison P, Sedgewick M, Riss G, Wyss A, Cardinault N, Duszka C, Goralczyk R, Groiler P. feedback regulation of β,β-carotene 15,15′-monooxygenase by retinoic acid in rats and chickens. J Nutr 2002; 132:3616–3622.

80. Yeum KJ, Lee-Kim YC, Yoon S, Lee KY, Park IS, Lee LS, Kim BS, Tang G, Russell RM, Krinsky NI. Similar metabolites formed from carotene by human gastric mucosal homogenates, lipoxygenase, or linoleic acid hydroperoxide. Arch Biochem Biophys 1995; 321:167–174.

81. Caris-Veyrat C, Amiot M-J, Ramasseul R, Marchon J-C. Mild oxidative cleavage of β,β-carotene by dioxygen induced by a ruthenium porphyrin catalyst: characterization of products and some possible intermediates. N J Chem 2001; 25:203–206.

14

Carotenoid Oxidative/Degradative Products and Their Biological Activities

Xiang-Dong Wang
Tufts University, Boston, Massachusetts, U.S.A.

I. INTRODUCTION

Carotenoids are a large family of plant pigments that may have specific biological activities in humans. More than 600 carotenoids have been isolated from nature. Substantial research has been done regarding the biological functions and metabolism of carotenoids, particularly for the major carotenoids (β-carotene, α-carotene, lycopene, cryptoxanthin, lutein, and zeaxanthin) found in human plasma and tissues. These carotenoids are important food components and there exists strong epidemiological evidence for their health benefits in terms of prevention of chronic diseases (e.g., cancer, cardiovascular disease, and age-related macular degeneration). The information on retinoid activity as the most important function of provitamin A carotenoids continues to accumulate. Other functions of carotenoids have also been defined, including antioxidant capabilities, enhancement of cellular gap junction communication, modulation of the immune system, inhibition of growth factor-induced cell proliferation, induction of apoptosis, and blocking of neoplastic transformation of normal cells. Several excellent chapters in this book will discuss these functions of carotenoids in detail.

There remains a remarkable discordance between the results of the observational epidemiological studies and the intervention trials using β-carotene as a potential chemopreventive agent (1). Clinical intervention trials conducted to determine the effect of β-carotene supplementation on the incidence of lung cancer in smokers found either no protective effect or a negative effect (2–7). However, supporting evidence for a protective role of fruits and vegetables rich in carotenoids in cancer prevention continues to be reported in human epidemiological studies (8–10) and intervention studies (11,12). A number of animal and laboratory studies have also shown that carotenoids can block certain carcinogenic processes and inhibit specific tumor cell growth (13–16). Recent in vivo and in vitro studies have provided useful information on the controversy regarding the chemopreventive versus the carcinogenic activity of carotenoids. One of the important aspects is that humans can absorb and accumulate significant amount of carotenoids in the tissues and these carotenoids can undergo extensive oxidation into various carotenoid metabolites. Therefore, both the beneficial and adverse effects of carotenoids may be due to their metabolites or decomposition products (Fig. 1). Understanding the molecular details behind the actions of these oxidative products may yield insights into both physiological and pathophysiological processes in human health and disease.

II. METABOLIC PRODUCTS OF CAROTENOIDS

The carotenoids are a class of lipophilic compounds with a polyisoprenoid structure. Most carotenoids contain a series of conjugated double bonds in the

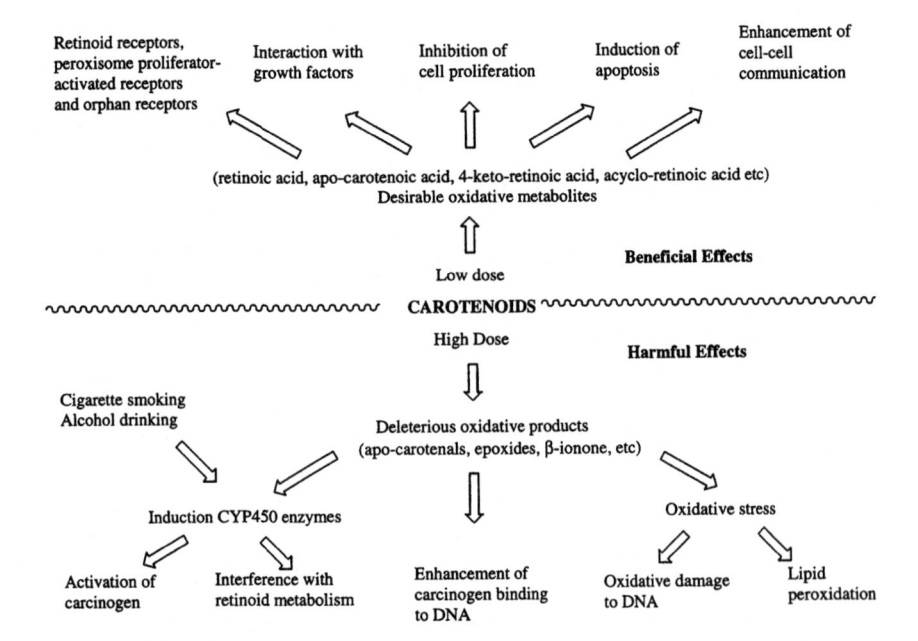

Figure 1 Simplified schematic illustration of possible mechanism(s) of carotenoids and their oxidative metabolites on their beneficial and detrimental effects to human health.

middle chain of the molecule, which are sensitive to oxidative modification and cis–trans isomerization. There are six major carotenoids (β-carotene, α-carotene, lycopene, cryptoxanthin, lutein, and zeaxanthin) that can be found routinely in human plasma and tissues. Among them, the most extensively studied is β-carotene, the most active precursor of vitamin A. β-Carotene is a symmetrical molecule with nine conjugated double bonds in its polyene chain (Fig. 2). Central cleavage of this molecule is a major pathway leading to vitamin A formation (17,18). This pathway has been substantiated by the cloning of the central cleavage enzyme, β-carotene 15,15'-dioxygenase, by two independent research groups using different species (19,20). Recent studies have further classified this enzyme as a nonheme iron monooxygenase (21,22). Retinal formed from β-carotene can be subsequently reduced to retinol or oxidized further to form retinoic acid (Fig. 2). Two excellent chapters in this book will discuss this topic in detail. An alternative pathway for carotenoid metabolism, the excentric cleavage pathway (or random cleavage) in mammals, has been a subject of controversy among scientists for several decades (18). One mechanism describing this excentric cleavage pathway, proposed by Glover in 1960 (23), suggests that oxidative cleavage of β-carotene starts at either end of chain with equal probability; the oxidative breakdown continues with removal of two-carbon units until the further oxidation is blocked by the methyl group at the C-13 position, which is at the β position with respect to the central carbon atom of β-carotene. Thus, β-carotene can yield one molecule of retinal via a series of β-apocarotenals of different chain lengths. This hypothesis was partially supported by Ganguly and coworkers in 1976 (24,25). They isolated significant amounts of β-apo-8'-, 10'-, and 12'-carotenal from the intestines of chickens given dietary β-carotene

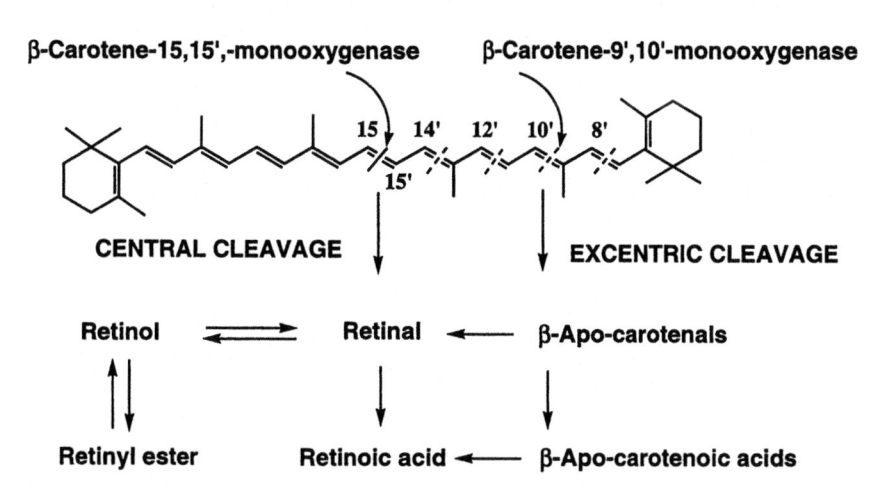

Figure 2 Metabolic pathway of β-carotene.

and suggested that excentric cleavage may have a role in β-carotene metabolism. Later in 1991, we provided evidence for a random cleavage of the β-carotene molecule and demonstrated that a series of homologous carbonyl cleavage products are produced, including retinal, retinoic acid, β-apo-14′-, 12′-, 10′-, and 8′-carotenals and β-apo-13-carotenone from β-carotene in tissue homogenates of humans, ferrets, and rats (26,27). Furthermore, we have isolated β-apo-12′-carotenal and β-apo-10′-carotenal as well as retinoids from ferret intestinal mucosa after perfusion of β-carotene in vivo (28,29). The production of β-apo-carotenals from β-carotene in rat intestinal mucosal homogenates continued for 60 min, whereas the appearance of retinal and retinoic acid was delayed, suggesting that β-apocarotenals may be intermediate compounds in the production of retinoids from β-carotene. Indeed, the perfusion of β-apo-14′-carotenal in ferrets increased the formation of apocarotenoic acid, retinoic acid, and retinol in vivo (30). We found that β-carotene, retinyl esters, retinol, and the less polar metabolites are absorbed into the lymph, whereas the more polar metabolites, including β-apo-carotenals, retinoyl-β-glucuronide, retinyl-β-glucuronide, and retinoic acid, are absorbed directly into the portal blood (31). These data indicate that the portal vein plays a role in β-carotene metabolism and that the differential absorption of β-carotene and its metabolites into lymph or portal blood is dependent on the polarity of the metabolites involved. However, the existence of the excentric cleavage pathway for β-carotene was not confirmed until a recent publication on the molecular identification of β-carotene 9′,10′-monooxygenase, which catalyzes the excentric cleavage of β-carotene at the 9′,10′ double bond, forming β-apo-10′-carotenal in humans and mice (32). Using the reported cDNA sequence for a carotene excentric cleavage enzyme from humans (NM031938), we have cloned a full-length carotene 9′,10′-monooxygenase in ferrets that encodes a protein of 540 amino acid and has 82% identity with human carotene 9′,10′-monooxygenase (33). This enzyme is expressed in the testis, liver, lung, prostate, intestine, stomach, and kidney of ferrets. Further investigation regarding the function and regulation of carotene 9′,10′-monooxygenase is needed.

In 1988, Napoli and Race (34) demonstrated that retinoic acid can be produced from β-carotene without formation of retinal as an intermediate compound. To ascertain if the production of retinoic acid occurred via the central cleavage pathway, involving direct oxidation of retinal to retinoic acid, or via the excentric pathway, involving oxidation of β-apocarotenals to retinoic acid, we used the inhibitor citral, which blocks the oxidation of retinal in human intestinal mucosa, in a set of experiments (30,35). We demonstrated that retinoic acid and β-apocarotenals were formed from the incubation of intestinal homogenate with β-carotene in both the presence and absence of citral. This proves that an excentric cleavage mechanism is involved in biosynthesis of retinoic acid from β-carotene, in addition to a central cleavage mechanism. Wang et al. (36)

demonstrated that the β-apocarotenals could be oxidized to the corresponding β-apocarotenoic acids, which are further oxidized through a process analogous to β oxidation to yield retinoic acid (Fig. 2). It is interesting that, similar to the small intestine, peripheral tissues (such as the lung, kidney, liver, and fat) of ferrets, rats, monkeys, and humans can also convert β-carotene to retinoic acid (26,34). The plasma concentration of retinoic acid increased after oral feeding of β-carotene in the rabbit (37) or after perfusion of β-carotene in ferrets (38). Thus, it is possible that increased dietary β-carotene or other provitamin A carotenoids may affect the steady-state concentration of retinoic acid in body fluids or tissues. The rapid metabolic clearance of retinoic acid from body fluids and tissue may increase the significance of local tissue conversion. A pathway similar to that of β-carotene may be involved in metabolism of other provitamin A carotenoids, such as α-carotene and cryptoxanthin, although this needs more investigation.

Lycopene has attracted attention due to its biological and physiochemical properties, especially related to its effects as the strongest antioxidant among the carotenoids. Lutein and zeaxanthin have an important role in protection against age-related macular degeneration. However, the metabolism of these carotenoids remains poorly understood. Relative to β-carotene, lycopene has the same molecular mass and chemical formula, but it has an open carbon-polyene chain without the β-ionone rings. Khachik et al. identified 5,6-dihydroxy-5,6-dihydrolycopene and epimeric 2,6-cyclolycopene-1,5-diols in human serum as two oxidative products of lycopene (39,40). Recently, using ferret as a model to mimic human carotenoid metabolism, we found that smoke exposure decreased plasma and lung lycopene concentrations in lycopene supplemented ferrets (41). Lycopene concentrations decreased by approximately 40% in plasma for both low-dose and high-dose lycopene-supplemented groups and 90% in lung tissue for both the low-dose and high-dose lycopene groups. Furthermore, we demonstrated that while all-*trans* lycopene is the predominant isomer in plasma and lung tissues of ferrets supplemented with lycopene (followed by 13-*cis*-lycopene and 9-*cis*-lycopene), smoke exposure appears to increase the cis isomers and decrease the trans isomers of lycopene in the lungs of ferrets. Very recently, we observed that the expression of ferret lung carotene 9′,10′-monooxygenase, which catalyzes the excentric cleavage of lycopene at the 9′,10′ double bond forming apo-10′-lycopenoids, was up-regulated by smoke exposure (33). The significance of this isomerization and formation of oxidative metabolites of lycopene is unclear and warrants further investigation. It has been shown that acycloretinoic acid is one autoxidation product of lycopene in toluene (42). Acycloretinoic acid inhibited the growth of HL-60 human promyelocytic leukemia cells (43) and human mammary cancer cells (44). However, it is not clear whether acycloretinoic acid can be produced from lycopene metabolism in cells and mammalian tissues. Similar concentrations of acycloretinoic acid and of lycopene are required for the inhibition of cell growth, which indicates that acycloretinoic acid may not be the active metabolite of lycopene (44). The non-provitamin A carotenoid canthaxanthin can generate two decomposition products, all-*trans*- and 13-*cis*-4-oxoretinoic acid (45). These metabolites have the same activity as canthaxanthin on enhancing cell–cell gap junctional communication in marine fibroblasts (45,46). It is interesting that 4-oxoretinoic acid has been shown to be a ligand of the nuclear receptor, RARβ (47). Whether canthaxanthin can regulate gene expression via this metabolite remains to be determined.

III. BIOLOGICAL ACTIVITIES OF CAROTENOID OXIDATIVE PRODUCTS

Carotenoids are shown to be regulators of cell differentiation, proliferation, and apoptosis, particularly in certain carcinoma cell lines, and these properties have been used as the rationale for using carotenoids for cancer chemoprevention. These biological activities of carotenoids are related to the function of intact carotenoids or their decomposition products, which can possess either more or less activity than their parent compounds, or have an entirely different function.

A. Beneficial Effects of Carotenoid Oxidative Products and Possible Mechanisms Involved

1. Retinoid-Dependent Activity of Carotenoid Metabolites

Retinoids, the most important oxidative products from provitamin A carotenoids, play an important role in several critical life processes, including vision, reproduction, metabolism, differentiation, hematopoiesis, bone development, and pattern formation during embryogenesis (48). Considerable evidence demonstrates that retinoids may be effective in the management of a variety of human chronic diseases, including cancer (49). The mechanism by which retinoids can elicit these effects resides in their ability to regulate gene expression at specific target sites within the body. It is important to point out that β-carotene and its excentric cleavage metabolites can serve as direct precursors for the all-*trans* and 9-*cis*-retinoic acid (30,34,36,50), which are ligands for retinoic acid receptor (RAR) and retinoid X receptor (RXR). Retinoid receptors function as ligand-dependent transcription factors and regulate gene expression by binding as dimeric complexes to the retinoic acid response element (RARE) and the retinoid X response element (RXRE), which are located in the 5' promoter region of susceptible genes. Therefore, the molecular mode of action of provitamin A carotenoids mediated by retinoic acid may involve several mechanisms: (a) transactivation through binding to RAREs in target gene promoters, thereby transcriptionally activating a series of genes with distinct antiproliferative activity; (b) transrepression of activator protein-1 (AP-1, composed of c-Jun and c-Fos), a transcription factor that mediates signals from growth factors, inflammatory peptides, oncogenes, and tumor promoters, thereby modulating cell proliferation; and (c) induction of apoptosis, thereby eliminating cells with unrepairable alterations in the genome or killing neoplastic cells. Since the down-regulation of retinoid receptors (loss or low expression of specific RARs and RXRs, e.g., RARβ as tumor suppressor) or "functional" down-regulation of retinoid receptors (lack of retinoic acid) could interfere with retinoid signal transduction and result in enhanced cell proliferation and potentially malignant transformation, up-regulation of retinoid receptor expression and function by provitamin A carotenoids may play a role in mediating the growth inhibitory effects of retinoids in cancer cells. This hypothesis was supported by recent animal studies reporting that both dietary and topical β-carotene prevents lung tumorigenesis in hamsters (14) and skin carcinoma formation in mice and induces retinoic acid receptor expression (15). Using the ferret model, we evaluated the effects of low-dose β-carotene supplementation (equivalent to an intake of 6 mg of β-carotene/day/70-kg person) on retinoic acid concentration, expression of RARs, proliferating cellular nuclear antigen (PCNA) expression, and histopathological changes in the lungs of cigarette smoke-exposed ferrets. We observed alveolar cell proliferation and keratinized squamous metaplasia in the lung tissue of ferrets with smoke exposure, but not in the low-dose β-carotene-supplemented groups with or without smoke exposure (51). Low-dose β-carotene supplementation in the smoke-exposed group partially prevented the decrease of lung retinoic acid levels, compared with the smoke exposure group alone. This supports the possibility that β-carotene, when given at a low dose, could act to supply adequate retinoic acid to the lung tissue of smoke-exposed ferrets. Recently, we have observed that the down-regulation of RARβ by smoke-borne carcinogens was completely reversed by treatments with either β-carotene or apo-14'-carotenoic acid in normal bronchial epithelium cells (52). This could be due to the conversion of β-carotene and apocarotenoic acid to retinoic acid, as RARβ can be induced by retinoic acid. This is supported by our further observation that the transactivation of the RARβ2 promoter by β-apo-14'-carotenoic acid appears to occur, in large part, via metabolism to the potent RAR ligand, all-*trans* retinoic acid (52). On the other hand, β-apo-13-carotenone, which is not an intermediate in the conversion of β-carotene to retinoic acid, had no transactivation activity of RAR (52,53). It will be interesting to investigate whether the biological activity of carotenoids or their metabolites are mediated through interaction with RXRs, PPAR, or other orphan receptors. Recent work has shown that the lack of RXRα in mouse epidermis results in hypersensitivity to chemical-carcinogen-induced skin carcinogenesis (54). Therefore, RXRs may function not only as heterodimeric partners of other nuclear receptors but as active transducers of tumor suppressive signals (49).

2.   Retinoid-Independent Activity of Carotenoid Metabolites

Carotenoid metabolites may possess their own biological activities, independent of retinoid signaling. β-Apocarotenoic acids are random cleavage products of β-carotene with chemical structures similar to that of all-*trans* retinoic acid. Recent studies show that β-apo-12′-carotenoic acid can inhibit the growth of HL-60 cells (55) whereas β-apo-14′-carotenoic acid can stimulate the differentiation of U937 leukemia cells (56) and inhibit the growth of breast cancer cells (57). These effects were not due to cellular conversion of β-apocarotenoid to retinoic acid because no retinoids were detected in the cells after treatment with apocarotenoids (57). Thus, it is possible that breakdown products of β-carotene may have a role in regulating cell function apart from their ability to be metabolized to retinoic acid. This is also supported by the finding that apocarotenoids have very low binding affinity to RAR (57). Although β-apo-14′-carotenoic acid can induce transcriptional activity of the RARβ2 promoter by its conversion to retinoic acid in the normal bronchial epithelial cells (52), it is possible that the conversion of β-carotene to retinoic acid is impaired in transformed cells. In terms of non-provitamin A carotenoids, it has been also shown that acycloretinoic acid, a possible metabolite of lycopene (42), inhibited the growth of HL-60 human promyelocytic leukemia cells (43) and human mammary cancer cells (44). The RAR does not mediate growth inhibition by acycloretinoic acid. It has been shown that this compound is not a ligand for RAR and RXR by chloramphenicol acetyltransferase assay (58).

Recent studies have shown that a higher intake of cooked tomatoes or lycopene was significantly associated with a lower circulating levels of insulin-like growth factors-1 (IGF-1) (59) and higher levels of IGF binding protein-3 (IGFBP-3) (60). Growth stimulation of MCF7 mammary cancer cells by IGF-1 was reduced by physiological concentrations of lycopene (61). Lycopene treatment also markedly reduced the IGF-1 stimulation of AP-1 binding and was associated with an increase in membrane-associated IGFBPs (61). The IGFs are mitogens that play a pivotal role in regulating cell proliferation, differentiation, and apoptosis (62). Several lines of evidence implicate IGF-1 and its receptor, IGF-IR, in lung cancer and other malignancies (63). IGFBP-3, one of the six members of the IGFBP family and a major circulating protein in human plasma (64), regulates the bioactivity of IGF-1 by sequestering IGF-1 from its receptor in the extracellular milieu, thereby inhibiting the mitogenic and antiapoptotic action of IGF-1. IGFBP-3 also inhibits cell growth and induces apoptosis independent of IGF-1 and its receptors (65,66). Furthermore, results from studies in lung cancer cell lines and human populations support a role of high levels of IGF-1 and low levels of IGFBP-3 in lung cancer (67–69). Since little is known regarding whether lycopene can inhibit smoke-induced lung carcinogenesis through modulation of IGF-1/IGFBP-3 levels, cell proliferation, and apoptosis, we have initiated studies to test the effectiveness of lycopene supplementation against lung preneoplastic lesions in our smoke-exposed ferrets (41). The results show that ferrets supplemented with lycopene and exposed to smoke had significantly higher plasma IGFBP-3 levels and a lower IGF-1/IGFBP-3 ratio than ferrets exposed to smoke alone. Both low-dose (equivalent 15 mg lycopene/day in human) and high-dose (60 mg lycopene/day in human) lycopene supplementations substantially inhibited smoke-induced squamous metaplasia and PCNA expression in the lungs of ferrets. No squamous metaplasia or PCNA overexpression was found in the lungs of control ferrets or those supplemented with lycopene alone. Furthermore, cigarette smoke exposure greatly increased BAD (a member of the BH3-only subfamily of Bcl-2) phosphorylation at both Ser 136 and Ser 112 and significantly decreased cleaved caspase-3 in the lungs of ferrets, as compared with controls. The elevated phosphorylation of BAD and down-regulated apoptosis induced by cigarette smoke in the lungs of ferrets was prevented by both low- and high-dose lycopene treatments (41). This study indicates that lycopene can exert its protective effects against smoke-induced lung carcinogenesis by up-regulating IGFBP-3, interrupting the signal transduction pathway of IGF-1, inhibiting cell proliferation, and promoting apoptosis (41). Investigation into whether this function is due to lycopene or its metabolites is underway in this laboratory.

B. Harmful Effects of Carotenoid Oxidative Products and Possible Mechanisms Involved

The failure of intervention studies to demonstrate a protective effect of supplemental β-carotene could be due to many factors. One biological explanation for the harmful effects of high-dose β-carotene supplementation in smokers has to do with the dosage used and the free radical-rich atmosphere in the lungs of cigarette smokers. This environment alters β-carotene metabolism and produces undesirable oxidative metabolites, which can facilitate the binding of metabolites of benzo[a]pyrene to DNA (70), induce carcinogen-activating enzymes (71,72), interfere with retinoid metabolism (72), down-regulate RARβ (51,73), induce oxidative stress (74,75), up-regulate AP-1 (c-Jun and c-Fos) activity (51,73), and enhance the induction of BALB/c 3T3 cell transformation by benzo[a]pyrene (76).

1. Detrimental Effects of Carotenoids are Related to the Carotenoid Dose Administered In Vivo and the High Accumulation of Carotenoids in Tissues

An important questions that remains to be answered is whether the beneficial versus detrimental effects of carotenoids are related to the carotenoid dose administered in vivo and the accumulation of carotenoids in a specific organ. Lowe et al. (77) demonstrated that β-carotene and lycopene protect against oxidative DNA damage (induced by xanthine/xanthine oxidase) in HT29 cells at relatively low concentrations (1–3 μM) but lose this capacity at higher concentrations (4–10 μM). Yeh and Hu (78) demonstrated that β-carotene and lycopene at a high concentration (20 μM) significantly enhanced levels of lipid-peroxidation induced by a lipid-soluble radical generator, AMVN [2,2'-azobis(2,4-dimethylvaleronitrile)]. We have examined whether there is a true hazard associated with high-dose β-carotene supplementation and smoking in an animal model (51,73). We evaluated the effects of high-dose β-carotene supplementation (equivalent to an intake of 30 mg of β-carotene/day/70-kg person) on retinoic acid level, RARβ expression, and histopathological changes in the lungs of cigarette smoke-exposed ferrets. Retinoic acid derived from either vitamin A or β-carotene acts on normal bronchial epithelium by inducing mucus and blocking squamous differentiation (79). Since squamous metaplasia occurs during the early stages of lung carcinogenesis, perturbations in retinoid signaling may contribute to lung carcinogenesis (80). A role for RARβ (which is induced by retinoic acid) as a tumor suppressor gene has been proposed (81). Recent in situ hybridization studies show that up to 50% of primary lung tumors lack RARβ expression and that loss of expression is an early event in lung carcinogenesis (82), although the molecular mechanism through which RARβ expression is lost is uncertain (49). Our results showed that alveolar cell proliferation and keratinized squamous metaplasia were observed in the lung tissue of the high-dose β-carotene-supplemented group with or without smoke exposure (51,73). These precancerous lesions in the lung tissue of the ferrets receiving high-dose β-carotene supplementation were associated with a low level of retinoic acid and down-regulated RARβ expression in the lung, as compared with the control group. We concluded that diminished retinoid signaling by the down-regulation of RARβ expression could be a mechanism for enhancement of lung tumorigenesis after high-dose β-carotene supplementation and cigarette smoke exposure. More significantly, smoke exposure in the high-dose β-carotene-supplemented group resulted in an even greater decrease in lung retinoic acid levels and accompanied an increase in oxidative metabolites of β-carotene. The dosages of β-carotene used in the ATBC and CARET studies were 20–30 mg/day for 2–8 years, and these doses are 10- to 15-fold higher than the average intake of β-carotene in a typical American diet (approximately 2 mg/day). Such a high dose of β-carotene in humans could result in an accumulation of a relatively high β-carotene level in lung tissue, especially after long periods of supplementation (Table 1). To test whether the outcome is due to differences in the levels of different carotenoids that accumulate in lung tissue or other organ, we recently conducted a study to evaluate the effects of lycopene supplementation at both a low dose and a high dose on blood and lung tissue

Table 1 Comparison of β-Carotene Doses, Plasma β-Carotene Levels, and Risk of Lung Cancer in Smokers and Smoke-Exposed Ferrets

β-Carotene	Intake (mg/day)	Plasma β-carotene increase (fold)	Risk of lung cancer
Observational studies (5–9 servings of fruits and vegetables)			
	~6	1.5–3	Decrease
Intervention studies			
ATBC	20	18	Increase
CARET	30	14	Increase
PHS (11% smoker)	50/other day	4	No effect
WHS (13% smoker)	50/other day	4	No effect
Ferret studies	30	21	Increase
	6	3	Decrease

Source: Adapted from Ref. 115.

lycopene levels in ferrets with or without cigarette smoke exposure (41). Ferrets in the low-dose lycopene group were supplemented with 1.1 mg/kg/day of lycopene, which is equivalent to an intake of 15 mg/day in humans. This dose of lycopene is slightly higher than the average intake of lycopene (9.4 ± 0.3 mg/day) in U.S. men and women (83). Ferrets in the high-dose lycopene group were supplemented with 4.3 mg/kg/day of lycopene, which is equivalent to 60 mg/day in humans and achievable from a diet high in enriched tomato products or supplements. We observed that the concentration of plasma lycopene (range from 226 to 373 nmol/L) in the ferret after low-dose lycopene supplementation was similar to the lycopene concentration (range 290–350 nmol/L) reported in humans (84,85). The lycopene concentration in the lungs of ferrets that were given a low dose of lycopene reached 342 nmol/kg which is within the range of lung lycopene concentration in normal humans (100–500 nmol/kg) (86). We also observed that the lycopene concentration in ferrets supplemented with a high dose of lycopene increased 3.4-fold in lung tissue and 1.6-fold in plasma, compared with ferrets supplemented with a low dose of lycopene. The observation that a higher increase in lycopene concentrations occurred in lung tissue than in plasma after lycopene supplementation also has been observed in humans (87). When the ferrets were supplemented with β-carotene at a dose of 30 mg/day, the concentration of β-carotene in the lungs of ferrets was 26 mmol/kg lung tissue, which was associated with an enhanced development of lung squamous metaplasia induced by cigarette smoke exposure (73). In contrast, in the lycopene study, the concentration of lycopene in the lungs was only 1.2 mmol/kg lung tissue in ferrets supplemented with lycopene at a dose of 60 mg/day, which caused no harmful effects but rather prevented the development of lung squamous metaplasia and cell proliferation induced by smoke exposure (41). These data suggest that the outcome of carotenoid supplementation depends on the carotenoid (or its metabolites), the dosage level, and the specific organs examined. This hypothesis is supported by recent β-carotene human intervention studies, which indicate that β-carotene may prevent gastric carcinogenesis and oral precancerous lesions (11,12). Unlike lung tissue, eliminating β-carotene though epithelial cells can prevent accumulation of excessive β-carotene in oral and gastric mucosa. Further-more, recent animal studies reported that both dietary and topical β-carotene failed to act as a tumor promoter in the AJ mouse model of lung cancer (88) and the two-stage model of skin tumorigenesis (15). It is important to point out there are a number of problems in extrapolating the data from these rodent models to human populations (89). Several animal studies have reported on the effects of carotenoids, but actual carotenoid levels in plasma and tissue are not described and the doses of carotenoids in the animal studies have been exceedingly high. For example, Kim et al. (90) provided evidence that lycopene decreased the incidence of lung tumors in B6C3F1 mice. However, enhancement of BaP-induced mutagenesis by lycopene was observed in the colon and lung of LacZ mice in a study by Guttenplan et al. (91). However, lycopene levels in lung tissue are not described in these studies.

2. Induction of Cytochrome P450 Enzymes by Excessive Carotenoid Metabolites Contributes to Carcinogenesis

Paolini et al. (71) showed a significant increase in several cytochrome P450 (CYP) enzymes (CYP1A1/2, CYP2A1, CYP2B1, and CYP3A1/2) in the lungs of rats supplemented with very high doses of β-carotene (500 mg/kg body weight). It has been reported that β-apo-8'-carotenal, an excentric cleavage product of β-carotene, but not β-carotene itself, is a strong inducer of CYP1A1 in rats (92). This study is particularly interesting because the formation of β-apo-8'-carotenal from β-carotene was threefold higher in lung extracts of smoke-exposed ferrets than from non-smoke-exposed ferrets (73). Induction of CYPs by either β-carotene oxidative cleavage products or cigarette smoke has two possible detrimental actions in lung tissue: (a) bioactivating carcinogens and (b) destroying retinoic acid, thereby enhancing lung carcinogenesis (Fig. 1). We recently carried out a study of whether the destruction of retinoic acid in the ferret lung after smoke alone or after high dose β-carotene (with or without smoke) treatment is due to CYP induction involved in the destruction of retinoic acid (72). Using retinoic acid as the substrate, we found that the formation of the polar metabolites including 18-hydroxyretinoic acid and 4-oxoretinoic acid increased 6- to 10-fold after incubation with smoke-exposed, high-dose β-carotene-supplemented, or both ferret lung microsomes, as compared with controls. Furthermore, this enhanced retinoic acid catabolism was substantially (~80%) inhibited by nonspecific CYPs inhibitors (disulfiram and liarozole), but were partially (~50%) inhibited by resveratrol (CYP1A1 inhibitor), α-naphthoflavone (CYP1A2 inhibitor), and antibodies against CYP1A1 and CYP1A2. Cigarette smoke exposure and/or pharmacological dose of β-carotene increased levels of CYP1A1 and 1A2 by three-to sixfolds but not levels of 2E1 and 3A1 in ferret lung tissue. These findings suggest that low levels of retinoic acid in the lung of ferrets exposed to cigarette smoke and/or a high-dose of β-carotene may be caused by the enhanced retinoic acid catabolism via induction of CYPs, CYP1A1 and CYP1A2 in particular, which provides a possible explanation for enhanced lung carcinogenesis seen with pharmacological dose of β-carotene supplementation in cigarette smokers.

An interaction between alcohol and β-carotene was observed in several human studies such that the high-dose β-carotene effect was more harmful in the lungs of the men who reported consuming larger amounts of alcohol (4,93). Although the mechanism for the interaction between alcohol and β-carotene enhances lung cancer development has not been elucidated, several reports regarding the potential harmful effects of β-carotene in the liver were reported (94,95). In baboons, consumption of ethanol together with β-carotene resulted in more hepatic injury than did consumption of either compound alone (95). Kessova et al. (94) demonstrated that β-carotene potentiates CYP2E1 induction by ethanol in rat liver. Recently, we have shown that CYP2E1 is the major cytochrome P450 enzyme responsible for the ethanol-enhanced catabolism of retinoic acid in hepatic tissue after treatment with alcohol (96). It seems that heavy alcohol intake may interfere with β-carotene and retinoic acid metabolism similar to that of cigarette smoke exposure (72), which may, at least in part, explain the associated adverse effects of β-carotene. This hypothesis was supported by our recent observation that chronic alcohol intake greatly interferes with the retinoid signaling pathway, producing an environment that may contribute to hepatocellular proliferation and carcinogenesis (97,98).

3. Enhancement of Carcinogen Binding to DNA by Carotenoid Cleavage Products

Several reports have appeared pertaining to the question of whether intact β-carotene or its metabolites can act as cocarcinogens. Carcinogenic metabolites of benzo[a]pyrene can bind to DNA and form DNA adducts, thereby damaging DNA (99). Salgo et al. (70) reported that β-carotene decreases the binding of metabolites of benzo[a]pyrene (one of the most important smoke-borne carcinogens) to DNA, whereas the high-performance liquid chromatography fractions containing β-carotene oxidative metabolites facilitate the binding of metabolites of benzo[a]pyrene to DNA. Although the oxidative metabolites were not identified, this study (70) provided a basis for the possible mechanism(s) for a harmful effect of the combination of smoking and β-carotene supplementation on initiation of carcinogenesis. Perocco et al. (76) showed that induction of BALB/ c 3T3 cell transformation by benzo[a]pyrene was markedly increased by the presence of β-carotene, although it is not clear whether the enhancement of cell transforming activity was due to β-carotene itself or to its metabolites. In general, these studies indicate that β-carotene itself can act as an anticarcinogen but that its oxidized products may facilitate carcinogenesis (Fig. 1).

4. Induction of Oxidative Stress by High-Dose β-Carotene and Its Oxidative Cleavage Products

One of the potential mechanisms for the results observed in the human β-carotene trials is that the presentation of high doses of β-carotene via supplements to the highly oxidative environment of the lung in smokers results in increased levels of oxidative metabolites of β-carotene, which may have detrimental effects (100–102). Indeed, the formation of β-apocarotenals and β-carotene 5,6,-epoxide increased two- to fivefold in the smoke-exposed ferrets versus the non-smoke-exposed ferrets (73,102). Recent studies have shown that carotenoid cleavage products, including apocarotenals and epoxides, inhibit mitochondrial respiration and elevate the accumulation of malondialdehyde in vitro (74,75). One possible mechanism to explain the instability of the β-carotene molecule is that exposure of lung cells to smoke results in increased lung cell oxidative stress and thereby causes a decrease in other antioxidants, such as vitamin C and vitamin E, which normally have a stabilizing effect on the unoxidized form of β-carotene (103,104). β-Carotene is capable of regenerating α-tocopherol from its radical (103,104). Conversely, vitamin E protect carotenoids from auto-xidation; the combination of β-carotene and α-tocopherol results in inhibition of free-radical-induced lipid peroxidation that is significantly greater than the sum of the individual inhibitions (105). In the absence of vitamin E, β-carotene can be cleaved randomly by enzyme-related radicals to produce β-apocarotenoids (106). A recent study by Palozza et al. (107) indicates that carotenoids may modulate cell growth by acting as intracellular redox agents depending on their redox potential and on the endogenous antioxidant environment. These data suggest that tocopherol may limit the pro-oxidant effects of carotenoids in biological systems. Moreover, we have shown that vitamin E enhances lymphatic transport of β-carotene and central cleavage of β-carotene to form vitamin A (rather than oxidative by-products) in vivo (28). It has also been reported that vitamin C is able to convert the β-carotene radical back to β-carotene and can help maintain β-carotene in its unoxidized form (103,104). The combination of β-carotene (20 mg/day) and vitamin E (50 mg/day) were not found to be protective against smoke-related lung cancer in the alpha-tocopherol, beta-carotene (ATBC) study.

However, vitamin C, which would facilitate both vitamin E recycling and β-carotene stability, was not used in the ATBC study. Epidemiological studies have shown that smokers have significantly lower plasma levels of vitamin C than nonsmokers (108). Similarly, passive smokers have reduced ascorbic acid concentrations in their plasma (109). It is particularly important to have broad antioxidant protection when using high doses of β-carotene in order to prevent the production of carotene excentric cleavage products and the subsequent cascade of events that may result from them (i.e., bioactivating carcinogens and destroying retinoic acid via induction of CYP enzymes, or facilitating the binding of benzo[a]pyrene metabolites to DNA). Both vitamins E and C can also inhibit cytochrome P450–mediated lipid peroxidation and carcinogen activation. However, in vitro work has shown that vitamin C can induce the decomposition of lipid hydroperoxides, which have the capacity to damage DNA (110). Thus, it will be important to examine whether vitamin C at varying doses could affect smoke-induced lung lesions, and whether these effects are protective or harmful. Possible protective effects of combined antioxidant supplementation in humans exposed to environmental tobacco smoke have been reported (111–113). These investigators reported that supplementation of the combined antioxidants resulted in a significant decrease in endogenous oxidative base damage in lymphocyte DNA in both smokers and nonsmokers. Recent study using a ferret model has show that β-carotene, used in combination with vitamins E and C, may have a possible chemopreventive effect against smoke-induced lung lesions (114). Results from these studies and the known biochemical interactions of β-carotene, vitamin E, and vitamin C suggest that this combination of nutrients may be an effective chemopreventive strategy against lung cancer in smokers.

IV. SUMMARY

To better understand both the beneficial and detrimental effects of carotenoids, greater knowledge of carotenoid metabolism and the biological effects of carotenoid metabolites is needed. In particular, knowledge of dose effects, tissue-specific effects, and possible adverse interaction with tobacco and alcohol is needed. Future research should provide more insight into the molecular mechanisms underlying the bioactivities of carotenoid metabolites and determine what dose of carotenoids (or its metabolites) or carotenoids combined with other antioxidants provides optimal protection while not increasing the risk of formation of undesirable metabolic by-products (especially in smokers and drinkers). This information is critically needed for future human studies involving carotenoids for prevention of lung cancer and cancers at other tissue sites.

REFERENCES

1. Mayne ST. Beta-carotene, carotenoids, and disease prevention in humans. FASEB J 1996; 10:690–701.
2. The Alpha-Tocopherol Beta-Carotene Cancer Prevention Study Group. The effect of vitamin E and beta carotene on the incidence of lung cancer and other cancers in male smokers. N Engl J Med 1994; 330:1029–1035.
3. Albanes D, Heinonen OP, Taylor PR, Virtamo J, Edwards BK, Rautalahti M, Hartman AM, Palmgren J, Freedman LS, Haapakoski J, Barrett MJ, Pietinen P, Malila N, Tala E, Liippo K, Salomaa ER, Tangrea JA, Teppo L, Askin FB, Taskinen E, Erozan Y, Greenwald P, Huttunen JK. Alpha-tocopherol and beta-carotene supplements and lung cancer incidence in the alpha-tocopherol, beta-carotene cancer prevention study: effects of base-line characteristics and study compliance. J Natl Cancer Inst 1996; 88:1560–1570.
4. Omenn GS, Goodman GE, Thornquist MD, Balmes J, Cullen MR, Glass A, Keogh JP, Meyskens FL Jr, Valanis B, Williams JH Jr, Barnhart S, Cherniack MG, Brodkin CA, Hammar S. Risk factors for lung cancer and for intervention effects in CARET, the Beta-Carotene and Retinol Efficacy Trial. J Natl Cancer Inst 1996; 88:1550–1559.
5. Omenn GS, Goodman GE, Thornquist MD, Balmes J, Cullen MR, Glass A, Keogh JP, Meyskens FL, Valanis B, Williams JH, Barnhart S, Hammar S. Effects of a combination of beta-carotene and vitamin A on lung cancer and cardiovascular disease. N Engl J Med 1996; 334:1150–1155.
6. Hennekens CH, Buring JE, Manson JE, Stampfer M, Rosner B, Cook NR, Belanger C, LaMotte F, Gaziano JM, Ridker PM, Willett W, Peto R. Lack of effect of long-term supplementation with beta carotene on the incidence of malignant neoplasms and cardiovascular disease. N Engl J Med 1996; 334:1145–1149.
7. Lee IM, Cook NR, Manson JE, Buring JE, Hennekens CH. Beta-carotene supplementation and incidence of cancer and cardiovascular disease: the women's health study. J Natl Cancer Inst 1999; 91:2102–2106.
8. Williams AW, Boileau TW, Zhou JR, Clinton SK, Erdman JW Jr. Beta-carotene modulates human prostate cancer cell growth and may undergo intracellular metabolism to retinol. J Nutr 2000; 130:728–732.
9. Feskanich D, Ziegler RG, Michaud DS, Giovannucci EL, Speizer FE, Willett WC, Colditz GA. Prospective study of fruit and vegetable consumption and risk of lung cancer among men and women. J Natl Cancer Inst 2000; 92:1812–1823.
10. Michaud DS, Feskanich D, Rimm EB, Colditz GA, Speizer FE, Willett WC, Giovannucci E. Intake of specific carotenoids and risk of lung cancer in 2 prospective US cohorts. Am J Clin Nutr 2000; 72:990–997.
11. Correa P, Fontham ET, Bravo JC, Bravo LE, Ruiz B, Zarama G, Realpe JL, Malcom GT, Li D, Johnson WD, Mera R. Chemoprevention of gastric dysplasia: randomized trial of antioxidant supplements and anti-helicobacter pylori therapy. J Natl Cancer Inst 2000; 92:1881–1888.
12. Mayne ST, Cartmel B, Baum M, Shor-Posner G, Fallon BG, Briskin K, Bean J, Zheng T, Cooper D, Friedman C, Goodwin WJ Jr. Randomized trial of supplemental beta-carotene to prevent second head and neck cancer. Cancer Res 2001; 61:1457–1463.

13. De Flora S, Bagnasco M, Vainio H. Modulation of genotoxic and related effects by carotenoids and vitamin A in experimental models: mechanistic issues. Mutagenesis 1999; 14:153–172.

14. Furukawa F, Nishikawa A, Kasahara K, Lee IS, Wakabayashi K, Takahashi M, Hirose M. Inhibition by beta-carotene of upper respiratory tumorigenesis in hamsters receiving diethylnitrosamine followed by cigarette smoke exposure. Jpn J Cancer Res 1999; 90:154–161.

15. Ponnamperuma RM, Shimizu Y, Kirchhof SM, De Luca LM. Beta-carotene fails to act as a tumor promoter, induces RAR expression, and prevents carcinoma formation in a two-stage model of skin carcinogenesis in male Sencar mice. Nutr Cancer 2000; 37:82–88.

16. Bishayee A, Sarkar A, Chatterjee M. Further evidence for chemopreventive potential of beta-carotene against experimental carcinogenesis: diethylnitrosamine-initiated and phenobarbital-promoted hepatocarcinogenesis is prevented more effectively by beta-carotene than by retinoic acid. Nutr Cancer 2000; 37:89–98.

17. Olson JA, Hayaishi O. The enzymatic cleavage of beta-carotene into vitamin A by soluble enzymes of rat liver and intestine. Proc Natl Acad Sci U S A 1965; 54:1364–1370.

18. Wang XD, Krinsky NI. The bioconversion of beta-carotene into retinoids. Subcell Biochem 1998; 30:159–180.

19. Wyss A, Wirtz G, Woggon W, Brugger R, Wyss M, Friedlein A, Bachmann H, Hunziker W. Cloning and expression of beta,beta-carotene 15,15'-dioxygenase. Biochem Biophys Res Commun 2000; 271:334–336.

20. von Lintig J, Wyss A. Molecular analysis of vitamin A formation: cloning and characterization of beta-carotene 15,15'-dioxygenases. Arch Biochem Biophys 2001; 385:47–52.

21. Leuenberger MG, Engeloch-Jarret C, Woggon WD. The reaction mechanism of the enzyme-catalyzed central cleavage of beta-carotene to retinal. Angew Chem Int Ed Engl 2001; 40:2613–2617.

22. Lindqvist A, Andersson S. Biochemical properties of purified recombinant human β-carotene 15,15'-monooxygenase. J Biol Chem 2002; 277:23942–23948.

23. Glover J. The conversion of beta-carotene into vitamin A. Vitam Horm 1960; 18:371–386.

24. Sharma RV, Mathur SN, Dmitrovskii AA, Das RC, Ganguly J. Studies on the metabolism of beta-carotene and apo-beta-carotenoids in rats and chickens. Biochim Biophys Acta 1976; 486:183–194.

25. Sharma RV, Mathur SN, Ganguly J. Studies on the relative biopotencies and intestinal absorption of different apo-beta-carotenoids in rats and chickens. Biochem J 1976; 158:377–383.

26. Wang XD, Tang GW, Fox JG, Krinsky NI, Russell RM. Enzymatic conversion of beta-carotene into beta-apo-carotenals and retinoids by human, monkey, ferret, and rat tissues. Arch Biochem Biophys 1991; 285:8–16.

27. Tang GW, Wang XD, Russell RM, Krinsky NI. Characterization of beta-apo-13-carotenone and beta-apo-14'-carotenal as enzymatic products of the excentric cleavage of beta-carotene. Biochemistry 1991; 30:9829–9834.

28. Wang XD, Marini RP, Hebuterne X, Fox JG, Krinsky NI, Russell RM. Vitamin E enhances the lymphatic transport of beta-carotene and its conversion to vitamin A in the ferret. Gastroenterology 1995; 108:719–726.

29. Hebuterne X, Wang XD, Smith DE, Tang G, Russell RM. In vivo biosynthesis of retinoic acid from beta-carotene involves and excentric cleavage pathway in ferret intestine. J Lipid Res 1996; 37:482–492.

30. Liu C, Wang XD, Russell RM. Biosynthesis of retinoic acid from beta-apo-14'-carotenal in ferret in vivo. J Nutr Biochem 1997; 8:652–657.

31. Wang XD, Krinsky NI, Marini RP, Tang G, Yu J, Hurley R, Fox JG, Russell RM. Intestinal uptake and lymphatic absorption of beta-carotene in ferrets: a model for human beta-carotene metabolism. Am J Physiol 1992; 263:G480–G486.

32. Kiefer C, Hessel S, Lampert JM, Vogt K, Lederer MO, Breithaupt DE, von Lintig J. Identification and characterization of a mammalian enzyme catalyzing the asymmetric oxidative cleavage of provitamin A. J Biol Chem 2001; 276: 14110–14116.

33. Hu K, Liu C, Krinsky NI, Russell RM, Wang XD. Cloning and characterization of carotene 9',10'-monooxygenase in ferrets (submitted).

34. Napoli JL, Race KR. Biogenesis of retinoic acid from beta-carotene. Differences between the metabolism of beta-carotene and retinal. J Biol Chem 1988; 263:17372–17377.

35. Wang XD, Krinsky NI, Tang GW, Russell RM. Retinoic acid can be produced from excentric cleavage of beta-carotene in human intestinal mucosa. Arch Biochem Biophys 1992; 293:298–304.

36. Wang XD, Russell RM, Liu C, Stickel F, Smith DE, Krinsky NI. Beta-oxidation in rabbit liver in vitro and in the perfused ferret liver contributes to retinoic acid biosynthesis from beta-apocarotenoic acids. J Biol Chem 1996; 271:26490–26498.

37. Folmani Y, Russell RM, Tang GW, Wolf DG. Rabbits fed on beta-carotene have higher serum levels of all-trans retinoic acid than those receiving no beta-carotene. Br J Nutr 1989; 62:195–201.

38. Wang XD, Krinsky NI, Russell RM. Retinoic acid regulates retinol metabolism via feedback inhibition of retinol oxidation and stimulation of retinol esterification in ferret liver. J Nutr 1993; 123:1277–1285.

39. Khachik F, Beecher GR, Smith JC Jr. Lutein, lycopene, and their oxidative metabolites in chemoprevention of cancer. J Cell Biochem Suppl 1995; 22:236–246.

40. Khachik F, Spangler CJ, Smith JC Jr, Canfield LM, Steck A, Pfander H. Identification, quantification, and relative concentrations of carotenoids and their metabolites in human milk and serum. Anal Chem 1997; 69:1873–1881.

41. Liu C, Lian F, Smith DE, Russell RM, Wang XD. Lycopene supplementation inhibits lung squamous metaplasia and induces apoptosis via up-regulating insulin-like growth factor-binding protein 3 in cigarette smoke-exposed ferrets. Cancer Res 2003; 63:3138–3144.

42. Kim SJ, Nara E, Kobayashi H, Terao J, Nagao A. Formation of cleavage products by autoxidation of lycopene. Lipids 2001; 36:191–199.

43. Nara E, Hayashi H, Kotake M, Miyashita K, Nagao A. Acyclic carotenoids and their oxidation mixtures inhibit the growth of HL-60 human promyelocytic leukemia cells. Nutr Cancer 2001; 39:273–283.

44. Ben-Dor A, Nahum A, Danilenko M, Giat Y, Stahl W, Martin HD, Emmerich T, Noy N, Levy J, Sharoni Y. Effects of acyclo-retinoic acid and lycopene on activation of the retinoic acid receptor and proliferation of mammary cancer cells. Arch Biochem Biophys 2001; 391:295–302.

45. Hanusch M, Stahl W, Schulz WA, Sies H. Induction of gap junctional communication by 4-oxoretinoic acid generated from its precursor canthaxanthin. Arch Biochem Biophys 1995; 317:423–428.

46. Nikawa T, Schulz WA, van den Brink CE, Hanusch M, van der Saag P, Stahl W, Sies H. Efficacy of all-*trans*-beta-carotene, canthaxanthin, and all-*trans*-, 9-*cis*-, and 4-oxoretinoic acids in inducing differentiation of an F9 embryonal carcinoma RAR beta-lacZ reporter cell line. Arch Biochem Biophys 1995; 316:665–672.

47. Pijnappel WW, Hendriks HF, Folkers GE, van den Brink CE, Dekker EJ, Edelenbosch C, van der Saag PT, Durston AJ. The retinoid ligand 4-oxo-retinoic acid is a highly active modulator of positional specification. Nature 1993; 366:340–344.

48. Chambon P. A decade of molecular biology of retinoic acid receptors. FASEB J 1996; 10:940–954.

49. Altucci L, Gronemeyer H. The promise of retinoids to fight against cancer. Nat Rev Cancer 2001; 1:181–193.

50. Wang XD, Krinsky NI, Benotti PN, Russell RM. Biosynthesis of 9-cis-retinoic acid from 9-cis-β-carotene in human intestinal mucosa in vitro. Arch Biochem Biophys 1994; 313:150–155.

51. Liu C, Wang XD, Bronson RT, Smith DE, Krinsky NI, Russell RM. Effects of physiological versus pharmacological beta-carotene supplementation on cell proliferation and histopathological changes in the lungs of cigarette smoke-exposed ferrets. Carcinogenesis 2000; 21:2245–2253.

52. Prakash P, Liu C, Hu KQ, Krinsky NI, Russell RM, Wang XD. Effects of beta-carotene, beta-apo-14′-carotenoic acid and benzo[a]pyrene on retinoic acid receptor β expression and growth of normal human bronchial epithelial cells. J Nutr 2004; 134 (in press).

53. Hu XM, White KM, Jacobsen NE, Mangelsdorf DJ, Canfield LM. Inhibition of growth and cholesterol synthesis in breast cancer cells by oxidation products of beta-carotene. Journal Nutrition Biochemistry 1998; 9:567–574.

54. Li M, Indra AK, Warot X, Brocard J, Messaddeq N, Kato S, Metzger D, Chambon P. Skin abnormalities generated by temporally controlled RXRalpha mutations in mouse epidermis. Nature 2000; 407:633–636.

55. Suzuki T, Matsui M, Murayama A. Biological activity of (all-E)-beta-apo-12′-carotenoic acid and the geometrical isomers on human acute promyelocytic leukemia cell line HL-60. J Nutr Sci Vitaminol (Tokyo) 1995; 41:575–585.

56. Winum JY, Kamal M, Defacque H, Commes T, Chavis C, Lucas M, Marti J, Montero JL. Synthesis and biological activities of higher homologues of retinoic acid. Farmaco 1997; 52:39–42.

57. Tibaduiza EC, Fleet JC, Russell RM, Krinsky NI. Excentric cleavage products of beta-carotene inhibit estrogen receptor positive and negative breast tumor cell growth in vitro and inhibit activator protein-1-mediated transcriptional activation. J Nutr 2002; 132:1368–1375.

58. Stahl W, von Laar J, Martin HD, Emmerich T, Sies H. Stimulation of gap junctional communication: comparison of acyclo-retinoic acid and lycopene. Arch Biochem Biophys 2000; 373:271–274.

59. Mucci LA, Tamimi R, Lagiou P, Trichopoulou A, Benetou V, Spanos E, Trichopoulos D. Are dietary influences on the risk of prostate cancer mediated through the insulin-like growth factor system? Br J Urol Int 2001; 87:814–820.

60. Holmes MD, Pollak MN, Willett WC, Hankinson SE. Dietary correlates of plasma insulin-like growth factor I and insulin-like growth factor binding protein 3 concentrations. Cancer Epidemiol Biomark Prev 2002; 11:852–861.

61. Karas M, Amir H, Fishman D, Danilenko M, Segal S, Nahum A, Koifmann A, Giat Y, Levy J, Sharoni Y. Lycopene interferes with cell cycle progression and insulin-like growth factor I signaling in mammary cancer cells. Nutr Cancer 2000; 36:101–111.

62. Yu H, Rohan T. Role of the insulin-like growth factor family in cancer development and progression. J Natl Cancer Inst 2000; 92:1472–1489.

63. Giovannucci E. Insulin-like growth factor-I and binding protein-3 and risk of cancer. Horm Res 1999; 51 (suppl 3):34–41.

64. Rechler M. Growth inhibition by insulin-like growth factor (IGF) binding protein-3—what's IGF got to do with it? Endocrinology 1997; 138:2645–2647.

65. Liu B, Lee HY, Weinzimer SA, Powell DR, Clifford JL, Kurie JM, Cohen P. Direct functional interactions between insulin-like growth factor-binding protein-3 and retinoid X receptor-alpha regulate transcriptional signaling and apoptosis. J Biol Chem 2000; 275:33607–33613.

66. Oh Y, Muller HL, Lamson G, Rosenfeld RG. Insulin-like growth factor (IGF)—independent action of IGF-binding protein-3 in Hs578T human breast cancer cells. Cell surface binding and growth inhibition. J Biol Chem 1993; 268:14964–14971.

67. Yu H, Spitz MR, Mistry J, Gu J, Hong WK, Wu X. Plasma levels of insulin-like growth factor-I and lung cancer risk: a case-control analysis. J Natl Cancer Inst 1999; 91:151–156.

68. London SJ, Yuan JM, Travlos GS, Gao YT, Wilson RE, Ross RK, Yu MC. Insulin-like growth factor I, IGF-binding protein 3, and lung cancer risk in a prospective study of men in China. J Natl Cancer Inst 2002; 94:749–754.

69. Hochscheid R, Jaques G, Wegmann B. Transfection of human insulin-like growth factor-binding protein 3 gene inhibits cell growth and tumorigenicity: a cell culture model for lung cancer. J Endocrinol 2000; 166:553–563.

70. Salgo MG, Cueto R, Winston GW, Pryor WA. Beta carotene and its oxidation products have different effects on microsome mediated binding of benzo[a]pyrene to DNA. Free Radic Biol Med 1999; 26:162–173.

71. Paolini M, Cantelli-Forti G, Perocco P, Pedulli GF, Abdel-Rahman SZ, Legator MS. Cocarcinogenic effect of beta-carotene. Nature 1999; 398:760–761.

72. Liu C, Russell RM, Wang XD. Exposing ferrets to cigarette smoke and a pharmacological dose of beta-carotene supplementation enhance in vitro retinoic acid catabolism in lungs via induction of cytochrome P450 enzymes. J Nutr 2003; 133:173–179.

73. Wang XD, Liu C, Bronson RT, Smith DE, Krinsky NI, Russell M. Retinoid signaling and activator protein-1 expression in ferrets given beta-carotene supplements and exposed to tobacco smoke. J Natl Cancer Inst 1999; 91:60–66.

74. Siems W, Sommerburg O, Schild L, Augustin W, Langhans CD, Wiswedel I. Beta-carotene cleavage products induce oxidative stress in vitro by impairing mitochondrial respiration. FASEB J 2002; 16:1289–1291.

75. Siems WG, Sommerburg O, Hurst JS, van Kuijk FJ. Carotenoid oxidative degradation products inhibit Na^+-K^+-ATPase. Free Radic Res 2000; 33:427–435.

76. Perocco P, Paolini M, Mazzullo M, Biagi GL, Cantelli-Forti G. Beta-carotene as enhancer of cell transforming activity of powerful carcinogens and cigarette-smoke condensate on BALB/c 3T3 cells in vitro. Mutat Res 1999; 440:83–90.

77. Lowe GM, Booth LA, Young AJ, Bilton RF. Lycopene and beta-carotene protect against oxidative damage in HT29 cells at low concentrations but rapidly lose this capacity at higher doses. Free Radic Res 1999; 30:141–151.

78. Yeh S, Hu M. Antioxidant and pro-oxidant effects of lycopene in comparison with beta-carotene on oxidant-induced damage in Hs68 cells. J Nutr Biochem 2000; 11:548–554.

79. Jetten AM, George MA, Smits HL, Vollberg TM. Keratin 13 expression is linked to squamous differentiation in rabbit tracheal epithelial cells and down-regulated by retinoic acid. Exp Cell Res 1989; 182:622–634.

80. Lotan R. Retinoids in cancer chemoprevention. FASEB J 1996; 10:1031–1039.

81. Houle B, Rochette-Egly C, Bradley WE. Tumor-suppressive effect of the retinoic acid receptor beta in human epidermoid lung cancer cells. Proc Natl Acad Sci USA 1993; 90:985–989.

82. Xu XC, Lee JS, Lee JJ, Morice RC, Liu X, Lippman SM, Hong WK, Lotan R. Nuclear retinoid acid receptor beta in bronchial epithelium of smokers before and during chemoprevention. J Natl Cancer Inst 1999; 91:1317–1321.

83. Dietary Reference Intakes: Vitamin A, Vitamin K and Micronutrients. Washington DC: National Academy Press, 2001.

84. Lu QY, Hung JC, Heber D, Go VL, Reuter VE, Cordon-Cardo C, Scher HI, Marshall JR, Zhang ZF. Inverse associations between plasma lycopene and other carotenoids and prostate cancer. Cancer Epidemiol Biomark Prev 2001; 10:749–756.

85. Vogt TM, Mayne ST, Graubard BI, Swanson CA, Sowell AL, Schoenberg JB, Swanson GM, Greenberg RS, Hoover RN, Hayes RB, Ziegler RG. Serum lycopene, other serum carotenoids, and risk of prostate cancer in US Blacks and Whites. Am J Epidemiol 2002; 155:1023–1032.

86. Schmitz HH, Poor CL, Wellman RB, Erdman JW Jr. Concentrations of selected carotenoids and vitamin A in human liver, kidney and lung tissue. J Nutr 1991; 121:1613–1621.

87. Hininger IA, Meyer-Wenger A, Moser U, Wright A, Southon S, Thurnham D, Chopra M, van Den Berg H, Olmedilla B, Favier AE, Roussel AM. No significant effects of lutein, lycopene or beta-carotene supplementation on biological markers of oxidative stress and LDL oxidizability in healthy adult subjects. J Am Coll Nutr 2001; 20:232–238.

88. Obermueller-Jevic UC, Espiritu I, Corbacho AM, Cross CE, Witschi H. Lung tumor development in mice exposed to tobacco smoke and fed beta-carotene diets. Toxicol Sci 2002; 69:23–29.

89. Cohen LA. A review of animal model studies of tomato carotenoids, lycopene, and cancer chemoprevention. Exp Biol Med (Maywood) 2002; 227:864–868.

90. Kim DJ, Takasuka N, Nishino H, Tsuda H. Chemoprevention of lung cancer by lycopene. Biofactors 2000; 13:95–102.

91. Guttenplan JB, Chen M, Kosinska W, Thompson S, Zhao Z, Cohen LA. Effects of a lycopene-rich diet on spontaneous and benzo[a]pyrene-induced mutagenesis in prostate, colon and lungs of the lacZ mouse. Cancer Lett 2001; 164:1–6.

92. Gradelet S, Leclerc J, Siess MH, Astorg PO. Beta-apo-8'-carotenal, but not beta-carotene, is a strong inducer of liver cytochromes P4501A1 and 1A2 in rat. Xenobiotica 1996; 26:909–919.

93. Albanes D, Virtamo J, Taylor PR, Rautalahti M, Pietinen P, Heinonen OP. Effects of supplemental beta-carotene, cigarette smoking, and alcohol consumption on serum carotenoids in the Alpha-Tocopherol, Beta-Carotene Cancer Prevention Study. Am J Clin Nutr 1997; 66:366–372.

94. Kessova IG, Leo MA, Lieber CS. Effect of beta-carotene on hepatic cytochrome P-450 in ethanol-fed rats. Alcohol Clin Exp Res 2001; 25:1368–1372.

95. Leo MA, Kim C-I, Lowe N, Lieber CS. Interaction of ethanol with β-carotene: delayed blood clearance and enhanced hepatotoxicity. Hepatology 1992; 15:883–891.

96. Liu C, Russell RM, Seitz HK, Wang XD. Ethanol enhances retinoic acid metabolism into polar metabolites in rat liver via induction of cytochrome P4502E1. Gastroenterology 2001; 120:179–189.

97. Chung J, Chavez PR, Russell RM, Wang XD. Retinoic acid inhibits hepatic Jun N-terminal kinase-dependent signaling pathway in ethanol-fed rats. Oncogene 2002; 21:1539–1547.

98. Chung J, Liu C, Smith DE, Seitz HK, Russell RM, Wang XD. Restoration of retinoic acid concentration suppresses ethanol-enhanced c-Jun expression and hepatocyte proliferation in rat liver. Carcinogenesis 2001; 22:1213–1219.

99. Hecht SS. Tobacco smoke carcinogens and lung cancer. J Natl Cancer Inst 1999; 91:1194–1210.

100. Mayne ST, Handelman GJ, Beecher G. Beta-carotene and lung cancer promotion in heavy smokers—a plausible relationship? J Natl Cancer Inst 1996; 88:1513–1515.

101. Arora A, Willhite CA, Liebler DC. Interactions of beta-carotene and cigarette smoke in human bronchial epithelial cells. Carcinogenesis 2001; 22:1173–1178.

102. Wang XD, Russell RM. Procarcinogenic and anticarcinogenic effects of beta-carotene. Nutr Rev 1999; 57:263–272.

103. Bohm FE, R. Land, E.J. McGarvey, D.J. Truscott T.G. Carotenoids enhance vitamin E antioxidant efficiency. J Am Chem Soc 1997; 119:621–622.

104. Bohm F, Edge R, McGarvey DJ, Truscott TG. Beta-carotene with vitamins E and C offers synergistic cell protection against NOx. FEBS Lett 1998; 436:387–389.

105. Palozza P, Krinsky NI. Beta-carotene and alpha-tocopherol are synergistic antioxidants. Arch Biochem Biophys 1992; 297:184–187.

106. Yeum KJ, dos Anjos Ferreira AL, Smith D, Krinsky NI, Russell RM. The effect of alpha-tocopherol on the oxidative cleavage of beta-carotene. Free Radic Biol Med 2000; 29:105–114.
107. Palozza P, Serini S, Torsello A, Di Nicuolo F, Piccioni E, Ubaldi V, Pioli C, Wolf FI, Calviello G. Beta-carotene regulates NF-kappaB DNA-binding activity by a redox mechanism in human leukemia and colon adenocarcinoma cells. J Nutr 2003; 133:381–388.
108. Schectman G, Byrd JC, Gruchow HW. The influence of smoking on vitamin C status in adults. Am J Public Health 1989; 79:158–162.
109. Tribble DL, Giuliano LJ, Fortmann SP. Reduced plasma ascorbic acid concentrations in nonsmokers regularly exposed to environmental tobacco smoke. Am J Clin Nutr 1993; 58:886–890.
110. Lee SH, Oe T, Blair IA. Vitamin C-induced decomposition of lipid hydroperoxides to endogenous genotoxins. Science 2001; 292:2083–2086.
111. Yong LC, Brown CC, Schatzkin A, Dresser CM, Slesinski MJ, Cox CS, Taylor PR. Intake of vitamins E, C, and A and risk of lung cancer. The NHANES I epidemiologic follow-up study. First National Health and Nutrition Examination Survey. Am J Epidemiol 1997; 146:231–243.
112. Howard DJ, Ota RB, Briggs LA, Hampton M, Pritsos CA. Oxidative stress induced by environmental tobacco smoke in the workplace is mitigated by antioxidant supplementation. Cancer Epidemiol Biomark Prev 1998; 7:981–988.
113. Duthie SJ, Ma A, Ross MA, Collins AR. Antioxidant supplementation decreases oxidative DNA damage in human lymphocytes. Cancer Res 1996; 56:1291–1295.
114. Chongviriyaphan N, Liu C, Lipman R, Russell RM, Wang XD. Beta-carotene in the presence of alpha-tocopherol and vitamin C pretects against lung squamous metaplasia in ferrets exposed to tobacco smoke (manuscript in preparation).
115. Wang XD. Mechanistic understanding of potential adverse effects of beta-carotene supplementation. In: Eisenbrand G, eds. Functional Food: Safety Aspects. Weinheim: Wiley-VCH, 2004: 189–215.

15

Conversion of Carotenoids to Vitamin A: New Insights on the Molecular Level

Johannes von Lintig
Universität Freiburg, Freiburg, Germany

The elucidation of the physiological roles played by vitamins has always been a major concern of nutritionists and biochemists. In humans, vitamin A deficiency (VAD) leads to night blindness in milder forms, whereas more severe progression can lead to corneal malformations, e.g., xerophthalmia. Besides visual defects, this deficiency affects the immune system, leads to infertility, and causes malformations during embryogenesis. The molecular basis for these diverse effects is found in the dual role exerted by vitamin A derivatives in animal physiology: In all visual systems, retinal or closely related compounds such as 3-hydroxyretinal serve as the chromophores of the visual pigments (rhodopsin) (1,2). In vertebrates, the vitamin A derivative retinoic acid (RA) is a major signal controlling a wide range of biological processes. RA is the ligand of two classes of nuclear receptors, the retinoic acid receptors (RARs) and the retinoid X receptors (RXRs) (3, 4; reviewed in 5 and 6). The active receptor complex, involved in processes as diverse as pattern formation during embryonic development, cell differentiation, and control of metabolic activity, is an RAR/RXR heterodimer that binds DNA regulatory sequences and regulates gene transcription in response to ligand binding. RXR is not only the heterodimer partner of the RAR receptor but also an obligate partner for other nuclear receptors (orphan receptors) controlling a wide range of activities in lipid metabolism (for recent review, see Ref. 7).

VAD is still a major problem leading to blindness and childhood mortality, particularly in developing countries (8). The demand for this vitamin can be satisfied by the natural content of animal or plant food sources. This phenomenon was first explained by Moore in 1930 (9). He described a conversion of β-carotene to vitamin A in the small intestine, providing the first evidence that a plant-derived carotenoid is the direct precursor for vitamin A in animals. Today we know that all naturally occurring vitamin A derives from carotenoids that exert provitamin A activity. In contrast to our wide and still-growing knowledge about the physiological functions of carotenoids and their retinoid derivatives, the molecular components involved in carotenoid metabolism have remained elusive. This chapter will focus on recent advances in this research field that provided the first molecular insights into animal carotenoid metabolism.

I. BIOCHEMICAL CHARACTERIZATION OF CAROTENOID CLEAVAGE ENZYMES IN CELL-FREE HOMOGENATES

A central cleavage mechanism at the C-15,C-15' carbon double bond for the conversion of β-carotene to vitamin A was initially proposed by Karrer (10). In 1954, Glover proposed an excentric cleavage reaction and a stepwise process, leading ultimately to only 1 mol vitamin A per mole of carotene consumed (11). Evidence for this excentric cleavage was provided by the observation that radioactive β-apocarotenals were converted in mammals to vitamin A esters with the release of "small" radioactive fragments (12).

Goodman and Huang (13) and Olson and Hyaishi (14) firstly described an enzymatic activity in cell-free homogenates from rat small intestine that catalyzed provitamin A conversion. These analyses showed that β-carotene is enzymatically cleaved at the central C-15,C-15' double bond, yielding two molecules of vitamin A aldehyde (retinal). The enzymatic activity depended on molecular oxygen and the enzyme was termed β,β-carotene 15,15'-oxygenase (BCO). The enzyme was reported to be soluble, to have a slightly alkaline pH optimum, and to be inhibited by ferrous iron chelators and by sulfhydryl-binding compounds, indicating that it contains a ferrous iron cofactor (15,16). Subsequently, this enzyme was also characterized in different mammalian species (17,18) and substrate specificity was determined for different β-carotene stereoisomers (19). Recent analyses dealing with the mode of action of BCO provided strong evidence that oxidative cleavage at the central (15,15') double bond is catalyzed in a monooxygenase mechanism via a transient carotene epoxide (20; see also Chapter 16). After the description of this enzyme it was generally assumed that the centric cleavage reaction constitutes the major step in vitamin A synthesis. However, the excentric cleavage of β-carotene was subsequently also demonstrated in cell-free homogenates of mammals (21,22). Furthermore, it was shown that the resulting long-chain apocarotenoids ($>C_{20}$)

are shortened to RA in a stepwise process that is most probably mechanistically related to β oxidation of fatty acids (23,24). Several endeavors were undertaken, and while highly enriched enzyme fractions could be obtained, all attempts to purify these enzymes to homogeneity failed. The lack of knowledge about the molecular structure of carotene oxygenases hindered more detailed investigations of this first crucial step in vitamin A metabolism.

II. OUT OF THE GREEN YONDER: MOLECULAR CLONING AND FUNCTIONAL CHARACTERIZATION OF β-CAROTENE-15,15′-OXYGENASES

Carotenoids have key biological functions in all major taxa. As shown in Figure 1, by oxidative cleavage of their ridge carbon backbone, diverse bioactive

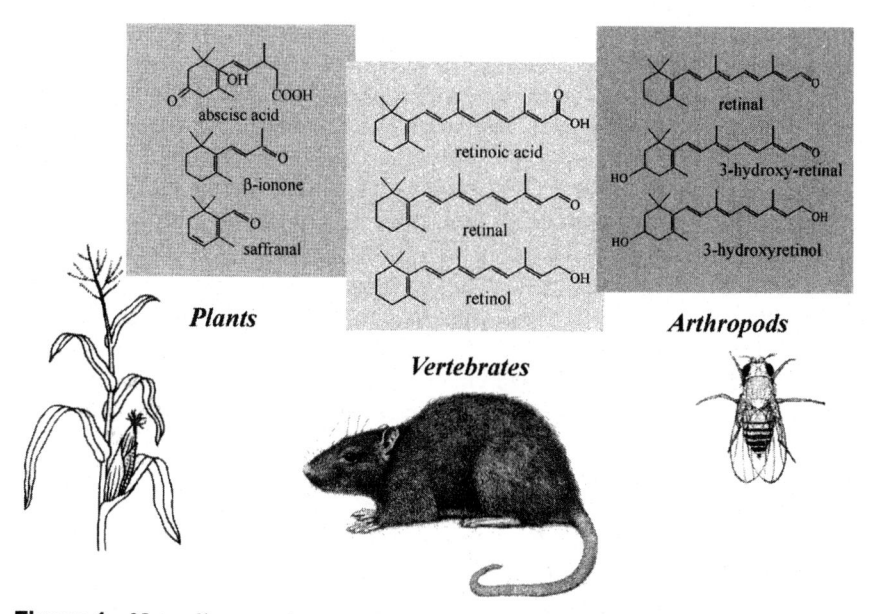

Figure 1   Naturally occurring apocarotenoids derived from C_{40} carotenoids in the plant and animal kingdom. In plants, a large subset of different apocarotenoids is found involved, for example, in growth regulation (abscisic acid) or the attraction of pollinating insect (β-ionone; safranal). In animals, mainly C_{20} apocarotenoids (vitamin A derivatives) are found. In all visual systems, retinal or closely related compounds such as 3-hydroxyretinal serve as the chromophores of the various visual pigments (1,2). In vertebrates, retinoic acid is an important signaling molecule binding to nuclear receptors involved in the regulation of target genes (6,7).

derivatives, such as vitamin A, the plant hormone abscisic acid, and several aroma compounds and apocarotenoid pigments, are synthesized (11,25–27). This diverse assortment of apocarotenoids found in nature results from the large number of carotenoids (more than 600), variations in the cleavage site, and modifications of the primary cleavage products. By analyzing the molecular basis of the abscisic acid-deficient phenotype of the maize *vp14* mutant, Schwartz and coworkers cloned for the first time a gene encoding a carotenoid-cleaving enzyme (25). The heterologously expressed and purified recombinant enzyme catalyzes the oxidative cleavage of 9-*cis*-epoxycarotenoids such as neoxanthin and violaxanthin to form xanthoxin, the direct precursor of abscisic acid (ABA). The re-combinant enzyme is soluble and depends on molecular oxygen and ferrous iron, thus having quite similar enzymatic properties as compared to the animal β,β-carotene 15,15′-oxygenase. Maize *vp14* belongs to an emerging gene family of putative carotenoid cleavage enzymes mainly found in plants and bacteria. In the meantime, new family members have been molecularly identified and functionally characterized, such as a carotenoid 9,10(9′,10′)-oxygenase with a broad substrate specificity and a zeaxanthin 7,8(7′,8′)-oxygenase from *Crocus* that is involved in the synthesis of safranal (28,29).

Due to the synthesis of apocarotenoids in all taxa, including retinal formation in green algae and halobacteria, we pursued the hypothesis that β-carotene cleavage in vitamin A metabolism is just a variation of this theme and is catalyzed by a related enzyme. To start, we established an efficient and reliable test system for the characterization of putative animal carotene oxygenases. For this purpose we equipped an *Escherichia coli* strain with a plasmid harboring the genes for β-carotene synthesis from the bacterium *Erwinia herbicola* (30). This *E. coli* strain becomes yellow by synthesizing β-carotene *de novo*. Then, upon introducing a gene encoding a β-carotene-cleaving enzyme, the resultant *E. coli* strain should be able to synthesize vitamin A at the expense of β-carotene and, therefore, should lose its yellow color. We searched the entire animal database and found several expressed *sequence tags* (ESTs) with weak sequence similarity to plant VP14, among them an EST fragment from the fruit fly *Drosophila melanogaster*. After cloning the corresponding full-length cDNA we expressed the encoded protein in the *E. coli* test system. Indeed, the resultant strain bleached, indicating that in the presence of the animal VP14-related enzyme retinoids are formed at the expense of β-carotene. The enzymatic properties of the recombinant purified *Drosophila* enzyme revealed that it exclusively catalyzed the centric cleavage of β-carotene to yield retinal. Thus, we molecularly identified and functionally characterized a β,β-carotene 15,15′-oxygenase (31).

Confirmation that this type of enzyme catalyzes the first step in vitamin A metabolism in metazoans more generally appeared shortly after we published our data. In an independent approach, Wyss and colleagues (32) succeeded in the molecular cloning and the functional characterization of a BCO from chicken. Their approach relied on partial protein purification, determination of peptide sequences, and use of this information to synthesize oligonucleotide primers to generate a partial cDNA and screen a cDNA library derived from small intestine. Amino acid sequence comparison between the *Drosophila* and chicken BCOs showed a overall similarity with several highly conserved regions and a significant similarity to some domains of the plant carotenoid oxygenase VP14 (33).

By sequence similarity to the identified genes from *Drosophila* and chicken, their counterparts from mouse and human were identified and functionally characterized (34–39). By the use of carotenoid-accumulating *E. coli* strains or by in vitro assays for enzymatic activity with the purified recombinant protein it was shown that these mammalian homologs catalyze exclusively the centric oxidative cleavage of β-carotene to yield retinal. Expression of the murine BCO in carotenoid-accumulating *E. coli* revealed the cleavage of carotenoid substrates such as β- and α-carotene but also lycopene, resulting in the last case in the formation of acyclic retinoids (34). However, the purified recombinant BCO catalyzes only the cleavage of carotenoid substrates with at least one unsubstituted β-ionone ring such as β-carotene and β-cryptoxanthin, and apparently no cleavage of lycopene and zeaxanthin could be detected (34,39). The K_m values for β-carotene were estimated to be in the range of $1-10\,\mu M$ for BCOs from the different species (31,34,37,39). BCO exhibits a slightly alkaline pH optimum, and enzymatic activity is sensitive to chelating agents such as o-phenanthroline and α,α'-bipyridyl, indicating that it depends on ferrous iron (37,39). Thus, the purified recombinant BCOs share biochemical properties that have already been described for the native BCOs. Purification of the recombinant BCO fusion proteins by affinity chromatography was achieved without the addition of detergents. This characteristic and the predicted amino acid sequences of the various BCOs indicate that we are dealing with hydrophilic proteins. Indeed, a cytosolic localization of the native BCO was recently demonstrated for its human representative (39). Therefore, in vitro tests for enzymatic activity must be conducted in the presence of detergents to mimic the interaction between the enzyme and its insoluble substrate. In vivo, however, the cytosolic localization of BCO may require specific binding proteins to deliver the carotenoid substrate as well as to bind the retinoid product, since both are highly lipophilic compounds. On the product side, three different types of cellular retinoid-binding proteins (CRBP I–III) have been characterized (40 and references therein). However, no direct protein–protein interaction between a recombinant murine BCO-GST fusion protein and CRBPs could be detected in pull-down experiments (37). Even though these results argue against a tight protein–protein interaction of CRBP with BCO, it seems likely that CRBPs may facilitate β-carotene cleavage by binding retinal. In mouse testis homogenates, an L-lactate dehydrogenase C was identified to interact specifically with BCO. So far, the exact physiological role of this type of alcohol dehydrogenase is not known, and there is no experimental evidence that this enzyme catalyzes either the oxidation or the reduction of aldehydes like retinal. It remains to be elucidated whether BCO may interact tissue specifically with a certain subset of proteins involved in retinoid metabolism, which then may control the metabolic flow of the primary cleavage product retinal either to retinol formation for vitamin A transport and storage or in the direction of RA formation for retinoid signaling.

To sum up, these investigations led to the molecular identification of β,β-carotene 15,15′-oxygenases from various metazoan species. The recombinant enzymes share common biochemical properties with the native BCOs from tissue homogenates. Based on its structural and biochemical properties, BCO from animals belongs to an ancient family of nonheme iron oxygenases heretofore described in plants and microorganisms.

III IN VERTEBRATES BOTH CENTRIC AND EXCENTRIC CAROTENOID-CLEAVAGE PATHWAYS EXIST

The dual function of vitamin A in vision (retinal) and in development and cell differentiation (RA) indicates that vertebrate retinoid metabolism is complex. This is reflected in a large subset of different retinoid-modifying enzymes, such as various retinoid-oxidizing enzymes as well as intracellular and extracellular retinoid-binding proteins. In vertebrates, there has long been a controversy over centric versus excentric cleavage of β-carotene in the synthesis of vitamin A. Evidence that in addition to a centric cleavage an excentric cleavage of carotenoids also occurs was provided by several investigations. Napoli and Race (41), for example, showed that, besides the formation of RA from retinal as the initial product of symmetrical β-carotene cleavage, RA is directly formed from β-carotene in cell-free homogenates. The first step in this alternative pathway might be the excentric cleavage of carotenoids, resulting in long-chain apocarotenoids that are subsequently shortened to yield RA (21,24).

In *Drosophila*, with vitamin A functions being restricted to vision, only one family member of nonheme iron carotenoid cleavage enzymes is found in the entire genome (42). However, in vertebrates, besides BCO, another protein with significant sequence identity, RPE65, exists, being specifically expressed in the retinal pigment epithelium (RPE) (43,44). Even though its function was not primarily linked with carotenoid metabolism, a role for RPE65 in retinoid metabolism of the eye was recently proposed based on mutant analysis. Although its exact biochemical function is not known, RPE65 seems to be required for the all-*trans* to 11-*cis* isomerization reaction that regenerates the 11-*cis*-retinal chromophore of rhodopsin in the visual cycle of the retina (45).

Besides RPE65, an additional *in silico*-predicted putative family member was found in the mouse database (35). Since this EST fragment possessed significant peptide sequence similarity to BCO, it represented a candidate for an enzyme catalyzing the excentric oxidative cleavage of carotenoids. Upon cloning the full-length cDNA, sequence analyses revealed that it encoded a protein of 532 amino acids. The deduced amino acid sequence shared approximately 40% sequence identity with BCO. Expression in the *E. coli* test system and in vitro assays for enzymatic activity revealed that this enzyme specifically catalyzed the cleavage of β-carotene at the C-9′,C-10′ double bond, resulting in the formation of one molecule of β-10′-apocarotenal and one molecule of β-ionone (35). To establish the occurrence of this type of carotene oxygenase in other vertebrates, we cloned cDNAs encoding this β,β-carotene 9′,10′-oxygenase (BCO-II) in humans and zebrafish. The molecular identification and functional

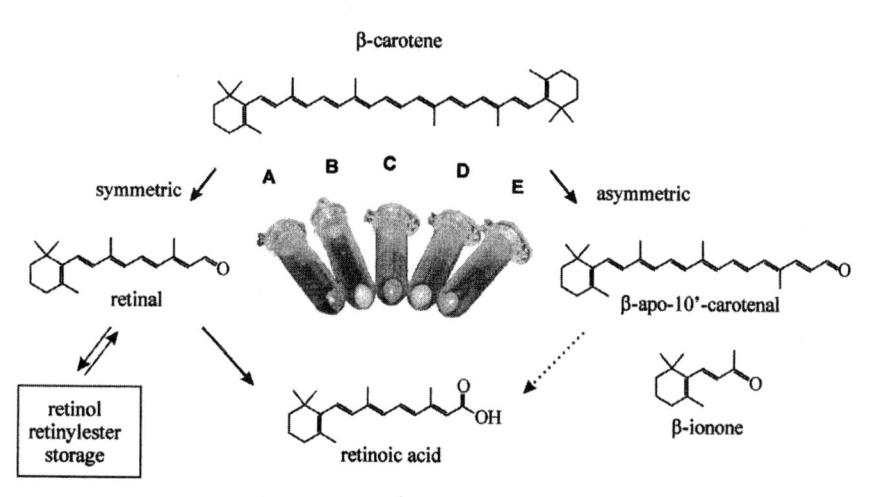

Figure 2 Overview of the symmetrical and the asymmetrical oxidative cleavage pathways of β-carotene in the mouse catalyzed by the β,β-carotene 15,15′-oxygenase (BCO) and β,β-carotene 9′,10′-oxygenase (BCO-II) activities, respectively. Center: colors of carotene synthesizing and accumulating *E. coli* strains expressing the two different types of carotene oxygenases compared to the controls. **A.** β-Carotene accumulating control strain. **B.** β-Carotene accumulating *E. coli* strain expressing mouse BCO. **C.** β-Carotene accumulating *E. coli* strain expressing mouse BCO-II. **D.** Lycopene accumulating *E. coli* strain expressing BCO-II. **E.** Lycopene accumulating control strain (for experimental details, see Ref. 35).

characterization of BCO-II in several vertebrate species provides strong evidence that both centric and excentric cleavage pathways for β-carotene exist in higher animals (Fig. 2).

On the level of the deduced amino acid sequences the two different types of animal carotene oxygenases possess several common structural features. Six histidine residues at conserved positions may be involved in the binding of the cofactor ferrous iron. In addition, there is a well-conserved domain EDDGVVLSSXVVS close to the C terminus that can be considered a BCO family signature sequence. Furthermore, sequence comparison revealed that the vertebrate BCOs have a higher degree of similarity to BCO-II and RPE65, so far both only found in vertebrates, than to its *Drosophila* ortholog. This indicates that the three vertebrate family members probably evolved from a common ancestor gene (Fig. 3). With the emerging number of sequences for carotenoid-cleaving enzymes from animals but also from plants being now

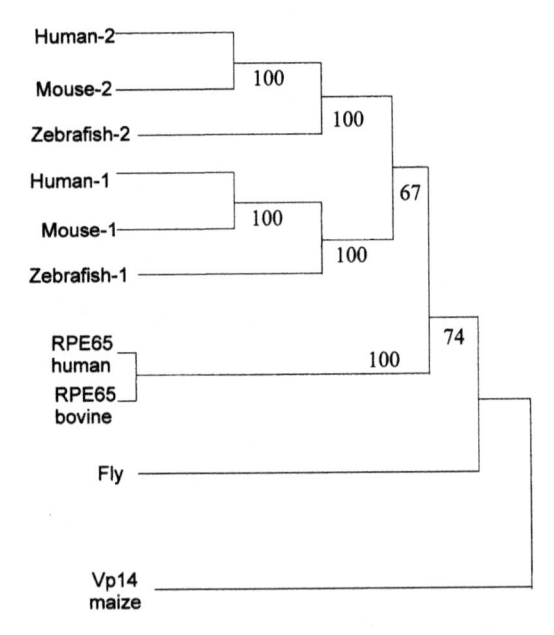

Figure 3 Phylogenetic tree calculation of the carotenoid cleaving nonheme iron oxygenase family. For the individual representatives the organism names are given, e.g., human-1 stands for β,β-carotene 15,15'-oxygenase and human-2 stands for β,β-carotene 9',10'-oxygenase. We used the deduced amino acid sequences for calculating the phylogenetic tree by a maximal parsimony analysis. The numbers at the branching points of the tree correspond to bootstrap values of 100 replicates.

available in the public database, this information can be used to define and narrow their catalytic domains and identify their active sites.

IV. INSECTS ARE SUITABLE MODELS TO IDENTIFY MOLECULAR PLAYERS IN METAZOAN CAROTENOID METABOLISM

The analyses described above led to the molecular cloning and functional characterization of BCOs from various metazoan species. However, no direct genetic evidence had yet been provided that this type of enzyme catalyzes the key step in vitamin A synthesis. Animal carotenoid metabolism follows a universal scheme. To become biologically active, dietary carotenoids must be first absorbed, then delivered to the site of action in the body, and in the case of provitamin A function metabolically converted. Invertebrates like *Drosophila* represent excellent models for the genetic dissection of this pathway since vitamin A is only needed for vision. The completed human and *Drosophila* genome projects have revealed that 60% of the genes of *Drosophila* possess homologs in the human genome. For a long time the fruit fly has served as a model for functional genomics, and a multitude of investigations led to the identification of genes involved in the visual process and the elucidation of their functions (for review, see Ref. 46). Among the various *Drosophila* mutants affected in their visual performance, the phenotype of five blind mutants could be assigned due to their characteristic electroretinograms to the so-called *neither inactivation nor afterpotential* (*nina*) phenotype. This phenotype is caused by a lack of functional visual pigments (rhodopsin) in the compound eyes of these fly mutants (47). The molecular reason for this phenotype was already determined for three of these five *nina* mutants. *ninaE* encodes the protein moiety (opsin) of the major *Drosophila* rhodopsin Rh1 (48). The *ninaA* gene encodes a molecular chaperone necessary for the maturation of Rh1 (49,50), whereas the *ninaC* gene encodes a class III myosin kinase necessary for the structural organization of the photoreceptor cells (47,51). The *ninaB* and *ninaD* mutants feature a characteristic not found in the three other *nina* mutants. Their visual performance can be rescued by feeding these flies retinal. Thus, the *ninaB* and *ninaD* genes were promising candidates to encode molecular components in the synthesis of the visual chromophore from dietary carotenoids, the sole source for vitamin A in *Drosophila* standard growth medium.

The *ninaB* mutations have been cytologically mapped on chromosome 3 to the position 87E-F in the *Drosophila* genome (52), coinciding with the physical localization of the *Drosophila* BCO gene. We performed detailed molecular analyses of this gene locus and found mutations in the BCO gene in two independent *ninaB* fly stocks which we showed to abolish the BCO function. Thus, the blind vitamin A-deficient phenotype of *ninaB* flies is caused by mutations in the BCO gene, providing the first direct genetic evidence that BCO actually catalyzes vitamin A synthesis in vivo (42). Since only this one representative of the nonheme iron carotenoid oxygenase gene family is encoded in the entire *Drosophila* genome, centric cleavage of carotenoids may represent the universal pathway for the synthesis of vitamin A in metazoans.

The *ninaB* gene is expressed exclusively in close spatial vicinity of the photoreceptor cells, indicating that carotenoids must be transported and delivered to BCO-expressing cells for vitamin A synthesis. In the second vitamin A-deficient *Drosophila* mutant, *ninaD*, the carotenoid content was shown to be significantly altered as compared to wild-type flies and ineffective in mediating visual pigment synthesis (53). Our molecular analyses revealed that this phenotype is caused by a defect in the uptake and body distribution of dietary carotenoids (54). The *ninaD* gene encodes a cellular surface receptor with significant sequence similarity to the mammalian class B scavenger receptors SR-BI and CD36. In *ninaD* flies, a nonsense mutation is found in the gene encoding this receptor, thus abolishing its function (54). Direct functional evidence for a role of the *ninaD* receptor in cellular carotenoid uptake was provided by P-element-mediated transformation of flies with a wild-type *ninaD* allele. Heat-shock-induced expression of the wild-type allele in the genetic background of *ninaD* flies resulted in the restoration of carotenoid uptake and visual pigment synthesis (54). Thus, these analyses provide genetic and functional evidence that the *ninaD* scavenger receptor is causally involved in the cellular uptake of carotenoids into target tissues.

There has been growing evidence that class B scavenger receptors, in particular SR-BI, are substantially involved in lipid metabolism, especially in cholesterol homeostasis in mammals (55,56). It was shown that these receptors mediate the bidirectional flux of unesterified cholesterol between circulating lipoproteins and the target cells (57,58). In insects, carotenoids are transported in the lipophorins of the hemolymph (59). These lipophorins are structurally related to the mammalian lipoprotein particles, also being transport vehicles for carotenoids (see Chapter 11). Insect in vitro systems provided evidence that the cellular uptake of lipids occurs by a flux between lipophorins and target cells. Like cholesterol exchange in mammals, the lipophorin particles are not necessarily internalized by receptor-mediated phagocytosis (60,61). One may speculate based on these results that the *ninaD* scavenger receptor mediates carotenoid uptake from lipophorins in a mechanistically similar manner.

It remains to be shown whether the cellular uptake of carotenoids is mediated by homologous receptors in mammals. Recently, it has been reported that in SR-BI-deficient mice vitamin E metabolism is impaired, resulting in an elevated plasma concentration of this vitamin (62). Together with the results from *Drosophila*, this finding may indicate that besides its crucial function in cholesterol homeostasis SR-BI may exert a role in the metabolism of fat-soluble vitamins of the isoprenoid substance class.

Insight into the molecular structure of a cellular carotenoid-binding protein (CBP) comes from the silkworm *Bombyx mori*. Tabunoki and colleagues (63) purified a lutein-binding protein from the silk gland of this insect and cloned the corresponding cDNA. This insect CBP has an apparent molecular mass of 33 kDA and binds carotenoids in a 1 : 1 molar ratio.

Sequence comparison revealed that CBP is a new member of the StAR protein family. In mammals these proteins are known as soluble protein carriers mediating the intracellular transport of lipids (for recent review, see Ref. 64). An example is the steroidogenic acute regulatory protein StAR/StarD1, which delivers cholesterol to mitochondrial P450 side chain cleavage enzymes in steroidogenic cells. The other family members are characterized by the 200- to 300-amino-acid StAR-related lipid transfer (START) domain with homology to StarD1. MLN64/StarD3 has been also shown in vitro to bind cholesterol, whereas Star2 binds phosphatidylcholine. There are several other family members of which the ligand is so far unknown (65). Based on the results from *B. mori*, these family members are putative candidates for cellular CBPs. Those proteins may be needed for delivering the lipophilic carotenoid substrates to BCO and/or for mediating the cellular transport of carotenoids in carotenoid-accumulating tissues.

Taken all together, these recent results coming from insects provide molecular insight into basic principles in animal carotenoid metabolism (Fig. 4). The identification of molecular players involved in cellular uptake, cellular transport, and metabolic conversion of carotenoids to retinoids may provide the key to understanding these processes as well in mammals.

V. GENE EXPRESSION OF CAROTENOID-OXYGENASES IN ADULT VERTEBRATES

Since the work of Moore (9) it has been known that vitamin A synthesis takes place in the small intestine in mammals. Subsequently, high BCO activity was also described in liver (15). After the molecular cloning of BCOs their tissue-specific steady-state mRNA levels were analyzed by reverse transcription-polymerase chain reaction (RT-PCR) and Northern blot analyses. In chicken, the tissue-specific expression patterns of BCO were analyzed by a combination of Northern blot and in situ hybridization experiments. Its mRNA was mainly localized in liver, in duodenal villi, as well as in tubular structures of the lung and the kidney (36). In the mouse, BCO mRNA was detectable in small intestine

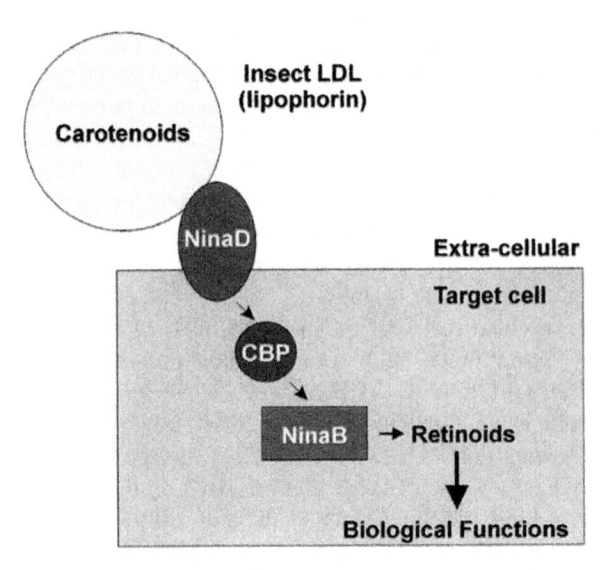

Figure 4 Schematic overview of the molecular players involved in insect carotenoid metabolism. The cellular uptake of carotenoids is mediated by the class II scavenger receptor *ninaD* from circulating lipophorins of the hemolymph (54). For the cellular transport specific carotenoid-binding proteins (CBP1) belonging to the StAR gene family exist (63). For retinoid synthesis carotenoids are converted by the BCO function encoded by the *ninaB* gene in *Drosophila* (42).

and liver but also in kidney, testis, uterine tissues, skin, and skeletal muscle (34,35,37). Analyses of BCO mRNA expression in humans revealed a comparable picture (39). Yan and colleagues (38) reported that BCO is preferentially expressed in the RPE of the human eye and only at much lower levels in other tissues. However, more recent results dealing with BCO expression in the eye showed only low mRNA levels in the RPE of humans and monkeys (66).

In mammals, a majority of provitamin A carotenoids are already converted to vitamin A in epithelial cells of the intestinal mucosa and are then transported to the liver for storage. However, the surprising result of all these current investigations is that BCO steady-state mRNA levels are quite high in peripheral nondigestive tissues. Testis, for example, requires retinoids for spermatogenesis, and vitamin A is needed for retinoid signaling in almost all tissues. Thus, BCO expression in peripheral tissues indicates that, besides an external vitamin A supply via the circulation, the provitamin A may contribute to local vitamin A demands. This inference is in agreement with the fact that in the circulation of mammals significant amounts of provitamin A carotenoids are present in addition to vitamin A derivatives. Interestingly, impairments in retinol transport caused by mutations leading to a loss of the RBP mainly affects the adult visual system in mice and humans (67,68). While the eyes have a tremendous demand for this vitamin, the amounts needed for retinoid signaling are much lower. Thus, it deserves to be investigated whether provitamin A carotenoids and the BCO function may contribute in peripheral tissues under certain physiological conditions and/or are essential to maintain retinoid-dependent biological processes.

Unlike vitamin A, high-dose supplementation of β-carotene in humans causes no hypervitaminosis A, indicating that β-carotene cleavage to vitamin A is tightly regulated. Several investigations with animal models showed that the vitamin A status of the individuals affects BCO enzymatic activity (69,70). Recent analyses provided evidence that BCO regulation in small intestine is mediated on the transcriptional level, possibly via a feedback regulation mechanism involving RA and its nuclear receptors (71). A role of retinoid signaling in the positive or negative regulation of retinoid-metabolizing enzymes on the transcriptional level has also been demonstrated for the retinal dehydrogenase, Aldh1, for the lecithin:retinol acyltransferase, LRAT, as well as for the RA-oxidizing enzyme CYP26 (72–74). More detailed analyses of BCO regulation now becomes feasible, including analyses of the BCO promoter, which will contribute to a better understanding of vitamin A homeostasis of the body, particularly under conditions in which carotenoids are the major source for this vitamin.

We also investigated the expression patterns of the excentric carotenoid-cleaving enzyme BCO-II in the mouse. BCO-II mRNA was expressed in the same tissues as BCO. In addition, low-abundance steady-state mRNA levels of BCO-II were present in spleen, brain, lung, and heart (35). The mRNA expression of both types of carotene oxygenases in the same tissues, e.g., small intestine and liver, confirms biochemical investigations and explains the observation of both centric and excentric cleavage activity in cell-free homogenates of the same tissue. However, it is not yet clear whether both enzymes are expressed in the same or in different cell types of these tissues, and this needs further elucidation.

Biological activities of β-apocarotenoids different from retinoids have been reported in various studies (e.g., 75,76). In vitro, BCO-II also catalyzed, besides β-carotene cleavage, the oxidative cleavage of lycopene (35). Favorable effects of lycopene, e.g., on certain kinds of cancers, have been repeatedly reported (77) (see also Chapter 18). Thus, besides being a putative precursor for RA formation in the case of β-carotene cleavage, it may be speculated that long-chain apocarotenoids per se may represent biologically active substances.

VI.   A VITAL ROLE OF BCO IN ZEBRAFISH EMBRYONIC DEVELOPMENT

Although animals convert carotenoids to vitamin A, it has been generally assumed that an external supply of dietary vitamin A maintains all retinoid-dependent physiological processes. Based on this supposition, a loss of the carotenoid oxygenase functions should have no consequences as long as dietary vitamin A is available. This seems valid for *Drosophila*, since the visual defects in the *ninaB* and *ninaD* mutants can be rescued at least under laboratory conditions by an external vitamin A supply (42,54). However, this question has not been fully answered for vertebrates, with a panoply of different vitamin A functions.

The vertebrate embryo is particularly sensitive to perturbations in its vitamin A levels. VAD results in embryonic malformations including hindbrain segmentation defects, neural crest cell death, absence of posterior branchial arches, as well as abnormalities of facial structures, limb buds, eyes, and somites (78–80). Using the zebrafish (*Danio rerio*) as an embryonic model, we addressed the question of whether BCO is needed for embryonic development. First, we demonstrated that BCO is expressed in clearly defined spatial compartments and translated into protein in zebrafish embryos (81). In addition, we demonstrated that the egg yolk of zebrafish contains, besides retinoids, significant amounts of β-carotene. To test whether there is an actual requirement for BCO during zebrafish embryonic development, we performed targeted gene knock-down experiments using morpholino *antisense* oligonucleotides. Loss of the BCO function resulted in abnormalities of the craniofacial skeleton, pectoral fins, and eyes, which are impairments well known from mammalian and zebrafish VAD embryos (81). Comparable impairments as caused by a BCO loss of function have been described in RA-deficient zebrafish *neckless* or *no-fin* mutants both caused by mutations in the retinal aldehyde dehydrogenase 2 (*raldh2*) gene or are provoked in wild-type embryos upon treatment with the retinal dehydrogenase inhibitor citral (81–84). Thus, these analyses suggest that provitamin A conversion is the prerequisite for RA signaling in several distinct developmental processes in zebrafish embryos and reveal a yet unexpected vital role of the provitamin in the development of a vertebrate species. The developmental use of the nontoxic provitamin instead of preformed yolk vitamin A for RA signaling processes may provide an additional control mechanism to finely balance retinoid levels at the cellular level in local tissue environments. Interestingly, embryonic expression of BCO has been also reported in mice, indicating that a developmental function of provitamin A may exist in mammals as well (34).

VII. CONCLUSIONS

The molecular identification of the different metazoan carotene oxygenases established the existence of an ancient family of nonheme iron oxygenases in animals. Via these enzymes animals have access to and can modulate their retinoids as needed for biological processes such as vision, cell differentiation, and development. With the increasing number of carotene oxygenases, this sequence information can be used to predict common structural features and to identify functional domains and active site residues. In the future, the biological role of these enzymes interlinking carotenoid and retinoid metabolism can be elucidated in more functional detail. This will include investigations dealing with biochemical, physiological, developmental, and medical aspects of carotenoids and their numerous derivatives. Furthermore, the identification of genes involved in carotenoid metabolism provides molecular markers to analyze genetic aspects of nutrient interactions and the basis to analyze genetic polymorphism in these genes within the population. The establishment of suitable animal model systems such as knockout mice in these genes may contribute to elucidating mechanisms underlying the pathogenesis of diseases as well as starting points for their prevention.

ACKNOWLEDGMENT

This work was supported by the German Research Foundation (DFG) by the Grant LI 956.

REFERENCES

1. Wald G. The molecular basis of visual excitation. Nature 1960; 219:800–807.
2. Vogt K. Is the fly visual pigment a rhodopsin. Z Naturforsch 1984; 39c:196–197.
3. Giguere V, Ong ES, Segui P, Evans RM Identification of a receptor for the morphogen retinoic acid. Nature 1987; 330:624–629.
4. Petkovich M, Brand NJ, Krust A, Chambon, P. A human retinoic acid receptor which belongs to the family of nuclear receptors. Nature 1987; 330:444–450.
5. Mangelsdorf DJ, Evans RM. The RXR heterodimers and orphan receptors. Cell 1995; 83:841–850.
6. Chambon P. A decade of molecular biology of retinoic acid receptors. FASEB J. 1996; 9:940–954.
7. Chawla A, Repa JJ, Evans RM, Mangelsdorf DJ. Nuclear receptors and lipid physiology: opening the X-files. Science 2001; 294:1866–1870.
8. Underwood B, Arthur P. The contribution of vitamin A to public health. FASEB J 1996; 9:1040–1048.

9. Moore T. Vitamin A and carotene. VI. The conversion of carotene to vitamin A in vivo. Biochem J 1930; 24:692–702.

10. Karrer P, Helfenstein A, Wehrli H, Wettstein, A. Über die Konstitution des Lycopins und Carotins. Helv Chim Acta 1930; 13:1084.

11. Glover J, Redfearn ER. The mechanism of the transformation of β-carotene into vitamin A in vivo. Biochem J 1954; 58:15.

12. Glover J. The conversion of β-carotene into vitamin A. Vitam Horm 1960; 18:371–386.

13. Goodman DS, Huang HS. Biosynthesis of vitamin A with rat intestinal enzyme. Science 1965; 149:879–880.

14. Olson JA, Hayaishi O. The enzymatic cleavage of beta-carotene into vitamin A by soluble enzymes of rat liver and intestine. Proc Natl Acad Sci U S A 1965; 54:1364–1370.

15. Goodman DS, Huang HS, Shiratori T. Mechanism of the biosynthesis of vitamin A from beta-carotene. J Biol Chem 1966; 241:1929–1932.

16. Fidge NH, Smith FR, Goodman DS. Vitamin A and carotenoids. The enzymic conversion of beta-carotene into retinal in hog intestinal mucosa. Biochem J. 1969; 114:689–694.

17. Lakshmanan MR, Chansang H, Olson JA. Purification and properties of carotene 15,15'-dioxygenase of rabbit intestine. J Lipid Res 1972; 13:477–482.

18. Nagao A, During A, Hoshino C, Terao J, Olson JA. Stoichiometric conversion of all trans-beta-carotene to retinal by pig intestinal extract. Arch Biochem Biophys 1996; 328:57–63.

19. Nagao A, Olson JA. Enzymatic formation of 9-cis, 13-cis, and all-trans retinals from isomers of beta-carotene. FASEB J 1994; 12:968–973.

20. Leuenberger MG, Engeloch-Jarret C, Woggon WD. The reaction mechanism of the enzyme-catalyzed central cleavage of beta-carotene to retinal. Angew Chem Int Ed Engl 2001; 40:2613–2617.

21. Wang XD, Tang GW, Fox JG, Krinsky NI, Russell RM. Enzymatic conversion of beta-carotene into beta-apo-carotenals and retinoids by human, monkey, ferret, and rat tissues. Arch Biochem Biophys 1991; 285:8–16.

22. Tang GW, Wang XD, Russell RM, Krinsky NI. Characterization of beta-apo-13-carotenone and beta-apo-14'-carotenal as enzymatic products of the excentric cleavage of beta-carotene. Biochemistry 1991; 30:9829–9834.

23. Sharma RV, Mathur SN, Ganguly J. Studies on the relative biopotencies and intestinal absorption of different apo-beta-carotenoids in rats and chickens. Biochem J 1976; 158:377–383.

24. Wang XD, Russell RM, Liu C, Stickel F, Smith DE, Krinsky NI. Beta-oxidation in rabbit liver in vitro and in the perfused ferret liver contributes to retinoic acid biosynthesis from beta-apocarotenoic acids. J Biol Chem 1996; 271:26490–26498.

25. Schwartz SH, Tan BC, Gage DA, Zeevaart JA, McCarty DR. Specific oxidative cleavage of carotenoids by VP14 of maize. Science 1997; 276:1872–1874.

26. Winterhalter P, Rouseff RL. Carotenoid-Derived Aroma Compounds. Washington, DC; American Chemical Society, 2002.

27. Buttery RG, Teranishi, R, Ling LC, Flath RA, Stern DJ. Quantitative studies on origins of fresh tomato volatiles. J Agric Food Chem 1988; 36:1257–1250.

28. Schwartz SH, Qin X, Zeevaart JA. Characterization of a novel carotenoid cleavage dioxygenase from plants. J Biol Chem 2001; 276:25208–25211.

29. Bouvier F, Suire C, Mutterer J, Camara B. Bouvier F, Suire C, Mutterer J, Camara B. Oxidative remodeling of chromoplast carotenoids: identification of the carotenoid dioxygenase CsCCD and CsZCD genes involved in crocus secondary metabolite biogenesis. Plant Cell 2003; 1:47–62.

30. Hundle BS, Alberti M, Nievelstein V, Beyer P, Kleinig H, Armstrong GA, Burke DH, Hearst JE. Functional assignment of Erwinia herbicola Eho10 carotenoid genes expressed in Escherichia coli. Mol Gen Genet 1994; 245:406–416.

31. von Lintig J, Vogt K. Filling the gap in vitamin A research. Molecular identification of an enzyme cleaving beta-carotene to retinal. J Biol Chem 2000; 275:11915–11920.

32. Wyss A, Wirtz G, Woggon WD, Brugger R, Wyss, M, Friedlein A, Bachmann H, Hunziker W. Cloning and expression of beta,beta-carotene 15,15'-dioxygenase. Biochem Biophys Res Commun 2000; 271:334–336.

33. von Lintig J, Wyss A. Molecular analysis of vitamin A formation: cloning and characterization of beta-15,15'-dioxygenases. Arch Biochem Biophys 2001; 385:47–52.

34. Redmond TM, Gentleman S, Duncan T, Yu S, Wiggert B, Gantt E, Cunningham FX Jr. Identification, expression, and substrate specificity of a mammalian beta-carotene 15,15'-dioxygenase. J Biol Chem 2001; 276:6560–6565.

35. Kiefer C, Hessel S, Lampert JM, Vogt K, Lederer MO, Breithaupt DE, von Lintig J. Identification and characterization of a mammalian enzyme catalyzing the asymmetric oxidative cleavage of provitamin A. J Biol Chem 2001; 276:14110–14116.

36. Wyss A, Wirtz GM, Woggon WD, Brugger R, Wyss M, Friedlein A, Riss G, Bachmann H, Hunziker W. Expression pattern and localization of beta,beta-carotene 15,15'-dioxygenase in different tissues. Biochem J 2001; 354:521–529.

37. Paik J, During A, Harrison EH, Mendelsohn CL, Lai K, Blaner WS. Expression and characterization of a murine enzyme able to cleave beta-carotene: the formation of retinoids. J Biol Chem 2001; 276:32160–32168.

38. Yan W, Jang GF, Haeseleer F, Esumi N, Chang J, Kerrigan M, Campochiaro M, Campochiaro P, Palczewski K, Zack DJ. Cloning and characterization of a human beta,beta-carotene-15,15'-dioxygenase that is highly expressed in the retinal pigment epithelium. Genomics 2001; 72:193–202.

39. Lindqvist A, Andersson S. Biochemical properties of purified recombinant human beta-carotene 15,15'-monooxygenase. J Biol Chem 2002; 277:23942–23948.

40. Vogel S, Mendelsohn CL, Mertz JR, Piantedosi R, Waldburger C, Gottesman ME, Blaner WS. Characterization of a new member of the fatty acid-binding protein family that binds all-trans-retinol. J Biol Chem 2001; 276:1353–1360.

41. Napoli JL, Race KR. Biogenesis of retinoic acid from beta-carotene. Differences between the metabolism of beta-carotene and retinal. J Biol Chem 1988; 263:17372–17377.

42. von Lintig J, Dreher A, Kiefer C, Wernet MF, Vogt K. Analysis of the blind *Drosophila* mutant ninaB identifies the gene encoding the key enzyme for vitamin A formation in vivo. Proc Natl Acad Sci U S A 2001; 98:1130–1135.

43. Hamel CP, Tsilou E, Pfeffer BA, Hooks JJ, Detrick B, Redmond TM. Molecular cloning and expression of RPE65, a novel retinal pigment epithelium-specific microsomal protein that is post-transcriptionally regulated in vitro. J Biol Chem 1993; 268:15751–15757.

44. Bavik C-O, Levy F, Hellman U, Wernstedt C, Eriksson U. The retinal pigment epithelial membrane receptor for plasma retinol-binding protein. Isolation and cDNA cloning of the 63-kDa protein. J Biol Chem 1993; 268:20540–20546.

45. Redmond TM, Yu S, Lee E, Bok D, Hamasaki D, Chen N, Goletz P, Ma JX, Crouch RK, Pfeifer K Rpe65 is necessary for production of 11-cis-vitamin A in the retinal visual cycle. Nat Genet 1998; 20:344–351.

46. Zuker CS. The biology of *Drosophila* vision. Proc Natl Acad Sci U S A 1996; 93:571–576.

47. Matsumoto H, Isono K, Pye Q, Pak WL. Gene encoding cytoskeletal proteins in *Drosophila* rhabdomeres. Proc Natl Acad Sci U S A 1987; 84:985–989.

48. O'Tousa JE, Baehr W, Martin RL, Hirsh J, Pak WL, Applebury ML. The *Drosophila* ninaE gene encodes an opsin. Cell 1985; 40:839–850.

49. Shieh BH, Stamnes MA, Seavello S, Harris GL, Zuker CS. The ninaA gene required for visual transduction in *Drosophila* encodes a homologue of cyclosporin A-binding protein. Nature 1989; 338:67–70.

50. Schneuwly S, Shortridge RD, Larrivee DC, Ono T, Ozaki M, Pak WL. *Drosophila* ninaA gene encodes an eye-specific cyclophilin (cyclosporine A binding protein). Proc Natl Acad Sci U S A 1989; 86:5390–5394.

51. Montell C, Rubin GM. The *Drosophila* ninaC locus encodes two photoreceptor cell specific proteins with domains homologous to protein kinases and the myosin heavy chain head. Cell 1988; 52:757–772.

52. Stephenson RS, O'Tousa J, Scavarda NJ, Randall LL, Pak WL. In: Cosens DJ, Vince-Price D, eds. The Biology of Photoreception. Cambridge, MA: Cambridge University Press, 1983:477–501.

53. Giovannucci DR., Stephenson RS. Identification and distribution of dietary precursors of the *Drosophila* visual pigment chromophore: analysis of carotenoids in wild type and ninaD mutants by HPLC. Vision Res 1999; 39:219–229.

54. Kiefer C, Sumser E, Wernet MF, Von Lintig J. A class B scavenger receptor mediates the cellular uptake of carotenoids in Drosophila. Proc Natl Acad Sci U S A 2002; 99:10581–10586.

55. Rigotti A, Trigatti BL, Penman M, Rayburn H, Herz J, Krieger M. A targeted mutation in the murine gene encoding the high density lipoprotein (HDL) receptor scavenger receptor class B type I reveals its key role in HDL metabolism. Proc Natl Acad Sci U S A 1997; 94:12610–12615.

56. Kozarsky KF, Donahee MH, Rigotti A, Iqbal SN, Edelman ER, Krieger M. Overexpression of the HDL receptor SR-BI alters plasma HDL and bile cholesterol levels. Nature 1997; 387:414–417.

57. Jian B, de la Llera-Moya M, Ji Y, Wang N, Phillips MC, Swaney JB, Tall AR, Rothblat GH. Scavenger receptor class B type I as a mediator of cellular cholesterol efflux to lipoproteins and phospholipid acceptors. J Biol Chem 1998; 273:5599–5606.

58. Yancey PG, de la Llera-Moya M, Swarnakar S, Monzo P, Klein SM, Connelly MA, Johnson WJ, Williams DL, Rothblat GH. High density lipoprotein phospholipid

composition is a major determinant of the bi-directional flux and net movement of cellular free cholesterol mediated by scavenger receptor BI. J Biol Chem 2000; 275:36596–36604.

59. Tsuchida K, Arai M, Tanaka Y, Ishihara R, Ryan RO, Maekawa H. Lipid transfer particle catalyzes transfer of carotenoids between lipophorins of *Bombyx mori.* Insect Biochem Mol Biol 1998; 28:927–934.

60. Tsuchida, K, Wells MA. Isolation and characterization of a lipoprotein receptor from the fat body of an insect, *Manduca sexta.* J Biol Chem 1990; 265:5761–5767.

61. Tsuchida K, Soulages JL, Moribayashi A, Suzuki K, Maekawa H, Wells MA. Purification and properties of a lipid transfer particle from *Bombyx mori:* comparison to the lipid transfer particle from *Manduca sexta.* Biochim Biophys Acta 1997; 337:57–65.

62. Mardones P, Strobel P, Miranda S, Leighton F, Quinones V, Amigo L, Rozowski J, Krieger M, Rigotti A. Alpha-tocopherol metabolism is abnormal in scavenger receptor class B type I (SR-BI)-deficient mice. J Nutr 2002; 132:443–449.

63. Tabunoki H, Sugiyama H, Tanaka Y, Fujii H, Banno Y, Jouni ZE, Kobayashi M, Sato R, Maekawa H, Tsuchida K. Isolation, characterization, and cDNA sequence of a carotenoid binding protein from the silk gland of Bombyx mori larvae. J Biol Chem 2002; 277:32133–32140.

64. Stocco DM, Clark BJ, Reinhart AJ, Williams SC, Dyson M, Dassi B, Walsh LP, Manna PR, Wang XJ, Zeleznik AJ, Orly J. Elements involved in the regulation of the StAR gene. Mol Cell Endocrinol 2001; 177:55–59.

65. Soccio RE, Adams RM, Romanowski MJ, Sehayek E, Burley SK, Breslow JL. The cholesterol-regulated StarD4 gene encodes a StAR-related lipid transfer protein with two closely related homologues, StarD5 and StarD6. Proc Natl Acad Sci U S A 2002; 99:6943–6948.

66. Bhatti RA, Yu S, Boulanger A, Fariss RN, Guo Y, Bernstein SL, Gentleman S, Redmond TM. Expression of beta-carotene 15,15′ monooxygenase in retina and RPE-choroid. Invest Ophthalmol Vis Sci 2003; 44:44–49.

67. Quadro L, Blaner WS, Salchow DJ, Vogel S, Piantedosi R, Gouras P, Freeman S, Cosma MP, Colantuoni V, Gottesman ME. Impaired retinal function and vitamin A availability in mice lacking retinol-binding protein. EMBO J 1999 Sep 1; 18(17):4633–4644.

68. Biesalski HK, Frank J, Beck SC, Heinrich F, Illek B, Reifen R, Gollnick H, Seeliger MW, Wissinger B, Zrenner E. Biochemical but not clinical vitamin A deficiency results from mutations in the gene for retinol binding protein. Am J Clin Nutr 1999; 69:931–936.

69. van Vliet T, van Vlissingen MF, van Schaik F, van den Berg H. Beta-carotene absorption and cleavage in rats is affected by the vitamin A concentration of the diet. J Nutr 1996; 126:499–508.

70. Parvin SG, Sivakumar B. Nutritional status affects intestinal carotene cleavage activity and carotene conversion to vitamin A in rats. J Nutr 2000; 130:573–577.

71. Bachmann H, Desbarats A, Pattison P, Sedgewick M, Riss G, Wyss A, Cardinault N, Duszka C, Goralczyk R, Grolier P. Feedback Regulation of beta,beta-Carotene

15,15′-monooxygenase by retinoic acid in rats and chickens. J Nutr 2002; 132:3616–3622.

72. Elizondo G, Corchero J, Sterneck E, Gonzalez FJ. Feedback inhibition of the retinaldehyde dehydrogenase gene ALDH1 by retinoic acid through retinoic acid receptor alpha and CCAAT/enhancer-binding protein beta. J Biol Chem 2000; 275:39747–39753.

73. Zolfaghari R, Ross AC. Lecithin:retinol acyltransferase from mouse and rat. J Lipid Res 2000; 41:2024–2034.

74. Yamamoto Y, Zolfaghari R, Ross AC. Regulation of CYP26 (cytochrome P450RAI) mRNA expression and retinoic acid metabolism by retinoids and dietary vitamin A in liver of mice and rats. FASEB J 2000; 14:2119–2127.

75. Tibaduiza EC, Fleet JC, Russell RM, Krinsky NI. Excentric cleavage products of beta-carotene inhibit estrogen receptor positive and negative breast tumor cell growth in vitro and inhibit activator protein-1-mediated transcriptional activation. J Nutr 2002; 132:1368–1375.

76. Siems W, Sommerburg O, Schild L, Augustin W, Langhans CD, Wiswedel I. Beta-carotene cleavage products induce oxidative stress in vitro by impairing mito-chondrial respiration. FASEB J 2002; 16:1289–1291.

77. Stahl W, Sies, H. Lycopene: a biologically important carotenoid for humans ? Arch Biochem Biophys 1996; 336:1–9.

78. Wilson JG, Roth, CB, Warkany J. An analysis of the syndrome of malformations induced by maternal vitamin A deficiency. Effects of restoration of vitamin A at various times during gestation. Am J Anat 1953; 85:189–217.

79. Maden M, Gale E, Kostetskii I, Zile M. Vitamin A-deficient quail embryo have half a hindbrain and other neural defects. Curr Biol 1996; 6:417–426.

80. White JC, Shankar VN, Highland M, Epstein ML, DeLuca HF, Clagett-Dame M. Defects in embryonic hindbrain development and fetal resorption resulting from vitamin A deficiency in the rat are prevented by feeding pharmacological levels of all-trans-retinoic acid. Proc Natl Acad Sci U S A 1998; 95:13459–13464.

81. Lampert JM; Holzschuh J, Hessel S, Driever W, Vogt K, von Lintig J. Provitamin A conversion via the beta,beta-carotene-15,15′-oxygenase is essential for pattern for-mation and differentiation during zebrafish embryogenesis. Development 2003; 130:2173–2186.

82. Begemann G, Schilling TF, Rauch G-J, Geisler R, Ingham PW. The zebrafish neckless mutation reveals a requirement for raldh2 in mesodermal signals that pattern the hindbrain. Development 2001; 128:3081–3094.

83. Grandel H, Lun K, Rauch GJ, Rhinn M, Piotrowski T, Houart C, Sordino P, Kuchler AM, Schulte-Merker S, Geisler R, Holder N, Wilson SW, Brand M. Retinoic acid signalling in the zebrafish embryo is necessary during pre-segmentation stages to pattern the anterior–posterior axis of the CNS and to induce a pectoral fin bud. Development 2002; 129:2851–2865.

84. Marsh-Armstrong N, McCaffery P, Gilbert W, Dowling JE, Drager UC. Retinoic acid is necessary for development of the ventral retina in zebrafish. Proc Natl Acad Sci U S A 1994; 91:7286–7290.

16

Enzymatic Versus Chemical Cleavage of Carotenoids: Supramolecular Enzyme Mimics for β-Carotene 15,15′-Monooxygenase

Wolf-D. Woggon and Mrinal K. Kundu
University of Basel, Basel, Switzerland

I. ENZYMATIC, CENTRAL CLEAVAGE OF β-CAROTENE

The central cleavage of β-carotene **1** is most likely the major pathway by which mammals produce the required retinoids (1), in particular, retinal **2**, which is essential for vision and is subsequently oxidized to retinoic acid **3** and reduced to retinol **4**. An alternative excentric cleavage of **1** has been reported involving scission of the double bond at C-7′/C-8′ producing β-8′-apocarotenal **5**, which subsequently undergoes bond scission and β oxidation leading to **3** (Fig. 1) (2). The significance of carotene metabolites such as **2**, **3**, and **4** to embryonic development and other vital processes such as skin and membrane protection is discussed elsewhere in this book.

The enzyme catalyzing retinal **2** formation has been known to exist in many tissues for quite some time. Only recently, however, the active protein was identified in chicken intestinal mucosa (3) following an improvement of a novel isolation and purification protocol and was cloned in *Escherichia coli* and BHK cells (4,5). Iron was identified as the only metal ion associated with the (overexpressed) protein in a $1:1$ stoichiometry, and since a chromophore is absent in the protein heme coordination and/or iron complexation by tyrosine can be excluded. The structure of the catalytic center remains to be elucidated by X-ray crystallography, but it can be predicted that the active site contains a mononuclear iron complex presumably consisting of histidines and carboxylic

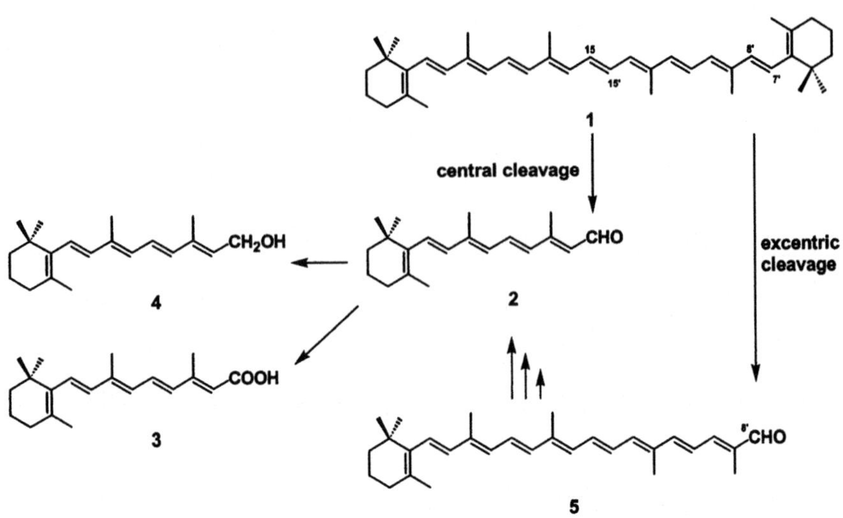

Figure 1   Central and excentric cleavage of β-carotene **1**.

acid residues. Furthermore, the enzymatic reaction mechanism was determined by incubating α-carotene **6**, a nonsymmetrical substrate of the enzyme, under a $^{17}O_2$ atmosphere in $H_2^{18}O$ followed by isolation and characterization of derivatives of cleavage products **2** and **7** (6). Accordingly, the enzyme cleaving the central double bond of **1** was found to be a nonheme iron monooxygenase and not dioxygenase as termed earlier (Fig. 2).

From the chemical point of view this enzymatic reaction is very unusual for various reasons: (a) the reaction proceeds completely regiospecific oxidizing only one E-configured, conjugated double bond out of nine in the linear part of the molecule; (b) the proposed mechanism implies a multistep sequence including epoxidation (see **8**), an epoxide hydrolase reaction, and C—C bond cleavage of the diol **9**. For each of these steps enzymatic reactions are known to exist. Epoxidation is known to be catalyzed by cytochromes P450 (7) as well as nonheme oxygenases (8). Epoxide hydrolases of bacterial origin have been developed so far as to become preparatively useful (9), and P450-catalyzed diol cleavage occurs during the side chain cleavage of cholesterol (10) and during the biosynthesis of biotin (11). However, a sequence of these three events catalyzed by a single enzyme seems to be quite unique, particularly when considering a nonheme monooxygenase as a cofactor with high-valence oxidation states for iron. Therefore, it is highly challenging to an organic chemist to design a synthetic catalyst that in principle can act the same way as the natural one does, to produce retinal **2** by selectively cleaving just the central C-15/C-15′ double bond

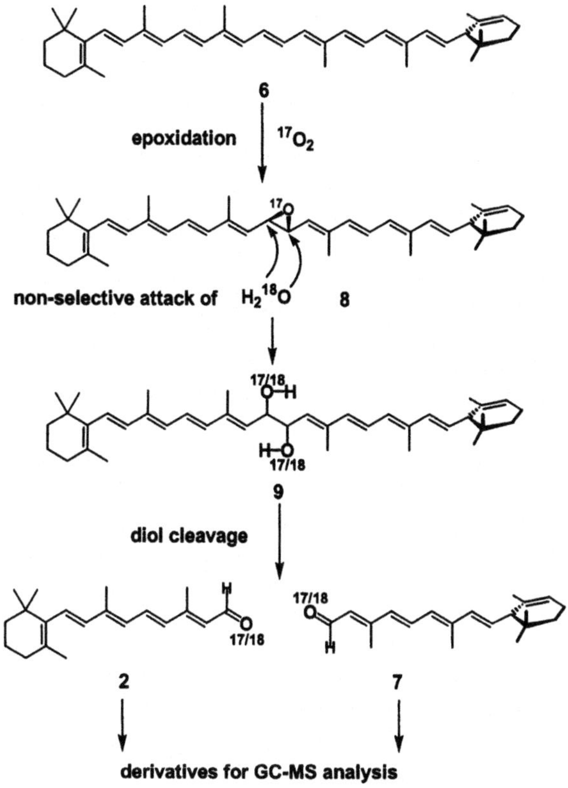

Figure 2 The reaction mechanism of the central cleavage of carotenoids.

of β-carotene **1**. Moreover, the mimic would definitely help to understand a plausible reaction pathway of this very special class of enzyme.

II. DESIGN AND SYNTHESIS OF ENZYME MIMICS OF β-CAROTENE 15,15'-MONOOXYGENASE

\In order to mimic such a regioselective system we envisaged to synthesize receptor **10** having the following fundamental criteria: (a) an association constant, K_a, of **1**–**10** that is orders of magnitude greater than that for retinal **2** so as to rule out any sort of product inhibition, (b) introduction of a reactive metal complex capable of cleaving E-configured double bonds; and (c) use of a co-oxidant that is not reactive to β-carotene **1** in the absence of the metal complex.

After initial molecular modeling studies using the MOLOC program (12), a supramolecular construct **10** consisting of two β-cyclodextrin moieties linked by a porphyrin spacer was designed for the binding of **1**. Each of the cyclodextrins was shown to be capable of binding one of the cyclohexenoid end groups of β-carotene **1**, leaving the porphyrin linker to span over the long polyene chain, which also shows, at least in static view, that the 15,15' double bond would be placed under the reactive metal center (Fig. 3). In the absence of **1**, different conformations of **10** are possible due to the rotation of the single bond around the ether linkages; in the presence of **1**, however, an induced fit should be observed yielding the inclusion complex **11**. Free-base porphyrins, such as **10** or its corresponding Zn complex **12**, display a characteristic fluorescence at around 600–650 nm, and the ability of carotenoids to quench this fluorescence was envisioned as a sensitive probe for the binding interaction of the two entities in an aqueous medium. It can be reasonably postulated that a cyclodextrin dimer such as **10** and **12** should be capable of providing a K_a for **1** in the region of 10^5–$10^7 \, M^{-1}$. Furthermore, one can expect K_a **(12)** $> K_a$ **(10)** due to conformational differences of the respective porphyrin macrocycles.

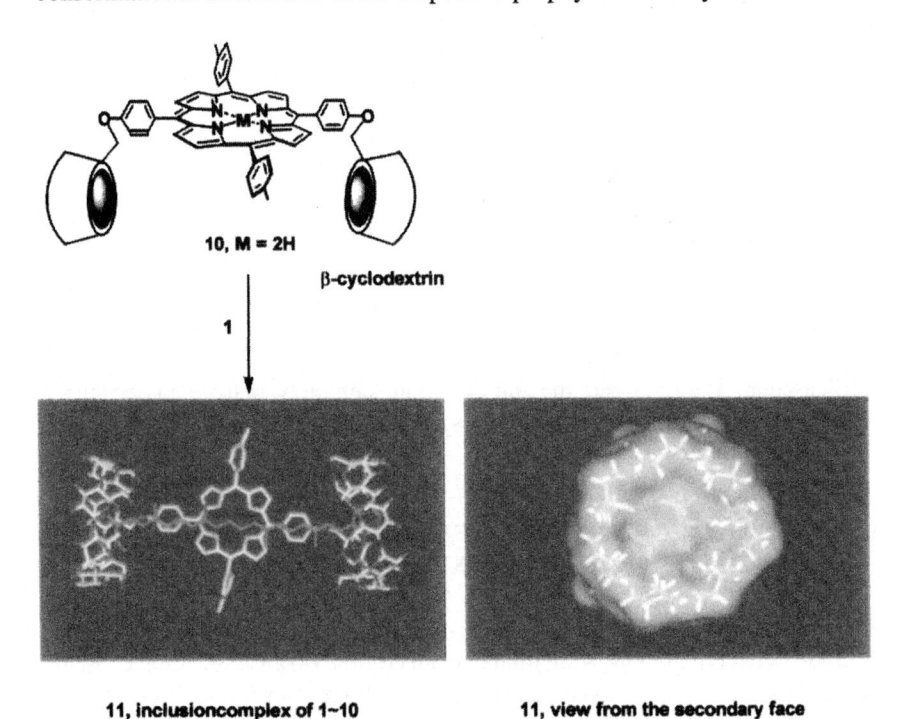

Figure 3 Inclusion complex of β-carotene **1** and the receptor **10**.

The syntheses of the receptors **10** and **12** were carried out by the treatment of bisphenol porphyrin **13** and its Zn complex **14**, respectively, with a large excess of β-cyclodextrin-6-O-monotosylate (CD-Tos) **15** using cesium carbonate as base in DMF (Fig. 4) (13). The synthesis was standardized under different conditions. Apart from cesium carbonate, a hindered organic base such as 1,8-diazabicycloundec-7-ene (DBU) was also found to be effective. However, DBU had to be used in large excess probably due to its inclusion in to the β-cyclodextrin cavity, rendering part of the base unavailable for the coupling reaction. The progress of the reaction was closely monitored by reverse-phase high-performance liquid chromatography (HPLC). It was noted that the reaction proceeds through the formation of mono-β-cyclodextrin porphyrins first and as the time progressed the appearance of the compound **10/12** was observed in the chromatogram; both the intermediates and **10/12** were easily detected by the characteristic Soret band at 420 nm.

The fluorescence quenching experiments (Fig. 5) revealed a binding constant K_a (**1–12**) = 8.3 × 10^6 M^{-1}. Due to its saddle-shaped conformation, the metal-free porphyrin **10** displays a smaller binding constant K_a (**1–10**) = 2.4 × 10^6 M^{-1} (13). This satisfied the first of our strategic criteria for mimicking the biological system, as the binding constant for retinal **2** to β-cyclodextrin is smaller by three orders of magnitude and hence no product inhibition should be expected after the oxidation of central double bond of β-carotene **1**.

For the choice of a metalloporphyrin capable of cleaving E-configured, conjugated double bonds, we chose a ruthenium porphyrin because preliminary experiments with (E,E)-1, 4-diphenyl-1,3-butadiene **17** and the complex **18** in the presence of *tert*-butylhydroperoxide (TBHP) looked promising, giving aldehydes **19** and **20** in good yield (Fig. 6) (14). The advantage of co-oxidants such as TBHP (or cumene hydroperoxide) is the inertness toward olefins in the absence of metal complexes. Accordingly, β-carotene **1** showed no degradation within 24 h when treated with excess of TBHP alone.

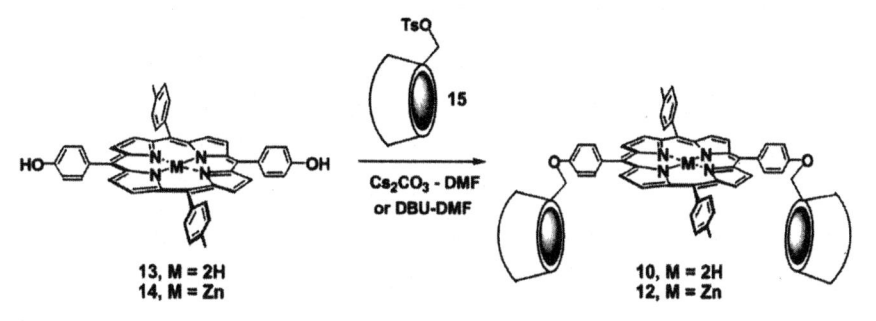

Figure 4 Syntheses of receptors **10/12**.

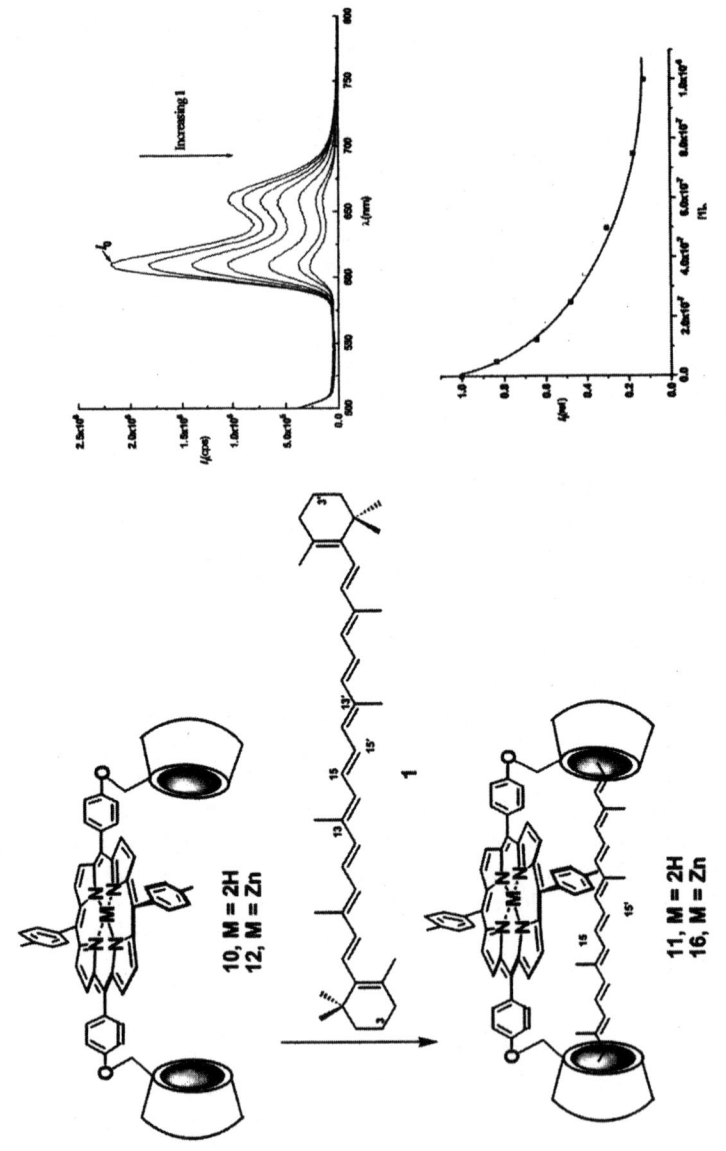

Figure 5 Quenching of the fluorescence of the receptors **10** and **12** on binding the substrate **1**, $\lambda_{exc} = 420$ nm, $\lambda_{em} = 654$ nm. Graph above: Overlayed fluorescence emission spectra of host **12** with increasing added concentrations of β-carotene **1**. Graph below: relative fluorescence intensities of aqueous solutions of **12** as a function of added β-carotene concentration. K_a was determined using a nonlinear least-squares fitting program (13).

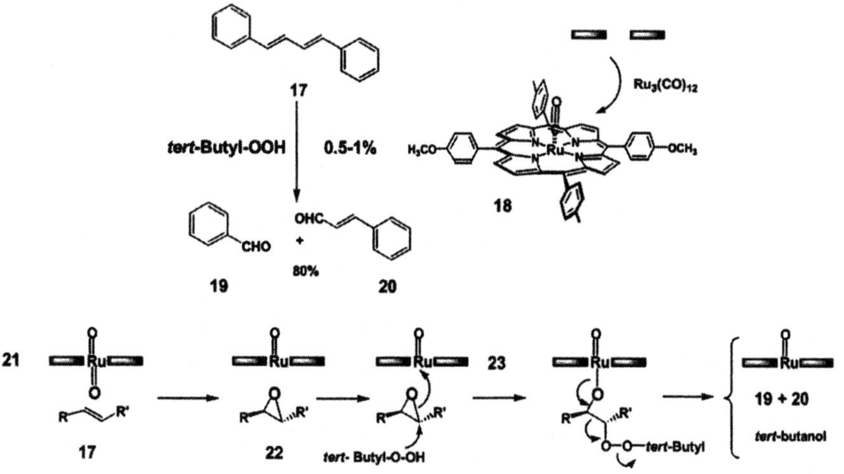

Figure 6 Ru porphyrin/TBHP-catalyzed double-bond cleavage.

A possible mechanism for this transformation, in principle also operating for the cleavage of carotenoids, involves O=Ru=O porphyrin **21**–catalyzed epoxidation to **22**, followed by nucleophilic attack of TBHP and ring opening with the assistance of **23**. Subsequent fragmentation yields the aldehydes (Fig. 6).

Finally, the synthesis of the biscyclodextrin Ru porphyrin receptor **24** was pursued in analogy to the preparation of **12** as described above, and the stage was set to attempt carotenoid cleavage. A biphasic system was established in which **1** was extracted from a 9:1 mixture of hexane and chloroform into water phase containing **24** (10 mol%) and TBHP. The reaction products, released from the receptor, were then extracted into the organic phase. Aliquots of these were subjected to HPLC conditions using a C_{30} reverse-phase column and detecting the signals at the respective wavelength of the formed apocarotenals and retinal, respectively, using a diode array UV-visible detector. Quantification was done by means of external calibration curves. The ratio of the reaction products is given in Figure 7. It is evident that **1** is not only cleaved at the central double bond but also at C-12′/C-11′ to give 12′-apocarotenal **25** and at C-10′/C-9′ to give 10′-apocarotenal **26** (13). The combined yield of aldehydes **2**, **25**, and **26** was 30%, which compares well with the efficiency of β-carotene 15,15′-monooxygenase giving retinal **2** in 20–25% yield (3).

At this point we considered two possible explanations leading to the cleavage of double bonds other than C-15/C-15′: (a) binding of β,β-carotene in an "unproductive" fashion, see **27** (Fig. 8), or (b) lateral movement of the substrate **1** within the two cyclodextrins rings, see **28**. The first possibility was investigated with the synthetic mono-bridged Ru porphyrin **29** (Fig. 8), for which

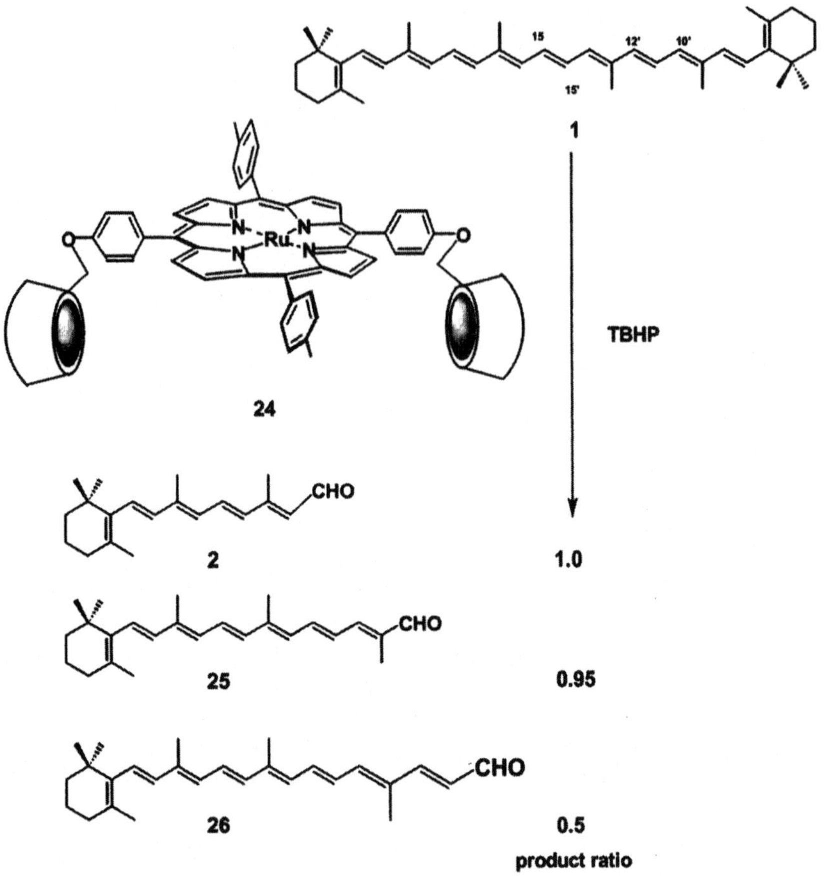

Figure 7 Cleavage of β-carotene **1** by **24**/TBHP.

the approach of **1** is only possible from one face (15). Reaction of β-carotene **1** with **29**/TBHP under the same conditions as described for **24** gave the same ratio of aldehydes **2**, **25**, and **26** as shown in Figure 7. Thus, it was concluded that the production of **25** and **26** is not due to substrate binding as shown in **27**, but rather due to the lateral movement of **1** within the cavities of the cyclodextrins (**28**, Fig. 8). Regarding the latter aspect, we reasoned that the selectivity of double-bond oxidation displayed by catalyst **24** should change if at least one of the end groups of the substrate **1** is exchanged for an equally hydrophobic substituent displaying different contacts with the interior of the β-cyclodextrin cavity. For this purpose, we chose cryptoxanthin derivatives **30** and **31**. Both compounds were oxidized with the same regioselectivity in favor of retinal **2** formation

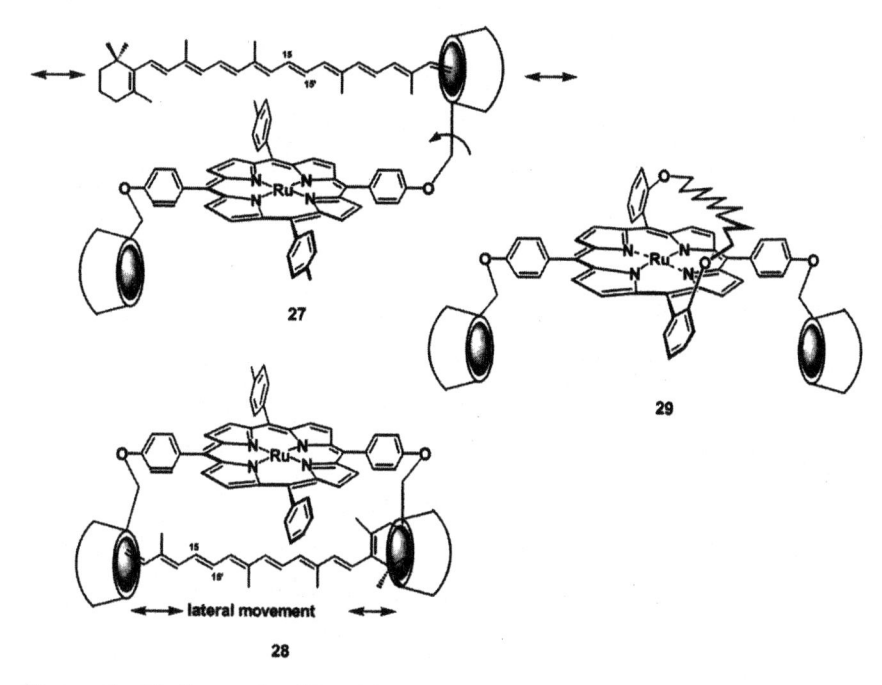

Figure 8 Binding modes, **27** and **28** of β,β-carotene **1** to the receptor **24**.

(Fig. 9) and are more selectively cleaved than β-carotene **1** (16). However, the best substrate was Phe-β-carotene **32**, a substrate analog of β-carotene 15,15′-monooxygenase (Fig. 9). Catalytic oxidation of **32** with the enzyme model **24**/ TBHP was indeed very regiospecific since only **2** and the corresponding Phe analog **33** were detected. This suggests that stronger hydrophobic interactions between the aromatic end group of **32** and the β-cyclodextrin cavity are responsible for stabilizing the 1 : 1 inclusion complex having the central double bond just under the reactive O=Ru=O center. In contrast, **1** slides within the cyclodextrin cavity exposing three double bonds rather than one to the reactive Ru=O. Determination of the binding constant of **32** to the receptor **10** supports this interpretation, i.e., K_a (**32**–**10**) = 5.0 × 10^6 M^{-1}, which is about two times larger than K_a (**1**–**10**) = 2.4 × 10^6 M^{-1}.

Thus, the supramolecular enzyme model **34** (Fig. 10), binding carotenoids purely by hydrophobic interactions, catalyzes the cleavage of these polyolefins in a way very similar to that of the enzyme β-carotene 15,15′-monooxygenase. However, the regioselectivity of the enzyme model depends on specific interactions of the end groups of carotenoids, reflected in different K_a values, with the hydrophobic interior surface of the β-cyclodextrins. In contrast, β-carotene 15,15′-monooxygenase exclusively catalyzes the bond scission of the central

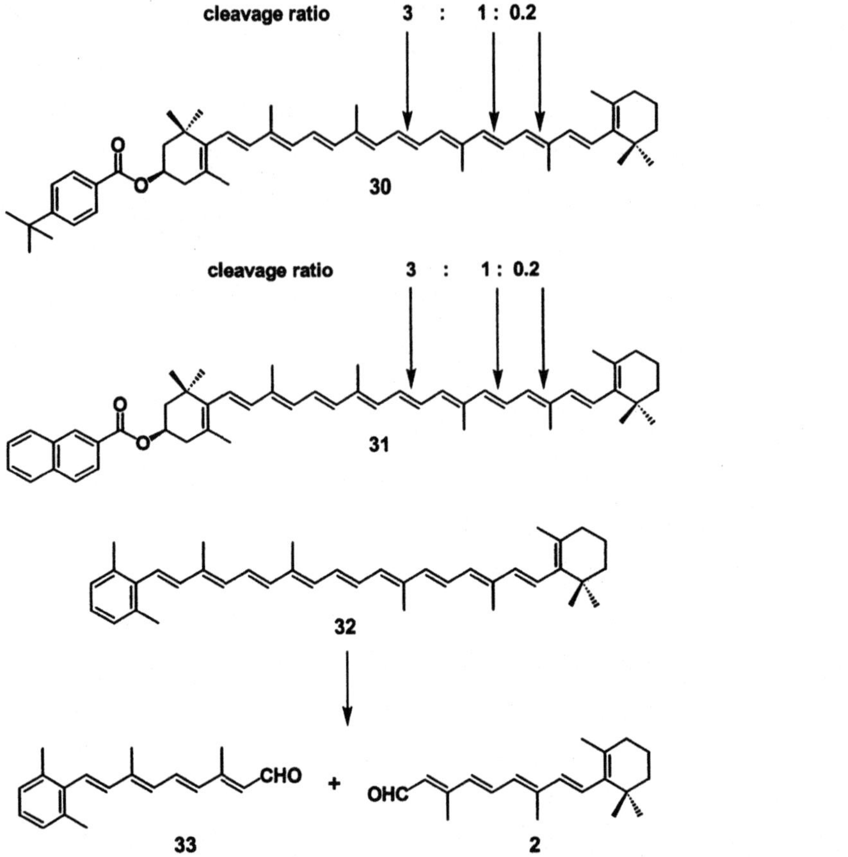

Figure 9 Oxidative cleavage of cryptoxanthin derivatives **30** and **31** and Phe-β-carotene **32** using the catalytic system **24**/TBHP.

double bond of all natural carotenoids investigated so far. Even artificial substrates such as **32** and **35**, lacking one methyl group in the polyene, are cleaved at the central double bond (Fig. 11) (17). Recently however, we observed two exceptions to the rule (18). The synthetic carotenoids **36** and **37**, originally designed as inhibitors, turned out to be substrates being cleaved at the C-14′/ C-15′ double bond. These results hint at hydrophobic interactions of the aromatic rings, placed in the center of the carotenoids, to aromatic residues of the ligand sphere of iron, most likely to the histidines. As a consequence, the substrate is "moved" within the active site by about 1.5 Å exposing the double bond adjacent to the usual one. Accordingly, hydrophobic interactions are significant to the regioselectivity of oxidation in both the enzyme and the enzyme mimic.

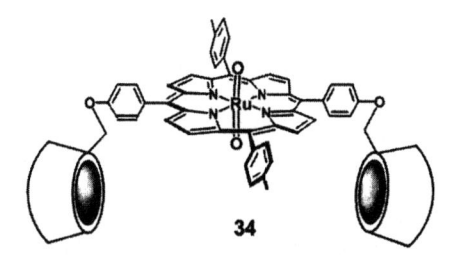

34

Figure 10 Structure of the supramolecular catalyst generated in situ from **24** and TBHP.

Even though cofactors of the enzyme and model compound are structurally and electronically very different the reaction sequences resemble each other, passing through an epoxide that opens to a diol or its equivalent, which subsequently fragments to aldehydes. To support our proposed mechanism of the enzymatic reaction (see Fig. 2), we attempted to prepare the central epoxide of β-carotene **38**. Since we had doubts that a building block with a doubly activated epoxide would survive a conventional synthesis of **38**, e.g., via Wittig reactions, we decided to employ catalyst **34** under optimized conditions for the generation and isolation of **38**. This approach was supported by the fact that, according to ¹H-NMR experiments (α-methylstyrene/**18**/TBHP), epoxide opening is the rate-determining step; thus, we had every reason to believe that the central epoxide of **1**, provided chemical stability, would accumulate within the first 1–2 h reaction time. First experiments with the established biphasic system and **1/34** indicated the formation of very small amounts of a compound displaying the expected UV ($\lambda_{max} \sim 330$ nm), correct mass (ESI-MS, m/z: 552), and ¹H NMR resonances corresponding to epoxide protons as reported (19). However, repeated HPLC purification did not furnish a spectroscopically pure compound in microgram quantities. We therefore abandoned the biphasic system, i.e., the excess of water, and turned to homogeneous reaction conditions. The most promising results have been obtained in DMF/**34**/TBHP. Actually an intense HPLC peak (about the same retention time as for the "epoxide" mentioned above) was observed displaying $\lambda_{max} = 332$ nm. Isolation of this compound and characterization by ESI-MS and two-dimensional NMR experiments led to assignment of the structure **39**, which in agreement with the UV displays a dominant retinyl ether chromophore, $J_{1,2} = 5.5$ Hz characteristic of a Z-configured double bond, and last but not least the absence of symmetry as expected for the epoxide **38**. Pursuing the same reaction in the NMR tube revealed in situ formation of **39** and excludes the possibility that **39** is an artifact obtained during workup/HPLC. The instantaneous reaction **38** to its isomer **39** can be explained by interaction of the O═Ru(IV) porphyrin with the epoxide **38**. Coordination of an epoxide to Ru was already evident during the formation of α-methylstyrene oxide (see above), but in the present case, given the

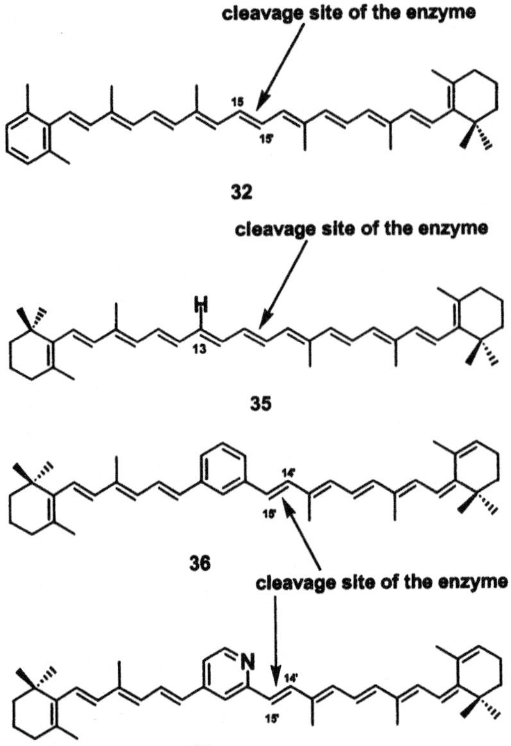

Figure 11 Regioselectivity of β-carotene 15,15′ monooxygenase action on nonnatural substrates.

highly activated epoxide, the system stabilizes by formation of a dihydro oxepin system (Fig. 12). A radical pathway, passing through intermediates **40** and **41**, seems to be most likely in particular since two double bonds are isomerized to adopt the Z configuration. In this context it is noteworthy that radical reaction have been invoked to explain the formation of both Z- and E-stilbene oxide from Z-stilbene using O=Ru=O tetramesityl porphyrin as catalyst (20).

III. CONCLUDING REMARKS

In this account the design and synthesis of a supramolecular enzyme mimic of β-carotene 15,15′-monooxygenase that binds carotenoids purely by hydrophobic interaction has been presented. Though structurally remote from the cofactor of

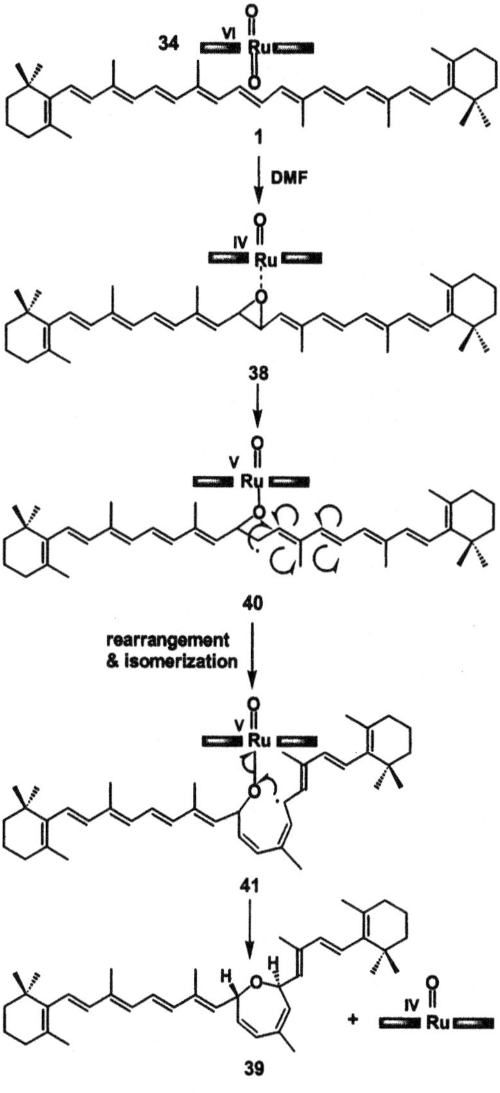

Figure 12 Ru-assisted transformation of the central epoxide **38** to the dihydro-oxepin **39**.

the corresponding protein the catalytic metal oxo center of this model has been shown to be efficient not only with respect to chemical reactivity but also regarding the regioselectivity of double-bond cleavage. Thus, our artificial system is one of the few enzyme mimics that catalyzes the transformation of unmodified, natural substrates of the respective enzyme.

Nevertheless there are some problems to solve regarding both the enzyme itself and the enzyme model. For example, we and others encountered difficulties in purifying the enzyme β-carotene 15,15' monooxygenase to full catalytic activity; somehow activity was lost during various chromatographic steps. The most likely explanation is the removal of the associated reductase required to reduce Fe(III) to Fe(II). Furthermore, the overexpressed protein must be crystallized, preferably in the presence of an inhibitor, in order to yield precise information about the cofactor. This certainly will not completely solve the problem of the unusual mechanism and related questions such as (a) those concerning the oxidation states of the Fe species that catalyzes the oxidative cleavage and (b) these concerning how the enzyme that obviously prefers rodlike substrates accommodates intermediates such as epoxides and diols. The "cofactor chemistry" of the enzyme mimic also needs further investigation of particular interest is the interaction of the Ru=O bond with E-configured double bonds, which obviously is quite different from approach of the corresponding Fe=O system. Also of interest is the Ru-assisted epoxide opening. Accordingly, the carotenoid adventure that began with one PhD student in our group in 1994 will continue.

REFERENCES

1. Britton G, Liaaen-Jensen S, Pfander H. Carotenoids today and challenge for the future. In: Britton G, Liaaen-Jensen S, Pfander S, eds. Carotenoids. Vol. 1A. Basel: Birkhäuser, 1995:13–26.
2. (a) Wang X-D, Tang G, Fox JG, Krinsky NI, Russell RM. Enzymatic conversion of beta-carotene into beta-apo-carotenals and retinoids by human, monkey, ferret, and rat tissues. Arch Biochem Biophys 1991; 258:8–16. (b) Yeum K-J, Dos Anjos Ferreira AL, Smith D, Krinsky NI, Russell RM. The effect of α-tocopherol on the oxidative cleavage of β-carotene. Free Radic Biol Med 2000; 29:105–114.
3. Wirtz G. Ueber die Substratspezifität und Reinigung der β-Carotin-15,15'-Dioxygenase. PhD dissertation, University of Basel, 1998.
4. Wyss A, Wirtz G, Woggon W-D, Brugger R, Wyss M, Friedlein A, Bachmann H, Hunziker W. Cloning and expression of β-carotene 15,15'-dioxygenase. Biochem Biophys Res Commun 2000; 271:334–336.
5. Wyss A, Wirtz G, Woggon W-D, Brugger R, Wyss M, Friedlein A, Bachmann H, Hunziker W. Expression pattern and localization of β-carotene 15,15'-dioxygenase in different tissues. Biochem J 2001; 354:521–529.
6. Leuenberger MG, Engeloch-Jarret C, Woggon W-D. The reaction mechanism of the enzyme-catalyzed central cleavage of β-carotene to retinal. Angew Chem Int Ed 2001; 40:2614–2617.
7. Woggon W-D. Cytochrome P450: significance, reaction mechanisms and active site analogues. In: Schmidtchen FP, ed. Bioorganic Chemistry, Models and Applications. Berlin: Springer-Verlag, 1996:39–96.

8. Ono T, Nakazono K, Kosaka H. Purification and partial characterization of squalene epoxidase from rat liver microsomes. Biochem Biophy Acta 1982; 709:84–90.

9. Drauz K, Waldmann H. Enzyme Catalysis in Organic Synthesis. Vol. 2. 2nd ed. Weinheim: Wiley-VCH, 2002.

10. Lieberman S, Lin YY. Reflections on sterol sidechain cleavage process catalyzed by cytochrome P450scc. J Steroid Biochem Mol Biol 2001; 78:1–14.

11. Stok JE, de Voss JJ. Expression, purification, and characterization of Biol: a carbon—carbon bond cleaving cytochrome P450 involved in biotin biosynthesis in *Bacillus subtilis*. Arch Biochem Biophys 2000; 384:351–360.

12. The MOLOC program was provided by F. Hoffmann–La Roche Inc., Basel.

13. French RR, Wirz J, Woggon W-D. A synthetic receptor for β-carotene. Towards an enzyme mimic for central cleavage. Helv Chim Acta 1998; 81:1521–1527.

14. French RR, Holzer P, Leuenberger MG, Woggon W-D. A supramolecular enzyme mimic that catalyzes the 15,15′ double bond scission of β-carotene. Angew Chem Int Ed 2000; 39:1267–1269.

15. French RR, Holzer P, Leuenberger MG, Nold MC, Woggon W-D. A supramolecular enzyme model catalyzing the central cleavage of carotenoids. J Inorg Biochem 2002; 88:295–304.

16. Holzer P. Ruthenium-Porphyrin-bis-Cyclodextrin-Komplexe als Supramolekulare Enzym-Modelle zur Regioselektiven Spaltung von Carotinoiden. PhD dissertation, University of Basel, 2002.

17. Wirtz GM, Bonemann C, Giger A, Müller RK, Schneider H, Schlotterbeck G, Schiefer G, Woggon W-D. The substrate specificity of β-carotene 15,15′-monooxygenase. Helv Chem Acta 2001; 84:2301–2315.

18. Leuenberger MG. The enzymatic cleavage of carotenoids: features and reaction mechanisms of the enzyme β-carotene 15,15′-monooxygenase. PhD dissertation, University of Basel, 2002.

19. Ben-Shabat S, Itagaki Y, Jockusch S, Sparrow JR, Turro NJ, Nakashi K. Formation of a nonaoxirane from A2E, a lipofuscin fluorophore related to macular degeneration, and evidence of singlet oxygen involvement. Angew Chem Int Ed 2002; 41:814–817.

20. Leung WH, Che CM. High-valent ruthenium(IV) and -(VI) oxo complexes of octaethylporphyrin. Synthesis, spectroscopy, and reactivities. J Am Chem Soc 1989; 111:8812–8818.

17
Relationship of Carotenoids to Cancer

Cheryl L. Rock
University of California, San Diego, La Jolla, California

I. INTRODUCTION AND KEY CONCEPTS

Cancer is a major health problem around the world (1). In the United States, cancer is the second leading cause of death, exceeded only by heart disease, with one of every four deaths in this country due to cancer (2,3). Over the past two decades, improvements in the five-year survival rates have been observed for some of the more common cancers in developed countries, presumably as a result of increased screening, earlier diagnosis, and improvements in initial treatments (3). As a result, there is an increasing population of cancer survivors, i.e., individuals who have successfully completed initial therapies but who are at increased risk for recurrence or new cancers, when compared with those who have not been diagnosed with cancer.

Carcinogenesis is a multistage process, resulting from multiple genetic and epigenetic events involving proto-oncogenes, tumor suppressor genes, and antimetastasis genes throughout progression (4). The cancer continuum extends from the earliest cellular changes, to a preneoplastic lesion, to a malignant tumor, and, finally, to metastasis. Although susceptibility to molecular and genetic changes in the process of carcinogenesis is likely linked to genetic or inherited factors, the epidemiological data, such as observations of cancer rates in migrant populations, strongly suggest that dietary factors play a role in approximately one-third of cancer cases (1,3).

Carotenoids exhibit several biological activities that could prevent or slow the progression of cancer. In addition to exhibiting antioxidant activity in vitro, carotenoids may influence carcinogenesis via effects on cell growth regulation, such as the inhibition of growth and malignant transformation and the promotion of apoptosis in transformed cells, similar to the effects of retinoids (5,6). The specific mechanisms by which carotenoids may reduce risk and progression of human cancers have not yet been elucidated, and the specific stages at which the biological activities of carotenoids may inhibit progression is unknown. Observational studies generally have examined the relationship between carotenoid intakes or tissue concentrations and various cancer indicators, such as the incidence of precursor lesions, diagnosis of cancer, or cancer deaths. The studies involving carotenoid supplements have tested the effect on cancer risk and progression in individuals who are at very high risk for cancer or in individuals who have already been diagnosed with precursor lesions or a primary cancer. Without knowledge of the specific mechanism or the point in the process at which carotenoids may exert a beneficial effect, interpreting the results of these epidemiological and clinical studies can be difficult.

An important consideration in the interpretation of observational studies that suggest associations between carotenoid intakes and cancer is that these compounds, whether quantified in the diet or assayed in tissue samples, reflect intake of vegetables and fruit, the major food sources of these compounds. These foods are complex, containing numerous constituents that have biological activities, so that assuming the specificity of a carotenoid association (or cause and effect) may be unwarranted. Conversely, vegetable and fruit intake may be considered a proxy for carotenoid intake. Plasma carotenoids are strongly and consistently associated with intake of vegetables and fruit in the diet in observational studies (7,8), and tissue concentrations increase in response to feeding or prescribing these foods (9–13) and in diet intervention studies that successfully promote increased vegetable and fruit intake (14–18). Another issue that is highly relevant to studies linking carotenoid intakes to cancer relates to the quality of the food content data. For these compounds, especially for the nonprovitamin A carotenoids, the quality of these data constrains the ability to accurately estimate carotenoid intakes in free-living populations. Improvements in the carotenoid database have occurred over the past few years (19), but the quality rating for food content data for these compounds remains low for most foods, indicating that data on carotenoid content are based on limited quantity and quality of assays. The actual amount of a carotenoid in a given food is influenced by genotype, plant maturity, climate, and other growing conditions, resulting in substantial inherent variability in the carotenoid content of the foods that are consumed and reported in the epidemiological studies (20) (see Chapter 11).

However, plasma concentrations of carotenoids are indicative of usual or habitual intakes of these compounds and are a more direct measure of exposure and potential biological activities in tissues. Thus, findings of an association between plasma or peripheral tissue carotenoid concentrations and risk for cancer are generally considered to be stronger support for the association when compared with findings based on dietary data alone.

This chapter summarizes results from major epidemiological studies and clinical trials relevant to the issue of whether carotenoids can influence the risk and progression of human cancers, with a focus on updating the findings presented in earlier reviews. The cancers highlighted are those for which available data and current evidence suggest a possible role for carotenoids or the major food sources of these compounds (vegetables and fruit) in their development and progression.

II. CAROTENOIDS AND LUNG CANCER

Lung cancer accounts for approximately 13% of the cancer diagnoses and is the major cause of cancer death in both men and women (31% and 25% of cancer deaths, respectively) in the United States (2,3). The incidence and death rates associated with lung cancer in men have been declining over the past decade, while death rates associated with lung cancer continue to increase in women (3).

Previous reviews of the overall association between nutritional factors and risk for lung cancer identified total vitamin A, β-carotene, and vegetables and fruit as the dietary factors most consistently associated with risk for lung cancer in earlier epidemiological studies (21–23). In fact, the strength and consistency of the inverse associations between intakes of β-carotene, yellow-orange and dark green vegetables, or plasma or serum β-carotene concentration, and risk for lung cancer provided strong support for the placebo-controlled clinical trials that tested the effect of β-carotene supplementation on lung cancer incidence in high-risk groups. The surprising results of these studies have been examined and reviewed in several commentaries from various perspectives (24–30).

As summarized in a 1996 review by Ziegler et al. (21), early observational studies consistently found the risk for lung cancer to be reduced in association with higher intakes of total vitamin A (inclusive of provitamin A carotenoids), vegetables (especially yellow-orange and dark green vegetables), and higher serum or plasma β-carotene. In a 1998 review conducted by the International Agency for Research on Cancer (IARC), all three of the cohort studies, all five of the case-control studies, and six of seven nested case-control studies that specifically examined the relationship between serum or plasma β-carotene and risk for lung cancer found lower circulating concentrations of β-carotene to be associated with increased risk (31). Relative risks (RRs) from the early observational studies of intakes and plasma concentrations typically indicated at least a 50% increase in risk in the lowest categories of carotenoid intake or serum β-carotene concentration, suggesting a substantial protective effect. Since those studies were published and reviewed, however, numerous observational studies have found protective associations between lung cancer risk and intakes or circulating concentrations of other carotenoids, as reviewed by Mayne (23). Specifically, more recent studies that have included analysis of associations with estimated intakes or serum concentrations of several carotenoids (and not simply quantifying β-carotene) have identified inverse relationships between lung cancer risk and intakes or blood levels of α-carotene, lutein, lycopene, and β-cryptoxanthin, in addition to inverse relationships between risk and intake (or serum levels) of β-carotene.

Since the last published review of this topic (23), the relationships between risk for lung cancer and intakes of carotenoids, carotenoid-rich vegetables and fruit, or circulating carotenoid concentrations have been examined within six cohorts and in two large case-control studies. Table 1 summarizes findings from the six most recent prospective studies. Findings from a multicenter case-control study of diet and lung cancer among nonsmokers (506 cases, 1045 controls) found protective effects for intakes of several items of interest, including tomatoes (odds ratio [OR] 0.5, 95% confidence interval [CI] 0.4, 0.6 for highest versus lowest tertile, $P = 0.01$ for trend), lettuce (OR 0.6, 95% CI 0.3–1.2, $P = 0.02$ for trend), carrots (OR 0.8, 95% CI 0.5, 1.1, not significant [NS]), total carotenoids (OR 0.8, 95% CI 0.6, 1.0, NS), and β-carotene (OR 0.8, 95% CI 0.6, 1.1, NS) (38). Darby et al. (39), in another large case-control study (1000 cases, 1500 controls), found intakes of carrots (relative risk [RR] 0.49, 95% CI 0.31, 0.78 for more than weekly versus never), tomato sauce (RR 0.69, 95% CI 0.55, 0.87 for few times per week or more versus never), and tomatoes (RR 0.74, 95% CI 0.57, 0.96 for 45+ g/day versus <16 g/day) to be significantly inversely associated with lung cancer risk. Intake of carotene, which was defined as β-carotene equivalents, had a significant protective association when adjusted for age and sex (RR 0.56, 95% CI 0.45, 0.71 for 2512 + µg/day versus <1305 µg/day, $P < 0.001$ for trend) but this protective effect was attenuated when smoking was added as an adjustment factor (RR 0.74, 95% CI 0.56, 0.96, $P = 0.06$ for trend) in that study. Thus, the more recent studies fairly consistently indicate that the early data relating β-carotene intake or serum concentration to lung cancer risk may have incorrectly encouraged a reductionist approach by focusing solely on β-carotene. Results from the more recent studies that involve the collection and examination of data relating to other carotenoids suggest that eating a variety of vegetables and fruits containing the various carotenoids, in addition to β-carotene, may help to lower the risk for lung cancer, particularly among smokers and others who are at high risk.

Two placebo-controlled studies have specifically tested the effect of β-carotene supplementation on lung cancer incidence as the primary focus, and two additional randomized trials involving β-carotene supplementation included lung cancer incidence or mortality among the major outcome variables (40–43). Characteristics and results of these studies are summarized in Table 2.

Table 1 Prospective Studies of Carotenoids and Risk for Lung Cancer, 2000–2002

Study	Subjects and key characteristics	Analytical approach	Years of follow-up	Relevant variables analyzed	Key findings	Comments
Voorrips et al., 2000 (32)	58,279 men aged 55–69 years at baseline (939 lung cancer cases), Netherlands Cohort Study on Diet and Cancer	Case-cohort analysis	6.3 years	Dietary α-carotene, β-carotene, lutein + zeaxanthin, β-cryptoxanthin, lycopene	Significantly protective effect on lung cancer incidence for lutein + zeaxanthin (RR 0.75, 95% CI 0.54, 1.03 for highest vs. lowest quintile, $P = 0.005$ for trend) and β-cryptoxanthin (RR 0.72, 95% CI 0.53, 0.98, $P = 0.0002$ for trend). Associations strongest among current smokers and weaker for former smokers.	Adjusted for age, family history, smoking, SES, energy intake; lutein + zeaxanthin association NS when adjusted for intakes of vitamin C and folate
Ratnasinghe et al., 2000 (33)	9142 Chinese tin miners, 40% provided baseline blood sample (339 confirmed lung cancer cases, 108 had a prediagnosis blood sample)	Nested case-control study	6 years	Serum α-carotene, β-carotene, lutein + zeaxanthin, and β-cryptoxanthin	In the total group, serum β-cryptoxanthin directly associated with increased risk of lung cancer (OR 2.9, 95% CI 1.4, 5.8 for highest vs. lowest tertile). Among non–alcohol drinkers (52% of sample), significant inverse relationship between serum lutein + zeaxanthin and lung cancer incidence (OR 0.4, 95% CI 0.2, 1.1 for highest vs. lowest tertile, $P = 0.04$ for trend). Among drinkers, significant direct relationship for serum β-carotene, lutein + zeaxanthin, and β-cryptoxanthin ($P < 0.04$ for trend).	Adjusted for age, sex, date of blood draw, radon and tobacco exposure

(continued)

Table 1 *Continued*

Study	Subjects and key characteristics	Analytical approach	Years of follow-up	Relevant variables analyzed	Key findings	Comments
Michaud et al., 2000 (34)	46,924 men in the Health Professionals Follow-up Study and 77,283 women in the Nurses' Health Study (275 and 519 new cancer cases, respectively)	Longitudinal pooled analysis	12 years	Dietary intakes of α-carotene, β-carotene, β-cryptoxanthin, lutein + zeaxanthin, lycopene	Significantly reduced risk of lung cancer with increased intake of α-carotene (RR 0.75, 95% CI 0.59, 0.96 for highest vs. lowest quintile) and total carotenoids (RR 0.68, 95% CI 0.49, 0.94). Marginally significant protective effects of lutein + zeaxanthin (RR 0.81, 95% CI 0.64, 1.01, $P = 0.06$ for trend) and β-cryptoxanthin (RR 0.82, 95% CI 0.65, 1.02, $P = 0.07$ for trend). Lycopene intake significantly protective for current smokers (RR 0.63, 95% CI 0.45, 0.88).	Adjusted for age, smoking status, age at start of smoking, energy intake, and time period
Yuan et al., 2001 (35)	18,244 men ages 45–64 years participating in a prospective study of diet and cancer in Shanghai, China (209 lung cancer cases)	Nested case-control study	12 years	Serum α-carotene, β-carotene, lutein + zeaxanthin, β-cryptoxanthin, and lycopene	Prediagnostic serum β-cryptoxanthin significantly inversely associated with risk for lung cancer (RR 0.45, 95% CI 0.22, 0.92 for highest vs. lowest quartile). Serum levels of other carotenoids significantly inversely associated with risk only when not adjusted for smoking status.	Adjusted for smoking status

Rohan et al., 2002 (36)	56,837 women aged 40–59 years enrolled in the Canadian National Breast Screening Study (196 lung cancer cases)	Case-cohort analysis	9–13 years	Dietary intakes of α-carotene, β-carotene, β-cryptoxanthin, lutein + zeaxanthin, lycopene	No associations between carotenoid intakes and risk of lung cancer. Analyses within strata defined by current smoking status also revealed no significant relationships.	Adjusted for age, study allocation, study center, smoking status, and intakes of energy, vitamin C, folate, and dietary fiber
Holick et al., 2002 (37)	27,084 male smokers aged 50–69 years who participated in the α-Tocopherol, β-Carotene Cancer Prevention Study (1644 lung cancer cases)	Longitudinal analysis, Cox proportional hazards models	14 years	Dietary intakes of α-carotene, β-carotene, β-cryptoxanthin, lutein + zeaxanthin, lycopene, and fruit and vegetables; serum β-carotene	Fruit and vegetable intake significantly inversely associated with risk for lung cancer (RR 0.73, 95% CI 0.62, 0.86 for highest vs. lowest quintile). Significantly lower risks of lung cancer also observed for highest vs. lowest quintiles of intakes of lycopene (28%), lutein + zeaxanthin (17%), β-cryptoxanthin (15%), and total carotenoids (16%), and serum β-carotene (19%).	Adjusted for age, years smoked, cigarettes per day, study group assignment, supplement use, plasma cholesterol, and intakes of energy and fat (intakes not used as adjustment factors for serum β-carotene)

CI, confidence interval; NS, not significant; HR, hazard ratio; OR, odds ratio; RR, relative risk; SES, socioeconomic status.

Table 2 Placebo-Controlled Studies that Tested the Effect of β-Carotene Supplementation on Lung Cancer Incidence or Mortality

Study	Subjects and key characteristics	Intervention	Dosage of β-carotene	Years of follow-up	Key findings	Comments
Blot et al., 1993 (40)	29,584 men and women aged 40–69 years in the general population of Linxian, China, 30% smokers	Factorial design of combination vitamin and mineral supplements, including β-carotene, vitamin E, and selenium	15 mg/ day	5 years	Significantly lower overall mortality (RR 0.91, 95% CI 0.84, 0.99) and cancer incidence (RR 0.87, 95% CI 0.75, 1.00) in the group receiving β-carotene (plus vitamin E and selenium). Also associated with reduced risk of lung cancer death (RR 0.55, 95% CI 0.26, 1.14).	Involved a combination supplement that included β-carotene
Alpha-Toco-pherol, Beta-Carotene Cancer Preven-tion Study Group 1994 (41)	29,133 male smokers aged 50 to 69 years in Finland, 100% smokers	Factorial design (2 × 2, β-carotene and α-toco-pherol)	20 mg/ day	5–8 years (median 6.1)	Significantly increased lung cancer incidence in subjects administered β-carotene (RR 1.16, 95% CI 1.02, 1.33). Increased overall mortality (8%) also associated with β-carotene supplementation.	Adverse effect stronger in subjects smoking >20 cigarettes/ day (RR 1.25, 95% CI 1.07, 1.46) vs. 5–19 cigarettes/day (RR 0.97, 95% CI 0.76, 1.23), and in those with higher alcohol intake (≥11 g/ day) (RR 1.35, 95% CI 1.01, 1.81) vs. lower intake (RR 1.03, 95% CI 0.85, 1.24)

| Omennetal., 1996 (42) | 18,314 male and female smokers, former smokers, and workers exposed to asbestos, 60% smokers | Compared placebo to β-carotene plus retinol | 30 mg/day | 4 years | Significantly increased lung cancer incidence in subjects administered β-carotene (plus retinol) (RR 1.28, 95% CI 1.04, 1.57). Increased overall mortality (17%) also associated with β-carotene supplementation. | Higher risk for lung cancer in association with β-carotene in the highest vs. lowest quartile of alcohol intake (RR 1.99, 95% CI 1.28, 3.09), and current smokers had higher risk for lung cancer than former smokers |
| Hennekens et al., 1996 (43) | 22,071 male physicians aged 40 to 84 years, 11% smokers | Factorial design (2 × 2, β-carotene and aspirin) | 50 mg every other day | 12 years | No difference in the incidence of total cancer or lung cancer or overall mortality. | |

CI, confidence interval; RR, relative risk.

As revealed in follow-up analysis and summarized in the table, incidence of lung cancer increased in response to β-carotene supplementation in two of the studies, and this surprising adverse effect was more likely to occur among smokers and in those reporting higher alcohol consumption (44–46). Another interesting observation in both of these trials was that study participants with lower baseline β-carotene intakes or serum concentrations exhibited higher lung cancer incidence during the study, regardless of study group assignment (41,44,45), which is in agreement with the findings from the observational studies. Fourteen-year follow-up of participants in the Alpha-Tocopherol, Beta-Carotene (ATBC) Study more recently identified an inverse association between baseline serum β-carotene concentration and risk for lung cancer (37), in addition to protective effects in association with higher (versus lower) baseline intakes of vegetables and fruit and other carotenoids (lycopene, lutein + zeaxanthin, β-cryptoxanthin).

Based largely on the results of the randomized trials involving β-carotene supplements, the current consensus is that these supplements are not advisable for the general population (22,47). The association between increased intake of vegetables and fruit that are good sources of the various carotenoids, including α-carotene, β-carotene, lycopene, lutein, and β-cryptoxanthin, and reduced risk for lung cancer also is evident in the clinical trial data. With regard to formulating public health guidelines, the latter strategy appears to be a better translation of the totality of the epidemiological evidence.

Also, evidence from the clinical trials indicates that smokers are at particular risk for increased risk for lung cancer in response to high doses and tissue concentrations of β-carotene. Results from both observational studies and the randomized trials suggest that higher levels of alcohol consumption also may be associated with increased likelihood of adverse, rather than beneficial, effects of higher carotenoid intakes. These observations are highly relevant to recent evidence from laboratory studies aimed at identifying the mechanisms by which β-carotene and the other carotenoids may influence the progression of cancer of the lung.

In tissue culture studies, β-carotene has been shown to induce both qualitative and quantitative changes in lung cancer cells that suggest benefits (48), so the issue of safety versus harm seems likely to relate to dosage and tissue concentration. The bioavailability of β-carotene from the most common supplement formulation is considerably higher than the bioavailability from foods, so the tissue response to a given amount of a carotenoid is much greater from most supplements compared to the response to food sources. To date, the most convincing evidence that explains how high doses (or high tissue concentrations) of β-carotene can increase risk for lung cancer, especially among smokers, is based on laboratory animal studies. In ferrets, the effect of β-carotene supplementation at doses equivalent to 30 mg/day and 6 mg/day in humans, with and without smoke exposure, has been examined, and these studies show detrimental effects at the high level (but not at the low level) of β-carotene administration (49,50). The effect involves depletion of tissue retinoic acid and interference in normal retinoid signaling, which appears to be linked to metabolic effects of high concentrations of the carotenoid oxidative cleavage products rather than a specific pro-oxidant effect in bronchial epithelial cells (51). Based on the biochemical characteristics of carotenoids and these cleavage products, one would expect that the cytochrome P450 enzymes are responsible for metabolizing these compounds, similar to the established role of these enzymes in metabolizing retinoids (52). These enzymes are induced by high doses and tissue concentrations of carotenoids and their metabolites (reviewed in Ref. 28). Alcohol also induces these metabolizing enzymes. Chronic alcohol consumption has been shown to promote decreased hepatic vitamin A in humans and laboratory animals (53), although the effect of alcohol on tissue carotenoid concentrations is more variable in human studies. Ethanol administration in animals, or heavy drinking in humans, has been observed to promote increased serum and liver β-carotene concentration (54,55). In free-living subjects, including the ATBC Study population, alcohol intake is typically inversely associated with serum carotenoid concentrations (56–59), but this relationship is likely mediated by lower intakes of carotenoid-rich foods among heavy drinkers.

As noted above, eating more vegetable and fruit sources of several carotenoids (β-carotene, α-carotene, lutein, β-cryptoxanthin, and lycopene) has been fairly consistently associated with reduced (and not increased) risk for lung cancer. The increased risk for lung cancer that was observed in the β-carotene supplement trials occurred in smokers and in association with blood concentrations that are well beyond that achieved from food sources, unless the diet is very unusual and the amounts eaten are extraordinary.

III. CAROTENOIDS AND BREAST CANCER

Breast cancer is the most common invasive cancer among women in developed countries. Breast cancer accounts for 31% of the incident cancers and 15% of the cancer deaths among women in this country, with 203,500 United States women likely diagnosed with breast cancer in 2002 (2). Although the steadily increasing incidence rate that characterized the 1980s has leveled off over the past decade (2,3), breast cancer continues to be very common. Meanwhile, mortality rates have been observed to be declining, especially in younger women, and this reduction in death rate is presumed to be due to both earlier detection and improvements in the initial treatments (2). As a result of the reduction in mortality rate concurrent with continued high incidence rates, the number of women in the United States who are breast cancer survivors is increasing.

Evidence from cell culture studies strongly suggests specific beneficial effects of both provitamin A and nonprovitamin A carotenoids on the development and progression of breast cancer (60–62). The effects are similar to the effects of retinoids in mammary cells, promoting normalization of cell growth regulation via differentiation or apoptosis when appropriate. Over the past few decades, at least 20 observational epidemiological studies have examined the relationship between risk for primary breast cancer and intakes of carotenoids, although the vast majority of these studies examined intake of β-carotene but not other carotenoids. In addition, the relationship between risk for breast cancer and intake of vegetables and fruits, or a dietary pattern that emphasizes these foods, has been examined in several studies.

In the past few years, two large observational studies addressed the relationship between breast cancer risk and intake of vegetables and fruit using combined and pooled data. These pooled studies were based on combinations of published observational studies with different study designs, and they produced somewhat divergent results. In a meta-analysis of 26 studies (21 case-control and five cohort studies) published from 1982 to 1997, the relationships between risk for breast cancer and intakes of vegetables, fruit, β-carotene, and vitamin C were examined (63). Intake of vegetables exhibited the strongest protective effect (RR 0.75, 95% CI 0.66, 0.85 for high versus low consumption), while the relationship with fruit intake was not significant (RR 0.94, 95% CI 0.74, 1.11) (63). Data from 11 of these studies allowed analysis of β-carotene intake, which was significantly inversely associated with risk (RR 0.82, 95% CI 0.76, 0.91 for approximately >7000 versus <1000 $\mu g/day$). Results from this meta-analysis are very similar to a summary based on 19 case-control and three cohort studies reported in 1997 (1), which found at least a 25% reduction in risk for breast cancer associated with higher vegetable and fruit intake in the majority of the studies and greater consistency for vegetable compared to fruit intake. In a pooled analysis of 7377 incident breast cancer cases from women enrolled in eight prospective cohort studies, the protective effect of total fruit and vegetable intake was found to be small and nonsignificant (RR 0.93, 95% CI 0.86, 1.00 for highest versus lowest quintiles) (64). Differences in the study designs and in the approaches used to estimate intake likely contribute to these inconsistent results. The pooled analysis that relied exclusively on data from cohort studies is based on studies with a better design because the dietary data were collected prior to diagnosis. However, the number of fruit and vegetable questions on the various instruments used to collect the dietary data across the cohort studies in the pooled analysis varied over fourfold, and combining widely disparate ranges of servings and types of vegetables and fruits may have limited the ability to identify a relationship with risk.

Using dietary data from the large Canadian National Breast Screening Study ($n = 56,837$), the association between intake of carotenoids and risk for primary breast cancer was recently explored in a large case-cohort study (1452 cases, 5239 noncases) (65). Significant relationships between intakes of the major carotenoids and risk were not observed in this cohort of women within the time frame of follow-up (8–13 years).

Fewer studies have examined the relationship between plasma or serum concentrations of carotenoids, a better indicator of carotenoids in peripheral tissues and a marker of vegetable and fruit intake, and risk for breast cancer. In the largest prospective study that examined this relationship (66), the odds ratio for the lowest versus highest quartile of total serum carotenoids was 2.31 (95% CI 1.35, 3.96), with serum concentrations of β-carotene (OR 2.21, 95% CI 1.29, 3.79), α-carotene (OR 1.99, 95% CI 1.18, 3.34), and lutein (OR 2.08, 95% CI 1.11, 3.90) inversely associated with risk. In a recent small study that also relied on prediagnostic serum carotenoids in the examination of the relationship between these compounds and risk for breast cancer (67), a protective association was found for serum β-carotene (OR 0.41, 95% CI 0.22, 0.79 for highest versus lowest quintile, $P = 0.007$ for trend), lycopene (OR 0.55, 95% CI 0.29, 1.06, $P = 0.04$ for trend), and total carotenoids (OR 0.55, 95% CI 0.29, 1.03, $P = 0.02$ for trend), adjusted for potentially influencing variables. Similarly, a recent small case-control study (153 cases, 151 controls) found significantly lower risk in higher versus lower pretreatment serum concentrations of β-carotene (OR 0.47, 95% CI 0.24, 0.91) (68), adjusted for other factors known to influence risk for breast cancer.

Thus, the observational epidemiological studies relating intakes of carotenoids or vegetables and fruit to risk for primary breast cancer are somewhat inconsistent and not entirely supportive. However, studies of associations based on serological data are more consistently supportive, with significant beneficial associations evident for several carotenoids, including α-carotene, β-carotene, lutein, and lycopene, when these compounds are examined.

An area of current interest is the potential effect of carotenoids or their major food sources, vegetables and fruit, on overall survival following the diagnosis of breast cancer. Despite encouraging 5-year survival rates, women who have been diagnosed with breast cancer and have completed initial surgical and medical treatments remain at considerable risk for recurrent cancer, new primary breast cancers, and early death compared with women who have not been diagnosed and treated for breast cancer.

The relationship between overall survival or recurrence and diet composition has been examined in 13 studies involving cohorts of women who had been diagnosed with breast cancer, and eight of these studies examined associations between intake of vegetables and fruit and/or β-carotene (69). Of these eight, three found a significant inverse association with risk of death, one found a trend for an association, and one found a significant inverse association in women with node-negative disease, who comprised 62% of that cohort (but not in the total group that included all stages of invasive breast cancer) (69,70). In the studies that found an inverse relationship with survival and intakes of vegetables and fruit and/or β-carotene, the magnitude of the protective effect was a 20–90% reduction in risk for death.

Two large multicenter randomized controlled trials are currently testing the effect of diet modification on survival following the diagnosis of breast cancer, and one of them, the Women's Healthy Eating and Living (WHEL) Study, is specifically testing the effect of increased intake of vegetables and fruit that are good sources of carotenoids and other phytochemicals and micronutrients on recurrence and survival. The WHEL Study participants are 3088 women who have been diagnosed with stage I (40%), stage II (55%), or stage IIIA (5%) invasive breast cancer and who were randomized into an intervention group or comparison group, following completion of initial therapies and within 48 months of diagnosis (71). Randomization was stratified by age, stage of tumor, and clinical site, and two-thirds of the women were under 55 years of age at randomization. The primary emphasis of the WHEL Study diet intervention is on increased vegetable and fruit intake, with daily dietary goals that include five vegetable servings, 16 ounces of vegetable juice, and three fruit servings. Plasma carotenoids are being quantified in serial blood samples as a biomarker of adherence to the high-vegetable and fruit diet. Feasibility study data demonstrate significantly increased plasma concentrations of α-carotene, β-carotene, and lutein in the intervention group (15,72,73). Participants will be followed in the WHEL Study for an average of 8 years (through 2006), and the study has 82% power to detect a 19% difference in breast cancer events over that time frame (71). A notable characteristic of the WHEL Study is that biological samples are collected from all study subjects at baseline and regular intervals, resulting in a sample specimen bank that can be linked to a considerable amount of detail on diet, lifestyle factors, and disease characteristics. An important and recognized feature of breast cancer is the heterogeneity on a molecular level, and variable cellular characteristics are anticipated to be among the determinants of response to the diet intervention.

Of relevance, a randomized clinical trial of fenretinide, also known as N-(4-hydroxyphenyl)retinamide (4-HPR), a synthetic retinoid with some metabolic and tissue storage characteristics that are similar to those of carotenoids, has been conducted to test for effects on risk for a second breast malignancy in premenopausal and postmenopausal women with early stage breast cancer. For the total group, the incidence of new cancers in the control and treatment arms was not statistically significant; however, possible beneficial effects were observed in the subgroup of premenopausal women (contralateral breast cancer: adjusted hazard ratio [HR] 0.66, 95% CI 0.41–1.07; ipsilateral breast cancer: adjusted HR 0.65, 95% CI0.46, 0.92) (74).

Thus, current evidence suggests a possible role for carotenoids or carotenoid-rich foods in reducing the risk and progression of breast cancer, with the most consistently supportive evidence from studies in which prediagnostic serological data are used to classify exposure. Results from a clinical trial that is testing whether consuming a carotenid-rich, high-vegetable and fruit diet can influence risk for recurrence and survival will be known within the next few years.

IV. CAROTENOIDS AND COLORECTAL CANCER

Colon cancer is the third most common cancer in men and women and also the third most common cause of cancer death in the United States and other developed countries (2,3). Colon and rectal cancers have a well-established and defined continuum of cellular changes and associated lesions that appear to occur in the stepwise process of developing an invasive tumor (75). Few studies to date have specifically examined the association between dietary factors, such as carotenoids, and the distinct tumor mutations that characterize colon carcinogenesis. However, cell culture studies have shown specific beneficial biological effects of carotenoids in colon cancer cell lines, and the mechanisms appear to involve both antioxidant and cell growth regulatory activities (76,77). Adenomatous polyps are considered the precursors of most large-bowel cancers (75), and the major clinical trials that tested the effect of dietary factors on the development and progression of colon cancer have focused on this point in the continuum, with the outcome being recurrent polyps. However, most adenomas do not develop into colon carcinomas, and the point at which the most important and modifiable molecular changes relevant to the biological activities of carotenoids has not been established.

As previously reviewed (1,78,79), numerous observational epidemiological studies have examined associations between intakes of carotenoids or their major food sources (vegetables and fruit) and the risk for colon cancer. The majority of the case-control studies, and studies based on prediagnosis serum carotenoid concentrations, found intakes of carotenoids and/or vegetables and fruit, and serum carotenoid concentration, to be associated with reduced risk. Since the last published review (79), a few notable observational epidemiological studies have examined the relationships between risk for colon cancer and intakes of carotenoids, vegetables and fruit. A large prospective study of the relationship between vegetable and fruit intake and incidence of colon and rectal cancers (involving 88,764 women and 47,325 men) did not find this association to be significant (80). A large case-control study addressed the relationship between estimated intakes of the specific carotenoid and risk for colon cancer (1993 cases, 2410 controls) (81). In that study, lutein was found to be inversely associated with colon cancer in both men and women (OR 0.83, 95% CI 0.66, 1.04 for upper versus lowest quintile, $P = 0.04$ for trend), while associations with the other carotenoids were not significant.

Based on the strength of the early epidemiological evidence, the effect of β-carotene supplementation on various possible biomarkers of colon carcinogenesis was examined in small samples of subjects, and two large randomized controlled trials tested the effect of β-carotene supplementation on the risk for recurrence of adenomatous polyps (82,83). Results of these two large placebo-controlled studies are summarized in Table 3. A significant beneficial effect of β-carotene supplementation was not observed in either of these trials.

Increased vegetable and fruit intake was among the dietary goals in the Polyp Prevention Trial (PPT), a large multicenter study that aimed to test the effect of multifaceted diet modification on the recurrence of colorectal adenomas. In the PPT, 2079 men and women with a history of adenomatous polyps were randomized to the diet intervention arm or control arm (84). The goals of the intervention were a diet low in fat (<20% of energy), high in fiber (18 g/ 1000 kcal/day), and high in vegetables and fruit (3.5 servings/1000 kcal/day). At study end, the intervention group had increased vegetable and fruit intake by an average of 1.1 servings/1000 kcal/day, and average reported intake of total carotenoids increased by on average approximately 50% (85). However, total plasma carotenoids were increased by only 5% by on average at study end, which is considerably lower than has been observed in response to high-vegetable and fruit diet interventions in other studies (14–18), including an intervention study aimed at a similar population (17). No effect on adenoma recurrence was observed in the PPT, when analyzed on the basis on study group assignment. However, the limited effect of the intervention on circulating carotenoids suggests that this study may not have adequately tested the effect of a high-vegetable and fruit intake. Also, in a secondary analysis of a subcohort of study participants ($n = 701$), average serum α-carotene, β-carotene, lutein, and total carotenoid concentrations at four time points during the study were found to be associated with decreased risk of polyp recurrence (OR 0.71, 0.76, 0.67, and 0.61, respectively, $P < 0.05$) (86).

Thus, whether intakes of carotenoids, vegetables, and fruit can influence risk for colon cancer remains unresolved. Results from the clinical trials that tested whether β-carotene supplementation can reduce risk for adenomatous polyp recurrence do not indicate any efficacy for that strategy. Increased knowledge of mechanisms, which would provide information about the stage at which carotenoids might influence the development and progression of colon cancer, would enable better interpretation of epidemiological studies and inform the design of intervention studies.

Table 3 Randomized Controlled Trials of β-Carotene Supplementation and Recurrence of Colorectal Adenomatous Polyps

Study	Subjects and key characteristics	Intervention	Dosage of β-carotene	Years of follow-up	Key findings	Comments
Greenberg et al., 1994 (82)	864 men and women with an adenomatous polyp diagnosed within 3 months and removed	Factorial design (2 × 2, β-carotene, vitamin C, and vitamin E)	25 mg/day	4 years	No treatment effect of β-carotene on incidence of new adenomatous polyps	
MacLennan et al., 1995 (83)	306 men and women with a history of adenomatous polyps that were removed	Factorial design (2 × 2, dietary fat reduction, wheat bran fiber, and β-carotene)	20 mg/day	2–4 years	No treatment effect of β-carotene on incidence of new adenomatous polyps	β-Carotene associated with nonsignificant higher incidence of new polyps (OR 1.5, 95% CI 0.9, 2.5) and large adenomas (OR 2.4, 95% CI 0.8, 7.0), and fewer adenomas with moderate or severe dysplasia (OR 0.6, 95% CI 0.2, 1.6)

CI, confidence interval; OR, odds ratio.

V. CAROTENOIDS AND CERVICAL CANCER

Cervical cancer is the second most common cancer for women worldwide (1). However, death rates from this cancer in women in developed countries are lower than many other common cancers due to the promotion and availability of screening procedures (2,3). Nonetheless, the human suffering and costs linked to this cancer remain high even in developed countries because for every case of invasive cervical cancer there are an estimated 50 cases of abnormal cervical smears that require monitoring, follow-up, and, often, ablative treatment procedures (87). Invasive cervical cancer arises from a progression of epithelial cell changes across a continuum of lesions classified as cervical intraepithelial neoplasia (CIN) I, II, III, and carcinoma in situ, which are earlier stages of this disease. HPV is now recognized as the causal agent for cervical cancer and the precursor lesions, although a number of other factors, including dietary factors, are believed to be important determinants of whether the HPV virus persists, disrupts cellular function, and enables progression of disease in the exposed individual.

Evidence for an association between carotenoids and risk for cervical neoplasia or cancer is relatively consistent in the early observational epidemiological studies, although HPV status was not considered in these earlier studies. As reviewed in 1996 (88), dietary carotenoids were inversely associated with risk for cervical neoplasia in five of 10 case-control studies, serum carotenoids were inversely associated with risk in four of five studies, and serum carotenoids were found to be protective in one cohort study. Recent epidemiological studies, in which HPV status is considered in the assessment of risk, have found mixed results. Ho et al. (89) did not observe a significant relationship between plasma β-carotene and risk for CIN in a large case-control study (378 cases, 366 controls), when adjusted for HPV status. In a smaller case-control study (147 cases, 191 controls) in which plasma carotenoids were quantified, adjusted plasma cryptoxanthin concentration was inversely associated with risk for cervical dysplasia (adjusted OR 0.3, 95% CI 0.1, 0.8 for highest versus lowest quartiles) (90). In a nested case-control study of dietary factors and risk for cytological abnormalities of the cervix in HPV-positive women (251 cases, 806 controls), a nonsignificant lower risk with higher dietary β-carotene intake was observed (91). A case-control study of Native American women (81 cases, 160 controls) revealed that increasing adjusted tertiles of serum α-carotene (OR 0.46, 95% CI 0.21, 1.00), β-cryptoxanthin (OR 0.39, 95% CI 0.17, 0.91), and lutein (OR 0.40, 95% CI 0.17, 0.95) were associated with increased risk of CIN (92).

Another approach in the examination of the relationship between carotenoid status and cervical cancer focuses on an earlier point in the cervix cancer continuum. The relationships between persistent HPV infection (rather than cytological abnormalities of the cervix) and serum carotenoids was examined in 123 low-income Hispanic women (93). In this cohort, adjusted mean concentrations of serum β-carotene, β-cryptoxanthin, and lutein were on average 24% lower ($P < 0.05$) among women who were HPV positive at two time points as compared with those who were HPV negative at both time points or positive at only one time point. More recently, higher levels of vegetable consumption were found to be associated with a 54% decreased risk of HPV persistence (adjusted OR 0.46, 95% CI 0.21, 0.97 for highest versus lowest tertile, $P = 0.033$ for trend) in a prospective cohort study in which women were examined at three time points (94). Also, a 56% reduction in risk for HPV persistence (adjusted OR 0.44, 95% CI 0.19, 1.01 for highest versus lowest tertile, $P = 0.046$ for trend) was found to be associated with plasma cis-lycopene concentration in that study.

Based on the strength and consistency of the earlier observational studies, five randomized controlled trials testing whether β-carotene supplements could increase the rate of regression of cervical dysplasia were initiated, and all have been completed (95–99). As shown in Table 4, none of these studies found a beneficial effect compared with placebo.

A better test of the associations observed in epidemiological studies, in which the carotenoids that are consumed are from food rather than supplements, involves testing the effect of a carotenoid-rich diet, which would provide the various carotenoids in addition to other micronutrients (e.g., vitamin C, folate). In a randomized clinical trial testing this strategy, 149 women with cervical dysplasia (63% CIN I, 37% CIN II) were enrolled and randomized to the diet intervention arm or control arm and followed for one year (18). The diet intervention efforts resulted in a substantial increase in plasma carotenoid and peripheral tissue concentrations, with plasma concentrations of total carotenoids increasing nearly twofold in the intervention group. This study was recently completed, and analysis of response is currently underway.

An important issue in the interpretation of clinical trials targeting women with CIN is that the stage at which carotenoids may influence the progression of cervical cancer is unknown. In vitro studies suggest that carotenoids can induce growth retardation in cervical dysplasia cell lines and apoptosis in HPV-infected cells (100). However, a carotenoid-rich diet may have a more meaningful clinical effect earlier in the HPV exposure and infection process, and thus, the earlier part of the continuum may be a more appropriate target for intervention. Overall, most intervention studies conducted to date in this area have been constrained by limited statistical power. The spontaneous regression rate for this condition typically falls in the range at which the number of subjects needed to detect a treatment effect is very high.

In summary, results from observational epidemiological studies quite consistently suggest a possible beneficial role for carotenoids and consumption of vegetables and fruit in the risk and progression of cervical cancer. However,

Table 4   Randomized Controlled Trials of β-Carotene Supplementation and Regression of Cervical Intraepithelial Neoplasia

Study	Subjects and key characteristics	Intervention	Dosage of β-carotene	Months or years of follow-up	Key findings	Comments
De Vet et al., 1991 (95)	278 women diagnosed with CIN I, II, and III	Compared placebo to β-carotene	10 mg/day	3 months	No effect on regression and progression	Dietary β-carotene included in secondary analysis (NS)
Fairley et al., 1996 (96)	111 women diagnosed with atypia, HPV, CIN I and II	Compared placebo to β-carotene	30 mg/day	12 months	No difference in the regression rate, cervical cytology, or amount of HPV DNA present	
Romney et al., 1997 (97)	69 women diagnosed with CIN I, II, and III	Compared placebo to β-carotene	30 mg/day	9 months	No effect on regression and progression	Outcome analysis adjusted for severity of CIN and type-specific persistent HPV infection and continual HPV infection with a high viral load at baseline and 9 months
Mackerras et al., 1999 (98)	141 women diagnosed with atypia, CIN I	Factorial design (2 × 2, β-carotene and vitamin C)	30 mg/day	2 years	Regression rate was nonsignificantly higher in those randomized to β-carotene (HR 1.58, 95% CI 0.86, 2.93, $P = 0.14$)	Possible interaction effect of β-carotene and vitamin C ($P = 0.052$), with 7 of the progressed lesions in those receiving both supplements versus a total of 6 in the other three study groups
Keefe et al., 2001 (99)	103 women diagnosed with CIN II and III	Compared placebo to β-carotene	30 mg/day	2 years	Overall regression rate was similar between treatment groups	CIN regression was negatively correlated with serum retinol concentrations

CIN, cervical intraepithelial neoplasia; HR, hazard ratio; HPV, human papillomavirus; NS, not significant.

consistent evidence from β-carotene supplement trials indicates that this approach is unlikely to affect rate of regression in women who present with a preneoplastic lesion. Results from a clinical trial testing the effect of a high-vegetable and fruit diet intervention on progression of abnormal cervical cell cytology will provide additional information about this association.

VI. CAROTENOIDS AND OVARIAN CANCER

Ovarian cancer is the fifth most common cancer in U.S. women, but it is the fourth most common cause of cancer death in this group, in part because it is not typically diagnosed in the early stages (2,3). Compared with the number of studies that have examined the associations between intakes of carotenoids, vegetables, and fruit and risk for many other cancers, relatively few epidemiological studies have addressed these associations in ovarian cancer. Of the case-control studies in which the relationships between risk for ovarian cancer and carotenoids (or their major food sources, vegetables and fruit) have been examined, six studies found protective effects of vegetable and fruit intake (101–106) and four studies found protective effects of carotenoid intake (102,107–109).

The most recent case-control study (549 cases, 516 controls) that examined the relationship between risk for ovarian cancer and dietary carotenoid intakes was a population-based study in which intakes of the individual carotenoids were estimated (109). Adjusted total carotenoid intake was significantly inversely related to risk (OR 0.55, 95% CI 0.36, 0.84 for highest versus lowest quintile). Among the individual dietary carotenoids examined, intakes of α-carotene (OR 0.60, 95% CI 0.39, 0.90 for highest versus lowest quintile), β-carotene (OR 0.58, 95% CI 0.38, 0.89), and lycopene (OR 0.53, 95% CI 0.35, 0.82) also exhibited significant inverse relationships with risk.

To date, the relationship between serum carotenoids and ovarian cancer risk has been examined in only one very small prospective study (110). In that study, serum micronutrients from 35 women who had been diagnosed with ovarian cancer over a 14-year period were compared with values from 67 control subjects from the cohort. Serum carotenoids were not found to be significantly associated with risk. No significant relationships between risk for ovarian cancer and adult dietary intakes of β-carotene and fruits and vegetables were found in a recent large cohort study (111), although adolescent intake of vegetables and fruit was found to be protective (RR 0.54, 95% CI 0.29, 1.03 for women who consumed ≥ 2.5 servings/day versus lower intakes). To date, no clinical trials have tested whether carotenoid supplementation or dietary modification can influence the risk and progression of ovarian cancer. Evidence linking intakes of carotenoids and their food sources to risk for ovarian cancer is limited, although intriguing, and more data about this relationship would be useful and informative.

VII. CAROTENOIDS AND PROSTATE CANCER

Prostate cancer is the most common cancer among men in the United States (2,3), accounting for 30% of the cancer diagnoses. Prostate cancer deaths currently account for 11% of cancer deaths among U.S. men, and mortality rates are currently declining (2). Due to the increasing interest in a possible role for lycopene in the risk and progression of prostate cancer, a considerable amount of evidence relating to that association has been collected and reported within the past few years, and the reader is referred to Chapter 20 for review of that relationship.

As recently reviewed (112–114), results from observational epidemiological studies relating prostate cancer risk to intakes of carotenoids, vegetables, and fruit have been notably inconsistent, with some studies actually finding a positive association rather than a protective or null association. Approximately nine studies to date have examined prostate cancer risk and total fruit and vegetable intake (112–115), and a protective association with risk was found in only two of these studies. The majority of the observational studies have examined associations with intakes of selected vegetables and fruits or carotenoids, with mixed results. Because lycopene is the major carotenoid in the diets of U.S. men, it has been suggested that lycopene may serve as a proxy of overall or total vegetable intake rather than indicating a specific role in prostate cancer progression (113). In fact, when adjusted for total vegetable and fruit intake, cruciferous vegetables, but not tomatoes and tomato products, were the vegetable subtype found to be significantly associated with risk in a recent large case-control study (628 cases, 602 controls) (115). In that study, the adjusted odds ratio for total vegetable intake was 0.65 (95% CI 0.45, 0.94, $P = 0.01$ for trend) for ≥ 28 servings versus < 14 servings/week, and the adjusted odds ratio for cruciferous vegetable intake was 0.59 (95% CI 0.39, 0.90, $P = 0.02$ for trend) for ≥ 3 servings/week versus < 1 serving/week. They also found a protective effect for lutein + zeaxanthin intake at a level of marginal significance (OR 0.68, 95% CI 0.45, 1.00 for > 2000 μg/day versus < 800 μg/day, $P = 0.09$ for trend), but intakes of other carotenoids were unrelated to risk.

Interestingly, a beneficial effect of β-carotene supplementation on prostate cancer risk was observed in a subgroup of participants in one of the large placebo-controlled supplement trials discussed earlier in relation to lung cancer (43,116,117). In that study, men were administered 50 mg β-carotene every other day and were followed for 12 years. Men in the lowest (versus highest) quartile for plasma β-carotene at baseline had a marginally significant ($P = 0.07$)

increased risk for cancer over the trial period. When the men in the lowest quartile for baseline plasma β-carotene concentration were compared according to study group assignment, a significant beneficial effect on risk for prostate cancer was observed in those administrated β-carotene versus placebo (RR 0.68, 95% CI 0.46, 0.99). In fact, those investigators are continuing to investigate the effect of β-carotene supplementation (50 mg every other day, with or without vitamin C, vitamin E, and a daily multiple vitamin formulation) in 15,000 U.S. men aged 55 years and older, with total and prostate cancer among the outcomes to be examined in the Physicians' Health Study (PHS) II (117). PHS II has 80% power to detect a 30% reduction in risk of prostate cancer for β-carotene and each of the other agents under study (117).

Thus, the possible link between carotenoids other than lycopene and prostate cancer risk remains an area of interest, although the early observational epidemiological studies focused on β-carotene and total vegetable and fruit intake have been fairly inconsistent. The results of PHS II should provide more useful information about the effect of β-carotene supplementation on prostate cancer risk.

VIII. CAROTENOIDS AND CANCER OF THE ORAL CAVITY, PHARYNX, AND LARYNX (HEAD AND NECK)

In 2002, 28,900 cancers of the oral cavity, pharynx, and larynx were expected to be diagnosed in the Unties States, and these cancers were expected to account for 7400 cancer deaths that year (2,3). Treatment failure for these cancers remains common, despite earlier detection and some improvements in the initial treatments, and the overall 5-year survival rate is approximately 56% (3). Thus, a useful strategy for primary and secondary prevention of these cancers is sorely needed.

As previously reviewed (112,118), substantial epidemiological, clinical, and laboratory evidence has suggested a possible role for carotenoids in the risk and progression of cancer of the oral cavity. To date, the majority of the case-control and cohort studies that have examined the relationships between intake of carotenoids, vegetables, and fruit and risk for these cancers have found a protective effect (112,118), even among high-risk groups, such as tobacco users. However, the most compelling evidence for a beneficial effect of β-carotene is from studies that have tested the effect of administering this carotenoid on intermediate end points relevant to these cancers (reviewed in Ref. 118). As previously summarized, the majority of the clinical studies testing the effect of β-carotene administration have shown significantly increased remission rates in patients with oral leukoplakia, a preneoplastic lesion that indicates increased risk for squamous cancers of the oral cavity. In addition, β-carotene has been shown to be protective in rodent models of oral carcinogenesis (31).

Based on the strength and consistency of the epidemiological and laboratory evidence, a placebo-controlled trial testing the effect of β-carotene supplementation on 264 men and women with a recent history of head and neck cancer was conducted (119). Study participants received 50 mg β-carotene/day or placebo and were followed for a median of approximately 4 years. The intervention had no effect on risk for the primary outcome, which was second primary tumors plus local recurrences (RR 0.90, 95% CI 0.56, 1.45), and no effect on total mortality was observed (RR 0.86, 95% CI 0.52, 1.42). Other end points examined were second head and neck cancer (RR 0.69, 95% CI 0.39, 1.25) and lung cancer, a common site of second primary cancer in these individuals (RR 1.44, 95% CI 0.62, 3.39). Although not significant, the point estimate for lung cancer is in agreement with the adverse effect of high-dose β-carotene supplements that was observed in the two β-carotene supplementation trials aimed at primary prevention of lung cancer (41,42). In contrast, the point estimate for head and neck cancer is in the direction of benefit, although the effect was not statistically significant.

IX. CAROTENOIDS AND OTHER CANCERS

Although early observational epidemiological studies have fairly consistently found a protective effect of dietary carotenoids, vegetables and fruits, and serum β-carotene concentration on risk for esophageal and stomach cancer (1,112), results from β-carotene supplement trials that focused on these cancers as primary outcomes are inconsistent. A randomized placebo-controlled study involving 3318 men and women with esophageal dysplasia (a precancerous condition) in China, who were administered 15 mg β-carotene/day plus a multivitamin and mineral formulation (versus placebo), found no beneficial effect on incidence of cancer of the esophagus (RR 0.90, 95% CI 0.70, 1.16) or stomach (RR 1.21, 95% 0.90, 1.64) (120). However, a population-based study conducted in the same region found a significant reduction in risk for stomach cancer (RR 0.79, 95% CI 0.64, 0.99), and a point estimate suggestive of a protective effect on risk for esophageal cancer (RR 0.96, 95% CI 0.78, 1.18), in 29,584 men and women administered 15 mg β-carotene/day plus vitamin E and selenium followed for a 5-year period (40). The effect of 30 mg β-carotene/day with or without vitamin C or *H. pylori* treatment (versus placebo) also was examined in 631 individuals in Columbia with a confirmed precancerous gastric lesion (multifocal nonmetaplastic atrophy or intestinal metaplasia), who were followed for 6 years (121). Regression rates were statistically significantly increased in association with β-carotene supplementation for both conditions (RR 5.1, 95% CI 1.7, 15.0, and RR 3.4, 95% CI 1.1, 9.8, respectively).

Finally, results from early observational epidemiological studies suggested that carotenoids could have a role in the prevention of skin cancer (1,112), which also resulted in a trial testing the effect of β-carotene supplementation (122). The randomized placebo-controlled trial tested the effect of β-carotene supplementation on recurrent nonmelanoma skin cancer in 1805 men and women with a history of basal cell and squamous cell cancers of the skin (122). Study subjects were administered 50 mg/day β-carotene or placebo and were followed for 5 years, but no beneficial effects of supplementation were observed.

X. SUMMARY AND CONCLUSIONS

A few themes are apparent in the current epidemiological and clinical evidence relating carotenoids and their major food sources, vegetables and fruit, to cancer. In most cases, the strongest and most consistent associations of reduced risk with higher intakes of carotenoids are found in the observational epidemiological studies, in which the protective effect is linked to food sources (and dosages and tissue concentrations of these compounds that are achievable via foods). In contrast, the clinical trials have largely involved high-dose β-carotene supplementation. Current evidence from the supplement trials certainly does not rule out a specific biological role for carotenoids in the risk and prevention of cancer, although the strategy of β-carotene supplementation has generally not been shown to be efficacious in reducing cancer outcomes in the vast majority of the trials that have tested that approach.

It should not be surprising that compounds with the diverse and potent biological activities of carotenoids could have differential effects across the ranges of dosage and tissue concentration that are achieved via foods versus highly concentrated (and often more bioavailable) formulations. Increased risk for lung cancer among smokers and heavy drinkers as a result of high intakes and tissue concentrations of β-carotene suggests a bell-shaped curve for the relationship between carotenoids and cancer. This type of relationship also is suggested by findings from animal model laboratory investigations.

More studies testing the effect of increased intake of carotenoid-rich vegetables and fruit on cancer outcomes, in which substantial changes in intake are achieved in the target population, would be informative and are unlikely to be associated with increased risk or adverse effects. In addition to being sources of the various carotenoids (β-carotene, α-carotene, lutein, zeaxanthin, β-cryptoxanthin, and lycopene), these foods are good sources of a variety of nutrients and non-nutrient constituents that either help to meet nutritional requirements or are established as being beneficial in reducing risk for diseases, such as folate and dietary fiber. Furthermore, these foods have other potential health benefits in the diet; for example, they are low in energy density, a characteristic that may help to reduce total energy intake and thus facilitate better weight control (another nutritional factor related to cancer risk).

Also, the point in the biological and cellular continuum of cancer at which an effect of β-carotene, other carotenoids, or increased vegetable and fruit intake has been tested in the clinical trials conducted to date is of necessity quite limited and finite, due largely to the limitations in resources allocated to test for effects. Increased knowledge of mechanisms and the identification of the stages of carcinogenesis at which intervention could affect molecular activities would be enormously useful in the interpretation of observational data and in designing clinical trials.

Laboratory evidence suggests that carotenoids may indeed reduce risk and progression of cancer, but differential genetic susceptibility is likely to result in variable response and outcome among humans with similar dietary intakes. Examination of the interactions between nutritional and genetic factors also would substantially refine the conduct and interpretation of epidemiological studies and clinical trials in this area.

Continued evaluation of the various carotenoids, including α-carotene, β-cryptoxanthin, lutein, and lycopene, in addition to β-carotene, in both observational epidemiological studies and clinical trials may help to identify food choices or dietary patterns that may be specifically linked to lower risk of cancer. Guidance toward increased vegetable and fruit intake as a prudent measure to reduce risk and progression of cancer could be better refined on the basis of these types of data (123,124). Results from ongoing clinical trials testing effects of intakes of carotenoids, vegetables, and fruit also will help to inform and refine the public health guidelines aimed at reducing cancer incidence and mortality.

REFERENCES

1. World Cancer Research Fund/American Institute for Cancer Research. Food, Nutrition and the Prevention of Cancer: A Global Perspective. Washington, DC: American Institute for Cancer Research, 1997.
2. Jemal A, Thomas A, Murray T, Thun M. Cancer statistics, 2002. CA Cancer J Clin 2002; 52:23–47.
3. Cancer Facts and Figures 2002. Atlanta: American Cancer Society, 2002.
4. Harris CC. Chemical and physical carcinogenesis: advances and perspectives for the 1990s. Cancer Res 1991; 51(Suppl):5023S–5044S.
5. Krinsky N. The antioxidant and biological properties of the carotenoids. Ann N Y Acad Sci 1998; 854:443–447.

6. Bertram JS. Carotenoids and gene regulation. Nutr Rev 1999; 57:182–191.

7. Polsinelli ML, Rock CL, Henderson SA, Drewnowski A. Plasma carotenoids as biomarkers of fruit and vegetable servings in women J Am Diet Assoc 1998; 98:194–196.

8. Campbell DR, Gross MD, Martini MC, Grandits GA, Slavin JL, Potter JD. Plasma carotenoids as biomarkers of vegetable and fruit intake. Cancer Epidemiol Biomark Prev 1994; 3:493–500.

9. Haegele AD, Gillette C, O'Neill C, Wolfe P, Heimendinger J, Sedlacek S, Thompson HJ. Plasma xanthophyll carotenoids correlate inversely with indices of oxidative DNA damage and lipid peroxidation. Cancer Epidemiol Biomark Prev 2000; 9:421–425.

10. Muller H, Bub A, Watzl B, Rechkemmer G. Plasma concentrations of carotenoids in healthy volunteers after intervention with carotenoid-rich foods. Eur J Nutr 1999; 38:35–44.

11. Paiva SAR, Yeum KJ, Cao G, Prior RL, Russell RM. Postprandial plasma carotenoid responses following consumption of strawberries, red wine, vitamin C or spinach by elderly women. J Nutr 1998; 128:2391–2394.

12. Yeum LK, Booth SL, Sadowski JA, Liu C, Tang G, Krinsky NI, Russell RM. Human plasma carotenoid response to the ingestion of controlled diets high in fruits and vegetables. Am J Clin Nutr 1996; 64:594–602.

13. Broekmans WMR, Klopping-Ketelaars IAA, Schuurman CRWC, Verhagen H, van den Berg H, Kok FJ, van Poppell G. Fruits and vegetables increase plasma carotenoids and vitamins and decrease homocysteine in humans. J Nutr 2000; 130:1578–1583.

14. Maskarinec G, Chan CLY, Meng L, Franke AA, Cooney RV. Exploring the feasibility and effects of a high-fruit and -vegetable diet in healthy women. Cancer Epidemiol Biomark Prev 1999; 8:919–924.

15. Rock CL, Flatt SW, Wright FA, Faerber S, Newman V, Kealey S, Pierce JP. Responsiveness of serum carotenoids to a high-vegetable diet intervention designed to prevent breast cancer recurrence. Cancer Epidemiol Biomark Prev 1997; 6:617–623.

16. Le Marchand L, Hankin JH, Carter FS, Essling C, Luffey D, Franke AA, Wilkens LR, Cooney RV, Kolonel LN. A pilot study on the use of plasma carotenoids and ascorbic acid as markers of compliance to a high fruit and vegetable dietary intervention. Cancer Epidemiol Biomark Prev 1994; 3:245–251.

17. Smith-Warner SA, Elmer PJ, Tharp TM, Fosdick L, Randall B, Gross M, Wood J, Potter JD. Increasing vegetable and fruit intake: randomized intervention and monitoring in an at-risk population. Cancer Epidemiol Biomark Prev 2000; 9:307–317.

18. Rock CL, Moskowitz A, Huizar B, Saenz CC, Clark JT, Daly TL, Chin H, Behling C, Ruffin MT. High vegetable and fruit diet intervention in premenopausal women with cervical intraepithelial neoplasia. J Am Diet Assoc 2001; 101:1167–1174.

19. Holden JM, Eldridge AL, Beecher GR, Buzzard IM, Ghagwat S, Davis CS, Douglass LW, Gebhardt S, Haytowitz D, Schakel S. Carotenoid content of U.S. foods: an update of the database. J Food Comp Anal 1999; 12:169–196.

20. Beecher GR, Khachik F. Analysis of micronutrients in foods. In: Moon TE, Micozzi MS, eds. Nutrition and Cancer Prevention: Investigating the Role of Micronutrients. New York: Marcel Dekker, 1991, pp 103–158.

21. Ziegler RG, Mayne ST, Swanson CA. Nutrition and lung cancer. Cancer Causes Control 1996; 7:157–177.

22. Albanes D. Beta-carotene and lung cancer: a case study. Am J Clin Nutr 1999; 69(suppl):1345S–1350S.

23. Mayne ST. Nutrition and lung cancer. In: Coulston AM, Rock CL, Monsen ER, eds. Nutrition in the Prevention and Treatment of Disease. San Diego: Academic Press, 2001, pp 387–396.

24. Van Zandwijk N. Chemoprevention of lung cancer. Lung Cancer 2001; 34(Suppl):S91–S94.

25. Vainio H. Chemoprevention of cancer: lessons to be learned from beta-carotene trials. Toxicol Lett 2000; 112–113:513–517.

26. Goodman GE. Lung cancer: prevention of lung cancer. Thorax 2002; 57:994–999.

27. Cooper DA, Eldridge AL, Peters JC. Dietary carotenoids and lung cancer: a review of recent research. Nutr Rev 1999; 57:133–145.

28. Pryor WA, Stahl W, Rock CL. Beta carotene: from biochemistry to clinical trials. Nutr Rev 2000; 58:39–53.

29. Mayne ST, Handelman GF, Beecher G. Beta-carotene and lung cancer promotion in heavy smokers—plausible relationship? J Natl Cancer Inst 1996; 88:1513–1515.

30. Erdman JW, Russell RM, Rock CL, Barua AB, Bowen PE, Burri BJ, Curran-Celentano J, Furr H, Mayne ST, Stacewicz-Sapuntzakis M. Beta-carotene and the carotenoids: beyond the intervention trials. Nutr Rev 1996; 54:185–188.

31. International Agency for Research on Cancer. IARC Handbooks of Cancer Prevention. Vol. 2, Carotenoids. New York: Oxford University Press, 1998.

32. Voorrips LE, Goldbohm RA, Brants HAM, Van Poppell GAFC, Sturmans F, Hermus JJ, Van den Brandt PA. A prospective study on antioxidant and folate intake and male lung cancer risk. Cancer Epidemiol Biomark Prev 2000; 9:357–365.

33. Ratnasinghe D, Forman MR, Tangrea JA, Qiao Y, Yao SX, Gunter EW, Barrett MJ, Giffen CA, Erozan Y, Tockman MS, Taylor PR. Serum carotenoids are associated with increased lung cancer risk among alcohol drinkers, but not among non-drinkers in a cohort of tin miners. Alc Alcohol 2000; 35:355–360.

34. Michaud DS, Feskanich D, Rimm EB, Colditz GA, Speizer FE, Willett WC, Giovannucci E. Intake of specific carotenoids and risk of lung cancer in 2 prospective US cohorts. Am J Clin Nutr 2000; 72:990–997.

35. Yuan JM, Ross RK, Chu XD, Gao YT, Yu MC. Prediagnostic levels of serum beta-cryptoxanthin and retinol predict smoking-related lung cancer risk in Shanghai, China. Cancer Epidemiol Biomark Prev 2001; 10:767–773.

36. Rohan TE, Jain M, Howe GR, Miller AB. A cohort study of dietary carotenoids and lung cancer risk in women (Canada). Cancer Causes Control 2002; 13:231–237.

37. Holick CN, Michaud DS, Stolzenberg-Solomon R, Mayne ST, Pietinen P, Taylor PR, Virtamo J, Albanes D. Dietary carotenoids, serum beta-carotene, and retinol and risk of lung cancer in the alpha-tocopherol beta-carotene cohort study. Am J Epidemiol 2002; 156:536–547.

38. Brennan P, Fortes C, Butler J, Agudo A, Benhamou S, Darby S, Gerken M, Jockel KH, Kreuzer M, Mallone S, Nyberg F, Pohlabeln H, Ferro G, Bottetta P. A multicenter case-control study of diet and lung cancer among non-smokers. Cancer Causes Control 2000; 11:49–58.

39. Darby S, Whitley E, Doll R, Key T, Silcocks P. Diet, smoking and lung cancer: a case-control study of 1000 cases and 1500 controls in south-west England. Br J Cancer 2001; 84:728–735.

40. Blot WJ, Li JY, Taylor PR, Guo W, Dawsey S, Want GQ, Yang CS, Zheng SF, Gail M, Li GY, Yu Y, Liu B, Tangrea J, Sun Y, Liu F, Fraumeni JF, Jr, Zhang YH, Li B. Nutrition intervention trials in Linxian, China: supplementation with specific vitamin/mineral combinations, cancer incidence, and disease-specific mortality in the general population. J Natl Cancer Inst 1993; 85:1483–1492.

41. The Alpha-Tocopherol, Beta Carotene Cancer Prevention Study Group. The effect of vitamin E and beta carotene on the incidence of lung cancer and other cancers in male smokers. N Engl J Med 1994; 330:1029–1035.

42. Omenn GS, Goodman GE, Thornquist MD, Balmes J, Cullen MR, Glass A, Keogh JP, Meyskens FL, Valanis B, Williams JH, Barnhart S, Hammar S. Effects of a combination of beta carotene and vitamin A on lung cancer and cardiovascular disease. N Engl J Med 1996; 334:1150–1155.

43. Hennekens CH, Buring JE, Manson JE, Stampfer M, Rosner B, Cook NR, Belanger C, LaMotte F, Gaziano JM, Ridker PM, Willett W, Peto R. Lack of effect of long-term supplementation with beta carotene on the incidence of malignant neoplasms and cardiovascular disease. N Engl J Med 1996; 334:1145–1149.

44. Albanes D, Heinonen OP, Taylor PR, Virtamo J, Edwards BK, Rautalahti M, Hartman AM, Palmgren J, Freedman LS, Haapakoski J, Barrett MJ, Pietinen P, Malila N, Tala E, Liipo K, Salomaa ER, Tangrea JA, Teppo L, Askin FB, Taskinen E, Erozan Y, Greenwald P, Huttunen JK. Alpha-tocopherol and beta-carotene supplements and lung cancer incidence in the alpha-tocopherol, beta-carotene cancer prevention study: effects of base-line characteristics and study compliance. J Natl Cancer Inst 1996; 88:1560–1570.

45. Omenn GS, Goodman GE, Thornquist MD, Balmes J, Cullen MR, Glass A, Keogh JP, Meyskens FL, Valanis B, Williams JH, Barnhard S, Cherniack MG, Brodkin CA, Hammar S. Risk factors for lung cancer and for intervention effects in CARET, the beta-carotene and retinol efficacy trial. J Natl Cancer Inst 1996; 88:1550–1559.

46. Cook NR, Lee IM, Manson JE, Buring JE, Hennekens CH. Effects of beta-carotene supplementation on cancer incidence by baseline characteristics in the Physicians' Health Study (United States). Cancer Causes Control 2000; 11:617–626.

47. Food and Nutrition Board, Institute of Medicine. Dietary Reference Intakes for Vitamin C, Vitamin E, Selenium, and Carotenoids. Washington, DC: National Academy Press, 2000.

48. Prakash P, Manfredi TG, Jackson CL, Gerber LE. Beta-carotene alters the morphology of NCI-H69 small cell lung cancer cells. J Nutr 2002; 132:121–124.

49. Wang XD, Liu C, Bronson RT, Smith DE, Krinsky NI, Russell RM. Retinoid signaling and activator protein-1 expression in ferrets given beta-carotene supplements and exposed to tobacco smoke. J Natl Cancer Inst 1999; 91:60–66.

50.   Russell RM. Beta-carotene and lung cancer. Pure Appl Chem 2002; 74:1461–1467.
51.   Arora A, Willhite CA, Liebler DC. Interactions of beta-carotene and cigarette smoke in human bronchial epithelial cells. Carcinogenesis 2001; 22:1173–1178.
52.   Roberts ES, Vaz AD, Coon MJ. Role of isozymes of rabbit microsomal cytochrome P-450 in the metabolism of retinoic acid, retinol, and retinal. Mol Pharmacol 1992; 41:4527–4533.
53.   Leo MA, Aleynik SI, Aleynik MK, Lieber CS. Beta-carotene beadlets potentiate hepatotoxicity of alcohol. Am J Clin Nutr 1997; 66:1461–1469.
54.   Leo MA, Kim CI, Lowe N, Lieber CS. Interaction of ethanol with beta-carotene: delayed blood clearance and enhanced hepatotoxicity. Hepatology 1992; 15:883–891.
55.   Ahmed S, Leo MA, Lieber CS. Interactions between alcohol and beta-carotene in patients with alcoholic liver disease. Am J Clin Nutr 1994; 60:430–436.
56.   Albanes D, Virtamo J, Taylor PR, Rautalahti M, Pietinen P, Heinonen OP. Effects of supplemental beta-carotene, cigarette smoking, and alcohol consumption on serum carotenoids in the alpha-tocopherol, beta-carotene cancer prevention study. Am J Clin Nutr 1997; 66:366–372.
57.   Brady WE, Mares-Perlman JA, Bowen P, Stacewicz-Sapuntzakis M. Human serum carotenoids concentrations are related to physiologic and lifestyle factors. J Nutr 1996; 126:129–137.
58.   Drewnowski A, Rock CL, Henderson SA, Shore AB, Fischler C, Galan P, Preziosi P, Hercberg S. Serum beta-carotene and vitamin C as biomarkers of vegetable and fruit intake in a community-based sample of French adults. Am J Clin Nutr 1997; 65:1796–1802.
59.   Rock CL, Thornquist MD, Kristal AR, Patterson RE, Cooper DA, Neuhouser ML, Neumark-Sztainer D, Cheskin LJ. Demographic, dietary and lifestyle factors differentially explain variability in serum carotenoids and fat-soluble vitamins: baseline results from the sentinel site of the Olestra Post-Marketing Surveillance Study. J Nutr 1999; 129:855–864.
60.   Sumantran VN, Zhang R, Lee DS, Wicha MS. Differential regulation of apoptosis in normal versus transformed mammary epithelium by lutein and retinoic acid. Cancer Epidemiol Biomark Prev 2000; 9:257–263.
61.   Rock CL, Kusluski RA, Galvez MM, Ethier SP. Carotenoids induce morphological changes in human mammary epithelial cell cultures. Nutr Cancer 1995; 23:319–333.
62.   Prakash P, Krinsky NI, Russell RM. Retinoids, carotenoids, and human breast cancer cell cultures: a review of differential effects. Nutr Rev 2000; 58:170–176.
63.   Gandini S, Merzenich H, Robertson C, Boyle P. Meta-analysis of studies on breast cancer risk and diet: the role of fruit and vegetable consumption and the intake of associated micronutrients. Eur J Cancer 2000; 36:636–646.
64.   Smith-Warner SA, Spiegelman D, Yaun SS, Adami HO, Beeson WL, van den Brandt PA, Folsom AR, Fraser GE, Freudenheim JL, Goldbohm RA, Graham S, Miller AB, Potter JD, Rohan TE, Speizer FE, Toniolo P, Willett WC, Wolk A, Zeleniuch-Jacquotte A, Hunter DJ. Intake of fruits and vegetables and risk of breast cancer: a pooled analysis of cohort studies. JAMA 2001; 285:769–776.

65. Terry P, Jain M, Miller AB, Howe GR, Rohan TE. Dietary carotenoids and risk of breast cancer. Am J Clin Nutr 2002; 76:833–888.
66. Toniolo P, Van Kappel AL, Akhmedkhanov A, Ferrari P, Kato I, Shore RE, Riboli E. Serum carotenoids and breast cancer. Am J Epidemiol 2001; 153:1142–1147.
67. Sato R, Helzlsouer KJ, Alberg AJ, Hoffman SC, Norkus EP, Comstock GW. Prospective study of carotenoids, tocopherols, and retinoid concentrations and the risk of breast cancer. Cancer Epidemiol Biomark Prev 2002; 11:451–457.
68. Ching S, Ingram D, Hahnel R, Belby J, Rossi E. Serum levels of micronutrients, antioxidants and total antioxidant status predict risk of breast cancer in a case control study. J Nutr 2002; 132:303–306.
69. Rock CL, Demark-Wahnefried W. Nutrition and survival after the diagnosis of breast cancer: a review of the evidence. J Clin Oncol 2002; 20:3302–3316.
70. Holmes MD, Stampfer MJ, Colditz GA, Rosner B, Hunter DJ, Willett WC. Dietary factors and the survival of women with breast carcinoma. Cancer 1999; 86:826–835.
71. Pierce JP, Faerber S, Wright F, Rock CL, Newman V, Flatt SW, Kealey S, Jones VE, Wasserman L, Caan BJ, Haan M, Gold E, Hollenbach KA, Jones L, Marshall JR, Ritenbaugh C, Stefanick ML, Thomson C, Natarajan L, Gilpin EA. A randomized trial of the effect of a plant based dietary pattern on breast cancer recurrence: the Women's Healthy Eating and Living (WHEL) Study. Control Clin Trials 2002; 23:728–756.
72. Pierce JP, Faerber S, Wright FA, Newman V, Flatt SW, Kealey S, Rock CL, Hryniuk W, Greenberg ER. Feasibility of a randomized trial of a high-vegetable diet to prevent breast cancer recurrence. Nutr Cancer 1997; 28:282–288.
73. McEligot AJ, Rock CL, Flatt SW, Newman V, Faerber S, Pierce JP. Plasma carotenoids are biomarkers of long-term high vegetable intake in women with breast cancer. J Nutr 1999; 129:2258–2263.
74. Veronesi U, De Palo G, Marubini E, Costa A, Formelli F, Mariani L, Decensi A, Camerini T, Del Turco MR, Di Mauro MG, Muraca MG, Del Vecchio M, Pinto C, D-Aiuto G, Boni C, Campa T, Magni A, Miceli R, Perloff M, Malone WF, Sporn MB. Randomized trial of fenretinide to prevent second breast malignancy in women with early breast cancer. J Natl Cancer Inst 1999; 91:1847–1856.
75. Boland CR. The biology of colorectal cancer. Cancer 1993;71(Suppl):4181–4186.
76. Palozza P, Serini S, Maggiano N, Angelini M, Boninsegna A, Di Nicuolo F, Ranelletti FR, Calviello G. Induction of cell cycle arrest and apoptosis in human colon adenocarcinoma cell lines by beta-carotene through down-regulation of cyclin A and Bcl-2 family proteins. Carcinogenesis 2002; 23:11–18.
77. Palozza P, Calviello G, Serini S, Maggiano N, Lanza P, Ranelletti FO, Bartoli GM. Beta-carotene at high concentrations induces apoptosis by enhancing oxy-radical production in human adenocarcinoma cells. Free Radic Biol Med 2001; 30:1000–1007.
78. Potter JD. Nutrition and colorectal cancer. Cancer Causes Control 1996; 7:127–146.
79. Slatttery ML, Caan BJ. Nutrition and colon cancer. In: Coulston AM, Rock CL, Monsen ER, eds. Nutrition in the Prevention and Treatment of Disease. San Diego: Academic Press, 2001, pp 357–372.

80. Michels KB, Giovannucci E, Joshipura KJ, Rosner BA, Stampfer MJ, Fuchs CS, Colditz GA, Speizer FE, Willett WC. Prospective study of fruit and vegetable consumption and incidence of colon and rectal cancers. J Natl Cancer Inst 2000; 92:1740–1752.
81. Slattery ML, Benson J, Curtin K, Ma KN, Schaeffer D, Potter JD. Carotenoids and colon cancer. Am J Clin Nutr 2000; 71:575–582.
82. Greenberg ER, Baron JA, Tosteson TD, Freeman DH, Beck GJ, Bond JH, Colacchio TA, Coller JA, Frankl HD, Haile RW, Mandel JS, Nierenberg DW, Rothstein R, Snover DC, Stevens MM, Summers RW, Van Stock RW. A clinical trial of antioxidant vitamins to prevent colorectal adenoma. N Engl J Med 1994; 331:141–147.
83. MacLennan R, Macrae F, Bain C, Battistutta D, Cahpuis P, Gratten H, Lambert J, Newland RC, Ngu M, Russell A, Ward M, Wahlqvist ML. Randomized trial of intake of fat, fiber, and beta carotene to prevent colorectal adenomas. J Natl Cancer Inst 1995; 87:1760–1766.
84. Schatzkin A, Lanza E, Corle D, Lance P, Iber F, Caan B, Shike M, Weissfeld J, Burt R, Cooper MR, Kikendall JW, Cahill J. Lack of effect of a low-fat, high-fiber diet on the recurrence of colorectal adenomas. N Engl J Med 2000; 342;1149–1155.
85. Lanza E, Schatzkin A, Daston C, Corle D, Freeman L, Ballard-Barbash R, Caan B, Lance P, Marshall J, Iber F, Shike M, Weissfeld J, Slattery M, Paskett E, Mateski D, Albert P. Implementation of a 4-y, high-fiber, high-fruit-and-vegetable, low-fat dietary intervention: results of dietary changes in the Polyp Prevention Trial. Am J Clin Nutr 2001; 74:387–401.
86. Steck-Scott S, Lanza E, Forman M, Sowell A, Borkowf C, Albert P, Schatzkin A. Relationship between serum carotenoids and polyp recurrence: results from the Polyp Prevention Trial. FASEB J 2001;15:A62.
87. Franco EL. Understanding the epidemiology of genital infection with oncogenic and nononcogenic human papillomaviruses: a promising lead for primary prevention of cervical cancer. Cancer Epidemiol Biomark Prev 1997; 6:759–761.
88. Potischman N, Brinton LA. Nutrition and cervical neoplasia. Cancer Causes Control 1996; 7:113–126.
89. Ho EYF, Palan PR, Basu J, Romney SL, Kadish AS, Mikhail M, Wassertheil-Smoller S, Runowicz C, Burk RD. Viral characteristics of human papillomavirus infection and antioxidant levels as risk factors for cervical dysplasia. Int J Cancer 1998; 78:594–599.
90. Goodman MT, Kiviat N, McDuffle K, Hankin JH, Hernandez B, Wilkens LR, Franke A, Kuypers J, Kolonel LN, Nakamura J, Ing G, Branch B, Bertram CC, Kamemoto L, Sharma S, Killeen J. The association of plasma micronutrients with the risk of cervical dysplasia in Hawaii. Cancer Epidemiol Biomark Prev 1998; 7:537–544.
91. Wideroff L, Potischman N, Glass AG, Greer CE, Greer E, Manos MM, Scott DR, Burk RD, Sherman ME, Wacholder S, Schiffman M. A nested case-control study of dietary factors and the risk of incident cytological abnormalities of the cervix. Nutr Cancer 1998; 30:130–136.

92. Schiff MA, Patterson RE, Baumgartner RN, Masuk M, van Asselt-King L, Wheeler CM, Becker TM. Serum carotenoids and risk of cervical intraepithelial neoplasia in Southwestern American Indian women. Cancer Epidemiol Biomark Prev 2001; 10:1219–1222.
93. Giuliano AR, Papenfuss M, Nour M, Canfield LM, Schneider A, Hatch K. Antioxidant nutrients: associations with persistent human papillomavirus infection Cancer Epidemiol Biomark Prev 1997; 6:917–923.
94. Sedjo RL, Roe DJ, Abrahamsen M, Harris RB, Craft N, Baldwin S, Giuliano AR. Vitamin A, carotenoids, and risk of persistent oncogenic human papillomavirus infection. Cancer Epidemiol Biomark Prev 2002; 11:876–884.
95. De Vet HCW, Knipschild PG, Willebrand D, Schouten HJ, Sturmans FJ. The effect of beta-carotene on the regression and progression of cervical dysplasia: a clinical experiment. Clin Epidemiol 1991; 44:273–285.
96. Fairley CK, Tabrizi SN, Chen S, Baghurst P, Young H, Quinn M, Medley G, McNeil JJ, Garland SM. A randomized clinical trial of beta carotene vs placebo for the treatment of cervical HPV infection. Int J Gynecol Cancer 1996; 6:225–230.
97. Romney SL, Ho GYF, Palan PR, Basu J, Kadish AS, Klein S, Mikhail M, Hagan RJ, Chang CJ, Burk RD. Effects of β-carotene and other factors on outcome of cervical dysplasia and human papillomavirus infection. Gynecol Oncol 1997; 65:483–492.
98. Mackerras D, Irwig L, Simpson JM, Weisberg E, Cardona M, Webster F, Walton L, Ghersi D. Randomized double-blind trial of beta-carotene and vitamin C in women with minor cervical abnormalities. Br J Cancer 1999; 79:1448–1453.
99. Keefe KA, Schell MJ, Brewer C, McHale M, Brewster W, Chapman JA, Rose GS, McMeeken DS, Lagerberg W, Peng WM, Wilczynski SP, Anton-Culver H, Meyskens FL, Berman ML. A randomized, double blind, phase III trial using oral beta-carotene supplementation for women with high-grade cervical intraepithelial neoplasia. Cancer Epidemiol Biomark Prev 2001; 10:1029–1035.
100. Muto Y, Fujii J, Shidoji Y, Moriwaki H, Kawaguchi T, Noda T. Growth retardation in human cervical dysplasia–derived cell lines by beta-carotene through down regulation of epidermal growth factor receptor. Am J Clin Nutr 1995; 62(Suppl):1535S–1540S.
101. Shu XO, Gao YT, Yuan JM, Ziegler RG, Brinton LA. Dietary factors and epithelial ovarian cancer. Br J Cancer 1989; 59:92–96.
102. Engle A, Muscat JE, Harris RE. Nutritional risk factors and ovarian cancer. Nutr Cancer 1991; 15:239–247.
103. Risch HA, Jain M, Marrett LD, Howe GR. Dietary fat intake and risk of epithelial ovarian cancer. J Natl Cancer Inst 1994; 86:1409–1415.
104. Kushi LH, Mink PJ, Folsom AR, Anderston KE, Zheng W, Lazovich D, Sellers TA. Prospective study of diet and ovarian cancer. Am J Epidemiol 1999; 149:21–31.
105. Parazzini F, Chatenoud L, Chiantera V, Benzi G, Surace M, La Vecchia C. Population attributable risk for ovarian cancer. Eur J Cancer 2000; 36:520–524.
106. Bosetti C, Negri E, Franceschi S, Pelucchi C, Talamini R, Montella M, Conti E, La Vecchia C. Diet and ovarian cancer risk: a case-control study in Italy. Int J Cancer 2001; 93:911–915.

107. Byers T, Marshall J, Graham S, Mettlin C, Swanson MA. A case-control study of dietary and nondietary factors in ovarian cancer. J Natl Cancer Inst 1983; 71:681–686.

108. Slattery ML, Schuman KL, West DW, French TK, Robison LM. Nutrient intake and ovarian cancer. Am J Epidemiol 1989; 130:497–502.

109. Cramer DW, Kuper H, Harlow BL, Titus-Ernstoff L. Carotenoids, antioxidants and ovarian cancer risk in pre- and postmenopausal women. Int J Cancer 2001; 94:128–134.

110. Helzlsouer KJ, Alberg AJ, Norkus EP, Morris JS, Hoffman SC, Comstock GW. Prospective study of serum micronutrients and ovarian cancer. J Natl Cancer Inst 1996; 88:32–37.

111. Fairfield KM, Hankinson SE, Rosner BA, Hunter DJ, Colditz GA, Willett WC. Risk of ovarian carcinoma and consumption of vitamins A, C, and E and specific carotenoids. Cancer 2001; 92:2318–2326.

112. Albanes D, Hartman TJ. Antioxidants and cancer: evidence from human observational studies and intervention trials. In: Papas AM, ed. Diet, Nutrition, and Health. Boca Raton: CRC Press, 1999, pp 497–544.

113. Kristal AR, Cohen JH. Tomatoes, lycopene, and prostate cancer: how strong is the evidence? Am J Epidemiol 2000; 151:124–127.

114. Kolonel LN. Nutrition and prostate cancer. In: Coulston AM, Rock CL, Monsen ER, eds. Nutrition in the Prevention and Treatment of Disease. San Diego: Academic Press, 2001, pp 373–386.

115. Cohen JH, Kristal AR, Stanford JL. Fruit and vegetable intakes and prostate cancer risk. J Natl Cancer Inst 2000; 92:61–68.

116. Cook NR, Stampfer MJ, Ma J, Manson JE, Sacks FM, Buring JE, Hennekens CH. Beta-carotene supplementation for patients with low baseline levels and decreased risks of total and prostate carcinoma. Cancer 1999; 86:1783–1792.

117. Christen WG, Gaziano JM, Hennekens CH. Design of Physicians' Health Study II—a randomized trial of beta-carotene, vitamins E and C, and multivitamins, in prevention of cancer, cardiovascular disease, and eye disease, and review of results of completed trials. Ann Epidemiol 2000; 10:125–134.

118. Mayne ST, Lippman SM. Cancer prevention: diet and chemopreventive agents. Retinoids, carotenoids and micronutrients. In: DeVita VT, Hellman S, Rosenberg SA, eds. Principles and Practice of Oncology, 6th ed. Philadelphia: Lippincott Williams & Wilkins, 2001, pp 575–590.

119. Mayne ST, Cartmel B, Baum M, Shor-Posner G, Fallon BG, Briskin K, Bean J, Zheng T, Cooper D, Friedman C, Goodwin WJ. Randomized trial of supplemental beta-carotene to prevent second head and neck cancer. Cancer Res 2001; 61:1457–1463.

120. Li JY, Taylor PR, Li B, Dawsey S, Wang GQ, Ershow AB, Guo W, Liu SF, Yang CS, Shen Q, Want W, Mark SD, Zou XN, Greenwald P, Wu YP, Blot WJ. Nutrition intervention trials in Linxian, China: multiple vitamin/mineral supplementation, cancer incidence, and disease-specific mortality among adults with esophageal dysplasia. J Natl Cancer Inst 1993; 85:1492–1498.

121. Correa P, Fontham ETH, Bravo JC, Bravo LE, Ruiz B, Zarama G, Realpe JL, Malcom GT, Li D, Johnson WD, Mera R. Chemoprevention of gastric

dysplasia: randomized trial of antioxidant supplements and anti-*Helicobacter pylori* therapy. J Natl Cancer Inst 2000; 92:1881–1888.

122. Greenberg ER, Baron JA, Stukel TA, Stevens MM, Mandel JS, Spencer SK, Elias PM, Lowe N, Nierenberg DW, Bayrd G, Vance JC, Freeman DH, Clendenning WE, Kwan T. A clinical trial of beta-carotene to prevent basal-cell and squamous-cell cancers of the skin. N Engl J Med 1990; 323:789–795.

123. Byers T, Nestle M, McTiernan A, Doyle C, Currie-Williams A, Gansler T, Thun M. American Cancer Society Guidelines on Nutrition and Physical Activity for Cancer Prevention: reducing the risk of cancer with healthy food choices and physical activity. CA Cancer J Clin 52:92–119, 2002.

124. Brown J, Byers T, Thompson K, Eldridge B, Doyle C, Williams AM. Nutrition during and after cancer treatment: a guide for informed choices by cancer survivors. CA Cancer J Clin 2002; 51:153–187.

18

Lycopene and Carcinogenesis

Eileen Ang
The University of Melbourne, Melbourne, Victoria, Australia

Elizabeth C. Miller and Steven K. Clinton
The Ohio State University, Columbus, Ohio, U.S.A.

I. INTRODUCTION

The belief that diet and nutrition contributes to cancer risk can be found in the writings of ancient scholars more than 2000 years ago. However, only in the last century did the application of the "scientific method" begin to provide experimental insight into the origins of cancer. At the present time, prominent investigators and expert committees continue to provide estimates, typically between 35% and 70%, regarding the proportion of the cancer burden attributable to diet and nutrition (1–3). Future research will likely confirm that many nutrients and nonnutrient substances found in the diet, as well as patterns of foods consumed, will modify cancer risk. The last decade has seen an emerging interest in the potential health benefits of tomato products (4) and lycopene, the carotenoid responsible for the familiar red color of tomatoes (5). Although entrepreneurs have been eager to market lycopene supplements and products enriched in lycopene to consumers based on hypothesized benefits, the scientific evidence has yet to establish a causal relationship between lycopene intake and risk of malignancy (6). However, accumulating evidence is especially suggestive that tomatoes may have cancer-preventive properties and that lycopene may be one of many components of tomatoes that participates in inhibiting carcinogenesis. It is imperative that funding agencies continue to support well-designed human and laboratory studies that address hypotheses focusing on tomatoes, lycopene, and carcinogenesis. This chapter will summarize the current state of knowledge regarding lycopene and cancer and serve as an entry point for those interested in pursuing research in this field.

II. CHEMISTRY

Investigators considering mechanisms whereby lycopene may influence the development of cancer must consider the unique chemical structure that determines its physical properties, reactivity, and, ultimately, biological impact (5). Lycopene is a highly unsaturated lipophilic 40-carbon carotenoid ($C_{40}H_{56}$) with a molecular weight of 536.85. The linear array of 11 conjugated and 2 unconjugated double bonds contributes to its susceptibility to oxidative degradation and isomerization by chemical and physical factors, including exposure to elevated temperature, light, oxygen, extremes in pH, and active surfaces (5,7,8). Lycopene lacks the β-ionone ring and therefore is devoid of any vitamin A activity. Lycopene exists in tomatoes and processed food predominantly in the all-trans configuration, i.e., the most thermodynamically stable form. As a polyene, *cis–trans* isomerization is possible, and approximately 10–20 different cis isomers are typically observed in blood and tissues of experimental animals (9,10) and humans (11,12). Isomerization to the *cis* configuration results in lower melting points, smaller extinction coefficients (which need to be considered during quantitative analysis of isomers to avoid underestimation), decreased color density (important in quality perception), a shift in λ_{max}, and the appearance of a new maximum (so-called *cis* peaks; useful in tentative identification of isomers) in the ultraviolet (UV) spectrum (13). The cis isomers most commonly found in human serum and tissue are thought to be 5-*cis*-, 9-*cis*-, 13-*cis*-, and 15-*cis*-lycopene, accounting for approximately 50–90% of total lycopene content in serum and tissue (11,12). While all-*trans* lycopene can theoretically be arranged in 2048 different geometrical configurations, steric hindrance allows only certain ethylenic groups of lycopene molecules to participate in *cis–trans* isomerization, and only about 72 lycopene *cis* isomers are structurally favorable (13,14). The biological significance of *cis* isomerization relative to biological functions, such as carcinogenesis, remains speculative, and the standardization of methods for the quantitative assessment of isomers in biological samples has not yet been well established. Much remains to be learned about lycopene digestion, absorption, intraorgan transport in the circulation, mechanisms of uptake by cells, intracellular localization, and the reactions that influence isomerization and degradation. The chemical characteristics of lycopene have a profound effect on each of these processes that will ultimately influence the role of dietary lycopene in the carcinogenic cascade.

III. LYCOPENE AND CANCER: ASSESSING THE PUBLISHED LITERATURE

Data regarding the role of lycopene in cancer risk have been derived from various types of investigations including epidemiological studies, human clinical investigations, rodent models, and cell culture systems (5). Each of these approaches has strengths and limitations, a review of which is beyond the scope of this chapter. However, several key considerations relevant to lycopene should be emphasized and considered as readers critically review the literature on lycopene and cancer risk.

Much of the epidemiological data regarding lycopene and cancer risk is derived from estimated consumption of lycopene containing foods reported using a diet assessment instrument, such as a food frequency questionnaire. Mathematically derived estimates of lycopene intake are calculated using a carotenoid database, such as provided by the U.S. Department of Agriculture (15). The average lycopene content of foods included in the database is derived from a number of samples that are representative of the marketed product. Unfortunately, the lycopene content of tomato-based food items can vary substantially due to differences among tomato strains, growing conditions, and food processing. In contrast to other major carotenoids, which are typically found in a diverse array of fruits and vegetables, lycopene is derived from a relatively limited number of foods. Thus, most diet assessment tools can include foods that account for lycopene intake (5). Tomatoes and tomato products (such as tomato soup, tomato juice, and tomato sauce) contribute to more than 85% of the dietary lycopene in the North American diet (16). In the United States, the estimated average daily lycopene consumption is approximately 3–4 mg/day and contributes to about 30–50% of total carotenoids in the diet (17,18). We can conclude that current diet assessment tools and techniques can provide an estimate of lycopene intake but that precision for any individual is difficult to achieve. Thus, large studies using well-tested instruments provide greater statistical power and instill a degree of confidence among readers that the cohort can categorize individuals into groups based on consumption of lycopene-containing foods, such as quartiles or quintiles.

Unfortunately, the intake of lycopene is not a precise index of the biologically relevant concentrations of lycopene in the blood or at a tissue, particularly when evaluating individuals. Rodents and humans, when assigned to consume specific amounts of lycopene, may show variable blood and tissue concentrations (9,10,19,20). The complexity of estimating the biologically relevant exposure to lycopene in epidemiological studies is due to the variability in bioavailability that occurs in part due to issues relating to the food and host factors. A detailed consideration of lycopene content of foods, absorption, bioavailability, metabolism, and tissue distribution is beyond the scope of this chapter. However, each of these issues is relevant to understanding the role of lycopene in carcinogenesis and should be considered as investigators review the literature. Bioavailability of lycopene from a food will be influenced by food processing, cooking techniques, and the presence of other components in the food or the meal (21–25). In turn, poorly understood host factors relative to digestive and absorptive processes, lipoprotein metabolism (critical transport vehicles for lycopene), and metabolic enzymes will influence the concentrations of lycopene that may reach a target tissue. Thus, it is not surprising that estimated lycopene intake and blood concentrations are often weakly correlated (26,27). A number of studies focus on the relationship between blood lycopene concentrations and cancer risk. Typically, plasma concentrations of lycopene are measured at one time point that may or may not represent long-term exposure. Within-person variation may be a source of error and weaken epidemiological associations. A recent study examined samples collected from 144 men collected 3–4 years apart and determined that total lycopene demonstrated a significant ($p < 0.001$) correlation of 0.63 over time (12). Thus, we feel that epidemiological studies of blood lycopene are a reasonable reflection of stable dietary patterns and metabolic processes over time in adults. However, readers should remain aware that blood lycopene is a biomarker of tomato product intake and thus cannot clearly differentiate between a mechanistic role of lycopene in cancer risk or other components found in the tomatoes.

Animal models of carcinogenesis provide an opportunity to conduct precisely controlled studies of dietary intake and risk of cancer. Interestingly, rats and mice, the most common species employed as experimental models, absorb lycopene poorly (9,10,28). However, increasing the dietary lycopene concentration to levels exceeding those found in typical human diets to overcome the poor absorption allows investigators to achieve blood and tissue concentrations similar to those found in humans (9–11). Recent studies in the ferret suggest that their absorption of lycopene may be more similar to that of humans, but the lack of carcinogenesis models in species other than rats and mice limits usefulness of these data (29). Readers should consider these issues when reviewing the literature, and investigators should carefully document lycopene content of the diet and report blood or tissue concentrations in order to aid in the interpretation of results.

The application of in vitro cell and organ culture systems are a valuable approach for understanding molecular mechanisms whereby lycopene may influence cancer cell biology. However, studies with carotenoids have technical concerns that should be addressed by all investigators. Pure lycopene in crystalline form is insoluble in aqueous media and each investigator must choose from a variety of approaches to deliver lycopene to the cells. The variable uptake of carotenoids by cells in culture should also be considered when different vehicles are used for in vitro delivery such as organic solvents, beadlets, or liposomes (30). Although largely unknown at present, it is important that future studies address the subcellular localization of lycopene within different intracellular compartments and how this may influence biological events. The in vivo physiological distribution of lycopene to cells most certainly is critically linked to lipoprotein metabolism, and we should strive to develop techniques that mimic this process with in vitro studies. In addition, the stability of the carotenoids under in vitro conditions is a concern. Ideally, investigators will consider the potential for degradation, oxidation, or metabolic conversion of the carotenoids to forms that influence outcomes examined.

In general, investigations in humans, rodents, and in vitro systems will benefit from including analytical studies of lycopene quantitation and metabolism. Opportunities exist for productive collaborations between epidemiologists and cancer biologists with experts in analytical chemistry. Critical insight into lycopene and cancer relationships will only be possible when biological mechanisms are coupled with precise analysis of lycopene chemistry.

IV. LYCOPENE AND CANCER: CAUSALITY

Scientific publications regarding lycopene and cancer are rapidly accumulating. This chapter is not an encyclopedic review of the literature but rather highlights the most intriguing and stimulating relationships that have emerged. Interestingly, scientists, regulatory agencies, marketers of food and supplement products, and organizations defining public health policy have differing opinions regarding the strength of the accumulated data relative to inference and causality (6). The discipline of public health policy continues to review criteria used to judge scientific evidence regarding dietary components and health or disease risk (31). In general, accepted categories of criteria that are used to assess a component relative to cancer risk include the following: consistency of results among studies, overall strength of the association, evidence for a biological gradient (dose–response), temporality (exposure precedes event), specificity, biological mechanisms, and, finally, experimental evidence from an intervention trial (31). These criteria should be considered as readers review the lycopene and cancer literature (6).

V. LUNG CANCER

The lung serves as a critical interface between the host and the ambient air and thus is particularly at risk for oxidative and ozone stress (32). Thus, the hypothesis that antioxidants may protect the lung from disease processes, including cancer, is appealing to investigators. Multiple antioxidant defense systems, including vitamins E and C, appear to be present in the lung tissue and secretions (32). The contribution of dietary carotenoids to the integrated host defense remains poorly defined.

Several dozen epidemiological studies of varying design and statistical power provide data relevant to tomato or lycopene intake and lung cancer risk (1,32,33). In general, the majority of case-control and cohort studies suggest a lower risk of lung cancer with greater exposure to lycopene or tomato products, with several of the studies reporting statistically significant results (34–36). Few studies in animal models of lung carcinogenesis have been completed with mixed results (37–39). Interestingly, lycopene catabolism appears to be accelerated by constituents in smoke (29,40). A recent study (29) where ferrets were exposed to tobacco smoke showed that lycopene supplementation prevented smoke-induced squamous metaplasia and positively impacted on other biomarkers associated with risk. A randomized trial of placebo versus a tomato-based juice with 23 mg of lycopene per serving consumed for 2 weeks demonstrated significant protection against ozone-induced lung inflammation and toxicity (32). Additional efforts should focus on lycopene interactions with tobacco/smoke constituents, other major etiological factors such as asbestos exposure, histological subtypes of lung cancer of varying etiology, and genetic polymorphisms influencing carcinogen metabolism. Until more definitive data are available, we conclude that diets rich in fruits and vegetables, particularly carotenoid-containing foods (including tomatoes), is the best way to minimize risk of lung carcinogenesis in parallel with avoidance of tobacco products (35).

VI. STOMACH/GASTRIC CANCER

Several studies have evaluated tomato products and lycopene in relation to gastric carcinoma risk and the majority show a trend toward lower risk with greater tomato product and lycopene exposure (1,33,41). However, these relationships have not yet been carefully examined in laboratory animal models or clinical studies. Lycopene interactions with etiological risk factors, such as chronic gastritis, exposure to nitrates, or *Helicobacter pylori* infection, remain to be addressed. Efforts should be directed to elucidating relationships between carcinogenesis of the gastric cardia and noncardia that are distinct disease processes and may demonstrate unique relationships with dietary variables.

VII. COLORECTAL CANCER

Although the results of epidemiological studies are mixed, the majority suggest a protective relationship between estimated lycopene exposure, tomato product consumption, or serum lycopene and colorectal cancer risk (1,33,41,42). Several rodent studies have examined colon carcinogenesis in response to lycopene treatment. Interestingly, tomato juice, but not pure lycopene, reduced colon cancer formation in the N-methylnitrosourea (MNU) model of colon carcinogenesis (43). Inhibition of aberrant crypt foci formation, a putative premalignant lesion, has been reduced in some studies (44–46). In general, the results are more supportive of a protective role for tomato products rather than lycopene per se although additional research is clearly necessary.

VIII. UPPER AERODIGESTIVE TRACT CANCER (ORAL CAVITY, PHARYNX, LARYNX, PROXIMAL ESOPHAGUS)

Collectively, these cancers are primarily related to tobacco and alcohol exposure although the modulation of risk by dietary and nutritional factors is probably a contributing variable (1). The majority of epidemiological studies support a protective role for diets rich in fruits and vegetables, including tomato products (1,33,47–49). Although fewer studies specifically examine a role for lycopene in carcinogenesis of the upper aerodigestive tissues (41,47–49), a recent representative study (50) reported a significant 33% lower risk of oral and pharyngeal cancer risk between the lowest and highest quintiles of estimated lycopene intake. Clarification of interactions between alcohol, constituents of tobacco smoke, and lycopene biology is a critical area of future investigation.

IX. PANCREATIC CANCER

There have been very few studies of lycopene or tomato products in relation to pancreatic cancer risk (1,33). Published research consists of three case-control studies, two nested case-control studies, and one cohort study (33,51). Although these studies support an inverse relationship between lycopene and risk of pancreatic cancer, it is premature to draw conclusions from such a limited portfolio of studies.

X. BLADDER CANCER

The majority of epidemiological studies fail to observe a relationship between tomato products, lycopene, and bladder cancer risk (1,33). Interestingly, tomato juice, but not lycopene, was shown to reduce bladder carcinogenesis in animal models (52,53).

XI. BREAST CANCER

Human studies investigating lycopene intake or blood concentrations and breast cancer risk have produced inconsistent results (1,33,41,54–57). One case-control report has been published investigating breast tissue concentrations of lycopene and breast cancer risk (58). Breast adipose concentrations of lycopene were significantly, inversely associated with risk (58). Two of three reported rodent studies suggest an inhibition of mammary carcinogenesis in lycopene treated animals (59–61). Several in vitro studies of human breast cancer cell lines suggest inhibitory effects on proliferation and survival, perhaps in part via alteration of insulin-like growth factor-1 (IGF-1) signaling pathways (62–66).

XII. CERVICAL CANCER

Cancer of the cervix is clearly related to human papilloma virus (HPV) infection. The possibility that a diet including tomatoes or lycopene may influence the response to the infection and modify risk is an intriguing hypothesis (1,33). Results of serological examination have been fairly consistent, suggesting that higher serum lycopene levels are associated with reduced risk of cervical premalignancy or cervical cancer (67–69). Two studies have investigated the association between serum lycopene concentrations or dietary lycopene consumption and risk of HPV infection (70,71). Among women enrolled in the Young Women's Health Study, a 56% reduction in risk of HPV persistence was reported in women with the highest plasma *cis*-lycopene concentrations (OR = 0.44, p = 0.046), although the trend did not attain statistical significance for dietary lycopene consumption (71). Conversely, there was no significant association between serum lycopene concentration and persistent HPV infection among a cohort of low-income Hispanic women (70). Because so few studies are available, additional efforts to address interrelationships between lycopene, other dietary variables, HPV infection, and cervical cancer risk are warranted.

XIII. OVARIAN CANCER

A literature search revealed only five studies (two case-control, one nested case-control, one meta-analysis, and one cohort study) that reported specific data regarding tomatoes or lycopene and ovarian cancer with variable conclusions (1,33,41,72–74). One recent, large case-control study reported that estimated dietary lycopene, particularly from tomato sauce, significantly reduced the risk of ovarian cancer, and the benefit was especially strong among premenopausal women (73). The Nurses' Health Study is the only prospective cohort study to evaluate estimated dietary lycopene consumption and risk of ovarian cancer, and no association was found (72). Thus, it is premature to conclude that tomatoes or lycopene influence ovarian cancer risk.

XIV. PROSTATE CANCER

Perhaps the strongest evidence for a relationship between lycopene and cancer risk is found in the prostate cancer literature that has been the subject of detailed reviews (5,6,75,76). The landmark reports from the prospective Health Professional's Follow-up Study (4,77) showed a significant association between the consumption of tomato products and estimated lycopene intake and a reduced risk of prostate cancer, and supported earlier, but less well-known, findings from the Seventh Day Adventists cohort (78). Estimated intake of lycopene (80% of which was derived from tomatoes and tomato products) was inversely related to prostate cancer risk when the highest quintile (median 19 mg lycopene/day) was compared with the lowest quintile (median 3 mg lycopene/day) (RR = 0.84, 95% CI = 0.73–0.96, p for trend = 0.003) (cumulative results from the updated analysis) (77). Several case-control studies also support a protective effect of tomatoes or tomato products (79–85). Several (86–88), but not all (89–91), studies suggest that higher plasma lycopene is associated with lower prostate cancer risk. The largest analysis of prospectively collected blood carotenoid patterns and risk of prostate cancer was conducted among the Physicians' Health Study cohort (86). Men in the highest quintile of plasma lycopene (>590 ng/mL) had a nonsignificant trend toward a lower risk of prostate cancer than men in the lowest quintile of plasma lycopene (OR, 0.75, p for trend = 0.12). The trend reached statistical significance when only prostate cancers with clinical stage C or D or Gleason score ≥7 were included (OR, 0.56, p for trend = 0.05). Overall, the epidemiological data supporting a protective relationship for tomato products and prostate cancer are fairly consistent, although not uniform (79,92), and support a possible role for lycopene in prostate carcinogenesis.

The detection of lycopene in the prostate (11) adds to the biological plausibility that lycopene may directly influence the malignant cascade. Two intervention studies have been reported regarding men with prostate cancer scheduled to undergo a prostatectomy. A 3-week food-based intervention containing 30 mg of lycopene per day was associated with increased prostate lycopene and a reduction in leukocyte and prostate tissue DNA damage compared with baseline measures (93–95). Another study involved consumption of 30 mg of lycopene per day as a tomato oleoresin supplement compared with a normal diet. Postsurgical prostate tissue specimens showed that men consuming the lycopene supplement had 47% greater prostatic lycopene and were less likely to have involvement of surgical margins (73% versus 18% of subjects, $p = 0.02$)

than controls (96). Large rodent studies in models of prostate carcinogenesis have not yet been published but are underway. Several in vitro studies suggest that lycopene may suppress proliferation and reduce viability of prostate cancer cells (97,98).

XV. LYCOPENE AND CARCINOGENESIS: MECHANISMS OF ACTION

Unlike some nutrients where a specific molecular target can be identified that mediates the biological events, lycopene will certainly have a much more complex and diverse array of mechanisms whereby it acts to influence risk of cancer. Indeed, the dominant theory regarding how lycopene may protect against carcinogenesis is related to its antioxidant properties (99,100). The oxidation of lipids, nucleic acids, and proteins is considered to be a component of the initiation and progression of many chronic diseases of aging including cancer and cardiovascular disease. It has been particularly challenging for investigators to characterize reliable and specific biomarkers of oxidative stress and exposure to antioxidants that can be employed in epidemiological, clinical, or animal studies (101). Thus, defining a role of lycopene in protecting cells from damage to critical macromolecules involved in the cancer cascade remains an elusive objective.

Other mechanisms whereby lycopene may influence cell biology related to cancer have also been proposed (5,100). Studies in cell culture systems suggest that exposure to lycopene may have antiproliferative and apoptotic effects or induce differentiation (66,100). The ability of lycopene to modify the cellular response to growth-promoting signals, such as IGF-I, has been considered (66,100). Considerable interest has been generated regarding the ability of carotenoids, including lycopene, to influence the expression of gap junctional proteins that direct intercellular communication and perhaps contribute to maintaining a differentiated cellular phenotype (96,102). Alterations in enzyme systems involved in carcinogen activation and degradation by lycopene have also been proposed (29). Although each of these concepts warrants continued investigation, clear mechanisms whereby lycopene may alter cancer risk have yet to be elucidated.

XVI. SUMMARY

The hypothesis that lycopene may demonstrate anticancer properties remains viable and warrants continued investigation in epidemiological, clinical, and laboratory studies. It is our opinion that the promotion of lycopene as a cancer-preventive agent is premature. In contrast, the data supporting a protective effect for a diet rich in fruits and vegetables is strong and should continue to be emphasized in current public health recommendations for cancer prevention. Although we cannot make a definitive claim regarding tomato products and cancer risk, the accumulated evidence supports consumption of tomato-based foods as a component of a healthy diet to prevent cancer. Understanding the role of lycopene in cancer will require additional investment in basic research devoted to the understanding of lycopene chemistry in biological systems, absorption, bioavailability, tissue distribution, metabolism, and mechanisms of action.

REFERENCES

1. World Cancer Research Fund. Food, Nutrition and the Prevention of Cancer: A Global Perspective. Washington, DC: American Institute for Cancer Research, 1997.
2. Block G, Patterson B, Subar A. Fruit, vegetables, and cancer prevention: a review of the epidemiological evidence. Nutr Cancer 1992; 18:1–29.
3. Doll R, Peto R. The causes of cancer: quantitative estimates of avoidable risks of cancer in the United States today. J Natl Cancer Inst 1981; 66:1191–1308.
4. Giovannucci E, Ascherio A, Rimm E, Stampfer M, Colditz G, Willett W. Intake of carotenoids and retinol in relation to risk of prostate cancer. J Natl Cancer Institute 1995; 87:1767–1776.
5. Clinton S. Lycopene: chemistry, biology, and implications for human health and disease. Nutr Rev 1998; 218:140–143.
6. Miller EC, Hadley CW, Schwartz SJ, Erdman JW Jr, Boileau TW-M, Clinton SK. Lycopene, tomato products, and prostate cancer prevention. Have we established causality? Pure Appl Chem 2002; 74:1435–1441.
7. Krinsky N. Overview of lycopene, carotenoids, and disease prevention. Proc Soc Exp Biol Med 1998; 218:95–97.
8. Krinsky N. The antioxidant and biological properties of the carotenoids. Ann NY Acad Sci 1998; 854:443–447.
9. Boileau T, Clinton S, Erdman J Jr. Tissue lycopene concentrations and isomer patterns are affected by androgen status and dietary lycopene concentration in male F344 rats. J Nutr 2000; 130:1613–1618.
10. Boileau T, Clinton S, Zaripheh S, Monaco M, Donovan S, Erdman J Jr. Testosterone and food restriction modulate hepatic lycopene isomer concentrations in male F344 rats. J Nutr 2001; 131:1746–1752.
11. Clinton S, Emenhiser C, Schwartz S, Bostwick D, Williams A, Moore B, Erdman J Jr. cis-trans lycopene isomers, carotenoids, and retinol in the human prostate. Cancer Epidemiol Biomark Prev 1996; 5:823–833.
12. Wu K, Schwartz S, Platz E, Clinton S, Erdman J Jr, Ferruzzi M, Willett W, Giovannucci E. Variations in plasma lycopene and specific isomers over time in a cohort of U.S. men. J Nutr 2003; 133:1930–1936.
13. Zechmeister L, Polgar A. Cis-trans isomerization and cis-peak effect in the alpha carotene set and in some other stereoisomeric sets. J Am Chem Soc 1944; 66:137–144.

14. Pauling L. Recent work on the configuration and electronic structure of molecules with some applications to natural products: isomerism and the structure of carotenoids. Fortschr Chem Org Naturstoffe 1939; 3:227–229.
15. Mangels A, Holden J, Beecher G, Forman M, Lanza E. Carotenoid content of fruits and vegetables: an evaluation of analytic data. J Am Diet Assoc 1993; 93:284–296.
16. Beecher G. Nutrient content of tomatoes and tomato products. Proc Soc Exp Biol Med 1998; 218:98–100.
17. Food and Nutrition Board, Institute of Medicine. Dietary Reference Intakes for Vitamin A, Vitamin K, Arsenic, Boron, Chromium, Copper, Iodine, Iron, Manganese, Molybdenum, Nickel, Silicon, Vanadium, and Zinc. Washington, DC: National Academy Press, 2002.
18. Forman M, Beecher G, Graubard B, Campbell W, Reichman M, Taylor P, Lanza E, Holden J, Judd J. The correlation between two dietary assessments of carotenoid intake and plasma carotenoid concentrations: application of a carotenoid food-composition database. Am J Clin Nutr 1993; 60:223–230.
19. Boileau A, Merchen N, Wasson K, Atkinson C, Erdman J Jr. cis-Lycopene is more bioavailable than trans-lycopene in vitro and in vivo in lymph-cannulated ferrets. J Nutr 1999; 129:1176–1181.
20. Hadley C, Clinton S, Schwartz S. The consumption of processed tomato products enhances plasma lycopene concentrations in association with a reduced lipoprotein sensitivity to oxidative damage. J Nutr 2003; 133:727–732.
21. Boileau T, Boileau A, Erdman J Jr. Bioavailability of all-trans and cis-isomers of lycopene. Exp Biol Med 2002; 227:914–919.
22. Williams A, Boileau T, Erdman J Jr. Factors influencing the uptake and absorption of carotenoids. Proc Soc Exp Biol Med 1998; 218:106–108.
23. Nguyen M, Schwartz S. Lycopene stability during food processing. Proc Soc Exp Biol Med 1998; 218:101–105.
24. Stahl W, Sies H. Uptake of lycopene and its geometrical isomers is greater from heat-processed than from unprocessed tomato juice in humans. J Nutr 1992; 122:2161–2166.
25. Gartner C, Stahl W, Sies H. Lycopene is more bioavailable from tomato paste than from fresh tomatoes. Am J Clin Nutr 1997; 66:116–122.
26. Freeman V, Meydani M, Yong S, Pyle J, Wan Y. Prostatic levels of tocopherols, carotenoids and retinol in relation to plasma levels and self-reported usual dietary intake. Am J Epidemiol 1999; 151:109–118.
27. Mayne S, Cartmel B, Silva F, Kim C, Fallon B, Briskin K, Zheng T, Baum M, Shor-Posner, G, Goodwin W Jr. Effect of supplemental beta-carotene on plasma concentrations of carotenoids, retinol, and alpha-tocopherol in humans. Am J Clin Nutr 1998; 68:642–647.
28. Cohen L. A review of animal model studies of tomato carotenoids, lycopene, and cancer chemoprevention. Exp Biol Med 2002; 227:864–868.
29. Liu D, Lian F, Smith D, Russell R, Wang X. Lycopene supplementation inhibits lung squamous metaplasia and induces apoptosis via up-regulating insulin-like growth factor-binding protein 3 in cigarette smoke exposed ferrets. Cancer Res 2003; 63:3138–3143.

30. Williams A, Boileau T-M, Clinton S, Erdman J Jr. Beta carotene stability and uptake by prostate cancer cells are dependent on delivery vehicle. Nutr Cancer 2000; 36:185–190.
31. Weed D. Causal and Preventive Inference. New York: Marcel Dekker, 1995:385–402.
32. Arab L, Steck-Scott S, Fleishauer A. Lycopene and the lung. Exp Biol Med 2002; 227:894–8990.
33. Giovannucci E. Tomatoes, tomato-based products, lycopene, and cancer: review of the epidemiologic literature. J Natl Cancer Inst 1999; 91:317–331.
34. Comstock G, Alberg A, Huang H, Wu K, Burke A, Hoffman S, Norkus E, Gross M, Cutler R, Morris J, Spate V, Helzlsouer K. The risk of developing lung cancer associated with antioxidants in the blood: ascorbic acid, carotenoids, alpha-tocopherol, selenium, and total peroxyl radical absorbing capacity. Cancer Epidemiol Biomark Prev 1997; 6:907–916.
35. Holick C, Michaud D, Stolzenberg-Solomon R, Mayne S, Pietinen P, Taylor P, Virtamo J, Albanes D. Dietary carotenoids, serum beta-carotene, and retinol and risk of lung cancer in the alpha-tocopherol, beta-carotene cohort study. Am J Epidemiol 2002; 156:536–547.
36. Michaud D, Feskanich D, Rimm E, Colditz G, Speizer F, Willett W. Intake of specific carotenoids and risk of lung cancer in 2 prospective US cohorts. Am J Clin Nutr 2000; 72:990–997.
37. Guttenplan J, Chen M, Kosinska W, Thompson S, Zhao Z, Cohen L. Effects of a lycopene-rich diet on spontaneous and benzo[a]pyrene-induced mutagenesis in prostate, colon and lungs of the lacZ mouse. Cancer Lett 2001; 164:1–6.
38. Hecht S, Kenney P, Wang M, Trushin N, Agarwal S, Rao A, Upadhyaya P. Evaluation of butylated hydroxyanisole, myo-inositol, curcumin, esculetin, resveratrol and lycopene as inhibitors of benzo[a]pyrene plus 4-(methylnitro-samino)-1-(3-pyridyl)-1-butanone-induced lung tumorigenesis in A/J mice. Cancer Lett 1999; 137:123–130.
39. Kim D, Takasuka N, Nishino H, Tsuda H. Chemoprevention of lung cancer by lycopene. Biofactors 2000; 13:95–102.
40. Handelman G, Packer L, Cross C. Destruction of tocopherols, carotenoids, and retinol in human plasma by cigarette smoke. Am J Clin Nutr 1996; 63:559–565.
41. La Vecchia C. Tomatoes, lycopene intake, and digestive tract and female hormone-related neoplasms. Exp Biol Med 2002; 227:860–863.
42. Malila N, Virtamo J, Virtanen M, Pietinen P, Albanes D, Teppo L. Dietary and serum alpha-tocopherol, beta-carotene and retinol, and risk for colorectal cancer in male smokers. Eur J Clin Nutr 2002; 56:615–621.
43. Narisawa T, Fukaura Y, Hasebe M, Nomura S, Oshima S, Sakamoto H, Inakuma T, Ishiguro Y, Takayasu J, Nishino H. Prevention of N-methylnitrosourea-induced colon carcinogenesis in F344 rats by lycopene and tomato juice rich in lycopene. Jpn J Cancer Res 1998; 89:1003–1008.
44. Narisawa T, Fukaura Y, Hasebe M, Ito M, Aizawa R, Murakoshi M, Uemura S, Khachik F, Nishino, H. Inhibitory effects of natural carotenoids, alpha-carotene, beta-carotene, lycopene and lutein, on colonic aberrant crypt foci formation in rats. Cancer Lett 1996; 107:137–142.

45. Wargovich M, Jimenez A, McKee K, Steele V, Velasco M, Woods J, Price R, Gray K, Kelloff G. Efficacy of potential chemopreventive agents on rat colon aberrant crypt formation and progression. Carcinogenesis 2000; 21:1149–1155.

46. Kim J, Araki S, Kim D, Park C, Takasuka N, Baba-Toriyama H, Ota T, Nir Z, Khachik F, Shimidzu N, Tanaka Y, Osawa T, Uraji T, Murakoshi M, Nishino H, Tsuda H. Chemopreventive effects of carotenoids and curcumins on mouse colon carcinogenesis after 1,2-dimethylhydrazine initiation. Carcinogenesis 1998; 19:81–85.

47. De Stefani E, Ronco A, Mendilaharsu M, Deneo-Pellegrini H. Diet and risk of cancer of the upper aerodigestive tract. II. Nutrients, Oral Oncol 1999; 35:22–26.

48. De Stefani E, Oreggia F, Boffetta P, Deneo-Pellegrini H, Ronco A, Mendilaharsu M. Tomatoes, tomato-rich foods, lycopene and cancer of the upper aerodigestive tract: a case-control in Uruguay. Oral Oncol 2000; 36:47–53.

49. De Stefani E, Brennan P, Boffetta P, Ronco A, Mendilaharsu M, Deneo-Pellegrini H. Vegetables, fruits, related dietary antioxidants, and risk of squamous cell carcinoma of the esophagus: a case-control study in Uruguay. Nutr Cancer 2000; 38:23–29.

50. Negri E, Franceschi S, Bosetti C, Levi F, Conti E, Parpinel M, La Vecchia C. Selected micronutrients and oral and pharyngeal cancer. Int J Cancer 2000; 86:122–127.

51. Abiaka C, Al-Awadi F, Al-Sayer H, Gulshan S, Behbehani A, Farghaly M, Negri E. Plasma micronutrient antioxidant in cancer patients. Cancer Detect Prev 2001; 25:245–253.

52. Okajima E, Ozono S, Endo T, Majima T, Tsutsumi M, Fukuda T, Akai H, Denda A, Hirao Y, Nishino H, Nir Z, Konishi Y. Chemopreventive efficacy of piroxicam administered alone or in combination with lycopene and beta-carotene on the development of rat urinary bladder carcinoma after N-butyl-N-(4-hydroxybutyl) nitrosamine treatment. Jpn J Cancer Res 1997; 88:543–552.

53. Okajima E, Tsutsumi M, Ozono S, Akai H, Denda A, Nishino H, Oshima S, Sakamoto H, Konishi Y. Inhibitory effect of tomato juice on rat urinary bladder carcinogenesis after N-butyl-N-(4-hydroxybutyl)nitrosamine initiation. Jpn J Cancer Res 1998; 89:22–26.

54. Levi F, Pasche C, Lucchini F, La Vecchia C. Dietary intake of selected micronutrients and breast-cancer risk. Int J Cancer 2001; 91:260–263.

55. Ronco A, De Stefani E, Boffetta P, Deneo-Pellegrini H, Mendilaharsu M, Leborgne F. Vegetables, fruits, and related nutrients and risk of breast cancer: a case-control study in Uruguay. Nutr Cancer 1999; 35:111–119.

56. Sato R, Helzlsouer K, Alberg A, Hoffman S, Norkus E, Comstock G. Prospective study of carotenoids, tocopherols, and retinoid concentrations and the risk of breast cancer. Cancer Epidemiol Biomark Prev 2002; 11:451–457.

57. Simon M, Djurie Z, Dunn B, Stephens D, Lababidi S, Heilbrun L. An evaluation of plasma antioxidant levels and the risk of breast cancer: a pilot case control study. Breast J 2000; 6:388–395.

58. Zhang S, Tang G, Russell R, Mayzel K, Stampfer M, Willett W, Hunter D. Measurement of retinoids and carotenoids in breast adipose tissue and a comparison of concentrations in breast cancer cases and control subjects. Am J Clin Nutr 1997; 66:626–632.

59. Nagasawa H, Mitamura T, Sakamoto S, Yamamoto K. Effects of lycopene on spontaneous mammary tumour development in SHN virgin mice. Anticancer Res 1995; 15:1173–1178.

60. Cohen L, Zhao Z, Pittman B, Khachik F. Effect of dietary lycopene on N-methylnitrosourea-induced mammary tumorigenesis. Nutr Cancer 1999; 34:153–159.

61. Sharoni Y, Giron E, Rise M, Levy J. Effects of lycopene-enriched tomato oleoresin on 7,12-dimethyl-benz[a]anthracene-induced rat mammary tumors. Cancer Detect Prev 1997; 21:118–123.

62. Prakash P, Russell R, Krinsky N. In vitro inhibition of proliferation of estrogen-dependent and estrogen-independent human breast cancer cells treated with carotenoids or retinoids. J Nutr 2001; 131:1574–1580.

63. Nahum A, Hirsch K, Danilenko M, Watts C, Prall O, Levy J, Sharoni Y. Lycopene inhibition of cell cycle progression in breast and endometrial cancer cells is associated with reduction in cyclin D levels and retention of p27(Kip1) in the cyclin E-cdk2 complexes. Oncogene 2001; 20:3428–3436.

64. Li Z, Wang Y, Mo B. The effects of carotenoids on the proliferation of human breast cancer cell and gene expression of bcl-2. Zhonghua Yu Fang Yi Xue Za Zhi 2002; 36:254–257.

65. Levy J, Bosin E, Feldman B, Giat Y, Miinster A, Danilenko M, Sharoni Y. Lycopene is a more potent inhibitor of human cancer cell proliferation than either alpha-carotene or beta-carotene. Nutr Cancer 1995; 24:257–266.

66. Karas M, Amir H, Fishman D, Danilenko M, Segal S, Nahum A, Koifmann A, Giat Y, Levy J, Sharoni Y. Lycopene interferes with cell cycle progression and insulin-like growth factor I signaling in mammary cancer cells. Nutr Cancer 2000; 36:101–111.

67. Kanetsky P, Gammon M, Mandelblatt J, Zhang Z, Ramsey E, Dnistrian A, Norkus E, Wright T Jr. Dietary intake and blood levels of lycopene: association with cervical dysplasia among non-Hispanic, black women. Nutr Cancer 1998; 31:31–40.

68. Nagata C, Shimizu H, Yoshikawa H, Noda K, Nozawa S, Yajima A, Sekiya S, Sugimori H, Hirai Y, Kanazawa K, Sugase M, Kawana T. Serum carotenoids and vitamins and risk of cervical dysplasia from a case-control study in Japan. Br J Cancer 1999; 81:1234–1237.

69. Batieha A, Armenian, H, Norkus E, Morris J, Spate V, Comstock G. Serum micronutrients and the subsequent risk of cervical cancer in a population-based nested case-control study. Cancer Epidemiol Biomark Prev 1993; 2:335–339.

70. Giuliano A, Papenfuss M, Nour M, Canfield L, Schneider A, Hatch K. Antioxidant nutrients: associations with persistent human papillomavirus infection. Cancer Epidemiol Biomark Prev 1997; 6:917–923.

71. Sedjo R, Roe D, Abrahamsen M, Harris R, Craft N, Baldwin S, and Giuliano A. Vitamin A, carotenoids, and risk of persistent oncogenic human papillomavirus infection. Cancer Epidemiol Biomark Prev 2002; 11:876–884.

72. Fairfield K, Hankinson S, Rosner B, Hunter D, Colditz G, Willett W. Risk of ovarian carcinoma and consumption of vitamins A, C, and E and specific carotenoids: a prospective analysis. Cancer 2001; 92:2318–2326.

73. Cramer D, Kuper H, Harlow B, Titus-Ernstoff L. Carotenoids, antioxidants and ovarian cancer risk in pre- and postmenopausal women. Int J Cancer 2001; 94:128–134.

74. McCann S, Moysich K, Mettlin C. Intakes of selected nutrients and food groups and risk of ovarian cancer. Nutr Cancer 2001; 39:19–28.

75. Miller EC, Giovannucci E, Erdman JW Jr, Bahnson R, Schwartz SJ, Clinton SK. Tomato products, lycopene, and prostate cancer risk. Urol Clin North Am 2002; 29:83–93.

76. Hadley C, Miller E, Schwartz S, Clinton S. Tomatoes, lycopene and prostate cancer: progress and promise. Exp Biol Med 2002; 227:869–880.

77. Giovannucci E, Rimm E, Liu Y, Stampfer M, Willett W. A prospective study of tomato products, lycopene, and prostate cancer risk. J Natl Cancer Inst 2002; 94:391–398.

78. Mills P, Beeson W, Phillips R, Fraser G. Cohort study of diet, lifestyle, and prostate cancer in adventist men. Cancer 1989; 64:598–604.

79. Cohen J, Kristal A, Stanford J. Fruit and vegetable intakes and prostate cancer risk. J Natl Cancer Inst 2000; 92:61–68.

80. Kolonel L, Hankin J, Whittemore A, Wu A, Gallagher R, Wilkens L, John E, Howe G, Paffenbarger R. Vegetables, fruits, legumes and prostate cancer: a multiethnic case-control study. Cancer Epidemiol Biomark Prev 2000; 9:795–804.

81. Schuman L, Mandel J, Radke A, Seal U, Halberg F. Some selected features of the epidemiology of prostatic cancer: Minneapolis–St. Paul, Minnesota case-control study, 1976–1979. Washington, DC: Hemisphere Publishing, 1982:345–354.

82. Key T, Silcocks P, Davey G, Appleby P, and Bishop D. A case-control study of diet and prostate cancer. Br J Cancer 1997; 76:678–687.

83. Tzonou A, Singorello L, Lagiou P, Wuu J, Trichopoulos D, Trichopoulou A. Diet and cancer of the prostate: a case-control study in Greece. Int J Cancer 1999; 80:704–708.

84. Norrish AE, Jackson RT, Sharpe SJ, Skeaff CM. Prostate cancer and dietary carotenoids. Am J Epidemiol 2000; 151:119–123.

85. Jain M, Hislop G, Howe G, Ghadirian P. Plant foods, antioxidants, and prostate cancer risk: findings from case-control studies in Canada. Nutr Cancer 1999; 34:173–184.

86. Gann P, Ma J, Giovannucci E, Willett W, Sacks F, Hennekens C, Stampfer M. Lower prostate cancer risk in men with elevated plasma lycopene levels: results of a prospective analysis. Cancer Res 1999; 59:1225–1230.

87. Lu Q, Hung J, Heber D, Go V, Reuter V, Cordon-Cardo C, Scher H, Marshall J, Zhang Z. Inverse associations between plasma lycopene and other carotenoids and prostate cancer. Cancer Epidemiol Biomark Prev 2001; 10:749–756.

88. Vogt T, Mayne S, Graubard P, Swanson C, Sowell A, Schoenberg J, Swanson G, Greenberg R, Hoover R, Hayes R, Ziegler R. Serum lycopene, other serum carotenoids, and risk of prostate cancer in US Blacks and Whites. Am J Epidemiol 2002; 155:1023–1032.

89. Hsing A, Comstock G, Abbey H, Polk B. Serologic precursors of cancer, retinol, carotenoids, and tocopherol and risk of prostate cancer. J Natl Cancer Inst 1990; 82:941–946.

90. Huang H, Alberg A, Norkus E, Hoffman S, Comstock G, Helzlsour K. Prospective study of antioxidant micronutrients in the blood and the risk of developing prostate cancer. Am J Epidemiol 2003; 157:335–344.

91. Nomura A, Stemmermann G, Lee J, Craft N. Serum micronutrients and prostate cancer in Japanese Americans in Hawaii. Cancer Epidemiol Biomark Prev 1997; 6:487–491.

92. Kristal A, Cohen J. Invited commentary: tomatoes, lycopene, and prostate cancer. How strong is the evidence? Am J Epidemiol 2000; 151:124–127.

93. Chen L, Stacewicz-Sapuntzakis M, Duncan C, Sharifi R, Ghosh L, Breemen R, Ashton D, Bowen P. Oxidative DNA damage in prostate cancer patients consuming tomato sauce-based entrees as a whole-food intervention. J Natl Cancer Inst 2001; 93:1872–1879.

94. Bowen P, Chen L, Stacewicz-Sapuntzakis M, Duncan C, Sharifi R, Ghosh L, Kim H, Christov-Tzelkov K, van Breemen R. Tomato sauce supplementation and prostate cancer: lycopene accumulation and modulation of biomarkers of carcinogenesis. Exp Biol Med 2002; 227:886–893.

95. van Breemen R, Xu X, Viana M, Chen L, Stacewicz-Sapuntzakis M, Duncan C, Bowen P, Sharifi R. Liquid chromatography-mass spectrometry of *cis*- and all-*trans*-lycopene in human serum and prostate tissue after dietary supplementation with tomato sauce. J Agric Food Chem 2002; 50:2214–2219.

96. Kucuk O, Sarkar F, Djuric Z, Sakr W, Pollak M, Khachik F, Banerjee M, Bertram J, Wood D Jr. Effects of lycopene supplementation in patients with localized prostate cancer. Exp Biol Med 2002; 227:881–885.

97. Kim L, Rao A, Rao L. Effect of lycopene on prostate LNCaP cancer cells in culture. J Med Food 2002; 5:181–187.

98. Kotake-Nara E, Kushiro M, Zhang H, Sugawara T, Miyashita K, Naga A. Carotenoids affect proliferation of human prostate cancer cells. J Nutr 2001; 131:3303–3306.

99. Matos H, Di Mascio P, Medeiros M. Protective effect of lycopene on lipid peroxidation and oxidative DNA damage in cell culture. Arch Biochem Biophys 2000; 383:56–59.

100. Heber D, Lu Q. Overview of mechanisms of action of lycopene. Exp Biol Med 2002; 227:920–923.

101. Mayne S. Antioxidant nutrients and chronic disease: use of biomarkers of exposure and oxidative stress status in epidemiologic research. J Nutr 2003; 133:933S–940S.

102. Stahl W, von Laar J, Martin H, Emmerich T, Sies H. Stimulation of gap junctional communication: comparison of acyclo-retinoic acid and lycopene. Arch Biochem Biophys 2000; 373:271–274.

19

Carotenoids and Eye Disease: Epidemiological Evidence

Julie A. Mares
University of Wisconsin–Madison Medical School, Madison, Wisconsin, U.S.A.

I. INTRODUCTION

The biological mechanisms by which carotenoids could protect the human eye against degenerative conditions of aging such as cataract and macular degeneration are described in chapter 22 (1). In the present chapter, epidemiologic evidence to evaluate a protective influence on these common eye conditions of aging and on other adult eye diseases is discussed. Epidemiology provides perspective about whether the influence of carotenoids on eye pathology can be generalized from the short term conditions used in experiments in culture dishes and in animals to longer time periods in people under a variety of environmental conditions and genetic make-ups. Further, results of epidemiologic studies form the basis to predict how important these influences are likely to be, relative to other general lifestyle or diet factors that influence disease risk. Evidence from both clinical trials and observations in large populations will be discussed.

II. AGE-RELATED MACULAR DEGENERATION

Age-related macular degeneration (AMD) is a degenerative condition of the central retina, or macula, that affects the center of the field of vision and the ability to see fine detail, such as is needed to read newspapers. Early signs of age-related maculopathy (ARM) are common, present in one-quarter of people older than 65 (2), and increase the risk for developing late AMD (3). The late form that affects vision is less common; about 7% of people 75 years of age and older can expect to develop late AMD over 10 years (3). This suggests that the process usually develops slowly over many years and that only some of the people who have early signs will actually develop the condition associated with severe loss of vision in their lifetime. Nevertheless, because medical interventions are currently of limited value in delaying the progression and cannot prevent the eventual loss of vision or provide a cure, AMD is the leading cause of legal blindness among older people (4).

Over the past 10 years, diet has been considered as one of several possible lifestyle changes (such as stopping smoking) that may delay the onset or progression AMD. The recent observation that high-dose antioxidants delay the progression from intermediate to late stages (5) heightens the interest in the possibility that the nutritional milieu can impact the natural history of age-related maculopathy. Carotenoids are one of several diet components previously reviewed (6) that are theorized to slow or prevent ARM.

Epidemiologic studies have investigated relationships of ARM to carotenoids that occur in eye tissues and the other most abundant carotenoids in systemic circulation. First discussed will be those carotenoids present in eyes [lutein and its structural isomer, zeaxanthin (9)] that compose macular pigment. These may protect the macula by absorbing light in the blue range and/or reducing free radical damage in rod outer segments (see Chapter 22) (1). People with AMD appear to have lower concentrations of macular pigment (10,11). These observations are consistent with lower levels of lutein and zeaxanthin in autopsy specimens of people with and without AMD (12). However, from these studies, it is not clear whether lower macular pigment contributes to or is a result of AMD. Epidemiological studies of newly developed (incident) AMD or early stages of age-related maculopathy can provide insights that strengthen or weaken the possibility of a causal association.

The overall body of evidence from epidemiologic studies to suggest the possibility that dietary lutein and zeaxanthin lower risk for AMD is inconsistent (Fig. 1). In one large case control study of incident cases of one form of late-stage AMD (neovascular and/or exudative macular degeneration), patients with this condition had lower levels of lutein and zeaxanthin in the diet (13) and blood (14). This comparison permitted the estimate that intake of lutein and zeaxanthin in high compared to low quintiles reduced the risk of this type of macular degeneration by more than twofold, and suggested that dietary lutein and/or zeaxanthin might have a large influence on risk for developing AMD.

Inferring a protective influence of dietary lutein and zeaxanthin requires consistent findings across epidemiological studies with different study samples and study designs to reduce the possibility that observations were the result of chance, of bias inherent in a particular study design, or of uncontrolled

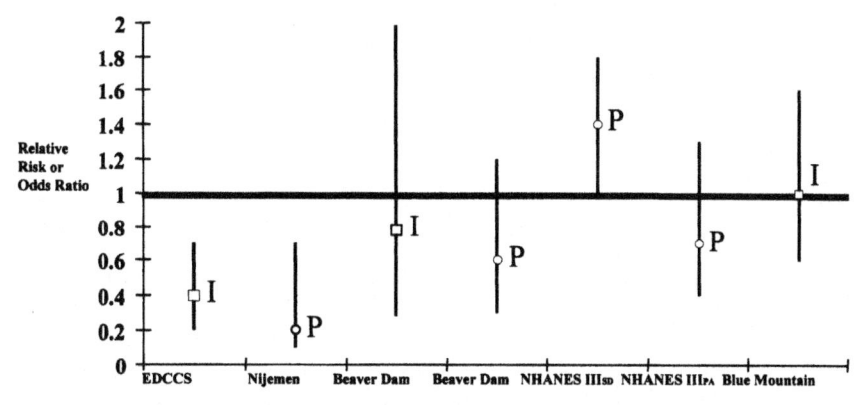

Figure 1   Adjusted risk ratios and 95% confidence intervals for early and/or late age-related maculopathy among people with dietary intakes of lutein and zeaxanthin in high versus low quintiles. P indicates prevalent maculopathy (determined in cross-sectional or retrospective studies) and I indicate incident maculopathy (determined in prospective studies). SD indicates soft drusen and PA indicates pigmentary abnormalities. The data are from the the Eye Disease Case-Control Study (EDCCS) (13), a case-control study conducted in Nijmegen, the Netherlands (15), the Beaver Dam Eye Study retrospective (17) and 5-year prospective analyses (18), the Third National Health and Nutrition Examination Survey (NHANES III) (16), and the Blue Mountains Eye Study (19).

confounding. To date, such evidence is lacking. Subsequently published epidemiological studies in four different samples (13–17) fail to support this initial observation of a protective relationship (Fig. 1) in the Eye Disease Case Control Study. Associations between levels of lutein and zeaxanthin in the blood and age-related maculopathy are also inconsistent across studies (Fig. 2) (12,13,16,18,19).

However, it is too early in the epidemiological investigations of relationships of lutein and zeaxanthin to project the lack of consistency as evidence for the lack of an important protective influence in the development of ARM. Inconsistency in study results at the early stages of developing epidemiological evidence might reflect limitations of study designs that are frequently employed in earlier stages of scientific investigation or limitations of the protective relationships to certain stages or types of disease. There is evidence to support the possibility that the inconsistency in results reflects several of these.

One possibility for the inconsistency may be that the protective influence of lutein and zeaxanthin may be limited to later stages of the disease, which are poorly represented by available studies. A recent study of the relationship between dietary lutein and zeaxanthin and ARM in a fifth population, the

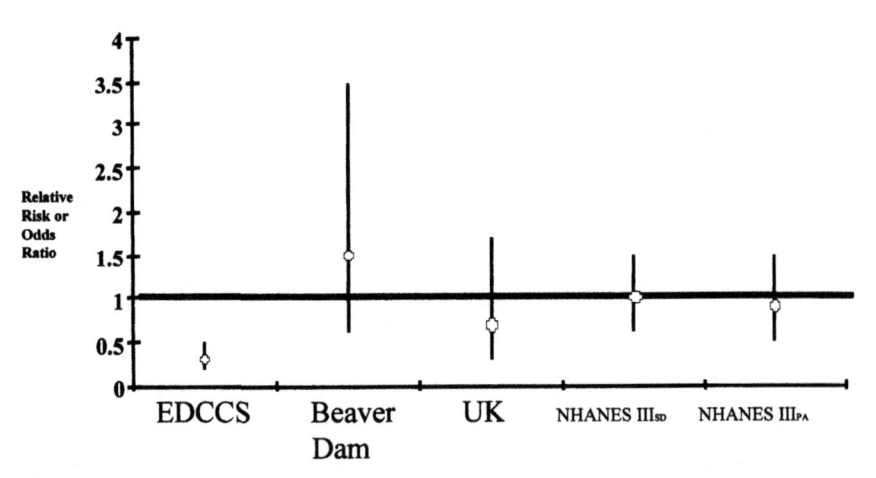

Figure 2 Adjusted risk ratios for early and/or late stages of age-related maculopathy among people with serum levels of lutein and zeaxanthin in high versus low quintiles. SD indicates soft drusen and PA indicates pigmentary abnormalities. The data are from the the Eye Disease Case-Control Study (EDCCS) (14); the Beaver Dam Eye Study nested case-control analysis (20), a case-control study in the United Kingdom (21), and the Third National Health and Nutrition Examination Survey (NHANES III) (18).

Atherosclerosis Risk in Communities (ARIC) study, supports this possibility (Mares-Perlman et al., unpublished manuscript). In this study, photographs of the retinal fundus were taken approximately 6 years after the collection of food frequency data, when subjects were between the ages of 45 and 65 years (22). Higher intake of lutein and zeaxanthin was not associated with the more common early sign of macular degeneration, soft drusen, the lipid- and mineral-rich deposit that often accompanies the condition (Fig. 3). However, the intake of lutein and zeaxanthin in high, compared to low, quintiles was associated with 40% lower odds for the presence of retinal pigment abnormalities, a less common and probably later manifestation of early AMD. This association remained after adjustment for other measured risk factors. There were too few cases of late AMD in this young sample to permit evaluation of relationships with this severe stage.

Associations of lutein and zeaxanthin intake by type of ARM across all studies are given in Figure 4. High intake is more often related to lower risk for late ARM and retinal pigment abnormalities, the less common of the two early stages of ARM. In contrast, high intake is related to higher odds for soft drusen, the most common early stage of ARM. These trends in data across many samples suggest that lutein may protect the retinal pigment epithelium against later degenerative changes but may not influence the accumulation of the lipid- and

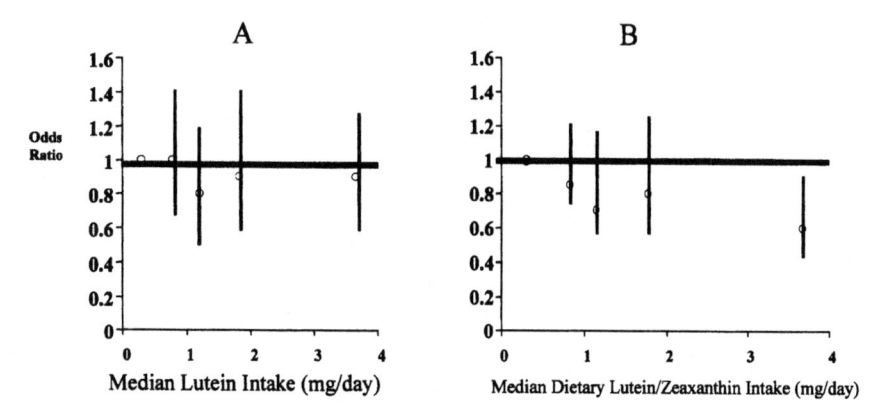

Figure 3 Quintile (lowest = referent) odds ratios and 95% confidence intervals for two types of early age-related maculopathy: (**A**) Soft drusen (494 cases) and (**B**) retinal pigmentary abnormalities (281 cases) in 1993–1996 among persons with dietary intakes of lutein and zeaxanthin in high versus low quintiles 6 years earlier (1988–1990) by median intake in quintiles in the Atherosclerosis Risk in Communities Study, after adjustment for age and energy intake (adjustment for blood pressure, blood cholesterol, and smoking did not influence the odds ratios) (Mares-Perlman et al., 2003, unpublished manuscript).

mineral-rich drusen. Additional studies in which these conditions are evaluated separately will permit more thoroughly investigation of this possibility.

A second reason for the inconsistency in early epidemiological studies could be that several of the study designs were cross-sectional (15,18,20,21) or retrospective (17), in which subjects' diets and eye photographs were obtained at the same time. If people have made changes in diet so that the diet assessed in the study reflects recent changes, rather than diet over the lifetime during which ARM may have slowly developed, then including such subjects would make associations between diet carotenoids and ARM hard to detect. If people with ARM or related conditions, such as cardiovascular disease or hypertension (which are related to higher risk of ARM in some studies), were more likely than those without these conditions to increase their intake of lutein-containing fruits and vegetables, then the risk ratios could be biased closer to unity. About half of people between the ages of 65 and 75 are likely to have encountered three or more chronic conditions. Therefore, they are more likely than middle-aged people to have made recent changes in diet to an attempt to improve health. Also, older people who survive long enough to be included in the sample are also likely to have better diets than those who have died. Therefore, a selective mortality bias is more likely to occur in cross-sectional studies that include older people. One strategy to evaluate whether bias as a result of diet change or selective mortality

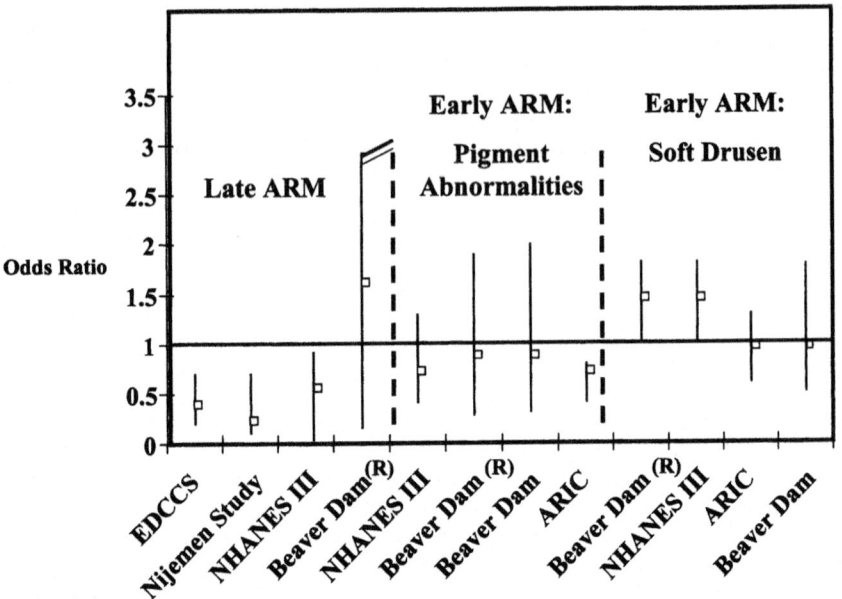

Figure 4 Odds ratios and 95% confidence intervals for late ARM and two types of early ARM among persons with dietary intakes of lutein and zeaxanthin in high versus low quintiles. The data include only studies that indicate risk ratios by type of ARM. They are from the the Eye Disease Case-Control Study (EDCCS) (11), a case-control study conducted in Nijmegen, the Netherlands (15), the Third National Health and Nutrition Examination Survey (NHANES III) (18), the Beaver Dam Eye Study retrospective analyses (R) (17), and 5-year prospective analyses (P) (16).

is likely to be influencing the risk ratios is to evaluate the associations in the youngest groups who are at risk for ARM.

When this was done in the Third National Health and Nutrition Examination Survey (18), associations of late ARM and pigmentary abnormalities were stronger and statistically significant in the youngest age groups at risk for these conditions, as observed in the younger cohort of the ARIC study. The distinctly higher risk for drusen among persons with high intake only in the oldest age group suggests that this association may be due to bias rather than a causal factor. High intake was also significantly related to lower odds for late ARM among people at earliest risk for this severe stage, after excluding persons older than 80 years (Fig. 5). This suggests that the biases may have contributed to an inability to observe protective associations in older people.

A third reason for inconsistency in relationships of dietary carotenoids to ARM in studies reported to date may be either that very low intakes may be needed to increase risk or that very high intakes are needed to decrease risk. Also, if the

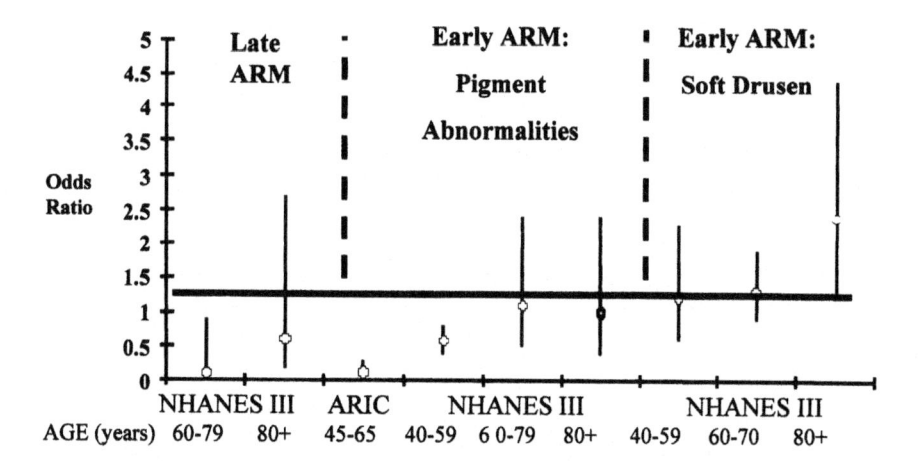

Figure 5 Adjusted risk ratios and 95% confidence intervals for early and/or late age-related maculopathy among people with dietary intakes of lutein and zeaxanthin in high versus low quintiles by type of maculopathy and age group. Data are from the Third National Health and Nutrition Examination Survey (NHANES III) (18) in the Atherosclerosis Risk in Communities Study (ARIC) (Mares-Perlman, unpublished data).

associations are modest, a wide range in intakes may be needed in order to detect the association above the noise due to measurement error or uncontrolled confounding. In support of this possibility, the intake of lutein and zeaxanthin is always associated with lower risk for late ARM or pigmentary abnormalities in those studies in which a substantial number of subjects had high intakes: at least 10% of the sample had lutein plus zeaxanthin intakes that were greater than about 3.5 mg/day (Fig. 6).

A fourth reason for inconsistency across studies may be the large number of physical attributes and lifestyles that might modify the ability to accumulate lutein and zeaxanthin. If unknown and not adjusted for, the noise may blur associations. While current studies indicate an ability to influence levels of macular pigment by increasing levels taken in from foods (23) or supplements (24,25), a large variability in levels in macular pigment is unexplained (25,26). Higher body fatness, which is related to lower macular pigment density in some studies (27–29), is an example. Body fat may influence the distribution of carotenoids in the body and the ability to accumulate carotenoids in the eye. Measurement and adjustment for body fat mass may clarify associations between lutein intake and AMD. The factors that influence the absorption and distribution of lutein and zeaxanthin are largely unknown. Clearly, a better understanding of factors that influence the absorption of lutein and zeaxanthin and accumulation in the retina will enhance our ability to measure and adjust for the factors that modify the relationship of dietary

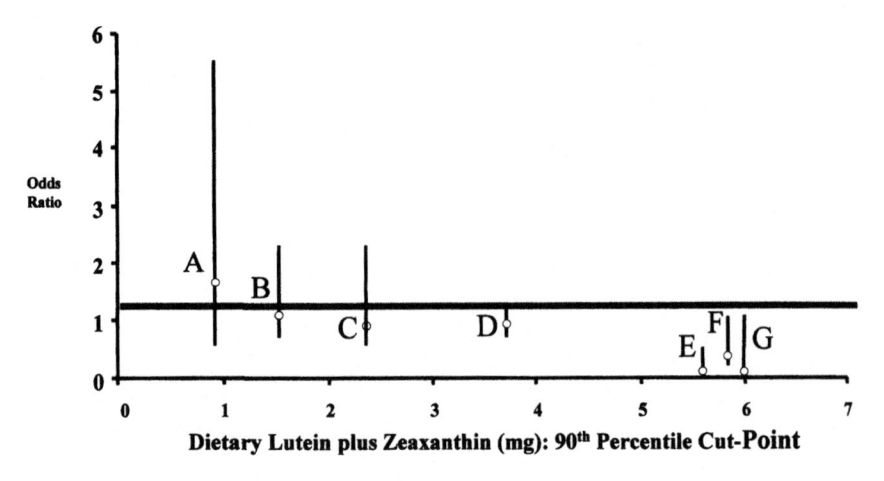

Limited to Late ARM and Pigmentary Abnormalities

Figure 6 Adjusted risk ratios and 95% confidence intervals for late age-related maculopathy and pigmentary abnormalities among people with dietary intakes of lutein and zeaxanthin in high versus low quintiles by level of lutein intake at the 90th percentile cutpoint. Data presented are limited to incident cases (EDCCS) or, in cross-sectional studies, to the earliest age groups at risk (late ARM: 60–70 years); pigmentary abnormalities (40–59 years in NHANES III and 45–65 years in ARIC). Data include only studies that present estimates of nutrient level and odds ratios by type of age-related maculopathy and are from the the Beaver Dam Eye Study retrospective analyses (17) for late ARM (A) and pigmentary abnormalities (B) or prospective analyses for pigmentary abnormalities (C) (16), the Atherosclerosis Risk in Communities Study (Mares-Perlman, unpublished data) for pigmentary abnormalities (D), the Eye Disease Case-Control Study (E) (13), and the Third National Health and Nutrition Examination Survey (18) for late ARM (ages 60 and older) (F) and pigmentary abnormalities (ages 40–59 years) (G).

lutein and zeaxanthin to ARM. Because it is possible to measure levels of macular pigment in vivo noninvasively, ongoing studies using this technique may provide more clues about the determinants of macular pigment. These determinants can be measured and adjusted for to improve future studies of associations of lutein and zeaxanthin intake to disease. Studies of levels of dietary carotenoids needed to increase macular pigment will also provide insights about the levels of intake that is needed to protect against macular degeneration (if it is, indeed, protective).

In summary, while the epidemiological evidence does not strongly support the idea that the intake of lutein plus zeaxanthin lowers the risk for developing AMD, the inconsistent observations may reflect bias or limitations of the protection to later stages of ARM or to very high intakes. Continued study of these associations in large prospective studies and/or other study designs that address these possibilities is expected to provide new insights about the possibility that higher intakes of these carotenoids may prevent or delay AMD.

Epidemiological studies have, also, not yet been able to address the possibility that the protective influence is limited to or is more marked with either the lutein or the zeaxanthin isomer. The scarcity of data on food composition of these two isomers precludes such investigations presently. Some insights may be provided when blood samples are used to estimate the relative intake of these two isomers from foods.

Several carotenoids that are absent in the eye but present in the blood may influence the oxidant load from environmental exposures such as cigarette smoke or inflammatory conditions. These may indirectly influence the development of macular degeneration by lowering the oxidation of low-density lipoprotein particles for which receptors exist in the retina (30). However, current evidence in epidemiological studies does not support this notion. While the dietary intake of one or more provitamin A carotenoids (β-carotene, α-carotene, β-cryptoxanthin) was related to lower prevalence of age-related maculopathy in a representative sample of the U.S. population (31) and to lower incidence (13,16) of various stages of ARM in some past studies, in the two latter studies this was no longer significant after control for the intake of carotenoids that are found in the retina (13) and fruits and vegetables, in general, in the other (16). Several studies find no associations with pro-vitamin A carotenoids in the diet (16,19,32) or blood (21,33–36). Moreover, retinol or preformed vitamin A, has not been related to ARM (13,16–18,30). Beta-carotene was one of several antioxidant nutrients in a supplement that was shown to lower the progression of intermediate to late-stage ARM, and may or may not have contributed to this benefit (5). Overall, there is not strong support in epidemiologic studies that pro-vitamin A carotenoids or vitamin A lower risk for ARM or slow its progression.

Lycopene, which has been detected in small quantities in the retina by some investigators (7) but not others (8,9), might protect against ARM because of its high ability to quench single oxygen (37). Low blood levels have been related to higher rates of ARM in two studies (33,35) but not others (14,21). Dietary levels have not been observed to be related to ARM (17,19,32). Therefore, epidemiological evidence to support a protective role of lycopene is not strong.

III. INHERITED RETINAL DEGENERATION

The possibility that eye carotenoids, lutein and zeaxanthin, may improve vision or slow other types of inherited retinal degeneration has only begun to be investigated. It is hypothesized that lutein and/or zeaxanthin may slow degeneration of vision in patients with retinitis pigmentosa, Usher's syndrome, or choroideremia, for the same reasons that they may protect against other degenerations in the eye.

However, only preliminary data in a small number of patients suggest that lutein supplementation slows vision loss in retinitis pigmentosa (37). This was not confirmed in a separate 6-month supplementation trial (38). Lutein supplementation for 6 months in patients with choroideremia also did not influence central vision (39). Differences in the effectiveness of lutein across studies might reflect a varied ability of people to accumulate retinal carotenoids in response to supplementation. The two latter studies indicated varied response of supplementation to macular pigment density enhancement following supplementation.

The influence of lutein and zeaxanthin from diet or supplements on the long-term natural history of inherited retinal degenerations is unknown. In one study (38) disease expression tended to be more severe in patients who had lower levels of macular pigment at the beginning of the study. This could reflect either a protective influence or a consequence of the disease. Because of the low prevalence of these conditions in the general population, epidemiological studies have a limited ability to gain insights about the magnitude of influence of intake of these carotenoids over the long term and the attributes that modify this influence. However, large multicentered studies that assess both past exposure to carotenoids and, prospectively, response to levels of carotenoids in the diet and in the macular pigment could provide better estimates.

IV. CATARACT

With age there is an increased propensity to develop opacities in the lens that eventually form cataracts, a condition that is present in over 50% of people older than 75 years (40). Carotenoids are some of several food components that may slow the development of cataracts, a condition for which surgery in the United States accounts for the largest single item cost in the Medicare budget (41).

As in the retina, lutein and zeaxanthin are the only detectable carotenoids in the lens (see Chapter 22). There is a small but consistent body of epidemiological evidence from prospective cohort studies that suggests that intakes of these carotenoids in high, compared with low quintiles, lowers risk for cataract surgery (42,43) or the incidence of nuclear cataract (44) the most common type of cataract for which cataract surgery is performed (45). These results (summarized in Fig. 7) are consistent with earlier studies of a lower prevalence of nuclear cataract among women (46) and men (47) with higher intake of lutein or zeaxanthin. They are also consistent with the finding of lower odds for cataract extraction associated with the intake of spinach in an Italian study (48). Moreover, there are two separate observations of higher lens density among people who have lower levels of these carotenoids in macular pigment (49,50).

Associations with blood levels have been investigated in only a few smaller studies. The incidence (51) or prevalence (52) of nuclear cataract was lower

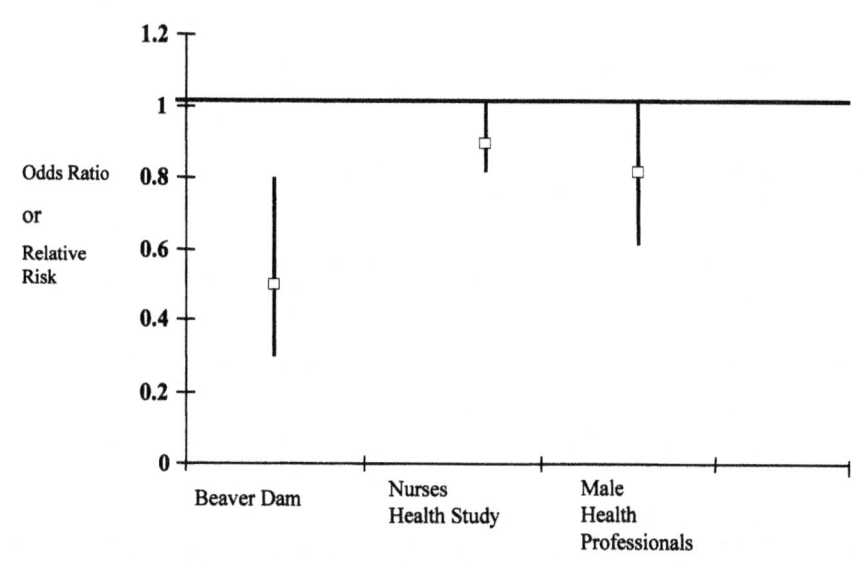

Figure 7 Risk ratios and 95% confidence intervals for nuclear cataract or cataract extraction in prospective cohort studies among persons with dietary lutein and zeaxanthin in high versus low quintiles. Data are from the Beaver Dam Eye Study (44) (using dietary estimates for the time period 10 years before baseline), the Male Health Professionals' Study (42), and the Nurses' Health Study (43).

among people with higher blood levels of these carotenoids, but in neither of these studies was this statistically significant. In two other studies, higher levels of lutein and zeaxanthin were associated with higher risk for prevalent cataract (53,54). However, temporal confounding is a possible explanation for direct associations, and this is supported by different associations between carotenoid intake at the time of cataract assessment and in earlier time periods (53).

Despite the results of several epidemiological studies that suggest a protective influence of lutein and zeaxanthin on lowering risk for cataract, there are no animal studies or clinical trials of lutein or zeaxanthin supplements that prove a protective effect of these carotenoids in the lens. The lower risk for cataract among people with high levels of lutein in the diet or retina may reflect other dietary attributes or lifestyles that are associated with high intake these carotenoids. Thus, more scientific evidence is needed that suggests a benefit of these carotenoids, independent of other aspects of diet that are more common in people who obtain them from food sources.

As with AMD, it is possible that carotenoids present in the blood, but not the lens, could influence cataract by lowering the oxidant burden in systemic circulation and, therefore, retaining blood antioxidants that are available to tissues.

High plasma concentrations of total carotenoids or β-carotene, the most abundant blood carotenoid, were associated with lower prevalence of some types of cataract in one study (55), but not several others (52,53,56–58). However, blood levels of carotenoids may not be good markers for levels of carotenoids in the diet or eye, as they are influenced by many factors that are poorly understood (59). Nevertheless, supplementation with β-carotene alone (60–62) or in combination with other nutrients (63,64) has not been associated with lower rates of cataract or cataract extraction, except in a subsample of subjects from one of two regions in one study (65), as part of a broad multinutrient supplement in an undernourished region of China (64) and among U.S. physicians who smoke (62). This could reflect a lack of influence of carotenoids that are not present in the lens except among persons exposed to high levels of oxidative stress or poor diets. Alternatively, the influence of carotenoids and other nutrients on lens opacities that develop over many years may require longer than the length of most clinical trials (up to 6 years) to observe.

In summary, a consistent body of evidence suggests that lutein and zeaxanthin may lower the risk for cataract extraction or the type of cataract that most often leads to extraction (nuclear cataract). There is not consistent evidence for a protective influence of β-carotene, but there is a possibility for a protective influence in limited subgroups of the population. Because of the high prevalence of cataracts and the aging population, even a modest lowering of risk of cataract with higher intakes of lutein and zeaxanthin could have a large impact on eye health and health care costs. The degree of risk reduction can be better estimated in long-term prospective studies across a variety of people. Also needed is evidence for a specific effect of these carotenoids rather than other dietary attributes that may protect against cataract, in clinical trials or even in animal experiments. The current evidence for associations of the status of other carotenoids that are not contained in eye tissues to the occurrence of cataract is inconsistent and, therefore, unsupportive to date.

V. DIABETIC EYE DISEASES

Common ocular complications of type I and type II diabetes involve the development of retinopathy and cataract of the lens. Carotenoid levels may be lower among people who develop diabetes and increase risk for these eye conditions, but the data needed to evaluate this possibility are limited. In a representative sample of the U.S. population, people with newly diagnosed diabetes had lower levels of serum carotenoids than those without this condition (66). Data to describe the relationship of carotenoid status to eye diseases commonly associated with diabetes are lacking.

In the only cross-sectional study of relationships between diabetic retinopathy and dietary carotenoids, people taking insulin who had a higher intake of

β-carotene were more likely to have retinopathy (67). However, because of the cross-sectional nature of this study, this result may be explained by increases in the intake of β-carotene or fruits and vegetables as a result of disease worsening, which also increases the risk for the development of diabetic retinopathy.

There are no published studies that describe the relationship of dietary carotenoids to cataracts in people with diabetes. However, in a small case-control study, patients with diabetes mellitus had higher lens optical density than controls (68), which may increase risk for cataract development. Patients with diabetes were also observed to have lower levels of macular pigment density (68). This may reflect lower availability of retinal carotenoids among people with diabetes or a compromise in the ability to take up retinal carotenoids. Data describing relationships of macular pigment density to the occurrence of both cataract and retinopathy in people with diabetes are needed to support the hypothesis that these or other dietary carotenoids correlated with their intake protect against these common complications of diabetes mellitus.

VI. SUMMARY AND CONCLUSIONS

In summary, there is evidence from epidemiological studies to support the possibility that lutein and zeaxanthin, the predominant carotenoids in the eye tissue, protect against the most common age-related eye conditions, i.e., macular degeneration and central cataract. Some studies suggest a large influence on risk but additional studies, particularly long-term prospective studies, are needed to better estimate the overall impact on risk. Continued research is also needed to rule out the possibility that what appear to be protective influences of lutein and zeaxanthin on risk for age-related macular degeneration and cataract do not reflect other aspects of diet or lifestyles of people with high levels of these carotenoids in their diets. Both clinical trials and large prospective studies (where the consistency of these patterns can be observed across groups of people who have and do not have other explanatory attributes) will be helpful. While clinical trials will provide definitive evidence of protection in specific, short-term circumstances, long-term prospective studies will contribute insights about protection over the long term and under a variety of circumstances. Ongoing studies of the determinants of levels of carotenoids in the eye, as reflected by macular pigment density, will also provide a greater understanding of the personal attributes that may influence the absorption of these carotenoids and uptake by eye tissues. This will improve risk estimates made in epidemiological studies and provide insights needed to recommend appropriate levels of intake based on individual characteristics.

There is a possibility that carotenoids may slow the progression or improve vision in people with less common inherited retinal degenerations, but this area of research is in its infancy. There is also the possibility that carotenoids may lower risk for the eye diseases of cataract and retinopathy that accompany diabetes mellitus. Yet the evidence is extremely limited and these possibilities have not been well investigated. The recent advances in ability to perform noninvasive measurements of retinal carotenoids will advance our understanding of the influence of predominant eye carotenoids on these eye diseases as well as the more common age-related eye diseases.

ACKNOWLEDGMENTS

This work is supported by National Institutes of Health, National Eye Institute grant EY013018 and 11722 and the Research to Prevent Blindness Lew S. Wasserman Award.

REFERENCES

1. Landrum JT, Bone RA. Mechanistic evidence for eye diseases and carotenoids. In this volume.
2. Klein R, Klein BEK, Jensen SC, Mares-Perlman JA, Cruickshanks KJ, Palta M. Age-related maculopathy in a multiracial United States population: the National Health and Nutrition Examination Survey III. Ophthalmology 1999; 106(6):1056–1065.
3. Klein R, Klein BEK, Tomany SC, Meure SM, Huang GH. Ten-year incidence and progression of age-related maculopathy: the Beaver Dam Eye Study. Ophthalmology 2002; 109(10):1767–1779.
4. National Society to Prevent Blindness Vision Problems in the US: Data Analyses. New York: National Society to Prevent Blindness, 1980:1–46.
5. Age-Related Eye Disease Study Research Group. A randomized, placebo-controlled, clinical trial of high-dose supplementation with vitamins C and E, beta-carotene, and zinc for age-related macular degeneration and vision loss: AREDS report no. 8. Arch Ophthalmol 2001; 119(10):1417–1436.
6. Mares-Perlman JA, Klein R. Diet and age-related macular degeneration. In: Taylor A, ed. Nutritional and Environmental Influences on the Eye. CRC Press: Boca Raton, FL, 1999:181–214.
7. Bernstein PS, Frederick K, Carvalho LS, Muir GJ, Zhao DY, Katz NB. Identification and quantitation of carotenoids and their metabolites in the tissue of the human eye. Eye Res 2001; 72:215–223.
8. Bone RA, Landrum JT, Friedes LM, Gomez CM, Kilbutn MD, Mendenez E, Vidal I. Distribution of stereo isomers in the human retina. Exp Eye Res 1997; 64:211–218.
9. Handelman GJ, Dratz EA, Reay CC, Van Kuijk JG. Carotenoids in the human macula and whole retina. Ophthalmol Vis Sci 1988; 29:850–855.

10. Beatty S, Henson, D. Macular pigment and age-related macular degeneration. Arch Ophthalmol 1999; 113:1518–1523.
11. Bernstein PS, Wintch SW. Resonance Raman measurement of macular carotenoids in normal subjects and in age-related macular degeneration patients. Ophthalmology 2002; 109(10):1780–1787.
12. Bone RA, Landrum JT, Mayne ST, Gomez CM, Tibor SE, Twaroska EE. Macular pigment in donor eyes with and without AMD: a case-control study. Invest Ophthalmol Vis Sci 2001; 42(1):235–240.
13. Seddon J, Ajani UA, Sperduto RD, Hiller R, Blair N, Burton TC, Farber MD, Gragoudas ES, Haller J, Miller DT. Dietary carotenoids, vitamins A, C, and E, and advanced age related macular degeneration. JAMA 1994; 272:1413–1420.
14. Eye Disease Case-Control Study Group. Antioxidant status and neovascular age-related macular degenration. Arch Ophthalmol 1993; 111:104–109.
15. Snellen ELM, Verbeek ALM, van den Hoogen GWP. Neovascular age-related macular degeneration and its relationship to antioxidant intake. Acta Ophthalmol Scand 2002; 80:368–371.
16. VandenLangenberg GM, Mares-Perlman JA, Klein R, Klein BE, Brady WE, Palta M. Associations between antioxidant and zinc intake and the 5-year incidence of early age-related maculopathy in the Beaver Dam Eye Study. Am J Epidemiol 1998; 148(2):204–214.
17. Mares-Perlman JA, Klein R, Klein BE. Association of zinc and antioxidant nutrients with age-related maculopathy. Arch Ophthalmol 1996; 114(8):991–997.
18. Mares-Perlman JA, Fisher AL, Klein R. Lutein and zeaxanthin in the diet and serum and their relation to age-related maculopathy in the Third National Health and Nutrition Examination Survey. Am J Epidemiol 2001; 153(5):424–432.
19. Flood V, Smith W, Wang J, Manzi F, Webb D, Mitchell P. Dietary antioxidant intake and incidence of early age-related maculopathy: the Blue Mountains Eye Study. Am Acad Ophthalmol 2002; 109(12) 2272–2277.
20. Mares-Perlman JA, Brady WE, Klein R. Serum antioxidants and age-related macular degeneration in a population-based case-control study. Arch Ophthalmol 1995; 113(12):1518–1523.
21. Sanders TAB, Haines AP, Wormald R, Wright LA, Obeid O. Essential fatty acids, plasma cholesterol, and matched control subjects. Am J Clin Nutr 1993; 57:428.
22. Klein R, Clegg L, Cooper LS, Hubbard LD, Klein BE, King WN, Folsom AR. Prevalence of age-related maculopathy in the Atherosclerosis Risk in Communities Study. Arch Ophthalmol 1999; 117(9):1203–1210.
23. Hammond BR, Johnson EJ, Russell RM, Krinsky NI, Yeum KJ, Edwards RB, Snodderly DM. Dietary modification of human macular pigment density. Invest Ophthalmol Vis Sci 1997; 38(9):1795–1801.
24. Landrum JT, Bone RA, Joa H, Kilburn MD, Moore LL, Sprague KE. A one year study of the macular pigment: the effect of 140 days of a lutein supplement. Eye Res 1997; 65:57–62.
25. Berendschot TJM, Goldbohm A, Klopping WAA, Van de Kratts J, Van Norel J, Van Norren D. Influence of lutein supplementation on macular pigment, assessed with two objective techniques. Invest Ophthalmol 2000; 41(11):3322–3326.

26. Curran-Celentano J, Hammond BR, Ciulla TA, Cooper DA, Pratt LM, Danis RB. Relation between dietary intake, serum concentrations, and retinal concentrations of lutein and zeaxanthin in adults in a Midwest population. Am J Clin Nutr 2001; 74:796–802.

27. Broekmans WM, Berendschot TT, Klopping-Ketelaars IA, DeVries AJ, Goldbohm RA, Tijburg LB, Kardinaal AF, Van Poppel G. Macular pigment density in relation to serum and adipose tissue concentrations of lutein and serum concentrations of zeaxanthin. Am J Clin Nutr 2002; 76(3):595–603.

28. Hammond BR, Ciulla TA, Snodderly DM. Macular pigment density is reduced in obese subjects. Invest Ophthalmol Vis Sci 2002; 43(1):47–50.

29. Johnson EJ, Hammond BR, Yeum KY, Qin J, Wang XD, Castaneda C, Snodderly DM, Russell R. Relation among serum and tissue concentrations of lutein and zeaxanthin and macular pigment density. Am J Clin Nutr 2000; 71:1555–1562.

30. Hayes KC, Lindsey S, Stephan ZF, Brecker D. Retinal pigment epithelium possesses both LDL and scavenger receptor activity. Invest Ophthalmol Vis Sci 1989; 30:225–232.

31. Goldberg J, Flowerdew J, Smith E, Brody JA, Tso MOM. Factors associated with age-related macular degeneration: an analysis of data from the First National Health and Nutrition Examination survey. Am J Epidemiol 1988; 128(4):700–710.

32. Smith W, Mitchell P, Webb K, Leeder S. Dietary antioxidants and age-related maculopathy. Ophthalmology: the Blue Mountains Eye Study. Ophthalmology 199; 106(4):761–767.

33. Simonelli F, Zarrilli F, Mazzeo S, Verde V, Romano N, Savoia M, Testa F, Franco Vitale D, Rinaldi M, Sacchetti L. Serum oxidative and antioxidant parameters in a group of Italian patients with age-related maculopathy. Clin Chim Acta 2002; 320(1–2):111–115.

34. West S, Vitale S, Hallfrisch J, Munoz B, Muller D, Bressler S, Bressler NM. Are antioxidants or supplements protective for age related macular degeneration? Arch Ophthalmol 1994; 112(2):222–227.

35. Mares-Perlman JA, Brady WE, Klein R, Klein BEK, Bowen P, Stacewicz-Sapuntazakis M, Palta M. Serum antioxidants and age related macular degeneration in a population-based case control study. Arch Ophthalmol 1995; 113(12):1518–1523.

36. Dimascio KS, Sies H. Lycopene as the most efficient biologic carotenoid singlet oxygen quencher. Arch Biochem Biophys 1989; 1:274.

37. Dagnelie G, Zorge IS, McDonald TM. Lutein improves visual function in some patients with retinal degeneration: a pilot study via the Internet. Optometry 2000; 71:147–164.

38. Aleman TS, Duncan JL, Bieber ML, DeCastro E, Marks DA, Gardner LM, Steinberg JD, Cideciyan AV, Maguire MG, Jacobson SG. Macular pigment and lutein supplementation in retinitis pigmentosa and usher syndrome. Invest Ophthalmol Vis Sci 2001; 42(8):1873–1881.

39. Duncan JL, Aleman TS, Gardner LM, De Castro E, Marks DA, Emmons JM, Bieber ML, Steinberg JD, Bennett J, Stone EM, Macdonald IM, Cideciyan AV, Maguire MG, Jacobson SG. Macular pigment and lutein supplementation in choroideremia. Eye Res 2002; 74:371–381.

40. Klein BEK, Klein R, Linton KLP. Prevalence of age-related lens opacities in a population: the Beaver Dam Eye Study. Ophthalmology 1992; 99:546–552.

41. Steinberg EP, Javitt JC, Sharkey PD. The content and cost of cataract surgery. Arch Ophthalmol 1993; 111:1041–1049.

42. Brown L, Rimm EB, Giovannucci EL, Chasan-Taber L, Seddo JM, Spiegelman D, Willett WC, Hankinson SE. A prospective study of carotenoid intake and risk of cataract extraction in U.S. men. Am J Clin Nutr 1999; 70:517–524.

43. Chasan-Taber L, Willett WC, Seddon JM, Stampfer MJ, Rosner B, Colditz GA, Speizer FE, Hankinson SE. A prospective study of carotenoid and vitamin A intake and risk of cataract extraction among U.S. women. Am J Clin Nutr 1999; 70:509–516.

44. Lyle BJ, Mares-Perlman JA, Klein BEK, Klein R, Greger JL. Dietary antioxidants and incidence of age-related nuclear cataracts. Am J Epidemiol 1999; 149:810–819.

45. Klein BEK, Klein R, Moss SE. Incident cataract surgery: the Beaver Dam Eye Study. Ophthalmology 1997; 4(4):573–580.

46. Jacques PF, Chylack LT, Hankinson SE, Khu P, Rogers G, Friend J, Tung W, Wolfe JK, Padhye N, Willett WC, Taylor A. Long-term nutrient intake and early age-related nuclear lens opacities. Arch Ophthalmol 2001; 119(7):1009–1019.

47. Mares-Perlman JA, Brady WE, Klein BEK, Klein R, Haus GJ, Palta M, Ritter LL, Shoff SM. Diet and nuclear lens opacities. Am J Epidemiol 1995; 141(4):322–334.

48. Tavani A, Negri E, La Vecchia C. Food and nutrient intake and risk of cataract. Ann Epidemiol 1996; 6(1):41–46.

49. Berendschot TJM, Broekmans WMR, Klopping-Ketelaars IAA, Kardinaal AFM, Can Poppel G, Van Norren D. Lens aging in relation to nutritional determinants and possible risk factors for age-related cataract. Arch Ophthalmol 2002; 120:1732–1737.

50. Hammond BR Jr, Wooten BR, Snodderly DM. Density of the human crystalline lens is related to the macular pigment carotenoid, lutein and zeaxanthin. Optometry Vis Sci 1997; 74(7):499–504.

51. Lyle BJ, Mares-Perlman JA, Klein BEK, Klein R, Palta M, Bowen PE, Greger JL. Serum carotenoids and tocopherols and incidence of age-related nuclear cataract. Am J Clin Nutr 1999; 69:272–277.

52. Gale CR, Hall NF, Phillips DIW, Martyn CN. Plasma antioxidant vitamins and carotenoids and age-related cataract. Am Acad Ophthalmol 2001; 108(11):1992–1998.

53. Mares-Perlman JA, Brady W, Klein BEK, Klein R, Palta M, Bowen P, Stacewicz-Sapuntzakis M. Serum carotenoids and tocopherols and severity of nuclear and cortical opacities. Invest Ophthalmol Vis Sci 1995; 36(2):276–288.

54. Olmedilla B, Granado F, Blanco I, Herrero C, Vaquero M, Millan I. Serum status of carotenoids and tocopherols in patients with age-related cataracts: a case-control study. J Nutr Health Aging 2002; 6(1):66–68.

55. Jacques PF, Hartz ST, McGandy RB, Sadowski JA. Nutritional status in persons with and without senile cataract: blood vitamin and mineral levels. Am J Clin Nutr 1988; 48:152–158.

56. Vitale S, West S, Hallfrisch J, Alston C, Wang F, Moorman C, Miller D, Singh V, Taylor HR. Plasma antioxidants and risk of cortical and nuclear cataract. Epidemiology 1993; 4(3):195–203.

57. Wong L, Ho SC, Coggon D, Cruddas AM, Hwang CH, Ho CP, Robertshaw AM, MacDonald DM. Sunlight exposure, antioxidant status, and cataract in Hong Kong fishermen. J Epidemiol Commun Health 1993; 47:46–49.

58. Knekt P, Heliovaara M, Rissanen A, Aromaa A, Aaran Ritva-Kaarina. Serum antioxidant vitamins and risk of cataract. BMJ 1992; 305:1392–1394.

59. Gruber M, Chappell R, Millen AE, Ficek T, Moeller SM, Iannaccone A, Kritchevsky SB, Mares-Perlman JA. Determinants of serum lutein/zeaxanthin in the Third National Health and Nutrition Survey. Am J Epidemiol (in review).

60. Teikari JM, Rautalahti M, Haukka J, Jarvinen P, Hartman AM, Virtamo J, Albanes D, Heinonen O. Incidence of cataract operations in Finnish male smokers unaffected by alpha tocopherol or beta carotene supplements. Clinical trial. J Epidemiol Commun Health 1998; 52(7):468–472.

61. Teikari JM, Virtamo J, Rautalahti M, Palmgren J, Liesto K, Heinonen OP. Long term supplementation with alpha-tocopherol and beta-carotene and age-related cataract. Acta Ophthalmol Scand 1997; 75(6):634–640.

62. Christen WG, Manson JE, Glynn RJ, Gaziano M, Sperduto RD, Buring JE, Hennekens CH. A randomized trial of beta carotene and age-related cataract in US physicians. Arch Ophthalmol 2003; 121:372–378.

63. Age-Related Eye Disease Research Group. A randomized, placebo-controlled, clinical trial of high-dose supplementation with vitamins C and E and beta carotene for age-related cataract and vision loss: AREDS report no 9. Arch Ophthalmol 2001; 119(10):1439–1452.

64. Sperduto RD, Hu Tian-Sheng, Milton RC, Zhao Jia-Liang, Everett DF, Cheng Qiu-Fang, Blot WJ, Bing Li, Taylor PR, Jung-Yao Li Dawsey S, Guo, Wan-De. The Linxian Cataract Studies. Arch Ophthalmol 1993; 111:1246–1252.

65. Chylack LT Jr, Brown NP, Bron A, Hurst M, Kopcke W, Thien U, Schalch W. The Roche European American Cataract Trial (REACT): a randomized clinical trial to investigate the efficacy of an oral antioxidant micronutrient mixture to slow progression of age-related cataract. Ophth Epidemiol 2002; 9(1):49–80.

66. Ford ES, Will JC, Bowman BA, Narayan KM. Diabetes mellitus and serum carotenoids: findings from the Third National Health and Nutrition Examination Survey. Am J Epidemiol 1999; 149(2):168–176.

67. Mayer-Davis EJ, Bell RA, Reboussin BA, Rushing J, Marshall JA, Hamman RF. Antioxidant nutrient intake and diabetic retinopathy: the San Luis Valley Diabetes Study. Ophthalmology 1998; 105(12):2264–2270.

68. Davis NP, Morland AB. Color matching in diabetes: optical density of the crystalline lens and macular pigments. Invest Ophthalmol 2002; 43(1):281–289.

20

Mechanistic Evidence for Eye Diseases and Carotenoids

John T. Landrum and Richard A. Bone
Florida International University, Miami, Florida, U.S.A.

I. INTRODUCTION

The existence of the macula lutea, or "yellow spot," in the human retina has been known since the end of the 18th century (1). The nature and identity of macular pigment carotenoids is now well established (2–8). It was recognized very early that the macula lutea filtered the light entering the eye prior to perception and thereby affected color matching (9). Walls suggested in the 1930s that the macular pigment might be responsible for reduction of chromatic aberration and improved visual acuity (10,11). In the early 1980s, it was postulated that the macular pigment might protect the structures of the retina lying posterior to itself by absorbing excess blue light (1,12). Our developing understanding of the etiologic development of age-related macular degeneration is further illuminating the significant role of the macular carotenoids in ocular health (13). The presence of carotenoids in lens and other ocular tissues is now also recognized (14). Whether it will be possible to establish a functional relationship between the presence of these carotenoids and maintenance of the health of the eye presents an unfinished challenge. This chapter will focus on carotenoids of the retina and lens where an evolving body of epidemiological data supports the premise that they play a role in maintaining ocular health (see Chapter 19).

II. ANATOMY OF THE EYE

The primate eye is a deceptively simple arrangement of optical components whose microanatomical architecture and physiological sophistication rival any biochemical/physiological system known. Figure 1A illustrates the major structures of the eye. Many diseases of the eye are associated with the functional health of individual localized structures (15).

A. Lens

The lens is principally composed of crystalline proteins formed as the living epithelial cells on the anterior face migrate radially and elongate during lens growth. A human lens has a typical volume of about 250 μL. A single layer of epithelial cells covers the front surface of the lens. The central, inner-most part of the lens is called the nucleus. A softer region, the cortex, surrounds this hard central region. The nuclear and cortical regions increase in size throughout life. The living, nucleated epithelial cells continually divide on the anterior face of the

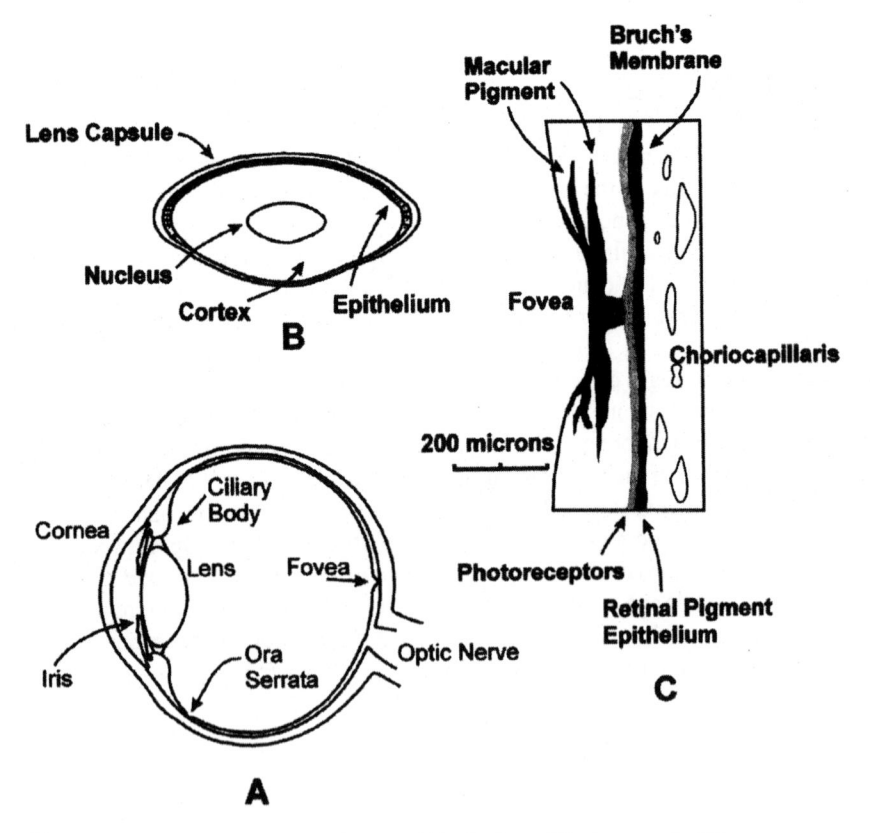

Figure 1   Anatomy of the human eye (A); the lens (B); the macula (C).

lens and the older epithelial cells are continually pushed toward the edges of the lens where they elongate, become anuclear, and add to the cortical layers. The inner cortical layers become more compact and harder with age and increase the inner nucleus of the lens (Fig. 1B). Lutein (L) and zeaxanthin (Z) are known components of the lens, but they are present at low concentrations, about 1×10^{-8} M (about 4 ng/lens) (14,16,17). There is evidence that about 75% of these carotenoids are found in the epithelial/cortical layers (18).

B. Retina

The neural retina contains the light-sensitive photoreceptors and lines the posterior, inner surface of the eye. The retina (about 1095 mm^2) extends from the posterior pole eccentrically forward to a junction with the ora serrata near the ciliary body. The retina is approximately $200-250 \text{ μm}$ in thickness and has several distinct layers. The inner layers include the neural axons. The outer portion of the retina is composed of three interacting layers: the photoreceptors (rods and cones), the retinal pigment epithelium, and the choriocapillaris. The retina contains, on average, a total of $150-200$ ng of carotenoids. Between 80% and 90% of these are the xanthophylls L and Z. Minor metabolites of L and Z have also been identified, but there is a striking absence of carotenes and the other carotenoids commonly detected in other human tissues (14,19).

1. Macula

The primate retina is distinguished from that of other vertebrates by the yellow pigmented fovea (the foveal pit is a well-known feature in birds but there is no pigmentation of the inner retinal layers) (Fig. 1C). The fovea is characterized by thinning of the inner retinal layers (about 150 μm) and a marked increase in the density of photoreceptors ($193,000 \text{ cones/mm}^2$, or about 30,000 total foveal cones) compared to the peripheral retina (20). This contributes to both the high resolution and the visual acuity associated with this part of the retina. The color-sensitive cones dominate in number relative to rods in the fovea and a small central region is rod free (21–23). The human macula is about 1.5 mm in diameter, corresponding to a visual angle of 3.2°. By way of illustration, the image of the full moon occupies a visual angle of about 0.5° and produces an image on the retina approximately 0.15 mm across.

2. Peripheral Retina

The peripheral retina is dominated by rods (20). Whereas the inner retinal layers of the macula are visibly colored by carotenoids, the peripheral retina has no discernible coloration. Modern analytical methods demonstrate that this region of the retina also contains the same two carotenoids, L and Z, found to dominate the macula, although at much lower concentrations (3,24).

3.   Retinal Pigment Epithelium/Choroid

The retinal pigment epithelium (RPE) is an extremely important tissue composed of a single layer of cells whose villi project inward and embrace the photoreceptor outer segments (Fig. 2). The RPE performs many essential tasks in support of photoreceptor visual function. All nutrients and oxygen must pass into the photoreceptors from the RPE, which is itself supported by the highly vascular capillary bed of the choroid. Typically, each RPE cell supports about 50 photoreceptors. The RPE functions actively in the visual cycle and is the site of *trans*-to-*cis* isomerization of retinal. The RPE villi phagocytose the older photoreceptor disks from the rods and cones, recycling membrane lipids, vitamin A, and other essential components. Loss of integrity between the photoreceptors and RPE, or direct damage to the RPE cells, results in loss of visual function. Throughout life, RPE cells accumulate increasing amounts of granular inclusions containing the autofluorescent age pigment lipofuscin (13). Analysis of the whole combined RPE/choroid for carotenoids shows that L and Z are present but at levels somewhat lower than those of the peripheral neural retina (14). Since higher levels of L and Z exist in the retina, it may be that the carotenoids in the RPE/choroid are a reflection of the transport process. However, recent reports suggest that L and Z may have a function in the RPE itself (13).

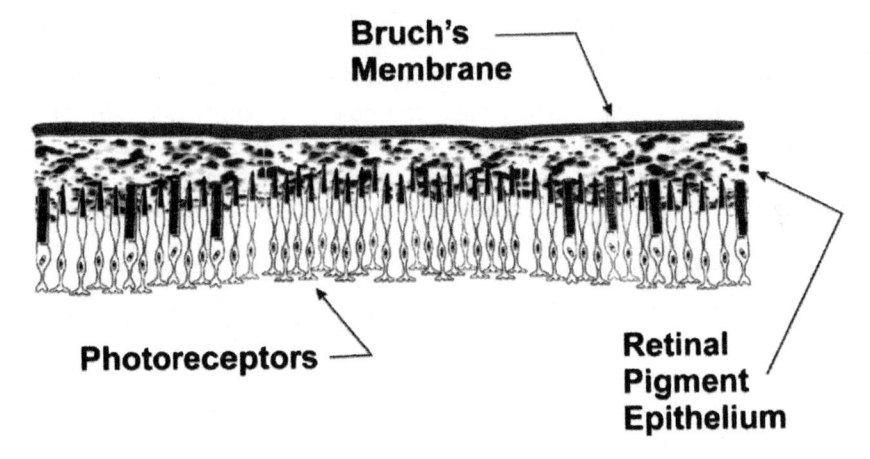

Figure 2   Photoreceptors and retinal pigment epithelium.

III. PHYSICAL AND CHEMICAL NATURE OF LUTEIN AND ZEAXANTHIN

Carotenoids may differ from one another in the length of the polyene chain, the structure of the end group, and the extent and nature of substitution on the end group (Fig. 3). The dominant ocular carotenoids, L and Z, are structural isomers having the formula $C_{40}H_{56}O_2$. They are remarkably similar to one another both in structure and in chemistry. L is more abundant in nature than Z. Despite their similarity, L and Z are not functionally equivalent, at least in the plant systems where they are synthesized (25). This may be true as well for the macular pigment. Understanding the separate roles that these carotenoids may have in ocular metabolism will depend on recognition of subtle differences in the topographic and/or electronic nature of these two molecules.

In addition to L and Z, minor carotenoids are present in certain ocular tissues (14). Some of these are metabolites of L and Z, and their formation may provide chemical insight into the nature of the processes that are occurring in the local environment where they are formed.

A. Carotenoid Structures

1. Zeaxanthin

Zeaxanthin is readily seen to be a structural relative of β-carotene (Fig. 3). The polyene chain contains nine conjugated double bonds, to which the β end groups are attached. Each β end group has an internal double bond between C-5 and C-6. This double bond is constrained by steric interactions from adopting a planar, fully conjugated conformation. In the X-ray structures of β-carotene and canthaxanthin, a dihedral angle of 40–53° is observed, and a similar geometry is thought to exist for Z (26,27). This nonplanar conformation has multiple consequences. It prevents significant $\pi - \pi$ overlap between the cyclohexene and the polyene chain, thereby influencing spectral properties, and it affects the relative orientation of the C-3 and C-3' hydroxyl groups. Thus, the preferred orientation of the OH can be expected to be a factor affecting the binding of the carotenoid with proteins and/or membranes (28,29) (see Chapter 7).

2. Lutein

Lutein possesses the ε-cyclohexene ring analogous to that seen in α-carotene (Fig. 3). The L molecule lacks the symmetry present in Z having one ε and one β ring. The ε ring of L is characterized by the presence of a double bond between the C-4 and C-5 carbons, and C-6 is a tetrahedral stereocenter. The cyclohexene ring can rotate about the C-6 to C-7 bond to assume a minimal energy conformation. The preferred conformation at the ε-ring/polyene chain junction is

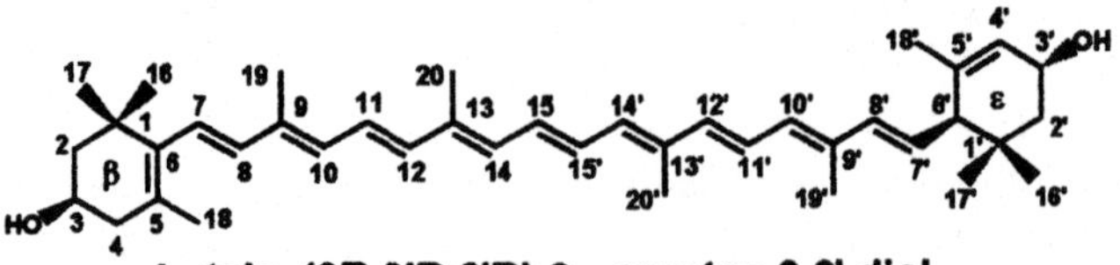

Lutein, (3R,3'R,6'R)-β,ε-caroten-3,3'-diol

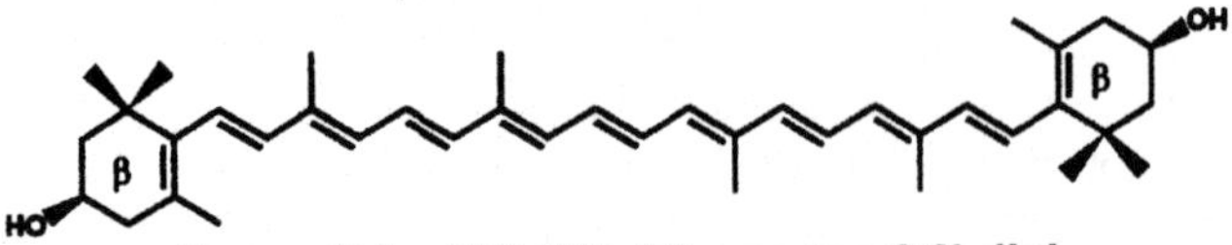

Zeaxanthin, (3R,3'R)-β,β-caroten-3,3'-diol

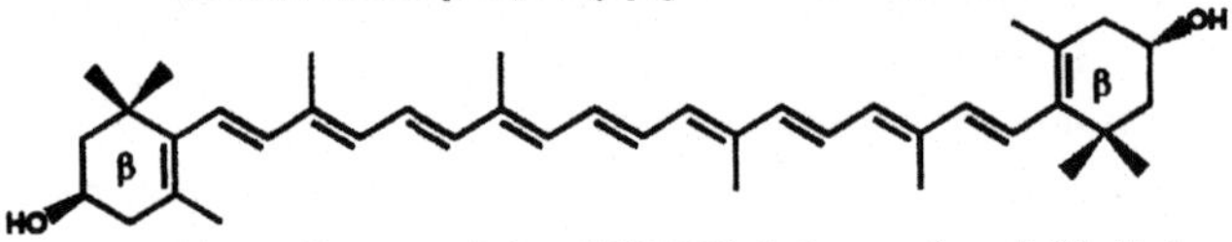

Meso-Zeaxanthin, (3R,3'S)-β,β-caroten-3,3'-diol

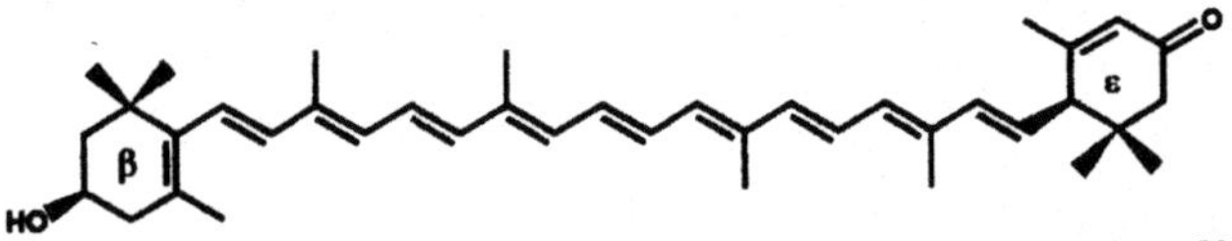

Dehydrolutein, (3R,6'R)-3-hydroxy-β,β-caroten-3'-one

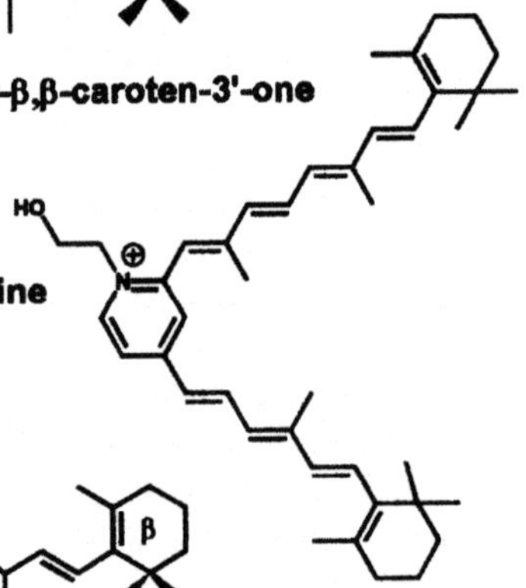

A2E, N-retinyl-N-retinylidene ethanolamine

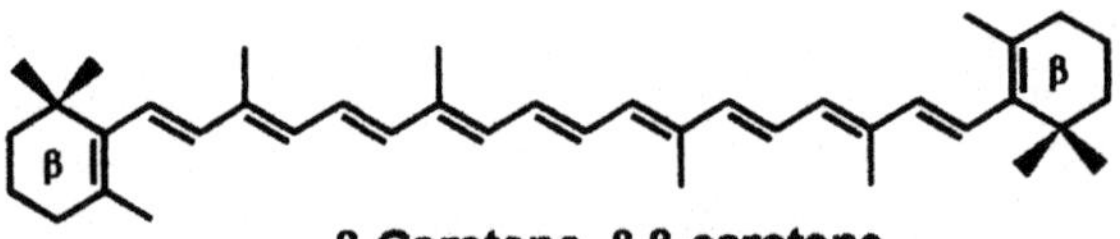

β-Carotene, β,β-carotene

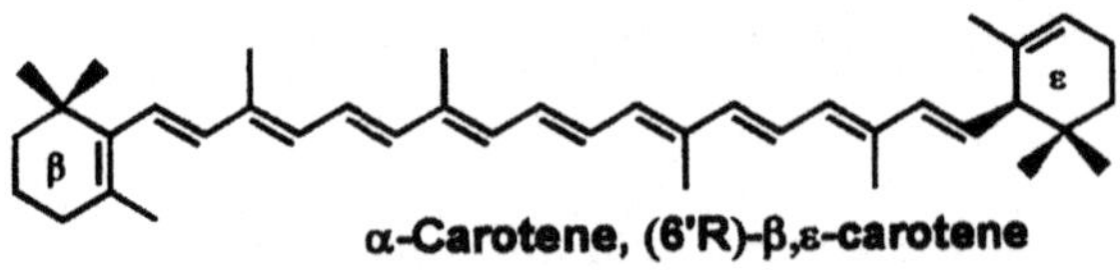

α-Carotene, (6'R)-β,ε-carotene

Figure 3 Structures of the principal carotenoids found in the human retina and the aging pigment, A2E, isolated from lipofuscin.

thought to be different from that adopted by the β ring and should direct the C-3′ hydroxyl group differently in L than in Z. It is the orientation of the hydroxyl groups of L or Z that is most likely to distinguish these molecules, modifying their ability to interact with xanthophyll-binding proteins (XBPs) and in their already noted preference for different average environments within bilipid membrane structures (28).

B. Spectroscopic Properties

The number of conjugated π bonds controls the absorption of visible light by alkenes. The greater the number of conjugated double bonds in a polyene system, the lower will be the transition energy and the longer the wavelength at maximal absorbance. L and Z have an extended chain of conjugation consisting of nine double bonds. Z contains two β rings and absorbs visible light at a somewhat longer wavelength than L. The spectra for L and Z, seen in Figure 4, are characteristic of the α- and β-carotene-bonding framework. Each carotenoid has three clearly discernible vibrational envelopes. The absorption envelope of Z extends significantly to longer wavelengths in comparison with L.

C. Solubility in Biological Tissues

The distinct difference between the polarities of the xanthophylls and the carotenes may be an important factor in their biological transport. It arises from

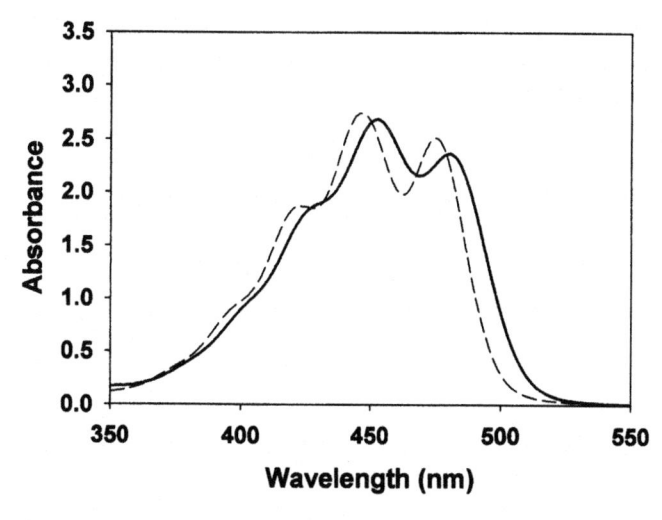

Figure 4 The UV/visible spectra of lutein (*dashed*) and zeaxanthin (*solid*) in ethanol.

the presence of the polar 3 and 3' hydroxyl groups. The xanthophylls are evenly distributed between the high-density and low-density lipoprotein fractions in human serum whereas the carotenes are found in greater amounts in the low-density lipoprotein fraction (30). Hydrophobic organic molecules, including carotenoids, are carried to the tissues in the blood by water-soluble lipoproteins. Once inside cells, they must be solubilized in membranes or lipid vesicles, or bound to proteins. Their movement within cells is consequently restricted to carrier vehicles that are hydrophobic in nature. Because of these factors and the high concentration of L and Z in the retina, the transport and localization of L and Z are thought to be regulated by specific transport proteins.

IV. CAROTENOIDS IN THE RETINA

Carotenoid occurrence in the human and primate eye is dominated by L and Z (31). The almost exclusive presence of these xanthophylls stands out in comparison to other tissues in the human body (19). The human retina is the single richest site of carotenoid accumulation in the human body. The total xanthophyll concentration of the human macula can vary by about one order of magnitude in the general population and is approximately 10^{-3} M in the central fovea. Fundus photographs that demonstrate the absence of macular pigmentation in carotenoid-depleted rhesus monkeys are solid experimental evidence that the macular pigment is of dietary origin (32). L and Z are specifically accumulated in this part of the eye by regulated active transport. An almost 10,000-fold higher concentration of carotenoids is present in the retina than in the blood. In addition to the L and Z, other minor carotenoid components are found in the retina. These too are xanthophylls, and evidence suggests that they are produced by metabolism of L and/or Z (14). A complete explanation of the mechanism by which L and Z are transported to the retina remains unknown, but such high concentrations strongly support the presence of specific XBPs capable of transporting carotenoids and possibly assisting in their cellular localization. A candidate for the XBP has recently been isolated (33).

A. Identity and Characterization of Retinal Carotenoids

1. Lutein

The identity of the two principal carotenoids present in the macula is now well established (2,7). L is the most abundant of the xanthophylls in the human diet and serum, and represents about 50% of the accumulated carotenoids in the retina. Full characterization of the macular carotenoids now includes high-performance liquid chromatography (HPLC) retention times of the macular components and their derivatives on several different chromatography stationary phases, comparison to authentic standards by co-injection, UV/visible spectroscopy, and mass spectroscopy (7,34,35).

The carotenoid concentration in the central macula is sufficiently high that it is clearly visible in the dissected retina. Its position within the inner layers was demonstrated by microspectrophotometry (1,36). The concentration of the carotenoids in the retina surrounding the macula is more than 100 times lower but is readily detectable even in the peripheral sections using HPLC (3,24). A striking characteristic of the carotenoid distribution is that L and Z are not present in identical proportions throughout the retina (Fig. 5) (3,8,24). The proportion of Z increases dramatically in the central macula, and Z is the dominant carotenoid in this part of the retina. In the peripheral regions of the retina, L is the dominant carotenoid.

2. Zeaxanthin and meso-(R,S)-zeaxanthin

L and Z exist in several stereoisomeric forms. Both L and Z are produced as a single stereoisomer by most higher plants (37,38). The consequence of the specificity of xanthophyll biosynthesis in plants is that the human diet includes, almost exclusively, ($3R,3'R$)-β,β-carotene-3,3'-diol (zeaxanthin) and ($3R,3'R,6'R$)-β, ε-carotene-3, 3'-diol (lutein). Minor sources of L and Z

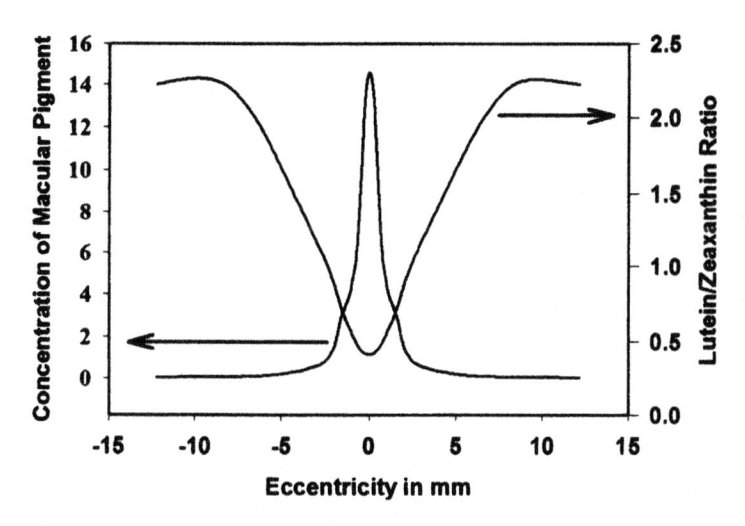

Figure 5 When plotted versus eccentric position (mm) relative to the fovea, the total carotenoid concentration is seen to peak at the fovea reaching a value 100 times that of the peripheral retina, whereas the lutein-to-zeaxanthin ratio exhibits a sharp minimum indicating the reversal of the dominance of lutein and zeaxanthin at the same location.

stereoisomers exist in the human diet (38). The central region of the macula contains a high proportion (about 30%) of the meso isomer of Z [(3R,3'S)-meso-β, β-carotene-3, 3'-diol, MZ] (34). MZ, whose UV-Vis spectrum is identical to that of Z, is not consistently detectable in other tissues or the serum. Current hypotheses to explain the presence of MZ suggest that it is converted from L within the eye (8,34,39,40). One hypothesis suggests that isomerization occurs by direct migration of the L ε-ring double bond with preservation of the configuration of the 3' carbon (39). An alternate pathway suggests that oxidation of the allylic L 3'-hydroxyl with loss of stereochemical configuration is followed by a reduction step leading to MZ formation (41).

3. Minor Carotenoids

Several other minor carotenoids present in the retina include dehydrolutein (Fig. 3), ε,ε-caroten-3,3-dione, and epilutein (14,39). While the significance of these carotenoids is unknown, they are thought to be products of L and/or Z oxidation within the retina. It is possible that they are absorbed from the blood where they are also observed.

B. Location of the Macular Carotenoids

1. The Inner Axons

The carotenoids found in the central region of the fovea are most concentrated in the photoreceptor axons of the Henle fiber layer. Microspectrophotometry of a retinal cross-section provides a clear image of the position of greatest carotenoid accumulation (Fig. 1C) (36). It is thought that the carotenoids are transported to this site from the choroid, passing across the RPE and the outer segments. The dichroic properties of carotenoids, which arise from their linear structure, gives some clue about the site they may occupy in these axons (42). The macular pigment, lying within the inner retinal layers, preferentially absorbs plane-polarized light that has a polarization perpendicular to the radially directed nerve axons. This gives rise to the entoptical phenomenon known as Haidinger's brushes (35,42). It can be deduced that the carotenoids are preferentially ordered, occupying sites within the nerve that are oriented perpendicularly to the nerve axon axis. The extent of this preference, while significant, has been determined to be a modest effect, (about 7%). It has been suggested that the carotenoids may either be concentrated in the bilipid membranes of the axons or be bound to proteins within the cell itself (42,43).

2. The Perifoveal Rods

Careful study of the carotenoid content of isolated rod outer segments has been independently accomplished in two research groups (44,45). Both groups have shown that L and Z are present in these structures in the perifoveal region. The L/Z ratios found in the outer segments maps the variation known to exist in the inner retinal layers (44). To date, the comparable analysis of the cone disks from the central macula has not been reported. These observations are consistent with the hypothesis that L and Z act as antioxidants when present in the photoreceptor outer segments.

3. Membranes

A membrane location is one possible site where L and Z may be accumulated in the nerve fibers. There is a growing body of knowledge about the preference for carotenoids to dissolve in membranes and their effects on membrane properties and structure (46,47). Z is incorporated into membranes, adopting a perpendicular orientation and spanning the bilipid layers. In contrast, L appears capable of occupying a wider range of environments within the membrane, and measurements indicate that the average angle of the L polyene axis to the plane of the membrane is nearly 23° (28). It remains to be established what significance these differences in membrane behavior have in the ocular distribution and functions of L and Z (29,46).

C. Xanthophyll-Binding Protein

The existence of a specific XBP that transports and possibly binds the carotenoids within the cells of the macula is widely accepted. Bernstein's report of a detergent-extractable XBP provides a solid basis for further investigation into the molecular mechanism of transport of the macular carotenoids (33). The XBP has a high affinity for carotenoids with hydroxylated cyclohexene ring end groups. A full understanding of the binding site and the factors influencing the expression of XBP will provide significant insight into the mechanism of carotenoid accumulation. Binding of L and Z to other cell proteins, most notably tubulin, has also been noted (43). The possibility exists that abnormalities in the expression of the XBP gene may be a cause or risk factor in retinal pathology.

D. Measurement of the Distribution of Carotenoids with Eccentricity

1. HPLC Postmortem Analysis

Using HPLC it has been possible to measure L and Z at various eccentricities across the retina. The total L and Z concentration drops by a factor of about 100 from the central fovea to the peripheral retina. As noted earlier, the proportion of Z plus MZ increases within the macula apparently due to an interconversion of L to MZ that occurs in this region. The role of MZ to retinal health is not established, but the consistent observation of its presence is supportive of the suggestion that it has a significant function.

2. Mature Retina

The average quantity of carotenoids in the mature retina has been separately measured by several groups (2,14,24,39). HPLC postmortem analysis and in vivo measurements using heterochromatic flicker photometry, the scanning ophthalmoscope, or other techniques have shown the amount of macular pigment to be either approximately constant or decreasing slightly with age (24,48–52). The measurement by resonance Raman spectroscopy shows a striking decrease in macular pigment with age (53). It will be important for further research to be completed that determines unambiguously the relationship that exists between age and macular pigment levels.

3. Neonatal Retina

An understanding of the development of the macular pigment during early life is lacking. A small number of fetal and neonatal retinas have been examined by HPLC (24). These studies indicate that macular pigmentation is not well developed until 2–3 years of age. The carotenoid content of the macula in the very young retina is dominated by L. This may indicate that the increase of foveal Z and specifically MZ is associated with developmental changes that take place early in life. The absence of MZ is consistent with the proposed slow formation of MZ from L, possibly including an oxidative process and keto intermediates. Because of the limited number of data available, it is not known to what extent accumulation of carotenoids occurs in the macula prior to foveal development. A careful mapping of the carotenoid distribution in neonates may provide useful insight into macular development and the process of carotenoid accumulation.

V. CAROTENOIDS IN THE LENS

The presence of carotenoids in the human lens was first reported by Yeum and has been confirmed by at least two other groups (16–18,54). The carotenoids L and Z are exclusively observed in almost equal amounts. The total mass of L and Z in the lens is typically about 4 ng (16). The concentration is an important factor influencing the potential function and role that a species may have in a physiological system. Based on the total analyzed mass of L and Z, the carotenoid concentration in the human lens is about 10 nM (10^{-8} M), assuming a homogeneous distribution. In vitro investigations of the antioxidant ability of carotenoids indicate that significant antioxidant function is not observed until carotenoid concentrations exceed about 100 times this value, approximately

10–100 μM (55,56). It is probable that the distribution of carotenoids in the lens is not uniform. In fact, the cortical layers contain as much as 75% of the carotenoids present in the lens (18). The living epidermis of the lens is a single cell layer having a thickness of approximately 15 μM (57). If the lens carotenoids are present chiefly in the epithelial cell layer, then carotenoid concentrations between 10^{-5} and 10^{-6} M exist within these cells. These are sufficiently high concentrations for physiological antioxidant function. Further study of the distribution of L and Z in lens is needed to determine what the epithelial concentration may be.

A. Light, Oxygen, and Generation of Reactive Oxygen Species

Where high oxygen levels and light are both present, as in the retina, the potential for photo-oxidation is very great. UV or blue light can be absorbed by highly conjugated, naturally occurring pigments, such as heme or A2E (Fig. 3), producing a triplet excited-state pigment molecule that efficiently transfers energy to molecular oxygen. The singlet oxygen and peroxyl species that result from photoactivation are highly reactive oxidants capable of damaging cellular structures and components (56,58,59). This mechanism is the underlying cause of erythema or sunburn of the skin, photokeratitis of the cornea, photic induction of cataract in the lens, and photochemical lesion on the retina (60,61) (see Chapter 22). Generally, photochemical processes require high-energy, short-wavelength light. Sunburn is caused by UV light [UVA (400–320 nm) and UVB (320–290 nm)]. UV light is a source of injury to the cornea and a risk factor for cataract in the lens (61). It is essentially all absorbed by the cornea and lens so that only visible blue light reaches the retina. Visible blue light with wavelengths ranging from 400 to 500 nm can also cause photochemical damage. Ham and Mueller determined that blue light, between 430 to 470 nm, poses the greatest hazard for the retina (62). The photochemistry of blue light also includes the activation of oxygen. Biological defenses against the reactive oxygen species (ROS) generated by light are well known. Singlet oxygen and other ROS can be intercepted by a variety of antioxidants at the cellular level when they are present in adequate concentrations (55,63–65). A rich arsenal of antioxidants is present in ocular tissues: vitamin C, vitamin E, glutathione peroxidase, and superoxide dismutase, in addition to the carotenoids L and Z (66).

B. Evidence of Photic Damage in the Eye

Evidence of the harmful effects of light on the eye and its tissues is abundant (61). Photokeratitis is the result of acute UV damage to the cornea; in the presence of high levels of oxygen, greater damage is observed than at low oxygen levels (61,67). Significant evidence has also accumulated demonstrating the deleterious effects of oxygen and light exposure on the lens and retina (68–72). The illumination of the eye during surgery can be of critical concern (73–75). High-intensity white light used during surgery has resulted in the production of photochemical lesions on the retina (76–81).

1. Cataract

The prevalence of cataract is greatest among aging individuals but can also be brought on by injury and/or steroid use (82). Three types of cataract are commonly described clinically: nuclear cataract (the most common), cortical cataract, and posterior subcapsular cataract (83–86). Cataract risk is related to exposure to UV radiation, a primary cause of ROS (87). That cataract occurs most commonly in the nuclear region of the lens is possibly due to lower levels of antioxidants in this region (18). The higher antioxidant levels in the cortical (as opposed to the nuclear) layer may scavenge ROS that initiate protein damage leading to cataract formation (18). Epidemiological studies have shown an association between the level of intake of the antioxidant vitamins C and E, the xanthophylls L and Z, and reduced risk of cataract (84,88,89). Recently, intake of L and Z were related to an approximately 20% lower risk of cataract extraction in men and women and a 50% lower risk of the development of nuclear cataract over 5 years (90–92) (see Chapter 19).

2. Age-Related Macular Degeneration

The single most prevalent disease of the retina is age-related macular degeneration (AMD) (93). Retinopathy is also associated with diabetes, and there are other diseases of the retina as well, including choroideremia and retinitis pigmentosa. Best's disease and Stargardt disease are genetically acquired maculopathies similar to AMD and occur early in life (15,94,95). The cause of early macular degeneration (Stargardt or Best's disease) is thought to be accelerated damage to the RPE (see below) that results from inadequate expression of proteins essential for the regulation of physiological events tied to oxidative metabolism (96). The occurrence of AMD is dependent on genetic (sex, race, eye color, and family history) and environmental factors (nutrition, light exposure, smoking) (93). Studies have shown that antioxidants can reduce the risk for the occurrence or progression of AMD (97). In addition, some studies have shown that there is a correlation between the intake and serum level of the xanthophylls, L and Z, and reduced odds ratios for neovascular AMD (98–100). Other studies have not revealed the same relationships, but this may be attributable to the relatively low intakes of L and Z by the subjects in these studies (101) (see Chapter 19). Macular pigment levels, as measured by HPLC, are associated with reduced odds for AMD (102). In a clinical trial, Richer has reported improvements in vision in patients consuming high levels of L and Z (in spinach) (103).

Despite a fundamental difficulty in assessing lifelong blue light exposure accurately, support for a relationship between light and AMD has developed (66,104,105). AMD is characterized by the appearance of structures called *drusen* that develop in the macular region of the retina. Drusen are the result of a buildup of insoluble, lipophilic material between the RPE cell layer and Bruch's membrane, the limiting barrier dividing the choriocapillaris from the retinal layers. In early stages of AMD, the drusen are small ($<$63 μm) and referred to as small, hard drusen, but in later stages the drusen are larger ($>$125 μm) and are referred to as confluent or soft drusen (106). [The terms "hard" and "soft" are observational terms and not intended to describe the physical nature of the deposits (107).] Microscopic study reveals that, due to the presence of drusen, the overlying RPE cell layer deforms and thins as it spreads to cover the resulting bulge. This thinning of the melanin-containing RPE layer results in an increase in the reflected light from the fundus and visible observation of the drusen (107,108). More importantly, deformation of the RPE cell layer damages the integrity of the contact between the microvilli of the RPE and the outer segments of the photoreceptors. Ultimately, complete separation between the photoreceptors and the RPE can occur. Photoreceptor cell death follows, resulting in permanent loss of vision. The time frame for this process is not well established and may vary significantly among individuals (107). The fundamental cause of the buildup of the drusen material may be the inability of the RPE cells to catabolize oxidized nonpolar membrane components present in the shed photoreceptor disks, e.g., polyunsaturated fatty acids. Monkeys raised on carotenoid-depleted diets show an absence of macular pigment and signs of retinal aging typical of early macular degeneration that are consistent with photic damage and drusen buildup (32).

In some AMD cases, the disruption of the RPE–photoreceptor integrity and the buildup of the drusen deposits are associated with neovascular intrusion of capillaries into the subretinal space. Fluid from these capillaries can accumulate between the choroid and the retina. There is a growing body of experimental evidence that supports the argument that AMD occurs, in part, due to the effects of the lipofuscin-associated chromophore, A2E (see Fig. 4), which specifically requires light exposure for its formation (109,110). The blue light–absorbing nature of the macular pigment can attenuate the amount of light reaching the RPE by as much as 40–90%. In turn, this should reduce the rate of formation of A2E and ROS. It has been demonstrated that L and Z reduce lipofuscin formation in cultured RPE cells (111). A2E is toxic and appears to damage mitochondrial function and integrity (112). When exposed to blue light A2E exhibits a phototoxic behavior that results in apoptotic cell death in cultured RPE cells (113,114). This phototoxicity is dramatically lowered by both phosphatidylglycerol and L (13,115). This observation suggests that at least some of the protective effects of L and Z may occur directly at the level of the RPE and are in addition to the ability of L and Z to absorb blue light. Experiments supplementing Japanese quail with Z also demonstrate that photoreceptors are protected in vivo from photic-induced apoptosis (116,117).

Further evidence of the protective function of the macular pigment exists in the pattern of photoreceptor loss. The greatest losses of photoreceptors occur in the region just beyond the fovea from 1.5° to 10° eccentricity. The region of highest pigmentation produces a protected zone in the central macula (20). Haegerstrom-Portnoy has shown that loss of short-wavelength cones is reduced in the region where macular pigment is most concentrated (118). Similar protection is observed for acute light exposure where the resulting lesion is less pronounced in the central macula (72,81). A condition known as Bull's eye maculopathy, associated with photosensitizing drugs, is characterized by a pattern of degeneration in which the macula is spared (75,119).

C. AMD and Blue Light

As described earlier, it appears that as A2E and lipofuscin build up within the RPE cells, blue light absorbed by this molecule may initiate the formation of singlet oxygen and ROS (72). Normal oxygen metabolism also generates ROS, even in the absence of light. It is probable that "dark" ROS production also contributes to AMD (120). ROS may damage any number of essential structures in RPE cells and the retina generally. However, the most noticeable result appears to be damage to the unsaturated lipid components of the shed photoreceptor disks, which are eliminated from the RPE through exocytosis and produce the extracellular deposits called drusen. The drusen, as they become sufficiently large, produce a mechanical barrier to nutrient and oxygen flow into the retina resulting in photoreceptor and RPE cell death and the secretion of vascular growth factors which in turn trigger the neovascular intrusion into the macula (108).

If this view of the disease process is correct, then retarding the oxidative events occurring in photoreceptor disks may have a dramatic influence on the development AMD. Reduction in the amount of blue light reaching the retina is one mechanism to accomplish this objective. Any factor that compromises the ability of the RPE to reduce the damage due to ROS might also be anticipated to contribute to development of AMD, e.g., smoking. Dietary changes altering the available vitamin E and C might be expected to be significant (97,121–123). Genetic defects, which result in incompetent or inadequate levels of the antioxidant proteins superoxide dismutase and glutathione peroxidase might be important contributors of AMD (124). Two forms of macular degeneration that are morphologically similar to AMD, Best's disease and Stargardt disease, are caused by genetic defects (95). In Stargardt disease the defect is known to occur in the *ABCR* gene responsible for transport of retinal to retinal dehydrogenase for conversion to retinol and subsequent transport from the disks in the photoreceptor to the RPE. Mice lacking a functional *ABCR* gene produce A2E at greatly accelerated rates (125).

VI. CAROTENOID SUPPLEMENTATION AND POTENTIAL THERAPEUTIC BENEFITS

Canthaxanthin (β,β-caroten-4,4'-dione), accumulation occurs in the retina when individuals consume large doses of this keto carotenoid (126,127). The carotenoid also accumulates in skin, resulting in a tanned appearance when high doses are consumed. High levels of carotenoids in the skin are known to be protective against erythema caused by light exposure (the mechanism for this is widely accepted to involve photogenerated singlet oxygen and free radicals), and canthaxanthin has been used as a treatment for erythropoietic porphyria (60,65,128). Accumulation of canthaxanthin can be accompanied by formation of carotenoid microcrystals within the retina which are noticeable during ophthalmic examination and lead to the term "gold dust retinopathy" (128,129). While there is no evidence that canthaxanthin causes a permanent deleterious effect in the retina, its use as a pharmaceutical has been curtailed. Canthaxanthin accumulation in the retina provided early evidence that retinal accumulation of carotenoids might be altered by dietary availability.

A. Range of MP Levels in the Normal Population

In normal Western populations, L and Z are consumed in relatively small amounts, 0–3 mg/day (130,131). Individuals whose diet is largely vegetarian may consume considerably greater amounts, and total L consumption can reach very high levels in some groups. Twenty six milligrams per day was estimated for some South Pacific Islanders (132). The upper quintile of consumption in a cohort of subjects in one major U.S. dietary study was estimated to be 6 mg/day (98). Since macular pigment is dietary in origin we expect that a relationship must exist between total dietary intake and macular pigment optical density (MPOD) values (133). Several studies have now been conducted in which MPOD values were measured for subjects whose dietary intake of carotenoids was assessed.

The average MPOD in the Western populations is in the range of 0.30–0.45 au (133–136). Dietary intake of L/Z and serum levels of these carotenoids correlate modestly with MPOD (137). Other factors in addition to intake or serum level may influence MPOD. Several supplementation trials of L and/or Z in humans have now been conducted (103,136, 138–154). Many have measured

MPOD levels in vivo, and the clear evidence that MPOD can be increased by supplements has emerged (133–137,139–141,144). We showed that the MPOD increases slowly during supplementation (140). This result is consistent with a process involving transport of the relatively large, lipophilic carotenoid molecule from the vascular choroid across the avascular neural layers of the fovea. Data now appear to support the hypothesis that the average rate of increase in the MPOD is related to serum concentration of L and Z (133,137). Comparison of results of different studies is complicated by a number of variables, including carotenoid source (food or commercial supplement), formulation, dosage, period of supplementation, and method of measurement of macular pigment. While nearly all subjects show a clear serum response to supplementation with L or Z, an MPOD response is not always observed, especially in short-term studies.

L supplements have been studied as potentially useful in a number of ocular pathologic conditions other than AMD, including choroideremia, retinitis pigmentosa, and cataract (144,145,153,155,156). Short-term supplementation in these studies has not had a dramatic effect.

B. Dietary Sources

Human dietary sources of the xanthophylls L and Z are primarily the dark green vegetables (157). L from vegetable sources is in the free, or unesterified, form. When present in fruits and flowers, the xanthophylls are primarily in the form of fatty acid diesters (158,159). The bioavailability of the xanthophylls depends on the availability of modest levels of fat consumed in the diet with the carotenoids. The fat is presumably needed to assist in solubilization of the carotenoids but may also influence lipase secretion and esterase activity thought to be required for cleavage of xanthophyll diesters (148). Currently L and Z are commercially available as dietary supplements. Commercial L is obtained by a hexane extraction of marigold blossoms (*Tagetes erecta*). L is sold either as a fatty acid diester or as an unesterified diol. Synthetic Z is also currently available.

VII. CONCLUSIONS

Carotenoids present in the retina are important contributors to long-term ocular health. The role of L and Z in reducing the rate of photo-oxidative stress in acute exposure to high-intensity light is clear, and the evidence that chronic or long-term photo-oxidative stress is involved in AMD continues to accumulate. A diet rich in L and Z can increase their concentration in the macula and may therefore have an influence on the rate of development of retinal damage associated with photo-oxidation and even the occurrence of AMD. Similarly, risk of cataract appears to be lowered by the presence of L and Z in the lens.

This epidemiological association has remained unsupported by direct study of the carotenoid content of the lens where only very low concentrations of the carotenoids have been detected. Further work is needed to determine whether a local concentration of L and Z in the lens epithelium could have a significant impact on the rate of photo-oxidation in the lens.

A number of other important questions must be answered to establish the details of L and Z function in the eye. These include the mechanisms of transport of L and Z into the eye, characterization of the proteins associated with this process, and the nature of the site(s) where L and Z are localized within cellular components of the eye. On a larger scale, clinical trials of L and Z are needed to determine the degree of protection they may provide against the onset of AMD.

ACKNOWLEDGMENTS

The authors thank Ms. Valerie Etienne-Leveille for her kind assistance and acknowledge support from the NIH NIGMS SCORE and RISE programs, NIH Grant GM08205.

REFERENCES

1. Nussbaum JJ, Pruett RC, Delori FC. Historic perspectives macular yellow pigment: the first 200 years. Retina 1981; 1:296–310.
2. Handelman GJ, Dratz EA, Reay CC, van Kuijk FJGM. Carotenoids in the human macula and whole retina. Invest Ophthalmol Vis Sci 1988; 29:850–855.
3. Snodderly DM, Handelman GJ, Adler AJ. Distribution of individual macular pigment carotenoids in central retina of macaque and squirrel monkeys. Invest Ophthalmol Vis Sci 1991; 32:268–279.
4. Brown PK, Wald G. Visual pigments in human and monkey retinas. Nature 1963; 200:37–43.
5. Wald G. Human vision and spectrum. Science 1945; 101:653–658.
6. Wald G. The photochemistry of vision. Documenta Ophthal 1949; 3:94–137.
7. Bone RA, Landrum JT, Tarsis SL. Preliminary identification of the human macular pigment. Vision Res 1985; 25:1531–1535.
8. Bone RA, Landrum JT, Friedes LM, Gomez CM, Kilburn MD, Menendez E, Vidal I, Wang W. Distribution of lutein and zeaxanthin stereoisomers in the human retina. Exp Eye Res 1997; 64:211–218.
9. Ruddock KH. Light transmission through the ocular media and macular pigment and its significance for psychophysical investigation. In: Jameson D, Hurvich LM, eds. Handbook of Sensory Physiology. Vol. 7. Berlin: Springer-Verlag, 1972:455–469.

10. Walls GL, Judd HD. The intraocular colour filters of vertebrates. Br J Ophthalmol 1933; 17:641–675, 705–725.
11. Reading VM, Weale RA. Macular pigment and chromatic aberration. J Opt Soc Am 1974; 64:231–234.
12. Kirschfeld K. Carotenoid pigments: their possible role in protecting against photooxidation in eyes and photoreceptor cell. Proc R Soc Lond B 1982; 216:71–85.
13. Shaban H, Richter C. A2E and blue light in the retina: the paradigm of age-related macular degeneration. Biol Chem 2002; 383:537–545.
14. Bernstein PS, Khachik F, Carvalho L, Muir G, Zhao D-Y, Katz N. Identification and quantitation of carotenoids and their metabolites in the tissues of the human eye. Exp Eye Res 2001; 72:215–223.
15. Yanoff M, Fine BS. Ocular Pathology. New York: Mosby, 2002:p 761.
16. Yeum K-J, Taylor A, Tang G, Russell RM. Measurement of carotenoids, retinoids, and tocopherols in human lenses. Invest Ophthalmol Vis Sci 1995; 36:2756–2761.
17. Bates CJ, Chen S-J, Macdonald A, Holden R. Quantitation of vitamin E and a carotenoid pigment in cataractous human lenses, and the effect of a dietary supplement. Int J Vitam Nutr Res 1996; 66:316–321.
18. Yeum K-J, Shang F, Schalch W, Russell RM, Taylor A. Fat-soluble nutrient concentrations in different layers of human cataractous lens. Curr Eye Res 1999; 19:502–505.
19. Schmitz HH, Poor CL, Wellman RB, Erdman JW Jr. Concentrations of selected carotenoids and vitamin A in human liver, kidney and lung tissue. J Nutr 1991; 121:1613–1621.
20. Curcio CA, Medeiros NE, Millican CL. Photoreceptor loss in age-related macular degeneration. Invest Ophthalmol Vis Sci 1996; 37:1236–1249.
21. Øesterberg G. Topography of the layer of rods and cones in the human retina. Acta Ophthalmol 1935; 13(Suppl 6):1–103.
22. Curcio CA, Millican CL, Allen KA, Kalina RE. Aging of the human photoreceptor mosaic: evidence for selective vulnerability of rods in central retina. Invest Ophthalmol Vis Sci 1993; 34:3278–3296.
23. Curcio CA, Sloan KR, Kalina RE, Hendrickson AE. Human photoreceptor topography. J Comp Neurol 1990; 292:497–523.
24. Bone RA, Landrum JT, Fernandez L, Tarsis SL. Analysis of the macular pigment by HPLC: retinal distribution and age study. Invest Ophthalmol Vis Sci 1988; 29:843–849.
25. Demmig-Adams B, Adams WW. The role of xanthophyll cycle carotenoids in the protection of photosynthesis. Trends Plant Sci 1996; 1:21–26.
26. Bart JCJ, MacGillavry CH. The crystal and molecular structure of canthaxanthin. Acta Crystallogr 1968; B24:1587–1606.
27. Senge MO, Hope H, Smith KM. Structure and conformation of photosynthetic pigments and related compounds. Z Naturforsch 1992; 47c:474–476.
28. Sujak A, Gabrielska J, Grudzinski W, Borc R, Mazurek P, Gruszecki WI. Lutein and zeaxanthin as protectors of lipid membranes against oxidative damage: the structural aspects. Arch Biochem Biophys 1999; 371:301–307.

29. Sujak A, Okulski W, Gruszecki WI. Organisation of xanthophyll pigments lutein and zeaxanthin in lipid membranes formed with dipalmitoylphosphatidylcholine. Biochim Biophys Acta 2000; 1509:255–263.

30. Erdman JW Jr, Bierer TL, Gugger ET. Absorption and transport of carotenoids. Ann NY Acad Sci 1993; 691:76–85.

31. Schalch W. Possible contribution of lutein and zeaxanthin, carotenoids of the macula lutea, to reducing the risk of age-related macular degeneration: a review. Hong Kong Journal of Ophthalmology 2001; 4:31–42.

32. Malinow MR, Feeney-Burns L, Peterson LH, L KM, Neuringer M. Diet-related macular anomalies in monkeys. Invest Ophthalmol Vis Sci 1980; 19:857–863.

33. Yemeleyanov AY, Katz N, Bernstein PS. Ligand-binding characterization of xanthophyll carotenoids to solubilized membrane proteins derived from human retina. Exp Eye Res 2001; 72:381–392.

34. Bone RA, Landrum JT, Hime GW, Cains A, Zamor J. Stereochemistry of the human macular carotenoids. Invest Ophthalmol Vis Sci 1993; 34:2033–2040.

35. Bone RA, Landrum JT, Cains A. Optical density spectra of the macular pigment in vivo and in vitro. Vision Res 1992; 32:105–110.

36. Snodderly DM, Auron JD, Delori FC. The macular pigment. II. Spatial distribution in primate retinas. Invest Ophthalmol Vis Sci 1984; 25:674–685.

37. Britton G. Overview of carotenoid biosynthesis. In: Britton G, Liaaen-Jensen S, Pfander H, eds. Carotenoids. Vol. 3. Basel: Birkhauser-Verlag, 1998:13–147.

38. Maoka T, Arai A, Shimizu M, Matsuno T. The first isolation of enantiomeric and meso-zeaxanthin in nature. Comp Biochem Physiol 1986; 83B:121–124.

39. Khachik F, Bernstein PS, Garland DL. Identification of lutein and zeaxanthin oxidation products in human and monkey retinas. Invest Ophthalmol Vis Sci 1997; 38:1802–1810.

40. Landrum JT, Bone RA, Moore LL, Gomez CM. Analysis of zeaxanthin distribution within individual human retinas. In: Packer L, ed. Methods in Enzymology. Vol. 299. San Diego: Academic Press, 1999:457–467.

41. Landrum JT, Bone RA. Lutein, zeaxanthin, and the macular pigment. Arch Biochem Biophys 2001; 385:28–40.

42. Bone RA, Landrum JT. Macular pigment in Henle fiber membranes: a model for Haidinger's brushes. Vision Res 1984; 24:103–108.

43. Bernstein P, Balashov N, Tsong ED, Rando R. Retinal tubulin binds macular carotenoids. Invest Ophthalmol Vis Sci 1997; 38:167–175.

44. Rapp LM, Seema SS, Choi JH. Lutein and zeaxanthin concentrations in rod outer segment membranes from perifoveal and peripheral human retina. Invest Ophthalmol Vis Sci 2000; 41:1200–1209.

45. Sommerburg OG, Siems WG, Hurst JS, Lewis JW, Kliger DS, van Kuijk FJGM. Lutein and zeaxanthin are associated with photoreceptors in the human retina. Cur Eye Res 1999; 19:491–495.

46. Sujak A, Gruszecki WI. Organization of mixed monomolecular layers formed with the xanthophyll pigments lutein or zeaxanthin and dipalmitoylphosphatidylcholine at the argon-water interface. Photochem Photobiol B 2000; 68:39–44.

47. Socaciu C, Jessel R, Haertel S, Diehl HA. Carotenoids in 1,2-dipalmitoyl-sn-glycero-3-phosphorylcholine liposomes: incorporation and effects on phase transition and vesicle size. J Med Biochem 2000; 4:71–82.
48. Chen S-J, Chang YC, Wu JC. The spatial distribution of macular pigment in humans. Curr Eye Res 2001; 23:422–434.
49. Beatty S, Murray I, Henson D, Carden D, Koh H, Boulton M. Macular pighment and risk for age related macular degeneration in subjects from a northern European population. Invest Ophthalmol Vis Sci 2001; 42:439–446.
50. Werner JS, Bieber M, Shefrin BE. Senescence of foveal and parafoveal cone sensitivities and their relations to macular pigment density. J Opt Soc Am A 2000; 17:1918–1932.
51. Delori FC, Goger DG, Hammond BR Jr, Snodderly DM, Burns SA. Macular pigment density measured by autofluorescence spectrometry: comparison with reflectometry and heterochromatic flicker photometry. J Opt Soc Am A 2001; 18:1212–1230.
52. Werner JS, Donnelly SK, Kliegl R. Aging and the human macular pigment density. Appended with translations from the work of Max Schultz and Ewald Hering. Vis Res 1987; 27:257–268.
53. Bernstein PS, Zhao D-Y, Wintch SW, Ermakov IV, McClane RW, Gellermann W. Resonance Raman measurement of macular carotenoids in normal subjects and in age-related macular degeneration patients. Ophthalmology 2002; 109:1780–1787.
54. Landrum JT, Bone RA, Kenyon E, Spargue K, Maya A. A preliminary study of the stereochemistry of human lens zeaxanthin. Invest Ophthalmol Vis Sci 1997; 38:S1026.
55. Viljanen K, Sundberg S, Ohshima T, Heinonen M. Carotenoids as antioxidants to prevent photooxidation. Eur J Lipid Sci Technol 2002; 164:353–359.
56. Beutner S, Bloedorn B, Frixel S, Hernandez-Blanco I, Hoffmann T, Martin H-D, Mayer B, Noack P, Ruck C, Schmidt M, Schulke I, Sell S, Ernst H, Haremza S, Seybold G, Sies H, Stahl W, Walsh R. Quantitative assessment of antioxidant properties of natural colorants and phytochemicals: carotenoids, flavonoids, phenols and indigoids. The role of β-carotene in antioxidant functions. J Sci Food Agric 2001; 81:559–568.
57. Taylor V, Al-Ghoul KJ, Lane CW, Davis VA, Kuszak JR, Costello MJ. Morphology of the normal human lens. Invest Ophthalmol Vis Sci 1996; 37:1396–1410.
58. Wright A, Hawkins CL, Davies MJ. Photo-oxidation of cells generates long-lived intracellular protein peroxides. Free Radic Biol Med 2003; 34:637–647.
59. Boulton M, Rozanowska M, Rozanowska B. Retinal photodamage. J Photochem and Photobiol B: Biology 2001; 64:144–161.
60. Mathews-Roth MM, Krinsky NI. Carotenoids affect development of UV-B induced skin cancer. Photochem Photobiol 1987; 46:507–509.
61. Young RW. The family of sunlight-related eye diseases. Opt Vis Sci 1994; 71:125–144.
62. Ham WT, Mueller HA, Ruffolo JJ, Millen JE, Cleary SF, Guerry RK, Guerry D. Basic mechanisms underlying the production of photochemical lesions in the mammalian retina. Curr Eye Res 1984; 3:165–174.

63. Krinsky NI. Antioxidant functions of carotenoids. Free Radic Biol Med 1989; 7:617–635.
64. Girotti AW. Photosensitized oxidation of membrane lipids: reaction pathways, cytotoxic effects, and cytoprotective mechanisms. J Photochem Photobiol B: Biol 2001; 63:103–113.
65. Mathews-Roth MM. Carotenoids quench evolution of excited species in epidermis exposed to UV-B (290-320 nm) light. Photochem Photobiol 1986; 43:91–93.
66. Beatty S, Koh H, Phil M, Henson D, Boulton M. The role of oxidative stress in the pathogenesis of age-related macular degeneration. Surv Ophthalmol 2000; 45:115–134.
67. Zuclich JA, Kurtin WE. Oxygen dependence of near-ultraviolet induced corneal damage. Photochem Photobiol 1977; 25:133–135.
68. Garner MH, Spector A. Sulfur oxidation in selected human cortical cataracts and nuclear cataracts. Exp Eye Res 1980; 31:361–369.
69. Augusteyn RC. Protein modification in cataract: possible oxidative mechanism. In: Duncan G, ed. Mechanisms of Cataract Formation in Human Lens. New York: Academic Press, 1981:72–115.
70. Varma SD. Scientific basis for medical therapy of cataracts by antioxidants. Am J Clin Nutr 1991; 53:335S–45S.
71. Varma SD, Chand D, Sharma YR, Kuck JRJ, Richards RD. Oxidative stress on lens and cataract formation: role of light and oxygen. Curr Eye Res 1984; 3:35–57.
72. Jaffe GJ, Irvine AR, Wood IS. Retinal phototoxicity from the operating microscope. The role of inspired oxygen. Ophthalmology 1988; 95:1130–1141.
73. Lawwill T, Crockett S, Currier G. Retinal damage secondary to chronic light exposure, thresholds and mechanisms. Documenta Ophthalmol 1977; 44:379–402.
74. Ham WT, Ruffolo JJ, Mueller HA, Clarke AM, Moon ME. Histologic analysis of photochemical lesions produced in rhesus retina by short-wavelength light. Invest Ophthalmol Vis Sci 1978; 17:1029–1035.
75. Weiter JJ, Delori FC, Dorey CK. Central sparing in annular macular degeneration. Am J Ophthalmol 1988; 106:286–292.
76. McDonald HR, Irvine AR. Light-induced maculopathy from the operating microscope in extracapsular cataract extraction and intraocular lens implantation. Ophthalmology 1983; 90:945–951.
77. Boldrey EE, Ho BT, Griffith RR. Retinal burns occurring at cataract extraction. Ophthalmology 1984; 91:1297–1302.
78. Hochheimer BF, d'Anna SA, Calkins JL. Retinal damage from light. Am J Ophthalmol 1979; 88:1039–1044.
79. Mainster MA, Ham WTJ, Delori FC. Potential retinal hazards. Ophthalmology 1983; 90:927–932.
80. McDonald HR, Harris MJ. Operating microscope induced retinal phototoxicity during pars plana vitrectomy. Arch Ophthalmol 1988; 106:521–523.
81. Michels M, Sternberg PJ. Operating microscope-induced retinal phototoxicity: pathophysiology, clinical manifestations and prevention. Surv Ophthalmol 1990; 34:237–252.

82. Leske MC, Wu S-Y, Nemesure B, Hennis A, Barbados ESG. Risk factors for incident nuclear opacities. Ophthalmology 2002; 109:1303–1308.

83. McCarty CA, Taylor HR. Recent developments in vision research: light damage in cataract. Invest Ophthalmol Vis Sci 1996; 37:1720–1723.

84. Jacques P, Taylor A, Hankinson SE, Willett WC, Mahnken B, Lee Y, Vaid K, Lahav M. Long-term vitamin C supplement use and prevalence of early age-related lens opacities. Am J Clin Nutr 1997; 66:911–916.

85. West SK, Duncan DD, Munoz B, Rubin GS, Fried LP, Bandeen-Roche K, Shein OD. Sunlight exposure and risk of lens opacities in population-based study. JAMA 1998; 280:714–718.

86. Delcourt D, Carrier I, Ponton-Sanchez A, Lacroux A, Cavacho MJ, Papoz L. Light exposure and the risk of cortical, nuclear and posterior subcapsular cataracts: the Pathologies Ocularis Liees a l'Age (OLA) study. Arch Ophthalmol 2000; 118:385–392.

87. Zigman S, Sutliff G, Rounds M. Relationships between human cataracts and environmental radiant energy. Lens Eye Tox Res 1991; 8:259–280.

88. Jacques P, Chylack LT Jr. Epidemiologic evidence of a role for the antioxidant vitamins and carotenoids in cataract prevention. Am J Clin Nutr 1991; 53:352S–355S.

89. Mares-Perlman JA, Klein BEA, Klein R, Ritter LL. Relation between lens opacities and vitamin and mineral supplement use. Ophthalmology 1994; 101:315–325.

90. Chasan-Taber L, Willett WC, Seddon JM, Stampfer MJ, Rosner B, Colditz GA, Speizer FE, Hankinson SE. A prospective study of carotenoid and vitamin A intakes and risk of cataract extraction in US women. Am J Clin Nutr 1999; 70:509–516.

91. Lyle B, Mares-Perlman J, Klein B, Klein R, Greger J. Antioxidant intake and risk of incident age-related nuclear cataracts in the Beaver Dam Eye Study. Am J Epidemiol 1999; 149:801–809.

92. Brown L, Rimm EB, Seddon JM, Giovannucci EL, Chasan-Taber L, Spiegelman D, Willett WC, Hankinson SE. A prospective study of carotenoids intake and risk of cataract extraction in US men. Am J Clin Nutr 1999; 70:517–524.

93. Age-Related Eye Disease Study Research Group. Risk factors associated with age-related macular degeneration. Ophthalmology 2000; 107:2224–2232.

94. Guggenheim J. Molecular genetics. New clues to the pathologies of retinal disease. Optom Today 1999; 39:38–42.

95. Allikmets R, Shroyer N, Singh N, Seddon JM, Lewis R, Bernstein PS, Peiffer A, Zabriske N, Li Y, Hutchinson a, Dean M, Lupski J, Lepper M. Mutation of the Stargardt disease gene (ABCR) in age-related macular degeneration. Science 1997; 277:1805–1807.

96. Weng J, Mata NL, Azarian SM, Tzakov RT, Birch DG, Travis GH. Insights into the function of Rim protein in photoreceptors and etiology of Stargardt disease from the phenotype in abcr knockout mice. Cell 1999; 98:13–23.

97. Age-Related Eye Disease Study Research Group. A randomized, placebo-controlled clinical trial of high-dose supplementation with vitamins C and E and beta-carotene for age-related cataract and vision loss: AREDS report no. 9. Arch Ophthalmol 2001; 119:1439–1452.

98. Seddon JM, Ajani UA, Sperduto RD, Hiller R, Blair N, Burton TC, Farber MD, Gragoudas ES, Haller J, Miller DT, Yannuzzi LA, Willett WC. Dietary carotenoids, vitamins A, C, and E and advanced age-related macular degeneration. JAMA 1994; 272:1413–1420.

99. Eye Disease Case-control Study Group. Antioxidant status and neovascular age-related macular degeneration. Arch Ophthalmol 1993; 111:104–109.

100. Mares-Perlman JA, Fisher AI, Klein R, Palta M, Block G, Millen AE, Wright JD. Lutein and zeaxanthin in the diet and serum and their relation to age-related maculopathy in the Third National Health and Nutrition Examination Survey. Am J Epidemiol 2001; 153:424–432.

101. Mares-Perlman JA, Brady WE, Klein R, Klein BEK, Bowen P, Stacewicz-Sapuntzakis M, Palta M. Serum antioxidants and age-related macular degeneration in a population-based case-control study. Arch Ophthalmol 1995; 113:1518–1523.

102. Bone RA, Landrum JT, Mayne ST, Gomez CM, Tibor SE, Twaroska EE. Macular pigment in donor eyes with and without AMD: a case-control study. Invest Ophthalmol Vis Sci 2001; 42:235–240.

103. Richer S. Atrophic ARMD—a nutrition responsive chronic disease. J Am Opt Assoc 1996; 67:6–10.

104. Smith W, Assink J, Klein R, Mitchell P, Klaver CCW, Klein BEK, Hofman A, Jensen S, Wang JJ, de Jong PTVM. Risk factors for age-related macular degeneration. Ophthalmology 2001; 108:697–704.

105. Cruickshanks KJ, Klein R, Klein BEK. Sunlight and age-related macular degeneration. Arch Ophthalmol 1993; 111:514–518.

106. Klein R, Davis MD, Magli YL, Segal P, Klein BEK, Hubbard LD. The Wisconsin age-related maculopathy grading system. Ophthalmology 1991; 98:1128–1134.

107. Sarks JP, Sarks SH, Killingsworth MC. Evolution of soft drusen in age-related macular degeneration. Eye 1994; 8:269–283.

108. Sarks SH. Ageing and degeneration in the macular region: a clinico-pathological study. Br J Ophthal 1976; 60:324–341.

109. Mata NL, Weng J, Travis GH. Biosynthesis of major lipofuscin fluorophore in mice and humans with ABCR-mediated retinal and macular degeneration. Proc Nat Acad Sci USA 2000; 97:7154–7159.

110. Mata NL, Tzekov RT, Liu X, Weng J, Birch DG, Travis GH. Delayed dark-adaptation and lipofuscin accumulation in abcr$^{+/-}$ mice: implication for involvement of ABCR in age-related macular degeneration. Invest Ophthalmol Vis Sci 2001; 42:1685–1690.

111. Sundelin SP, Nilsson SEG. Lipofuscin-formation in retinal pigment epithelial cells is reduced by antioxidants. Free Radic Biol Med 2001; 31:217–225.

112. Suter M, Reme CE, Grimm C, Wenzel A, Jaattela M, Esser P, Kociok N, Leist M, Richter C. Age-related macular degeneration: the lipofuscin component A2E detaches pro-apoptotic proteins from mitochondria and induces apoptosis in mammalian retinal epithelial cells. J Biol Chem 2000; 275:39625–39630.

113. Sparrow JR, Nakanishi K, Parish CA. The lipofuscin fluorophore A2E mediates blue light-induced damage to retinal pigmented epithelial cells. Invest Ophthalmol Vis Sci 2000; 41:1981–1989.

114. Sparrow JR, Cai B. Blue light-induced apoptosis of A2E-containing RPE: involvement of caspase-3 and protection by Bcl-2. Invest Ophthalmol Vis Sci 2001; 42:1356–1362.
115. Shaban H, Borras C, Vina J, Richter C. Phosphatidylglycerol potently protects human retinal pigment epithelial cells against apoptosis induced by A2E, a compound suspected to cause age-related macular degeneration. Exp Eye Res 2002; 75:99–108.
116. Thomson LR, Toyoda Y, Langner A, Delori FC, Garnett KM, Craft NE, Nichols CR, Cheng KM, Dorey CK. Elevated retinal zeaxanthin and prevention of light-induced photoreceptor cell death in quail. Invest Ophthalmol Vis Sci 2002; 43:3538–3549.
117. Thomson LR, Toyoda Y, Delori FC, Garnett KM, Wong Z-Y, Nichols CR, Cheng KM, Craft NE, Dorey CK. Long term dietary supplementation with zeaxanthin reduces photoreceptor death in light-damaged Japanese quail. Exp Eye Res 2002; 75:529–546.
118. Haegerstrom-Portnoy G. Short-wavelength-sensitive-cone sensitivity loss with aging: a protective role for macular pigment? J Opt Soc Am 1988; 5:2140–2144.
119. Bernstein HN, Ginsberg G. The pathology of chloroquine retinopathy. Arch Ophthalmol 1964; 71:238–245.
120. Esposito E, Rotilio D, Matteo V, Giulio C, Cacchio M, Algeri S. A review of specific dietary antioxidants and the effects on biochemical mechanisms related to neurodegenerative processes. Neurobiol Aging 2002; 23:719–735.
121. Organisciak DT, Wang HM, Li ZY, Tso MO. The protective effect of ascorbate in retinal light damage of rats. Invest Ophthalmol Vis Sci 1985; 26:1580–1588.
122. Friedrichson T, Kalbach HL, Buck P, van Kuijk FJGM. Vitamin E in macular and peripheral tissues of the human eye. Curr Eye Res 1995; 14:693–701.
123. Hunt DF, Organisciak DT, Wang HS, Wu RL. Alpha-tocopherol in the developing rat retina: a high pressure liquid chromatographic analysis. Curr Eye Res 1984; 3:1281–1288.
124. Delcourt D, Cristol JP, Leger CL, Descomps B, Papoz L. Associations of anti-oxidant enzymes with cataract and age-related macular degeneration. The POLA study. Ophthalmology 1999; 106:215–222.
125. Sun H, Nathans J. ABCR, the ATP-binding cassette transporter responsible for Stargardt macular dystrophy, is an efficient target of all-trans-retinal-mediated photooxidative damage in vitro. Implications for retinal disease. J Biol Chem 2001; 276:11766–11774.
126. Daicker B, Schiedt K, Adnet JJ, Bermond P. Canthaxanthin retinopathy: an investigation by light and electron microscopy and physicochemical analysis. Graefe's Arch Clin Exp Ophthalmol 1987; 225:189–197.
127. Goralczyk R, Buser S, Bausch J, Bee W, Zühlke U, Barker FM. Occurrence of birefringent retinal inclusions in cynomolgus monkeys after high doses of canthaxanthin. Invest Ophthalmol Vis Sci 1997; 38:741–752.
128. de Sélys R, Decroix J, Frankart M, Hassoun A, Willcox D, Pirard C, Bourlond A. Erythropoietic protoporphyria. Ann Dermatol Venereol 1988; 115:555–560.
129. McGuinness R, Beaumont P. Gold dust retinopathy after the ingestion of canthaxanthin to produce skin-bronzing. Med J Aust 1985; 143:622–623.

130. Nebeling LC, Forman MR, Graubard BI, Snyder RA. The impact of lifestyle characteristics on carotenoid intake in the United State: The 1987 National Health Interview Survey. Am J Public Health 1997; 87:268–271.

131. Nebeling LC, Forman MR, Graubard BI, Snyder RA. Changes in carotenoid intake in the United State: The 1987 and 1982 National Health Interview Surveys. J Am Diet Assoc 1997; 97:991–996.

132. Le Marchand L, Hankin JH, Bach F, Kolonel LN, Wilkens LR, Stacewicz-Sapuntzakis M, Bowen P, Beecher GR, Laudon F, Baque P, Daniel R, Seruvati L, Henderson B. An ecological study of diet and lung cancer in the South Pacific. Int J Cancer 1995; 63:18–23.

133. Bone RA, Landrum JT, Guerra LH, Ruiz CA. Lutein and zeaxanthin dietary supplements raise macular pigment density and serum concentration of these carotenoids. J Nutr 2003; 133:992–998.

134. Broekmans WMR, Berendschot TTJM, Klöpping-Ketelaars IA, de Vries AJ, Goldbohm RA, Tijburg LB, Kardinaal AF, Poppel Gv. Macular pigment density in relation to serum and adipose tissue concentrations of lutein and serum concentrations of lutein and serum concentrations of zeaxanthin. Am J Clin Nutr 2002; 76:595–603.

135. Hammond BR, Caruso-Avery M. Macular pigment optical density in a southwestern sample. Invest Ophthalmol Vis Sci 2000; 41:1492–1497.

136. Berendschot TTJM, Goldbohm RA, Klöpping WAA, van de Kraats J, van Norel J, van Norren D. Influence of lutein supplementation on macular pigment, assessed with two objective techniques. Invest Ophthalmol Vis Sci 2000; 41:3322–3326.

137. Bone RA, Landrum JT, Dixon Z, Chen Y, Llerena CM. Lutein and zeaxanthin in eyes, serum and diet of human subjects. Exp Eye Res 2000; 71:239–245.

138. Falsini B, Piccardi M, Iarossi G, Fadda A, Merendino E, Valentini P. Influence of short-term antioxidant supplementation on macular function in age-related maculopathy. A pilot study including electrophysiologic assessment. Ophthalmology 2003; 110:51–60.

139. Hammond BR Jr, Johnson EJ, Russell RM, Krinsky NI, Yeum K-J, Edwards RB, Snodderly DM. Dietary modification of human macular pigment density. Invest Ophthalmol Vis Sci 1997; 38:1795–1801.

140. Landrum JT, Bone RA, Joa H, Kilburn MD, Moore LL, Sprague KE. A one year study of the macular pigment: the effect of 140 days of a lutein supplement. Exp Eye Res 1997; 65:57–62.

141. Landrum JT, Bone RA, Kilburn MD. The macular pigment: a possible role in protection from age-related macular degeneration. In: Sies H, ed. Advances in Pharmacology. Vol. 38. San Diego: Academic Press, 1997:537–556.

142. Olmedilla B, Granado F, Southon S, Wright AJA, Blanco I, Gil-Martinez E, van den Berg H, Thurnham D, Corridan B, Chopra M, Hininger I. A European multicentre, placebo-controlled supplementation study with a-tocopherol, caroten-rich palm oil, lutein or lycopene: analysis of serum responses. Clin Sci 2002; 102:447–456.

143. Richer S. ARMD—pilot (case series) environmental intervention data. J Am Optom Assoc 1999; 70:24–36.

144. Aleman T, Duncan J, Bieber M, de Castro E, Marks D, Gardner L, Steinberg J, Cideciyan A, Maguire M, Jacobson S. Macular pigment and lutein supplementation in retinitis pigmentosa and Usher syndrome. Invest Ophthalmol Vis Sci 2001; 42:1873–1887.

145. Olmedilla B, Granado F, Blanco I, Vaquero M, Cjigal C. Lutein in patients with cataracts and age-related macular degeneration: a long-term supplementation study. J Sci Food Agric 2001; 81:904–909.

146. Olmedilla B, Granado F, Gil-Martinez E, Blanco I. Supplementation with lutein (4 months) and alpha-tocopherol (2 months) in separate or combined oral doses, in control men. Cancer Lett 1997; 114:179–181.

147. Kostic D, White WS, Olson JA. Intestinal absorption, serum clearance, and interactions between lutein and beta-carotene when administered to human adults in separate or combined oral doses. Am J Clin Nutr 1995; 62:604–610.

148. Roodenburg AJC, Leenen R, van het Hof KH, Weststrate JA, Tijburg LBM. Amount of fat in the diet affects bioavailability of lutein esters but not of alpha-carotene, beta-carotene, and vitamin E in humans. Am J Clin Nutr 2000; 71:1187–1193.

149. Granado F, Olmedilla B, Gil-Martinez E, Blanco I. Lutein ester in serum after lutein supplementation in human subjects. Br J Nutr 1998; 80:445–449.

150. Khachik F, Beecher GR, Smith JC Jr. Lutein, lycopene, and their oxidative metabolites in chemoprevention of cancer. Cell Biochem Suppl 1995; 22:236–246.

151. O'Neill ME, Thurnham D. Intestinal absorption of beta-carotene, lycopene and lutein in men and women following a standard meal: response curves in the triacylglycerol-rich lipoprotein fraction. Br J Nutr 1998; 79:149–159.

152. Schweitzer D, Lang GE, Beuermann B, Remsch H, Hammer M, Thamm E. Objective determination of optical density of xanthophyll after supplementation of lutein. Ophthalmologe 2002; 99:270–275.

153. Duncan JL, Aleman TS, Gardner LM, De Castro E, Marks DA, Emmons JM, Bieber ML, Steinberg JD, Bennett J, Stone EM, Macdonald IM, Cideciyan AV, Maguire MG, Jacobson SG. Macular pigment and lutein supplementation in choroideremia. Exp Eye Res 2002; 74:371–381.

154. Bowen P, Herbst-Espinosa S, Hussain E, Stacewicz-Sapuntzakis M. Esterification does not impair lutein bioavailability in humans. J Nutr 2002; 132:3668–3667.

155. Dagnelie G, Zorge IS, McDonald TM. Lutein improves visual function in some patients with retinal degeneration: a pilot study via the Internet. Opt Vis Sci 2000; 71:147–164.

156. Granado F, Olmedilla B, Blanco I. Serum depletion and bioavailability of lutein in type I diabetic patients. Eur J Nutr 2002; 41:47–53.

157. Hart DJ, Scott KJ. Development and evaluation of an HPLC method for the analysis of carotenoids in foods, and the measurement of the carotenoid content of vegetables and fruits commonly consumed in the UK. Food Chem 1995; 54:101–111.

158. Goodwin TW. The Biochemistry of the Carotenoids. Vol. 1. London: Chapman and Hall, 1980:377.

159. Piccaglia R, Marotti M, Grandi S. Lutein and lutein ester content in different types of *Tagetes patula* and *T. erecta*. Ind Crops Prod 1998; 8:45–51.

21
Heart and Vascular Diseases

Howard D. Sesso and J. Michael Gaziano
*Brigham and Women's Hospital and Harvard Medical School, and
VA Boston Healthcare System, Boston, Massachusetts, U.S.A.*

I. INTRODUCTION

One of the more consistent findings in nutritional epidemiology research is that those who consume higher amounts of fruits and vegetables tend to have lower rates of heart and vascular diseases, including coronary heart disease and stroke (1–5). Data from short-term dietary intervention trials largely confirm these findings, suggesting that diets emphasizing fruit and vegetable intake lead to improvements in coronary risk factors and reduce cardiovascular mortality (6–8). For example, use of the Dietary Approaches to Stop Hypertension (DASH) diet, in part emphasizing increases in fruit and vegetable intake, resulted in improvements in blood pressure (6) and possibly high-density lipoprotein (HDL) cholesterol (9). The precise mechanisms for these apparent protective effects are not entirely clear; however, much attention has been focused on the notion that micronutrients with antioxidant properties might be responsible for the associated lower rates of chronic diseases.

Carotenoids are plant derived fat-soluble pigments efficient in quenching singlet oxygen and free radicals (10). Carotenoids are stored in the liver or adipose tissue, and are lipid-soluble by becoming incorporated into plasma lipoprotein particles during transport (11). For these reasons, carotenoids are considered to fall into the antioxidant family of dietary factors through which may reduce the risk of chronic diseases such as heart and vascular disease, cancer, and diabetes.

In this review of carotenoids and vascular diseases, we will initially discuss some of the proposed biological mechanisms through which carotenoids may be associated with heart and vascular diseases. We will then provide a summary of the epidemiological evidence concerning the effect of both dietary and blood carotenoids—including α-carotene, β-carotene, lycopene, lutein/zeaxanthin, and β-cryptoxanthin—on the risk of heart and vascular disease. Next, the evidence from the primary and secondary prevention trials of β-carotene supplementation using heart and vascular disease as an end point will be provided. Finally, we will summarize the evidence on carotenoids and the risk of heart and vascular disease, suggesting some future directions for research in this area.

II. BIOLOGICAL MECHANISMS

Basic research provides a plausible mechanism by which dietary antioxidants, including carotenoids, might reduce the risk of atherosclerosis through inhibition of oxidative damage. Data from in vitro and in vivo studies suggest that oxidative damage to low-density lipoprotein (LDL) promotes several steps in atherogenesis (12), including endothelial cell damage (13,14), foam cell accumulation (15–17) and growth (18,19), and synthesis of autoantibodies (20). In addition, animal studies suggest that free radicals may directly damage arterial endothelium (21), promote thrombosis (22), and interfere with normal vasomotor regulation (23). In vitro data have demonstrated the possible role of these antioxidants in preventing or retarding various steps in atherogenesis by inhibiting oxidation of LDL or other free radical reactions.

Another mechanism by which carotenoids may reduce the risk of heart and vascular diseases includes inflammation. In recent years evidence has begun to accumulate that C-reactive protein is associated with the carotenoids. Data from the cross-sectional Third National Health and Nutrition Survey showed that nonsmoking subjects in the upper 15% of C-reactive protein distribution had significantly lower serum α-carotene, β-carotene, lutein/zeaxanthin, β-cryptoxanthin, and lycopene levels (24). In a study of elderly nuns, aged 77–99 years, the authors also found that elevated C-reactive protein levels were associated with significantly lower plasma α-carotene ($p = 0.02$), β-carotene ($p = 0.02$), lycopene ($p = 0.03$), and total carotenoid ($p = 0.01$) concentrations (25). Additional data on how elevated carotenoid levels may reduce atherosclerotic progression and clinically manifested heart and vascular diseases remain to be elucidated.

III. TOTAL CAROTENOID INTAKE AND RISK OF HEART AND VASCULAR DISEASES

The promising results for fruit and vegetable intake and the association with heart and vascular diseases have led to the assumption that total or individual dietary carotenoid intake must also be inversely associated with the risk of coronary heart disease and stroke. The abundance of carotenoids in a wide array of fruits and vegetables supports this claim; however, several other dietary factors found in many fruits and vegetables may also explain these results.

Early evidence of the potential benefits of dietary carotenoids on the risk of vascular disease came from several studies. Rimm et al. (26) examined data in a large cohort of men in the Health Professionals' Follow-up Study, finding an inverse association between total dietary carotenoid intake and a lower risk of coronary artery disease. The multivariate relative risks for increasing quintiles of carotene intake were 1.00 (ref.), 0.92, 0.91, 0.86, and 0.71 (p, trend = 0.03). Upon stratification by smoking status, the inverse association strengthened among former and current smokers. In a cohort study of 5133 Finnish men and women aged 30–69 years, a similar inverse association was noted for dietary carotenoid intake, particularly in the highest tertile (27). A community-based study of 1299 elderly men and women in Massachusetts had a follow-up of 4.75 years (28). Using a score based on the intake of carotene-containing fruits and vegetables, the multivariate relative risks of cardiovascular death for increasing quartiles of carotene-containing fruits and vegetables were 1.00 (ref.), 0.77, 0.63, and 0.59 (p, trend = 0.014). Finally, in a cohort study of 747 Massachusetts residents age 60 and older, the combined intake of the five primary dietary carotenoids was associated with a possible lower risk of coronary heart disease mortality after up to 12 years of follow-up (29). Subjects in the upper quintile of dietary carotenoid intake had a nonsignificant 36% reduction in coronary heart disease mortality compared with those in the lowest quintile of intake.

More recent studies on dietary carotenoids and vascular disease have tended to calculate a total dietary carotenoid value, typically summed from intake estimates of α-carotene, β-carotene, lycopene, lutein/zeaxanthin, and β-cryptoxanthin. Two separate papers analyzed data from more than 34,000 postmenopausal women in the Iowa Women's Health Study for the association between dietary carotenoid intake and coronary heart disease death or stroke death over 7 years (30,31). Dietary carotenoid intake was not associated with the risk of coronary heart disease death, with multivariate relative risks for increasing quintiles of 1.00 (ref.), 1.26, 1.18, 1.04, and 1.03 (p, trend = 0.71) (30). For stroke death, there was a similar lack of association for dietary carotenoids in multivariate models (p, trend = 0.88), but it was attenuated from age-adjusted models in which a suggestion of a decreased risk of stroke death for higher quintiles of carotenoid intake was present (31).

IV. SERUM AND PLASMA CAROTENOIDS AND RISK OF HEART AND VASCULAR DISEASES

Additional support for the hypothesis that carotenoids and vascular diseases are associated comes from a multitude of studies examining plasma or serum levels of carotenoids and the subsequent risk of cardiovascular disease. The nested case-control study, in which cases and controls are selected and matched from an existing cohort study, is the preferred study design to efficiently examine this hypothesis because it uses prospective data. Traditional case-control studies have also been instrumental in building the literature on this hypothesis, but tend to be more vulnerable to bias and error.

We next provide details on some of the more recent studies that have been published examining the relation between plasma and serum carotenoids and the risk of vascular disease. The Rotterdam Study was a nested case-control study examining major serum carotenoids in 108 pairs of Dutch subjects with an average follow-up of 5.8 years for cases of aortic atherosclerosis (32). Although no significant linear trends were found for each carotenoid of interest, likely due in part to the small number of cases in each quartile, there was a possible association with serum lycopene and aortic atherosclerosis. Compared with the lowest quartile of serum lycopene, higher quartiles had multivariate relative risks of 0.89, 0.78, and 0.66 (p, trend $= 0.28$).

A case-control study of 104 cases of myocardial infarction and 106 unmatched controls revealed lower levels of lycopene and β-cryptoxanthin among cases, although the result was only adjusted for plasma cholesterol (33). A small cohort study of 638 initially elderly (aged 65–85 years) Dutch men and women found that β-cryptoxanthin and lutein were inversely associated with all-cause mortality (34). Ford and Giles published data from a large cross-sectional analysis of serum carotenoids and the prevalence of angina pectoris using data from the National Health and Nutrition Examination Survey III (35). Among 11,327 middle-aged and older men and women, higher quartiles of α-carotene, β-carotene, and β-cryptoxanthin were all inversely associated with the prevalence of angina (all p, trend < 0.05). Finally, D'Odorico et al. (36) examined plasma carotenoids and risk of atherosclerosis in the carotid arteries in 392 middle-aged Italian men and women followed for approximately 5 years. Of the five major carotenoids, only a combined measure of α- and β-carotene was associated with a lower incidence of atherosclerotic lesions in the carotid arteries ($p = 0.04$).

V. INDIVIDUAL CAROTENOIDS AND RISK OF HEART AND VASCULAR DISEASES

Most of the promising initial observational studies of carotenoids focused on dietary, serum, and plasma β-carotene, ultimately leading to the initiation of several large primary and secondary prevention trials of heart and vascular disease using β-carotene supplementation (detailed in Section VI below). However, following the disappointing results from trials of β-carotene supplementation, research has focused on other specific major carotenoids that may be in part responsible for the apparent benefit supported by high levels of fruit and vegetable intake.

A limited number of epidemiological investigations have simultaneously considered the major carotenoids and risk of heart and vascular disease. A recent study examined multiple dietary carotenoids and the risk of coronary artery disease among 73,286 women in the Nurse's Health Study, with 12 years of follow-up (37). In overall multivariate models, potential inverse associations were noted for α-carotene and β-carotene, but not for lutein/zeaxanthin, lycopene, or β-cryptoxanthin. The relative risks of coronary artery disease for increasing quintiles of α-carotene were 1.00 (ref.), 0.89, 0.69, 0.89, and 0.74 (p, trend = 0.05); for β-carotene the relative risks were 1.00 (ref.), 0.93, 0.91, 0.80, and 0.80 (p, trend = 0.04). Results stratified by baseline smoking status for each carotenoid did not appear to mediate the overall associations. In a parallel cohort of 43,738 male health professionals followed for approximately 8 years, during which 328 strokes occurred (210 ischemic, 70 hemorrhagic, 48 unclassified), there was generally no association between α-carotene, β-carotene, and lycopene with the risk of stroke (38). However, the pattern of relative risks for increasing quintiles of β-carotene intake suggested a possible non-linear association that was not explored in greater detail, with relative risks of 1.00 (ref.), 0.75, 0.83, 0.76, and 0.77 (p, trend $>$0.2). Higher quintiles of dietary lutein were associated with lower risks of total stroke, with multivariate relative risks of 1.00 (ref.), 0.89, 0.88, 0.87, and 0.70 (p, trend = 0.06). Results were similar for lutein and the risk of ischemic stroke.

In terms of other observational data, β-carotene and lycopene have generated a large proportion of interest for their respective roles in the prevention of heart and vascular diseases, whereas other carotenoids—lutein/zeaxanthin, α-carotene, and β-cryptoxanthin—have been studied less extensively. Studies often consider these three carotenoids as part of a larger study of dietary or plasma carotenoids in relation to heart and vascular diseases, but few have exclusively focused on these specific carotenoids. In certain respects, this is not surprising given the strong correlations among the major carotenoids in the diet and blood (39). We now detail some of the observational studies focusing on specific major carotenoids in the diet and the blood for their associations with heart and vascular diseases.

A. β-Carotene

For decades β-carotene has been the most widely studied individual carotenoid for its possible association with heart and vascular disease risk. This has not been without reason, as β-carotene is one of the most abundant carotenoids and has provitamin A activity (40). Initial studies examining β-carotene, often in the context of fruit and vegetable intake, provided compelling evidence for a potential inverse association with the risk of heart and vascular diseases (41–44). Prospective epidemiological data continue to emerge in support of β-carotene. For example, data in 4802 men and women free of baseline cardiovascular disease from the Rotterdam Study indicated that those in increasing tertiles of dietary β-carotene intake had multivariate relative risks of 1.00 (ref.), 0.72, and 0.55 (p, trend = 0.013) (32).

B. Lycopene

While the majority of research to date regarding dietary, plasma, and adipose lycopene has focused on its potential role in the prevention of prostate cancer (45), burgeoning support has emerged for an additional role in the prevention of heart and vascular diseases. Because lycopene is found in high concentrations in a relatively small number of plant foods (tomato, watermelon, pink grapefruit, papaya, apricot), it may have greater appeal for targeted prevention efforts since tomato-based foods are the predominant food source. More than 80% of lycopene intake in the United States is from tomato products, including ketchup, tomato juice, and tomato sauces (46). Lycopene has significant antioxidant potential in vitro and has been hypothesized to play a prominent role in preventing cardiovascular disease (47–49).

Two reports from the EURAMIC study suggest that intimal wall thickness and the risk of myocardial infarction are reduced in persons with higher adipose tissue concentrations of lycopene (50,51). Another study of 520 middle-aged Finnish men and women as part of the Antioxidant Supplementation in Atherosclerosis Prevention study noted similar significant decreases in intimal wall thickness among men with higher plasma lycopene, but not among women (52). Finally, a recently published study among 1028 middle-aged Finnish men found that those in the lowest quartile of serum lycopene had a significantly greater mean intima–media thickness of the common carotid artery, with a trend across quintiles (53). Other studies report possible inverse associations of higher serum lycopene levels and a reduced risk of myocardial infarction (54,55), cardiovascular disease (55–57), carotid atherosclerosis (58,59), and aortic atherosclerosis (32).

To date, data are particularly lacking in women with regard to plasma lycopene levels and the risk of heart and vascular disease. In a prospective, nested case-control study of 483 cases of cardiovascular disease and 483 age- and smoking-matched controls free of cardiovascular disease during an average of 7 years follow-up, plasma lycopene was measured (60). The multivariate relative risks of total cardiovascular disease for women in increasing quartiles of plasma lycopene were 1.00 (ref.), 0.94, 0.62, and 0.67 (p, trend = 0.05). This pattern in relative risks suggested a threshold effect in which women in the upper half of plasma lycopene had a significant 34% reduction in cardiovascular disease risk. For cardiovascular disease excluding angina, an L-shaped association was apparent as women in the upper three quartiles had a significant multivariate 50% risk reduction compared with those in the lowest quartile of plasma lycopene.

In addition to the data on dietary lycopene and other carotenoids presented earlier, more recent data also exist on the association between dietary lycopene and the risk of cardiovascular disease in the Women's Health Study, a cohort of more than 39,000 female health professionals with 7.2 years of follow-up (61). Women in increasing quintiles of lycopene had multivariate relative risks of cardiovascular disease of 1.00 (ref.), 1.11, 1.14, 1.15, and 0.90 (p, trend $= 0.34$). For the consumption of tomato-based products, women consuming 1.5 to fewer than 4, 4 to fewer than 7, 7 to fewer than 10, and 10 or more servings per week had relative risks (95% CIs) of cardiovascular disease of 1.02, 1.04, 0.68, and 0.71 (p, trend $= 0.029$) compared to women consuming fewer than 1.5 servings per week. Results from this study indicate that although dietary lycopene was not strongly associated with the risk of cardiovascular disease, the possible inverse associations noted for higher levels of tomato-based products suggest that dietary lycopene may still have a role in heart and vascular disease prevention.

Small-scale human dietary intervention studies demonstrate the ability of various tomato products to increase plasma lycopene levels in middle-aged, healthy subjects (49,62,63). Some (49,63), but not all (62), of these studies with either lycopene-containing foods or lycopene supplementation have demonstrated potential short-term improvements in LDL oxidation. However, lycopene supplementation over the course of several weeks did not result in reductions of LDL cholesterol levels, despite improvements in LDL oxidation (49). Whether these apparent short-term benefits translate into long-term improvements in health, manifested by a reduction in the risk of heart and vascular diseases, remains unknown.

C. Lutein/Zeaxanthin

Lutein/zeaxanthin is found in a wide variety of fruits and vegetables, including cooked spinach, lettuce, broccoli, peas, lima beans, oranges and orange juice, celery, string beans, and squash (64). Lutein, contained mostly in dark green vegetables (64,65), has been found to protect against the development or progression of atherosclerosis. Studies have shown that lutein is effective in reducing the impact of adhesion molecules along aortic endothelial cells, reflecting a possible role in the development of atherosclerosis (66). Data from the Health Professionals' Follow-up Study, consisting of 43,738 male health professionals followed for approximately 8 years, reported that higher quintiles of dietary lutein were associated with lower risks of total stroke, with multivariate relative risks of 1.00 (ref.), 0.89, 0.88, 0.87, and 0.70 (p, trend $= 0.06$) (38).

The authors reported results for ischemic stroke that closely paralleled the overall stroke data.

Two other key studies have provided support for a role of lutein/zeaxanthin. First, 480 men and women aged 40–60 years from the Los Angeles Atherosclerosis Study were followed for 18 months for the progression of intima–media thickness of the common carotid arteries (67). Subjects in increasing quintiles of plasma lutein had a smaller progression of atherosclerosis (p, trend = 0.0007). A second observational study that examined carotid intima–media thickness included 231 case-control pairs from the Atherosclerosis Risk in Communities study cohort (58). Both lutein/zeaxanthin (odds ratio per standard deviation increase: 0.76, 95% CI: 0.59–0.95) and β-cryptoxanthin (odds ratio per standard deviation increase: 0.75, 95% CI: 0.59–0.94) were significantly and inversely associated with carotid intima–media thickness.

D. α-Carotene and β-Cryptoxanthin

The food sources of α-carotene tend to closely parallel those for β-carotene. Carrots alone—whether raw or cooked—accounted for a whopping 55% of α-carotene intake in the Framingham Heart Study (68). In contrast, carrots were responsible for 37% of β-carotene intake. Based the foods and beverages listed in the Willett semiquantitative food frequency questionnaire, there are only three major food contributors to dietary β-cryptoxanthin intake: orange juice (46.8%), oranges (32.4), and peaches (14.2%) (68). This presents a unique advantage similar to that for lycopene intake, with a limited number of food sources allowing for an improved ability to isolate whether β-cryptoxanthin itself or some other dietary component in oranges and/or peaches may be important in the prevention of heart and vascular diseases. However, comprehensive data are not yet available on the association of either α-carotene or β-cryptoxanthin with heart and vascular diseases.

VI. TRIALS OF β-CAROTENE SUPPLEMENTATION

Based on a strong evidence base from observational studies detailed earlier, several large clinical trials, such as the Physicians' Health Study (PHSI) (69), were initiated and completed in examining the effect of β-carotene supplementation. Many of these clinical trials were designed to study the promise of β-carotene supplementation for reducing the risk of other diseases (e.g., cancer, eye disease), with heart and vascular disease a secondary outcome. Other ongoing primary [Physicians' Health Study II (70) and the Supplementation en Vitamines et Mineraux Antioxydants (SUVIMAX) study (71)] and secondary [Women's Antioxidant Cardiovascular Study (72)] prevention trials continue to test β-carotene supplementation and the risk of heart and vascular diseases. Therefore, we now focus our discussion on the completed primary and secondary prevention trials that have included β-carotene either as an individual study agent or as part of an antioxidant cocktail for the risk of heart and vascular disease.

A. β-Carotene: Primary Prevention Trials in Subjects Without Heart and Vascular Disease

Results from large-scale randomized trials of β-carotene in the primary prevention of heart and vascular disease have largely been disappointing, indicating either no association or a weak positive association. The results from three clinical trials suggest that β-carotene supplementation was not associated with the risk of heart and vascular diseases. The Skin Cancer Prevention Study randomized 1805 men and women with a history of skin cancer to 50 mg of β-carotene daily or placebo (73). After a median follow-up of 8.2 years, there was no association of β-carotene supplementation with cardiovascular mortality (relative risk, 1.15; 95% CI, 0.81–1.63). Next, the Alpha-Tocopherol, Beta-Carotene (ATBC) Cancer Prevention Study was a large-scale randomized trial of antioxidant vitamins in a well-nourished population. This 2 × 2 factorial trial tested the effect of synthetic vitamin E (50 mg/day) and β-carotene (20 mg/day) among 29,133 Finnish male smokers aged 50–69 years. There was a possible increase in ischemic heart disease mortality (relative risk, 1.12; 95% CI, 1.00–1.25) and no association with the risk of angina (relative risk, 1.06; 95% CI, 0.97–1.16) among those assigned to β-carotene (74).

Two other primary prevention trials examining β-carotene as an individual study agent reveal a null association with the risk of heart and vascular diseases. First, the PHS I was a randomized, double-blind, placebo-controlled trial of β-carotene (50 mg on alternate days) and low-dose aspirin among 22,071 U.S. male physicians aged 40–84 years (75). After 12 years, there were no differences in cardiovascular mortality (relative risk, 1.09; 95% CI, 0.93–1.27), myocardial infarction (relative risk, 0.96; 95% CI, 0.84–1.09), stroke (RR, 0.96; 95% CI, 0.83–1.11), or a composite of the three end points (relative risk, 1.00; 95% CI, 0.91–1.09) associated with β-carotene assignment. A trial complementing the PHS I, the Women's Health Study, evaluated the effect of β-carotene (50 mg on alternate days), vitamin E, and low-dose aspirin on the development of cardiovascular disease in 39,876 healthy female health professionals (76). While the vitamin E and aspirin components of the trial are continuing, the β-carotene arm was terminated after just over a mean of 2 years follow-up, largely in response the null findings on β-carotene reported in the PHS I. β-Carotene supplementation had no effect on cardiovascular mortality (relative risk, 1.17; 95% CI, 0.54–2.53), myocardial infarction (relative risk, 1.08; 95% CI,

0.56–1.27), stroke (relative risk, 1.42; 95% CI, 0.96–2.10), or a composite of these endpoints (relative risk, 1.14; 95% CI 0.87–1.49). Smoking status did not modify the null association between β-carotene supplementation and the risk of heart and vascular diseases.

B. β-Carotene: Secondary Prevention Trials in Subjects with Heart and Vascular Disease

β-Carotene supplementation has been less well studied in secondary prevention than in primary prevention settings. Although no data are yet available from randomized trials specifically designed to answer whether β-carotene supplementation alone (as opposed to in combination with other antioxidants) is effective in secondary prevention of heart and vascular diseases, subgroup analyses in some of the aforementioned primary prevention trials allow an empirical examination of this issue.

In the ATBC trial, 1862 men had a baseline history of myocardial infarction and were randomized to β-carotene supplementation for 6 years. Among this subgroup of men, β-carotene was associated with a potential reduction in the risk of nonfatal myocardial infarction (relative risk, 0.67; 95% CI, 0.44–1.02), but a nonsignificant increased risk of fatal coronary heart disease (relative risk, 1.58; 95% CI, 1.05–2.40) (77). In PHS I, 333 men reported a history of chronic stable angina or a coronary revascularization procedure prior to randomization. Among those in the β-carotene group, a reduction (relative risk, 0.46, 95% CI 0.24–0.85) in the risk of major cardiovascular events was observed after 5 years, and a persistent though attenuated reduction was also found after 12 years (relative risk, 0.71, 95% CI 0.47–1.07) (78).

C. β-Carotene as Part of a Combination Intervention

Other primary prevention trials have considered β-carotene as part of a nutrient combination. While informative, it is difficult to extrapolate the findings for a mixture of several nutrients to the individual effects of β-carotene supplementation. There are three primary and three secondary prevention trials of heart and vascular disease that have been completed and published.

First, the Cancer Prevention Trial was a primary prevention trial conducted in a poorly nourished population in China that was at high risk for upper gastrointestinal cancers, presumably due to a low intake of micronutrients (79). Nearly 30,000 men and women were randomized to a cocktail of synthetic vitamin E (30 mg daily), β-carotene (15 mg daily), and selenium (50 μg daily). Participants taking this antioxidant cocktail had a relative risk of 0.90 (95% CI, 0.76–1.07) for cerebrovascular mortality and 0.91 (95% CI, 0.84–0.99) for total mortality compared with those on placebo. Second, the β-Carotene and Retinol

Efficacy Trial (CARET) evaluated a combined treatment of β-carotene (30 mg/ day) and retinol (25,000 IU/day) among 18,314 men and women at elevated risk of lung cancer due to cigarette smoking and/or occupational exposure to asbestos (80). After 4 years, there was a borderline significant increased risk of cardiovascular death (relative risk, 1.26; 95% CI, 0.99–1.61) among individuals assigned to β-carotene and retinol. Finally, the Age-Related Eye Disease Study Group (AREDS) reported that an antioxidant cocktail of β-carotene, vitamin C, and vitamin E randomized to 4757 middle-aged and older subjects was not related to the risk of cardiovascular disease (relative risk, 1.06; 95% CI, 0.84–1.33) (81).

The HDL-Atherosclerosis Treatment Study (HATS) (82), the Heart Protection Study (HPS) (83), and the Multivitamins and Probucol (MVP) study (84) are each secondary prevention trials investigating β-carotene supplementation as part of a mixture of antioxidants, with results favoring no association between β-carotene and the risk of secondary events. In HATS, 160 men and women with coronary artery disease were randomly assigned in a 2×2 factorial design to simvastatin plus niacin, or to an antioxidant combination (800 IU of vitamin E, 1000 mg of vitamin C, 25 mg of natural β-carotene, and 100 µg selenium). After a mean follow-up of 14 months, 21% of subjects taking the antioxidant combination developed cardiovascular disease versus 24% in the placebo group ($p > 0.05$) (82). In the Heart Protection Study (HPS), a 2×2 factorial design tested a daily antioxidant cocktail (600 mg of synthetic vitamin E, 250 mg of vitamin C, and 20 mg of β-carotene) and simvastatin (40 mg) among 20,536 men and women with angina, stroke, claudication, or diabetes. Main-effects analyses showed neither a beneficial nor a deleterious effect of the antioxidant cocktail on cardiovascular outcomes over 5 years of follow-up (83). Finally, in the MVP study, a combination of vitamin C (1000 mg/day), vitamin E (1400 IU/day), and β-carotene (100 mg/day) had no effect on the rate and severity of restenosis (84).

VII. CONCLUSIONS

Although more than 600 carotenoids have been identified (85), the majority of research in nutrition has focused on the five most common carotenoids: α-carotene, β-carotene, lycopene, lutein/zeaxanthin, and β-cryptoxanthin. Carotenoids may prevent heart and vascular disease in a number of ways. In addition to the established antioxidant mechanisms, other explanations include an association between carotenoids and inflammatory markers such as C-reactive protein or other biomarkers of vascular disease. Studies that examine fruit and vegetable intake have overwhelmingly supported a cardioprotective role. Recently published observational studies continue to support total carotenoids and individual carotenoids—measured from dietary intake, supplement use, plasma, and serum—in the prevention of heart and vascular diseases.

β-Carotene is the most studied carotenoid, whose early promising results spawned several large primary and secondary prevention trials that have provided null results for heart and vascular diseases. Two possible explanations for the discrepancy between the observational and trial evidence are an insufficient duration or dose of β-carotene supplementation, limiting its effects on the development of heart and vascular disease. Meta-analyses of β-carotene supplementation must be considered in the context of all studies indicated in Section VI above, carefully differentiating between trials that examine individual β-carotene supplementation versus those that include β-carotene as part of an antioxidant cocktail. More research is needed to understand how β-carotene, other carotenoids, vitamins, and minerals all interact when consumed either as a supplement or in the diet.

Significant progress has been made in the last decade on the other major carotenoids besides β-carotene—α-carotene, lycopene, lutein/zeaxanthin, and β-cryptoxanthin—in support of a possible inverse association with the risk of heart and vascular diseases. In particular, more studies are needed on lycopene and lutein/zeaxanthin in terms of their potential roles in the prevention of heart and vascular disease. Lycopene (tomatoes) and β-cryptoxanthin (oranges) have a limited number of food sources compared with their carotenoid counterparts. This makes lycopene and β-cryptoxanthin promising carotenoids whose intake can be increased with relatively simple dietary recommendations. Additional data from interventions of dietary approaches focused on increasing total or specific carotenoid intake can provide critical information on the biological mechanisms supporting the observational findings for carotenoids and a possible reduced risk of heart and vascular disease.

REFERENCES

1. Joshipura KJ, Hu FB, Manson JE, Stampfer MJ, Rimm EB, Speizer FE, Colditz G, Ascherio A, Rosner B, Spiegelman D, Willett WC. The effect of fruit and vegetable intake on risk for coronary heart disease. Ann Intern Med 2001; 134:1106–1114.
2. Mozaffarian D, Kumanyika SK, Lemaitre RN, Olson JL, Burke GL, Siscovick DS. Cereal, fruit, and vegetable fiber intake and the risk of cardiovascular disease in elderly individuals. JAMA 2003; 289:1659–1666.
3. Bazzano LA, He J, Ogden LG, Loria CM, Vupputuri S, Myers L, Whelton PK. Fruit and vegetable intake and risk of cardiovascular disease in US adults: the first National Health and Nutrition Examination Survey Epidemiologic Follow-up Study. Am J Clin Nutr 2002; 76:93–99.
4. Liu S, Manson JE, Lee IM, Cole SR, Hennekens CH, Willett WC, Buring JE. Fruit and vegetable intake and risk of cardiovascular disease: the Women's Health Study. Am J Clin Nutr 2000; 72:922–928.

5. Joshipura KJ, Ascherio A, Manson JE, Stampfer MJ, Rimm EB, Speizer FE, Hennekens CH, Spiegelman D, Willett WC. Fruit and vegetable intake in relation to risk of ischemic stroke. JAMA 1999; 282:1233–1239.

6. Sacks FM, Svetkey LP, Vollmer WM, Appel LJ, Bray GA, Harsha D, Obarzanek E, Conlin PR, Miller ER, 3rd, Simons-Morton DG, Karanja N, Lin PH. Effects on blood pressure of reduced dietary sodium and the Dietary Approaches to Stop Hypertension (DASH) diet. DASH-Sodium Collaborative Research Group. N Engl J Med 2001; 344:3–10.

7. de Lorgeril M, Salen P, Martin JL, Monjaud I, Delaye J, Mamelle N. Mediterranean diet, traditional risk factors, and the rate of cardiovascular complications after myocardial infarction: final report of the Lyon Diet Heart Study. Circulation 1999; 99:779–785.

8. Trichopoulou A, Costacou T, Bamia C, Trichopoulos D. Adherence to a mediterranean diet and survival in a greek population. N Engl J Med 2003; 348:2599–2608.

9. Obarzanek E, Sacks FM, Vollmer WM, Bray GA, Miller ER, 3rd, Lin PH, Karanja NM, Most-Windhauser MM, Moore TJ, Swain JF, Bales CW, Proschan MA. Effects on blood lipids of a blood pressure-lowering diet: the Dietary Approaches to Stop Hypertension (DASH) Trial. Am J Clin Nutr 2001; 74:80–89.

10. Young AJ, Lowe GM. Antioxidant and prooxidant properties of carotenoids. Arch Biochem Biophys 2001; 385:20–27.

11. Parker RS. Carotenoids in human blood and tissues. J Nutr 1989; 119:101–104.

12. Steinberg D, Parthasarathy S, Carew TE, Khoo JC, Witztum JL. Beyond cholesterol. Modifications of low-density lipoprotein that increase its atherogenicity. N Engl J Med 1989; 320:915–924.

13. Hessler JR, Morel DW, Lewis LJ, Chisolm GM. Lipoprotein oxidation and lipoprotein-induced cytotoxicity. Arteriosclerosis 1983; 3:215–222.

14. Yagi K. Increased serum lipid peroxides initiate atherogenesis. Bioessays 1984; 1:58–60.

15. Quinn MT, Parthasarathy S, Steinberg D. Endothelial cell-derived chemotactic activity for mouse peritoneal macrophages and the effects of modified forms of low density lipoprotein. Proc Natl Acad Sci USA 1985; 82:5949–5953.

16. Schaffner T, Taylor K, Bartucci EJ, Fischer-Dzoga K, Beeson JH, Glagov S, Wissler RW. Arterial foam cells with distinctive immunomorphologic and histochemical features of macrophages. Am J Pathol 1980; 100:57–80.

17. Gerrity RG. The role of the monocyte in atherogenesis: I. Transition of blood-borne monocytes into foam cells in fatty lesions. Am J Pathol 1981; 103:181–190.

18. Fogelman AM, Shechter I, Seager J, Hokom M, Child JS, Edwards PA. Malondialdehyde alteration of low density lipoproteins leads to cholesteryl ester accumulation in human monocyte-macrophages. Proc Natl Acad Sci USA 1980; 77:2214–2218.

19. Goldstein JL, Ho YK, Basu SK, Brown MS. Binding site on macrophages that mediates uptake and degradation of acetylated low density lipoprotein, producing massive cholesterol deposition. Proc Natl Acad Sci USA 1979; 76:333–337.

20. Salonen JT, Yla-Herttuala S, Yamamoto R, Butler S, Korpela H, Salonen R, Nyyssonen K, Palinski W, Witztum JL. Autoantibody against oxidised LDL and progression of carotid atherosclerosis. Lancet 1992; 339:883–887.

21. Beckman JS, Beckman TW, Chen J, Marshall PA, Freeman BA. Apparent hydroxyl radical production by peroxynitrite: implications for endothelial injury from nitric oxide and superoxide. Proc Natl Acad Sci USA 1990; 87:1620–1624.

22. Marcus AJ, Silk ST, Safier LB, Ullman HL. Superoxide production and reducing activity in human platelets. J Clin Invest 1977; 59:149–158.

23. Saran M, Michel C, Bors W. Reaction of NO with O2-. implications for the action of endothelium-derived relaxing factor (EDRF). Free Radic Res Commun 1990; 10:221–226.

24. Kritchevsky SB, Bush AJ, Pahor M, Gross MD. Serum carotenoids and markers of inflammation in nonsmokers. Am J Epidemiol 2000; 152:1065–1071.

25. Boosalis MG, Snowdon DA, Tully CL, Gross MD. Acute phase response and plasma carotenoid concentrations in older women: findings from the nun study. Nutrition 1996; 12:475–478.

26. Rimm EB, Stampfer MJ, Ascherio A, Giovannucci E, Colditz GA, Willett WC. Vitamin E consumption and the risk of coronary heart disease in men. N Engl J Med 1993; 328:1450–1456.

27. Knekt P, Reunanen A, Jarvinen R, Seppanen R, Heliovaara M, Aromaa A. Antioxidant vitamin intake and coronary mortality in a longitudinal population study. Am J Epidemiol 1994; 139:1180–1189.

28. Gaziano JM, Manson JE, Branch LG, Colditz GA, Willett WC, Buring JE. A prospective study of consumption of carotenoids in fruits and vegetables and decreased cardiovascular mortality in the elderly. Ann Epidemiol 1995; 5:255–260.

29. Sahyoun NR, Jacques PF, Russell RM. Carotenoids, vitamins C and E, and mortality in an elderly population. Am J Epidemiol 1996; 144:501–511.

30. Kushi LH, Folsom AR, Prineas RJ, Mink PJ, Wu Y, Bostick RM. Dietary antioxidant vitamins and death from coronary heart disease in postmenopausal women. N Engl J Med 1996; 334:1156–1162.

31. Yochum LA, Folsom AR, Kushi LH. Intake of antioxidant vitamins and risk of death from stroke in postmenopausal women. Am J Clin Nutr 2000; 72:476–483.

32. Klipstein-Grobusch K, Launer LJ, Geleijnse JM, Boeing H, Hofman A, Witteman JC. Serum carotenoids and atherosclerosis. The Rotterdam Study. Atherosclerosis 2000; 148:49–56.

33. Ruiz Rejon F, Martin-Pena G, Granado F, Ruiz-Galiana J, Blanco I, Olmedilla B. Plasma status of retinol, alpha- and gamma-tocopherols, and main carotenoids to first myocardial infarction: case control and follow-up study. Nutrition 2002; 18:26–31.

34. De Waart FG, Schouten EG, Stalenhoef AF, Kok FJ. Serum carotenoids, alpha-tocopherol and mortality risk in a prospective study among Dutch elderly. Int J Epidemiol 2001; 30:136–143.

35. Ford ES, Giles WH. Serum vitamins, carotenoids, and angina pectoris: findings from the National Health and Nutrition Examination Survey III. Ann Epidemiol 2000; 10:106–116.

36. D'Odorico A, Martines D, Kiechl S, Egger G, Oberhollenzer F, Bonvicini P, Sturniolo GC, Naccarato R, Willeit J. High plasma levels of alpha- and beta-carotene are associated with a lower risk of atherosclerosis: results from the Bruneck study. Atherosclerosis 2000; 153:231–239.

37. Osganian SK, Stampfer MJ, Rimm E, Spiegelman D, Manson JE, Willett WC. Dietary carotenoids and risk of coronary artery disease in women. Am J Clin Nutr 2003; 77:1390–1399.

38. Ascherio A, Rimm EB, Hernan MA, Giovannucci E, Kawachi I, Stampfer MJ, Willett WC. Relation of consumption of vitamin E, vitamin C, and carotenoids to risk for stroke among men in the United States. Ann Intern Med 1999; 130:963–970.

39. Michaud DS, Giovannucci EL, Ascherio A, Rimm EB, Forman MR, Sampson L, Willett WC. Associations of plasma carotenoid concentrations and dietary intake of specific carotenoids in samples of two prospective cohort studies using a new carotenoid database. Cancer Epidemiol Biomark Prev 1998; 7:283–290.

40. Pryor WA, Stahl W, Rock CL. Beta carotene: from biochemistry to clinical trials. Nutr Rev 2000; 58:39–53.

41. Acheson RM, Williams DR. Does consumption of fruit and vegetables protect against stroke? Lancet 1983; 1:1191–1193.

42. Vollset SE, Bjelke E. Does consumption of fruit and vegetables protect against stroke? Lancet 1983; 2:742.

43. Gey KF, Stahelin HB, Eichholzer M. Poor plasma status of carotene and vitamin C is associated with higher mortality from ischemic heart disease and stroke: Basel Prospective Study. Clin Invest 1993; 71:3–6.

44. Armstrong BK, Mann JI, Adelstein AM, Eskin F. Commodity consumption and ischemic heart disease mortality, with special reference to dietary practices. J Chronic Dis 1975; 28:455–469.

45. Giovannucci E, Rimm EB, Liu Y, Stampfer MJ, Willett WC. A prospective study of tomato products, lycopene, and prostate cancer risk. J Natl Cancer Inst 2002; 94:391–398.

46. Clinton SK. Lycopene: chemistry, biology, and implications for human health and disease. Nutr Rev 1998; 56:35–51.

47. Arab L, Steck S. Lycopene and cardiovascular disease. Am J Clin Nutr 2000; 71:1691S–1695S.

48. Fuhrman B, Elis A, Aviram M. Hypocholesterolemic effect of lycopene and beta-carotene is related to suppression of cholesterol synthesis and augmentation of LDL receptor activity in macrophages. Biochem Biophys Res Commun 1997; 233:658–662.

49. Agarwal S, Rao AV. Tomato lycopene and low density lipoprotein oxidation: a human dietary intervention study. Lipids 1998; 33:981–984.

50. Kohlmeier L, Kark JD, Gomez-Gracia E, Martin BC, Steck SE, Kardinaal AF, Ringstad J, Thamm M, Masaev V, Riemersma R, Martin-Moreno JM, Huttunen JK, Kok FJ. Lycopene and myocardial infarction risk in the EURAMIC study. Am J Epidemiol 1997; 146:618–626.

51. Gomez-Aracena J, Sloots J, Garcia-Rodriguez A, et al. Antioxidants in adipose tissue and myocardial infarction in a Mediterranean area. Nutr Metab Cardiovasc Dis 1997; 7:376–382.

52. Rissanen T, Voutilainen S, Nyyssonen K, Salonen R, Salonen JT. Low plasma lycopene concentration is associated with increased intima-media thickness of the carotid artery wall. Arterioscler Thromb Vasc Biol 2000; 20:2677–2681.

53. Rissanen TH, Voutilainen S, Nyyssonen K, Salonen R, Kaplan GA, Salonen JT. Serum lycopene concentrations and carotid atherosclerosis: the Kuopio Ischaemic heart disease risk factor study. Am J Clin Nutr 2003; 77:133–138.

54. Street DA, Comstock GW, Salkeld RM, Schuep W, Klag MJ. Serum antioxidants and myocardial infarction. Are low levels of carotenoids and alpha-tocopherol risk factors for myocardial infarction? Circulation 1994; 90:1154–1161.

55. Rissanen TH, Voutilainen S, Nyyssonen K, Lakka TA, Sivenius J, Salonen R, Kaplan GA, Salonen JT. Low serum lycopene concentration is associated with an excess incidence of acute coronary events and stroke: the Kuopio Ischaemic heart disease risk factor study. Br J Nutr 2001; 85:749–754.

56. Schmidt R, Fazekas F, Hayn M, Schmidt H, Kapeller P, Roob G, Offenbacher H, Schumacher M, Eber B, Weinrauch V, Kostner GM, Esterbauer H. Risk factors for microangiopathy-related cerebral damage in the Austrian stroke prevention study. J Neurol Sci 1997; 152:15–21.

57. Kristenson M, Zieden B, Kucinskiene Z, Elinder LS, Bergdahl B, Elwing B, Abaravicius A, Razinkoviene L, Calkauskas H, Olsson AG. Antioxidant state and mortality from coronary heart disease in Lithuanian and Swedish men: concomitant cross sectional study of men aged 50. BMJ 1997; 314:629–633.

58. Iribarren C, Folsom AR, Jacobs DR Jr, Gross MD, Belcher JD, Eckfeldt JH. Association of serum vitamin levels, LDL susceptibility to oxidation, and autoantibodies against MDA-LDL with carotid atherosclerosis. A case-control study. The ARIC study investigators. Atherosclerosis risk in communities. Arterioscler Thromb Vasc Biol 1997; 17:1171–1177.

59. McQuillan BM, Hung J, Beilby JP, Nidorf M, Thompson PL. Antioxidant vitamins and the risk of carotid atherosclerosis. The Perth Carotid Ultrasound Disease Assessment study (CUDAS). J Am Coll Cardiol 2001; 38:1788–1794.

60. Sesso HD, Buring JE, Norkus EP, Gaziano JM. Plasma lycopene, other carotenoids, and retinol and the risk of cardiovascular disease in women. Am J Clin Nutr 2004; 79:47–53.

61. Sesso HD, Liu S, Gaziano JM, Buring JE. Dietary lycopene, tomato-based food products and cardiovascular disease in women. J Nutr 2003; 133:2336–2341.

62. Dugas TR, Morel DW, Harrison EH. Dietary supplementation with beta-carotene, but not with lycopene, inhibits endothelial cell-mediated oxidation of low-density lipoprotein. Free Radic Biol Med 1999; 26:1238–1244.

63. Bub A, Watzl B, Abrahamse L, Delincee H, Adam S, Wever J, Muller H, Rechkemmer G. Moderate intervention with carotenoid-rich vegetable products reduces lipid peroxidation in men. J Nutr 2000; 130:2200–2206.

64. Mangels AR, Holden JM, Beecher GR, Forman MR, Lanza E. Carotenoid content of fruits and vegetables: an evaluation of analytic data. J Am Diet Assoc 1993; 93:284–296.

65. Mares-Perlman JA, Millen AE, Ficek TL, Hankinson SE. The body of evidence to support a protective role for lutein and zeaxanthin in delaying chronic disease. Overview. J Nutr 2002; 132:518S–524S.

66. Martin KR, Wu D, Meydani M. The effect of carotenoids on the expression of cell surface adhesion molecules and binding of monocytes to human aortic endothelial cells. Atherosclerosis 2000; 150:265–274.

67. Dwyer JH, Navab M, Dwyer KM, Hassan K, Sun P, Shircore A, Hama-Levy S, Hough G, Wang X, Drake T, Merz CN, Fogelman AM. Oxygenated carotenoid lutein and progression of early atherosclerosis: the Los Angeles atherosclerosis study. Circulation 2001; 103:2922–2927.

68. Tucker KL, Chen H, Vogel S, Wilson PW, Schaefer EJ, Lammi-Keefe CJ. Carotenoid intakes, assessed by dietary questionnaire, are associated with plasma carotenoid concentrations in an elderly population. J Nutr 1999; 129:438–445.

69. The Steering Committee of the Physicians' Health Study Research Group. Final report on the aspirin component of the ongoing physicians' health study. N Engl J Med 1989; 321:129–135.

70. Christen WG, Gaziano JM, Hennekens CH. Design of physicians' health study II— a randomized trial of beta-carotene, vitamins E and C, and multivitamins, in prevention of cancer, cardiovascular disease, and eye disease, and review of results of completed trials. Ann Epidemiol 2000; 10:125–134.

71. Hercberg S, Preziosi P, Briancon S, Galan P, Triol I, Malvy D, Roussel AM, Favier A. A primary prevention trial using nutritional doses of antioxidant vitamins and minerals in cardiovascular diseases and cancers in a general population: the SU.VI.MAX study—design, methods, and participant characteristics. Supplementation en Vitamines et Mineraux AntioXydants. Controled Clin Trials 1998; 19:336–351.

72. Manson JE, Gaziano JM, Spelsberg A, Ridker PM, Cook NR, Buring JE, Willett WC, Hennekens CH. A secondary prevention trial of antioxidant vitamins and cardiovascular disease in women. Rationale, design, and methods. The WACS research group. Ann Epidemiol 1995; 5:261–269.

73. Greenberg ER, Baron JA, Karagas MR, Stukel TA, Nierenberg DW, Stevens MM, Mandel JS, Haile RW. Mortality associated with low plasma concentration of beta carotene and the effect of oral supplementation. JAMA 1996; 275:699–703.

74. Rapola JM, Virtamo J, Haukka JK, Heinonen OP, Albanes D, Taylor PR, Huttunen JK. Effect of vitamin E and beta carotene on the incidence of angina pectoris. A randomized, double-blind, controlled trial. JAMA 1996; 275:693–698.

75. Hennekens CH, Buring JE, Manson JE, Stampfer M, Rosner B, Cook NR, Belanger C, LaMotte F, Gaziano JM, Ridker PM, Willett W, Peto R. Lack of effect of long-term supplementation with beta carotene on the incidence of malignant neoplasms and cardiovascular disease. N Engl J Med 1996; 334:1145–1149.

76. Lee IM, Cook NR, Manson JE, Buring JE, Hennekens CH. Beta-carotene supplementation and incidence of cancer and cardiovascular disease: the Women's Health Study. J Natl Cancer Inst 1999; 91:2102–2106.

77. Rapola JM, Virtamo J, Ripatti S, Huttunen JK, Albanes D, Taylor PR, Heinonen OP. Randomised trial of alpha-tocopherol and beta-carotene supplements on incidence of major coronary events in men with previous myocardial infarction. Lancet 1997; 349:1715–1720.

78. Gaziano JM, Manson JE, Ridker PM, Buring JE, Hennekens CH. Beta carotene therapy for chronic stable angina [abstract]. Circulation 1990; 82(4 Suppl III):202.

79. Blot WJ, Li JY, Taylor PR, Guo W, Dawsey S, Wang GQ, Yang CS, Zheng SF, Gail M, Li GY, et al. Nutrition intervention trials in Linxian, China: supplementation with specific vitamin/mineral combinations, cancer incidence, and disease-specific mortality in the general population. J Natl Cancer Inst 1993; 85:1483–1492.

80. Omenn GS, Goodman GE, Thornquist MD, Balmes J, Cullen MR, Glass A, Keogh JP, Meyskens FL, Valanis B, Williams JH, Barnhart S, Hammar S. Effects of a combination of beta carotene and vitamin A on lung cancer and cardiovascular disease. N Engl J Med 1996; 334:1150–1155.

81. A randomized, placebo-controlled, clinical trial of high-dose supplementation with vitamins C and E and beta carotene for age-related cataract and vision loss: AREDS report no. 9. Arch Ophthalmol 2001; 119:1439–1452.

82. Brown BG, Zhao XQ, Chait A, Fisher LD, Cheung MC, Morse JS, Dowdy AA, Marino EK, Bolson EL, Alaupovic P, Frohlich J, Albers JJ. Simvastatin and niacin, antioxidant vitamins, or the combination for the prevention of coronary disease. N Engl J Med 2001; 345:1583–1592.

83. MRC/BHF Heart Protection Study of antioxidant vitamin supplementation in 20,536 high-risk individuals: a randomised placebo-controlled trial. Lancet 2002; 360:23–33.

84. Tardif JC, Cote G, Lesperance J, Bourassa M, Lambert J, Doucet S, Bilodeau L, Nattel S, de Guise P. Probucol and multivitamins in the prevention of restenosis after coronary angioplasty. Multivitamins and Probucol Study Group. N Engl J Med 1997; 337:365–372.

85. Holden JM, Eldridge AL, Beecher GR, Buzzard IM, Bhagwat S, Davis CS, Douglass LW, Gebhardt S, Haytowitz D, Schakel S. Carotenoid content of US foods: an update of the database. J Food Comp Anal 1999; 12:169–196.

22
Carotenoids in Systemic Protection Against Sunburn

Wilhelm Stahl and Helmut Sies
Heinrich-Heine-Universität, Düsseldorf, Germany

I. INTRODUCTION

Directly and indirectly, the sun provides the energy supporting life on earth. All foods and fuels are ultimately derived from plants using solar energy in the process of photosynthesis. The sun releases the majority of its energy as visible light, but infrared (IR) and ultraviolet (UV) rays are also significant parts of the solar spectrum (1). According to the range of wavelengths, UV light is divided into UVA (320–400 nm), UVB (280–320 nm), and UVC (100–280 nm). The spectrum of visible light ranges from 400 to 700 nm. While UVC light is mainly absorbed by the ozone layer, UVB and UVA rays reach the terrestrial surface. Exposure to visible and UV light may interfere with essential biochemical functions in living organisms and damage biologically important structures like DNA, lipids, and proteins (2–4). In DNA, UV radiation leads to the formation of thymidine dimers, photo-oxidation products, and single-strand breaks. Animals and plants have developed various strategies of defense against light-induced damage (5). Photosynthetic organisms make use of carotenoids for photoprotection of reaction centers and pigment–protein antennae via energy dissipation (6). Absorption and reflection of light provide other mechanisms of defense (7). An adaptive response of human skin toward irradiation with sunlight is pigmentation and thickening of the stratum corneum. The epidermal pigment melanin provides protection, lowering the radiant energy by the absorption of UV light.

   Light-induced damage in exposed tissues is involved in the pathobiochemistry of several human diseases of skin and eye (4,8). Sun exposure may cause skin disorders including premature aging, photoallergic and phototoxic reactions, and skin cancer (9–12). Polymorphous light eruption (PLE) is the most common sun-induced skin disorder with an estimated prevalence of 10–20%, characterized by an intermittent skin reaction to UVA irradiation (9,13). The formation of reactive oxygen species following UV radiation, which may interfere with signal transduction pathways involved in the regulation of proinflammatory genes, is considered to be one of the causes of PLE.

Chemical substances including certain active ingredients of sunscreen and skin care products may trigger photoallergic and phototoxic reactions (14). Sunlight affects the immune status not only of the skin but of the entire organism. Visible light (400–700 nm) can penetrate epidermal and dermal layers of the skin and may directly interact with circulating lymphocytes, modulating immune function. In contrast to visible light, in vivo exposure to UVB and UVA radiation can alter normal human immune function only by a skin-mediated response (3,15).

II. SUNBURN

The most common adverse reaction to solar radiation is the so-called sunburn reaction or solar erythema. Sunburn is defined as an injury to the skin with erythema, tenderness, and sometimes painful blistering following overexposure to UV radiation (16). The erythema starts to develop a few hours after irradiation, culminating about 18–24 h following irradiation. It should be noted that "erythema" is a nonspecific term generally used to define the redness of the skin that may result from a variety of causes. Thus, UV-induced erythema should be correctly used to describe the sunburn reaction, which is caused by an increased blood flow in the affected area. Direct and indirect damage due to photochemical reactions ultimately leads to vasodilation and edema. DNA damage and the activation of inflammatory pathways are involved in activation of the response.

UVB rays are considered to be the major cause of sunburn, DNA damage, and development of skin cancer. Irradiation with the highly erythematogenic UVB induces a series of complex events including the production of inflammatory mediators, alteration of vascular responses, and an inflammatory cell infiltrate. Damage to proteins and DNA accumulates within skin cells, and characteristic morphological changes occur in keratinocytes and other skin cells. When a cell becomes irreversibly damaged by UV exposure, cell death follows via apoptotic mechanisms leading to the appearance of so-called sunburn cells in the epidermis (17,18). Enzymatic and nonenzymatic antioxidants effectively suppress sunburn cell formation, suggesting that reactive oxygen species play a role in the progression of UVB-induced apoptosis.

UVB radiation acts as a local immunosuppressant damaging the Langerhans cells in the epidermis. Immunological studies on individuals subjected to extended UVB irradiation show additional systemic immunosuppression (3,19).

The UV dose required to produce UV-induced erythema varies depending on the skin type; different skin types are often categorized following the Fitzpatrick skin type scale (20). This system denotes six different skin types classified according to skin, hair, and eye color, and reaction to sun exposure. It ranges from skin type I, with white or freckled skin, green or light blue eyes, red hair, and high sensitivity to sunlight, to skin type VI with black skin, dark brown eyes, and black hair experiencing sunburn almost never. Recent studies have shown that skin response to UV rays can also be predicted, to a good approximation, by skin colorimetry (45).

Interindividual differences also determine the minimal erythema dose (MED). The MED is the lowest dose of UV radiation that will produce a barely detectable erythema 24 h after exposure (21). Its value differs between individuals and depends on the skin type and the actual endogenous protection by melanin (tanning). There are several strategies for sun protection, including avoidance of sun exposure, use of protective clothing and sunscreens, and tanning by increasing the content of melanin in the epidermis (22).

III. CHEMISTRY AND ANTIOXIDANT ACTIVITY OF CAROTENOIDS

Reactive oxygen species are generated in the skin following UV exposure. Subsequent structural damage by oxidation and interferences with cellular signaling pathways are thought to contribute to the adverse effects of sun exposure (9,24). There is evidence from in vivo and in vitro studies that antioxidants may be useful in protecting the skin against this type of damage (22,23,25). Hydrophilic and lipophilic antioxidants have been applied topically for sun protection. For systemic sun protection, vitamins C and E as well as carotenoids were investigated.

The physicochemical and biochemical properties of carotenoids make them suitable candidates for endogenous sun protection (26). Carotenoids contain an extended system of conjugated double bonds that makes them efficient scavengers of singlet molecular oxygen ($^1O_2$) via physical or chemical quenching (27–30). Physical quenching is the dominating process in the interaction of carotenoids with singlet oxygen. It involves the transfer of excitation energy from $^1O_2$ to the carotenoid, which is subsequently dissipated as thermal energy. In the process of physical quenching, the carotenoid remains intact and can undergo further cycles of singlet oxygen quenching. Carotenoids are the most efficient natural $^1O_2$ quenchers. Among the natural carotenoids present in human blood and skin, lycopene exhibits the highest quenching rate constant (30).

Most carotenoids also efficiently scavenge peroxyl radicals, especially at low oxygen tension (26,31,32). The intermediate radical is stabilized via the system of conjugated double bonds. The interaction of carotenoids with free radicals has been studied in various model systems. Mixtures of carotenoids are more effective than single compounds (33). Such a synergistic effect was most pronounced when lycopene or lutein was present in the mixture. Under specific conditions carotenoids may also act as pro-oxidants (34–36). Pro-oxidant properties have been discussed in the context of adverse effects observed upon β-carotene supplementation at high levels (37,38).

In homogeneous solutions carotenoids tend to isomerize and form a mixture of all-trans, mono- and poly-cis isomers (39). The predominant configuration in nature is all-trans, but several cis isomers have been identified in human blood and skin (43). It should be noted that cis isomers of carotenoids with absorption maxima in the visible range of the spectrum exhibit an additional absorption maximum in the UV range. The extent of absorption depends on the position of the cis double bond within the molecule.

IV. SKIN CAROTENOIDS

At present, our knowledge of transport and distribution of intact carotenoids in skin is limited. The carotenoid pattern in human skin is similar to that found in blood and most tissues and is dominated by β-carotene, lycopene, lutein, zeaxanthin, and cryptoxanthin (40–42). Xanthophylls carrying a hydroxyl group can occur as carotenol fatty acid esters, but only small amounts of carotenol esters have been detected in human skin and blood (43,44). Carotenoids contribute measurably and significantly to normal human skin color, in particular the appearance of "yellowness" as defined objectively by means of chromametry using the three-dimensional color system (L, a, and b values) (45). The L value is a parameter for lightness of skin, and the b value (blue/yellow axis) is indicative of pigmentation. Such measurement of skin color, in particular of the b value, may potentially be an additional tool for monitoring the carotenoid status. Positive a values (red/green axis) are a measure for redness of the skin. Consuming high amounts of carotenoids may result in a discoloration of the skin that turns orange or yellow. Such a condition is known as carotenodermia and is accompanied by hypercarotenemia (increased blood carotene levels). It affects the palm, sole, tip of the nose and nasolabial fold, extending gradually over the entire body. Carotenodermia has been reported after excessive ingestion of carotene-rich foods or carotenoid-containing supplements and was associated with an increased uptake of β-carotene, lycopene, and canthaxanthin (23,46,47).

The levels of carotenoids vary in different areas of the skin. By means of reflection spectroscopy, higher basal values were measured in the skin of the forehead, palm of the hand, and dorsal skin, while lower levels were found in the skin of the arm and back of the hand (48). Upon treatment with β-carotene in doses of 24 mg/day, increases in carotenoid skin levels were detected in all areas. In facial skin, mean β-carotene values of about 0.1–0.3 nmol/g wet tissue were measured by means of HPLC; lutein and α-carotene concentrations were lower. Higher levels at about 1.5 nmol/g wet tissue were found when subcutaneous fat was included in sample analyses. Interestingly, β-carotene plasma levels and content in oral mucosal epithelium are skin type associated (49). Lowest levels were determined in skin type I, highest in skin type IV. A similar skin type-dependent increase in β-carotene was measured in oral mucosa epithelium. The reasons for these differences are not known.

V. INTERVENTION STUDIES IN HUMANS TO PREVENT SUNBURN (SOLAR ERYTHEMA)

Specific carotenoid supplements that mainly contain β-carotene are widely used as so-called oral sun protectants. It has been claimed that an increased supply with carotenoids contributes to the prevention of UV-dependent diseases. There is increasing evidence from human studies that an elevated intake of carotenoids, even from different sources, ameliorates a primary reaction of the skin after exposure to sunlight, namely, sunburn or the UV-induced erythema. However, the studies available are limited in number and differ in study design, making comparison difficult. Although most of the studies revealed moderate protection upon intervention with carotenoids, no beneficial effects were described in other reports. Facing safety concerns regarding the application of high doses of β-carotene, the discussion about suitable dose levels for prevention is still controversial.

β-Carotene has successfully been introduced as a photoprotectant in the management of erythropoietic protoporphyria by Mathews-Roth (50), who was also among the first researchers to investigate sun-protective effects of this compound in healthy individuals. In a clinical trial, the effects of oral β-carotene on the responses of skin to solar radiation were investigated (51). Over a period of 10 weeks healthy volunteers received 180 mg of β-carotene per day. After intervention the participants were exposed to natural sunlight for up to 2 h; the MED and the degree of erythema were evaluated as an indicator of protection. Compared to the placebo control, the threshold MED was significantly higher in the group that received β-carotene; no signifcant difference between groups was found in the degree of erythema.

Light-protective effects of β-carotene in combination with canthaxanthin were tested in patients with light-sensitive psoriasis and PLE; patients with vitiligo but otherwise normal light sensitivity were used as controls (52). MED was used as a measure for sensitivity. In all groups MED was increased after treatment, although the effect was most pronounced in patients with psoriasis and PLE. The authors (52) noted that maximal serum concentrations of carotenoids were reached after 2–6 weeks of treatment but the maximal protection factor was not estimated before 8–16 weeks of intervention.

Several other studies, different in dosing and duration of treatment, investigated the effects of carotene supplementation against UV-induced sunburn. It is interesting to note that in the studies in which protection was observed, supplementation with carotenoids lasted for at least 10 weeks. In the studies reporting no protective effects the treatment period was only 3–4 weeks (53,54).

Supplementing β-carotene for 3 weeks at a dose of 90 mg/day led to elevated levels of this carotenoid in plasma and skin. However, the treatment provided no clinically or histologically detectable protection when skin was irradiated with 3 MED to provoke a sunburn reaction (53). No protection against UV-induced erythema was found when volunteers received 150 mg/day of an carotenoid mixture that contained β-carotene and canthaxanthin over 4 weeks (54). Erythema was challenged with UVA, UVB, or psoralen UV treatment. MED values before and after carotenoid supplementation did not significantly differ although the serum levels of carotenoids increased during the study.

In several other investigations with longer duration of supplementation, protective effects against sunburn were observed. After pretreatment with 30 mg of β-carotene per day for 10 weeks, and an additional 13 days during sun exposure, the development of erythema induced by natural sunlight was lower under supplementation with β-carotene than in a placebo control group (55). Additional protection was achieved in the β-carotene group by the application of a topical sunscreen cream. The authors concluded that presupplementation with β-carotene before and during exposure to sunlight in combination with a topical sunscreen is more efficient than the sunscreen alone.

Lee et al. (56) reported a modest protective effect against UVA- and UVB-induced erythema when supplementing a natural carotenoid mixture. The carotenoid mix, which contained mainly β-carotene and only small amounts of α-carotene, cryptoxanthin, zeaxanthin, and lutein, was given for 24 weeks. At the beginning of the experiment a dose of 30 mg carotenoids per day was applied; the dose was increased every 8 weeks to reach a final dose of 90 mg/day. The MED after treatment was 1.5-fold higher than the MED before treatment, which indicates a protective effect mediated by carotenoids. During the study the serum levels of α- and β-carotene increased. The amount of lipid hydroperoxides in serum decreased during the study in a dose-dependent manner: compared to the starting level, it was about 40% lower at a dose of 90 mg carotenoids per day.

A similar carotenoid mixture was applied in a study where the protective effects of carotenoids alone or in combination with tocopherol were investigated (57). Carotenoids were supplied with an algal product (Betatene from Dunaliella) which contained mainly β-carotene (all-trans and 9-cis isomers) but also small amounts of α-carotene, cryptoxanthin, zeaxanthin, and lutein. The carotenoid supplement delivering 25 mg total carotenoids per day and a combination of the supplement (25 mg carotenoids per day) with vitamin E (R,R,R-α-tocopherol; 500 IU/day) was ingested over 12 weeks. At day 0, week 4, 8, and 12, erythema was induced with a solar-light simulator; β-carotene and α-tocopherol serum levels and carotenoid levels in skin were determined at the same time. Light-induced erythema was significantly diminished from week 8 on; suppression of erythema formation was more pronounced when the combination of carotenoids and tocopherol was applied. However, the difference between carotenoid treatment and application of the antioxidant mixture was statistically not significant. Serum levels of β-carotene and α-tocopherol increased during supplementation and reached a plateau after 4 weeks of treatment. Other mixtures of antioxidants, including β-carotene as a constituent, have also been investigated (58). An antioxidant combination supplying 4.8 mg β-carotene, 20 mg vitamin E, 120 mg vitamin C, 50 μg selenium (25 mg selenium yeast), 50 mg standardized tomato extract, and 50 mg standardized grape seed extract per day was given to 8 volunteers for 16 weeks. Light sensitivity was assessed by determining the MED. No difference regarding light sensitivity between the antioxidant supplement and the placebo group was found in this study. However, treatment with antioxidants slowed down both development and grade of UVB-induced erythema.

Based on the results of two intervention trials in individuals at high risk for lung cancer, concerns about the safety of supplementation with higher doses of β-carotene have been raised (59,60). In these studies, β-carotene was applied in doses of 20 and 30 mg/day alone or in combination with α-tocopherol or retinol for several years. Thus, it was investigated whether a high dose of β-carotene can be substituted by a mixture of carotenoids in sun protection (61). The erythema-protective effect of β-carotene (24 mg/day from an algal source) was compared to that of a 24-mg carotenoid mix composed of β-carotene, lutein, and lycopene (8 mg/day each) and a control group. Supplementation lasted 12 weeks and carotenoid levels in serum and skin, as well as erythema intensity, were measured before and 24 h after irradiation with a solar light simulator, both at baseline and after 6 and 12 weeks of treatment. β-Carotene serum levels increased in the β-carotene group, whereas in the mixed-carotenoid group the serum levels of all three carotenoids were elevated after treatment; no change was found in the control group. The intake of either β-carotene or a mixture of carotenoids led to similar increases in total carotenoids in skin from week 0 to week 12; no change of total carotenoids in skin was determined in the control group. The intensity of erythema 24 h after irradiation was diminished in both groups receiving carotenoids; it was significantly lower than baseline after 12 weeks of supplementation. Based on the results of this study (61), it was concluded that long-term supplementation for 12 weeks with 24 mg of a carotenoid mix supplying similar amounts of β-carotene, lutein, and lycopene ameliorates UV-induced erythema in humans, and that this effect is comparable to the treatment with 24 mg of β-carotene alone.

VI. PROTECTION BY DIETARY INTERVENTION

Protective effects may also be achieved employing dietary sources rich in carotenoids. Tomato contains high amounts of carotenoids, and the major carotenoid pigment in the tomato is lycopene. Lycopene is the acyclo analog of β-carotene and a very efficient antioxidant. Processed tomato products contain even higher amounts of carotenoids than tomatoes; therefore, tomato paste was selected for an intervention with a natural dietary source rich in carotenoids to protect against UV-induced erythema in humans (62).

Volunteers ingested tomato paste (40 g/day, equivalent to 16 mg lycopene/day) together with olive oil to improve bioavailability over a period of 10 weeks; controls received olive oil only. Serum levels of lycopene and total carotenoids in skin increased after the intake of tomato paste; no changes were observed in the control group. Erythema was induced by irradiation of dorsal skin with a solar light simulator at day 0, week 4, and week 10 of the study. At week 10, erythema formation was significantly lower in the group consuming the tomato paste than in the control group. No significant difference was found at week 4 of treatment. This study demonstrates that protection against UV light-induced erythema can be achieved by ingestion of a commonly consumed dietary source of lycopene. In addition to lycopene, other carotenoids are present in the tomato, e.g., phytoene and phytofluene. The levels of both these compounds increase in serum upon consumption of tomato products. They have characteristic absorption maxima in the UVA and UVB range (39) wich might contribute to UV-protective effects of tomato products.

VII. CONCLUSION

Oral supplementation with β-carotene and combinations of carotenoids provides moderate protection against UV-induced erythema (sunburn reaction). Apparently, intake for several weeks is required to obtain measurable protection. In the studies where protection was observed, treatment with carotenoids was for at least 10 weeks, whereas only a 3- to 4-week supplementation was applied in the studies showing no effects. Carotenoids may be used to increase the basal protection and thus increase the defense against UV light-mediated damage to skin. The protective effect is not sufficient to prevent damage following extensive sun exposure (sunbathing, skiing, etc.); here the additional use of a topical sunscreen is recommended. However, more than 70% of the average erythemal UV exposure does not occur during vacation time (63). Thus, systemic sun protection is a valuable concept in long-term protection against skin damage from solar radiation (64).

ACKNOWLEDGMENT

Our research is supported by the Deutsche Forschungsgemeinschaft (SFB 503/ B1; Si 255/11-3). H.S. is a Fellow of the National Foundation for Cancer Research (NFCR), Bethesda, MD.

REFERENCES

1. Seidlitz HK, Thiel S, Krins A, Mayer H. Solar radiation at the earth's surface. In: Giacomoni PU, ed. Sun Protection in Man. Amsterdam: Elsevier, 2001:705–738.
2. Wenk J, Brenneisen P, Meewes C, Wlaschek M, Peters T, Blaudschun R, Ma W, Kuhr L, Schneider L, Scharffetter-Kochanek K. UV-induced oxidative stress and photoaging. Curr Probl Dermatol 2001; 29:83–94.
3. Berneburg M, Krutmann J. Photoimmunology, DNA repair and photocarcinogenesis. J Photochem Photobiol B 2000; 54:87–93.
4. Packer L, Valacchi G. Antioxidants and the response of skin to oxidative stress: vitamin E as a key indicator. Skin Pharmacol Appl Skin Physiol 2002; 15:282–290.
5. Demmig-Adams B, Adams WW III. Antioxidants in photosynthesis and human nutrition. Science 2002; 298:2149–2153.
6. Frank HA, Young AJ, Britton G, Cogdell RJ. The Photochemistry of Carotenoids. London: Kluwer Academic, 1999.
7. Ortonne JP. Photoprotective properties of skin melanin. Br J Dermatol 2002; 146:7–10.
8. Pinnell SR. Cutaneous photodamage, oxidative stress, and topical antioxidant protection. J Am Acad Dermatol 2003; 48:1–19.
9. Krutmann J. Ultraviolet A radiation-induced biological effects in human skin: relevance for photoaging and photodermatosis. J Dermatol Sci 2000; 23:S22–S26.
10. Murphy GM. Diseases associated with photosensitivity. J Photochem Photobiol B 2001; 64:93–98.
11. Wlaschek M, Tantcheva-Poor I, Naderi L, Ma W, Schneider LA, Razi-Wolf Z, Schuller J, Scharffetter-Kochanek K. Solar UV irradiation and dermal photoaging. J Photochem Photobiol B 2001; 63:41–51.
12. Balin AK, Allen RG. Oxidative stress and skin cancer. In: Cutler RG, Rodriguez H, eds. Critical Reviews of Oxidative Stress and Aging: Advances in Basic Science, Diagnostics and Intervention. River Edge, NJ: World Scientific, 2003:955–965.
13. Naleway AL. Polymorphous light eruption. Int J Dermatol 2002; 41:377–383.

14. Gould JW, Mercurio MG, Elmets CA. Cutaneous photosensitivity diseases induced by exogenous agents. J Am Acad Dermatol 1995; 33:551–573.
15. Roberts JE. Light and immunomodulation. Ann NY Acad Sci 2000; 917:435–445.
16. Clydesdale GJ, Dandie GW, Muller HK. Ultraviolet light induced injury: immunological and inflammatory effects. Immunol Cell Biol 2001; 79:547–568.
17. Cesarini JP. Sunburn and apoptosis. In: Altmeyer P, Hoffmann K, Stücker M, eds. Skin Cancer and UV Radiation. Berlin: Springer-Verlag, 1997:94–101.
18. Kulms D, Schwarz T. Molecular mechanisms of UV-induced apoptosis. Photodermatol Photoimmunol Photomed 2000; 16:195–201.
19. Cesarini JP. Sunburn and apoptosis. In: Altmeyer P, Hoffmann K, Stücker M, eds. Skin Cancer and UV Radiation. Berlin: Springer-Verlag, 1997:94–101.
20. Andreassi L, Flori ML, Rubegni P. Sun and skin. Role of phototype and skin colour. Adv Exp Med Biol 1999; 455:469–475.
21. Orentreich D, Leone A-S, Arpino G, Burack H. Sunscreens: practical applications. In: Giacomoni PU, ed. Sun Protection in Man. Amsterdam: Elsevier, 2001:535–559.
22. Boelsma E, Hendriks HF, Roza L. Nutritional skin care: health effects of micronutrients and fatty acids. Am J Clin Nutr 2001; 73:853–864.
23. Stahl W, Sies H. Protection against solar radiation–protective properties of antioxidants. In: Giacomoni PU, ed. Sun Protection in Man. Amsterdam: Elsevier Science, 2001:561–572.
24. Klotz LO, Holbrook NJ, Sies H. UVA and singlet oxygen as inducers of cutaneous signaling events. Curr Probl Dermatol 2001; 29:95–113.
25. Thiele J, Dreher F, Packer L. Antioxidant defense systems in skin. In: Elsner P, Maibach H, eds. Cosmeceuticals. New York: Marcel Dekker, 2000:145–187.
26. Krinsky NI. The antioxidant and biological properties of the carotenoids. Ann NY Acad Sci 1998; 854:443–447.
27. Foote CS, Denny RW. Chemistry of singlet oxygen. VII. Quenching by beta-carotene. J Am Chem Sci 1968; 90:6233–6235.
28. Edge R, McGarvey DJ, Truscott TG. The carotenoids as anti-oxidants—a review. J Photochem Photobiol B Biol 1997; 41:189–200.
29. Baltschun D, Beutner S, Briviba K, Martin HD, Paust J, Peters M, Röver S, Sies H, Stahl W, Steigel A, Stenhorst F. Singlet oxygen quenching abilities of carotenoids. Liebigs Ann 1997; 1887–1893.
30. Di Mascio P, Kaiser S, Sies H. Lycopene as the most efficient biological carotenoid singlet oxygen quencher. Arch Biochem Biophys 1989; 274:532–538.
31. Kennedy TA, Liebler DC. Peroxyl radical scavenging by beta-carotene in lipid bilayers. J Biol Chem 1992; 267:4658–4663.
32. Burton GW, Ingold KU. ß-Carotene: an unusual type of lipid antioxidant. Science 1984; 224:569–573.
33. Stahl W, Junghans A, de Boer B, Driomina E, Briviba K, Sies H. Carotenoid mixtures protect multilamellar liposomes against oxidative damage: synergistic effects of lycopene and lutein. FEBS Lett 1998; 427:305–308.
34. Young AJ, Lowe GM. Antioxidant and prooxidant properties of carotenoids. Arch Biochem Biophys 2001; 385:20–27.

35. Eichler O, Sies H, Stahl W. Divergent optimum levels of lycopene, beta-carotene and lutein protecting against UVB irradiation in human fibroblasts. Photochem Photobiol 2002; 75:503–506.
36. Biesalski HK, Obermueller-Jevic UC. UV light, beta-carotene and human skin: beneficial and potentially harmful effects. Arch Biochem Biophys 2001; 389:1–6.
37. Wang XD, Russell RM. Procarcinogenic and anticarcinogenic effects of beta-carotene. Nutr Rev 1999; 57:263–272.
38. Omaye ST, Krinsky NI, Kagan VE, Mayne ST, Liebler DC, Bidlack WR. Beta-carotene: friend or foe? Fundam Appl Toxicol 1997; 40:163–174.
39. Britton G. Structure and properties of carotenoids in relation to function. FASEB J 1995; 9:1551–1558.
40. Wingerath T, Stahl W, Sies H. Beta-cryptoxanthin selectively increases in human chylomicrons upon ingestion of tangerine concentrate rich in beta-cryptoxanthin esters. Arch Biochem Biophys 1995; 324:385–390.
41. Biesalski HK, Hemmes C, Hopfenmüller W, Schmid C, Gollnick HPM. Effects of controlled exposure of sunlight on plasma and skin levels of beta-carotene. Free Radic Res 1996; 24:215–224.
42. Peng Y-M, Peng Y-S, Lin Y, Moon T, Baier M. Micronutrient concentrations in paired skin and plasma of patients with actinic keratoses: effect of prolonged retinol supplementation. Cancer Epidemiol Biomark Prev 1993; 2:145–150.
43. Wingerath T, Sies H, Stahl W. Xanthophyll esters in human skin. Arch Biochem Biophys 1998; 355:271–274.
44. Granado F, Olmedilla B, Gil-Martinez E, Blanco I. Lutein ester in serum after lutein supplementation in human subjects. Br J Nutr 1998; 80:445–449.
45. Alaluf S, Heinrich U, Stahl W, Tronnier H, Wiseman S. Dietary carotenoids contribute to normal human skin color and UV photosensitivity. J Nutr 2002; 132:399–403.
46. La Placa M, Pazzaglia M, Tosti A. Lycopenaemia. J Eur Acad Dermatol Venereol 2000; 14:311–312.
47. Gupta AK, Haberman HF, Pawlowski D, Shulman G, Menon IA. Canthaxanthin. Int J Dermatol 1985; 24:528–532.
48. Stahl W, Heinrich U, Jungmann H, von Laar J, Schietzel M, Sies H, Tronnier H. Increased dermal carotenoid levels assessed by noninvasive reflection spectrophotometry correlate with serum levels in women ingesting Betatene. J Nutr 1998; 128:903–907.
49. Gollnick HP, Siebenwirth C. Beta-carotene plasma levels and content in oral mucosal epithelium is skin type associated. Skin Pharmacol Appl Skin Physiol 2002; 15:360–366.
50. Mathews-Roth MM. Carotenoids in erythropoietic protoporphyria and other photosensitivity diseases. Ann NY Acad Sci 1993; 691:127–138.
51. Mathews-Roth MM, Pathak MA, Parrish JA, Fitzpatrick TB, Kass EH, Toda K, Clemens W. A clinical trial of the effects of oral beta-carotene on the responses of human skin to solar radiation. J Invest Dermatol 1972; 59:349–353.
52. Wennersten G, Swanbeck G. Treatment of light sensitivity with carotenoids. Acta Dermatovener 1974; 54:491–499.

53. Garmyn M, Ribaya-Mercado JD, Russell RM, Bhawan J, Gilchrest BA. Effect of beta-carotene supplementation on the human sunburn reaction. Exp Dermatol 1995; 4:104–111.
54. Wolf C, Steiner A, Hönigsmann H. Do oral carotenoids protect human skin against ultraviolet erythema, psoralen phototoxicity, and ultraviolet-induced DNA damage? J Invest Dermatol 1988; 90:55–57.
55. Gollnick HPM, Hopfenmüller W, Hemmes C, Chun SC, Schmid C, Sundermeier K, Biesalski HK. Systemic beta carotene plus topical UV-sunscreen are an optimal protection against harmful effects of natural UV-sunlight: results of the Berlin–Eilath study. Eur J Dermatol 1996; 6:200–205.
56. Lee J, Jiang S, Levine N, Watson RR. Carotenoid supplementation reduces erythema in human skin after simulated solar radiation exposure. Proc Soc Exp Biol Med 2000; 223:170–174.
57. Stahl W, Heinrich U, Jungmann H, Sies H, Tronnier H. Carotenoids and carotenoids plus vitamin E protect against ultraviolet light-induced erythema in humans. Am J Clin Nutr 2000; 71:795–798.
58. Greul AK, Grundmann JU, Heinrich F, Pfitzner I, Bernhardt J, Ambach A, Biesalski HK, Gollnick H. Photoprotection of UV-irradiated human skin: an antioxidative combination of vitamins E and C, carotenoids, selenium and proanthocyanidins. Skin Pharmacol Appl Skin Physiol 2002; 15:307–315.
59. Omenn GS, Goodman GE, Thornquist MD, Balmes J, Cullen MR, Glass A, Keogh JP, Meyskens FL, Valanis B, Williams JH, Barnhart S, Cherniack MG, Brodkin CA, Hammar S. Risk factors for lung cancer and for intervention effects in CARET, the beta-carotene and retinol efficacy trial. J Natl Cancer Inst 1996; 88:1550–1559.
60. The ATBC Study Group. The effect of vitamin E and beta carotene on the incidence of lung cancer and other cancers in male smokers. N Engl J Med 1994; 330:1029–1035.
61. Heinrich U, Gärtner C, Wiebusch M, Eichler O, Sies H, Tronnier H, Stahl W. Supplementation with beta-carotene or a similar amount of mixed carotenoids protects humans from UV-induced erythema. J Nutr 2003; 133:98–101.
62. Stahl W, Heinrich U, Wiseman S, Eichler O, Sies H, Tronnier H. Dietary tomato paste protects against ultraviolet light-induced erythema in humans. J Nutr 2001; 131:1449–1451.
63. Godar DE, Wengraitis SP, Shreffler J, Sliney DH. UV doses of Americans. Photochem Photobiol 2001; 73:621–629.
64. Sies H, Stahl W. Nutritional protection against skin damage from sunlight. Ann Rev Nutr 2004; 24: (in press).

23
Carotenoids and Immune Responses

David A. Hughes
Institute of Food Research, Norwich, Norfolk, England

Previous chapters in this volume have described numerous epidemiological studies, in vitro experiments, animal studies, and clinical trials that show a protective role for carotenoids in protecting against cancer. One suggested mechanism for this effect is that they can enhance immune function and, therefore, the body's tumor surveillance mechanisms.

I. OXIDATIVE STRESS AND THE IMMUNE SYSTEM

In plants, carotenoids serve two essential functions: as accessory pigments in photosynthesis, and in photoprotection. These functions are achieved through the chemical structure of carotenoids, which allows the molecules to absorb light and to quench singlet oxygen and free radicals.

Oxidative stress, arising from cumulative damage caused by reactive oxygen species (ROS), is present throughout life and is believed to be a major contributor to the aging process (1). The immune system is especially vulnerable to oxidative damage because many immune cells produce these reactive compounds as part of the body's defense mechanisms to destroy invading pathogens. Higher organisms have evolved a variety of antioxidant defense systems either to prevent the generation of ROS or to intercept any that are generated. Enzymes such as catalase and glutathione peroxidase can safely decompose peroxides, particularly hydrogen peroxide produced during the "respiratory burst" involved in killing invading microorganisms, whereas superoxide dismutase intercepts or "scavenges" free radicals. However, the food we eat provides us with a large amount of our body's total supply of antioxidants in the form of various essential micronutrients and "nonnutrients," including the carotenoids.

The immune system appears to be particularly sensitive to oxidative stress. Immune cells rely heavily on cell–cell communication, particularly via membrane-bound receptors, to work effectively. Cell membranes are rich in polyunsaturated fatty acids (PUFAs), which, if peroxidized, can lead to a loss of membrane integrity, altered membrane fluidity (2), and alterations in intracellular signaling and cell function. It has been shown that exposure to ROS can lead to a reduction in cell membrane receptor expression (3). In addition, the production of relatively large amounts of ROS by phagocytic immune cells, resulting from respiratory burst activity, can damage the cells themselves if they are not sufficiently protected by antioxidants (4).

II. ANIMAL STUDIES

As stated above, because the immune system has a major role in preventing the development of cancer it has been suggested that β-carotene, and possibly other carotenoids present in the diet, may enhance the function of immune cells involved in detecting and eliminating tumor cells. Indeed, as stated in an earlier review on this topic by Bendich (5), the possibility that carotenoids could enhance immune function was first put forward in the 1930s. Green and Mellanby (6), using vitamin A-deficient rats, showed that dietary carotenoids could overcome bacterial infections, and in 1931 it was reported that dietary supplementation with carotenoids could reduce the number and severity of respiratory infections in children (7). At the time it was concluded that these beneficial effects were due to vitamin A derived from the carotenoids, and it was not until the 1950s that this was refuted. Investigators at the Karolinska Institute, who were attempting to extract an antibacterial substance from nonpathogenic bacteria, discovered that the tomato juice being used in the culture media contained an effective antibacterial agent, which transpired to be lycopene (8). These workers showed that both synthetic all-*trans* lycopene and natural, tomato-extracted lycopene could increase the resistance of mice infected with *Klebsiella pneumoniae*, whereas vitamin A was ineffective. β-Carotene was effective, but not as potent as lycopene or other non-provitamin A carotenoids such as crocetin, bixin, and crocin (8). Because of an inability to determine the mechanisms of action of the carotenoids at that time, the research was abandoned (5), and it was not until the publication of the major review article on β-carotene and cancer in *Nature* by Peto and colleagues in 1981 (9) that researchers returned to examine the influence of carotenoids on immune responses in earnest.

In 1986 Bendich and Shapiro examined the effect of dietary supplementation with placebo, β-carotene, or canthaxanthin (used as a non-provitamin A carotenoid comparator) on the ex vivo mitogen-stimulated T-cell (the cell type involved in orchestrating adaptive immune responses) and B-cell (the cell type involved in antibody production) proliferative responses in rats. The proliferation of both cell types was enhanced when the diets contained either of the carotenoids (10), despite the fact that the animals were well nourished, healthy, and presumably immunocompetent. Serum and tissue analysis showed that the canthaxanthin was not converted to vitamin A, and it was therefore concluded that the immunoenhancement seen was due to a carotenoid effect separate from any provitamin A activity. More recently, it has been shown that lycopene can increase T helper cell numbers ($CD4^+$, which stimulate immune responses) and normalize T-cell differentiation caused by tumorigenesis in mice (11).

Animal studies have also shown that β-carotene can influence aspects of tumor surveillance. There is now ample evidence that β-carotene has cancer-preventive activity in experimental animals, based on models of skin carcinogenesis in mice and buccal pouch carcinogenesis in hamsters (12). Natural killer (NK) cells can kill virally infected cells and tumor cells. Homozygous mice, genetically deficient in NK cell activity, grow tumors and develop leukemia more rapidly than do heterozygous littermates with normal NK cell function. In athymic mice where, in the absence of T lymphocytes, NK cells have a greater responsibility, it has been shown that β-carotene can induce a significant activation of NK cells, resulting in an increased cytolysis of tumor cell targets (13). Macrophages detect tumor cells and present tumor antigens to lymphocytes, and in hamsters pretreated with or given β-carotene or cryptoxanthin following tumor induction, the tumoricidal properties of macrophages and secretion of the macrophage cytokine tumor necrosis factor-α were increased (14,15).

There has been some recent interest in the possibility that carotenoids might provide a supportive treatment in *Helicobacter pylori* infection (16). Mice fed meals rich in astaxanthin, a carotenoid found in seafood, particularly salmon, showed significantly lower colonization levels and had lower inflammation scores compared with untreated mice and astaxanthin also inhibited the in vitro growth of *H. pylori* (17). It is thought that the host immune response to this infection might be of importance with regard to the clinical outcome, e.g., to explain why only a proportion of infected individuals develop peptic ulcers. Neutrophil infiltration results in excessive free radical generation, which initiates a membrane peroxidation cascade that leads to mucosal damage. The immune response is polarized to a T helper type 1 (Th1) cell response (these cells are involved in stimulating cell-mediated immune responses) with release of the proinflammatory cytokine, interferon-γ, which activates phagocytic cells and also contributes to mucosal damage (18). It has been shown that mice treated with astaxanthin showed a significant increase in interleukin (IL)-4 release, suggesting a shift to a Th2 cell response (these cells are involved in enhancing antibody production). It was suggested that the observed shift of the Th1/Th2 balance following treatment was probably the result of the down-regulation of Th1 cells and up-regulation of Th2 cells by astaxanthin; although another possible mechanism of action is that it neutralizes reactive free oxygen metabolites in the mucosa (19). Further studies are required both to elucidate the relative importance of Th1 versus Th2 cells in the immune response to *H. pylori* and to describe the effect and mechanism of action of carotenoids in this condition.

III. HUMAN STUDIES

A. Effects of β-Carotene

Repeated exposure to ultraviolet (UV) light markedly suppresses immune function (20). Because photoprotection is one of the major functions of carotenoids in nature, several studies have assessed the ability of β-carotene to protect the immune system from UV-induced free radical damage. In one study, a group of young males were placed on a low-carotenoid diet (<1.0 mg/day total carotenoids) and given either placebo or 30 mg β-carotene/day for 28 days prior to periodic exposure to UV light. Delayed-type hypersensitivity (DTH) responses were significantly suppressed in the placebo group after UV treatments and the suppression was inversely proportional to plasma β-carotene concentrations in this group (21), but no significant suppression of DTH responses was seen in the β-carotene-treated group. In a later study, the same research team studied a group of healthy older males, again given either 30 mg β-carotene or placebo for 28 days prior to periodic exposure to UV light. They again observed a suppression of DTH response following UV exposure, but in this age group the extent of the protective effect of β-carotene appeared less than had been observed with the younger men (22). The authors suggest that this might have been due either to a reduced plasma response to supplementation in the older age group and/or to higher plasma vitamin E levels than was observed in the younger men. These workers also observed that stronger DTH responses were associated with higher plasma β-carotene concentrations in both UV- and non-UV-exposed individuals. The ability of β-carotene to protect against the harmful effects of natural UV-sunlight has also been demonstrated by exposing healthy female students to time- and intensity-controlled sunlight exposure; a Berlin-based study involved taking volunteers to the Red Sea and exposing areas of their skin to the sunlight by lifting discretely placed flaps in their specially designed swim-suits (23)!

A number of studies have examined the effect of β-carotene on immune function by measuring changes in the numbers of lymphocyte subpopulations and on the expression of cell activation markers. However, because of the large variation in intakes of β-carotene and the duration of supplementation, a variety of results have been obtained and it is extremely difficult to make adequate comparisons between the different studies. Indeed, doses ranging from dietary achievable levels of 15 mg/day up to pharmacological doses of 300 mg/day have been provided over periods of 14 days to 12 years. What seems common to many studies, however, is that more marked changes are observed in those involving older individuals. This might be predicted, given that a reduction in the body's ability to mount an immune response is a recognized feature of ageing— "immunosenescence" (24). For example, there have been reported increases in the numbers of CD4$^+$ lymphocytes (T "helper" cells that stimulate cell-mediated immune responses) or in the ratio of CD4$^+$ to CD8$^+$ cells (T "suppressor" cells that inhibit responses), and in the percentages of lymphocytes expressing markers of cell activation, such as IL-2 receptors and transferrin receptors (25,26), particularly in older individuals. The potential for increasing the numbers of CD4$^+$ cells led to the suggestion that β-carotene might be useful as an immunoenhancing agent in the management of human immunodeficiency virus (HIV) infection. Preliminary studies have shown a slight but insignificant increase in CD4$^+$ numbers in response to β-carotene (60 mg/day for 4 weeks) in patients with acquired immune deficiency syndrome (AIDS) (27), but long-term effectiveness in managing HIV infection or AIDS has not been reported.

Other studies have been unable to confirm the increase in T-cell-mediated immunity in healthy individuals following β-carotene supplementation. Santos and colleagues (28) have recently reported the results of two studies in the elderly: a short-term, high-dose study (90 mg/day for 21 days) in women and a longer term, lower dose trial (50 mg/alternate days for 10–12 years) in men. The conclusion of both studies was that there was no significant difference in T-cell function as assessed by DTH response, lymphocyte proliferation, IL-2 production, and composition of lymphocyte subsets. However, these investigators also examined the effect of β-carotene supplementation on NK cell activity in the longer term trial with male volunteers. Supplementation with β-carotene resulted in significantly greater NK cell activity compared with subjects of a similar age given placebo treatment (Fig. 1) (29). This study also highlighted the reduction in NK cell activity that is observed with age but, interestingly, the increase in NK cell activity observed in older men (65–86 years) following β-carotene supplementation restored it to the level seen in a group of younger males (51–64 years). The mechanism for this remains unknown, but it was not due to an increase in the percentage of NK cells or to an increase in IL-2 production. The authors suggest that β-carotene may be acting directly on one or more of the lytic stages of NK cell cytotoxicity, or on NK cell activity-enhancing cytokines other than IL-2, such as IL-12. This suggestion still awaits confirmation.

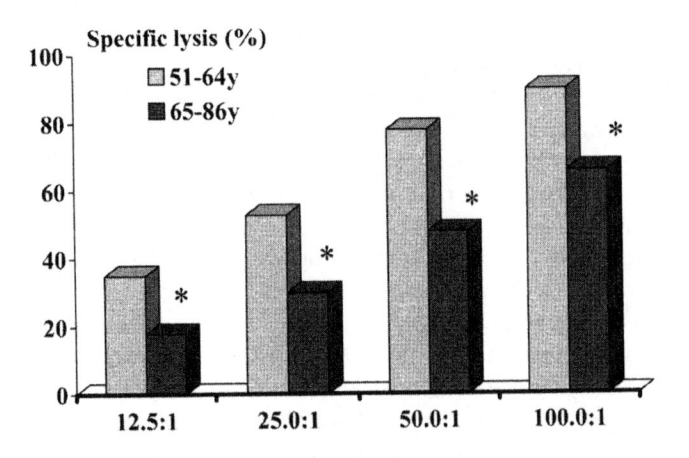

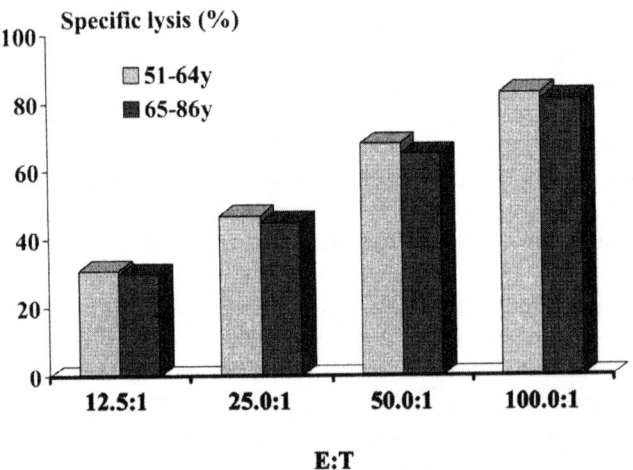

Figure 1 Natural killer cell activity in different age groups of subjects consuming placebo or β-carotene. Natural killer cell activity was determined at several effector to target cell ratios ($E:T$) using effector cells from subjects consuming placebo ($n = 17$ for 51–64 y and $n = 13$ for 65–86 y) or β-carotene ($n = 21$ for 51–64 y and $n = 8$ for 65–86 y). Data are expressed as % target cell lysis; * = $p < 0.05$. (Reprinted from Santos et al. (29) © American Journal of Clinical Nutrition, American Society for Clinical Nutrition.)

Since antigen-presenting cells initiate cell-mediated immune responses, we have investigated whether β-carotene supplementation can influence the function of human blood monocytes, the main antigen-presenting cell type present in the bloodstream. A prerequisite for this function is the expression of major histocompatibility complex (MHC) class II molecules (HLA-DR, HLA-DP, and HLA-DQ) (30), which are present on the majority of human monocytes. The antigenic peptide is presented to the T helper lymphocyte within a groove of the MHC class II molecule (Fig. 2). Since the degree of immune responsiveness of an individual has been shown to be proportional to both the percentage of MHC class II-positive monocytes and the density of these molecules on the cell surface (31), it is possible that one mechanism by which β-carotene may enhance cell-mediated immune responses is by enhancing the cell surface expression of these molecules. In addition, cell-to-cell adhesion is critical for the initiation of a primary immune response, and it has been shown that the intercellular

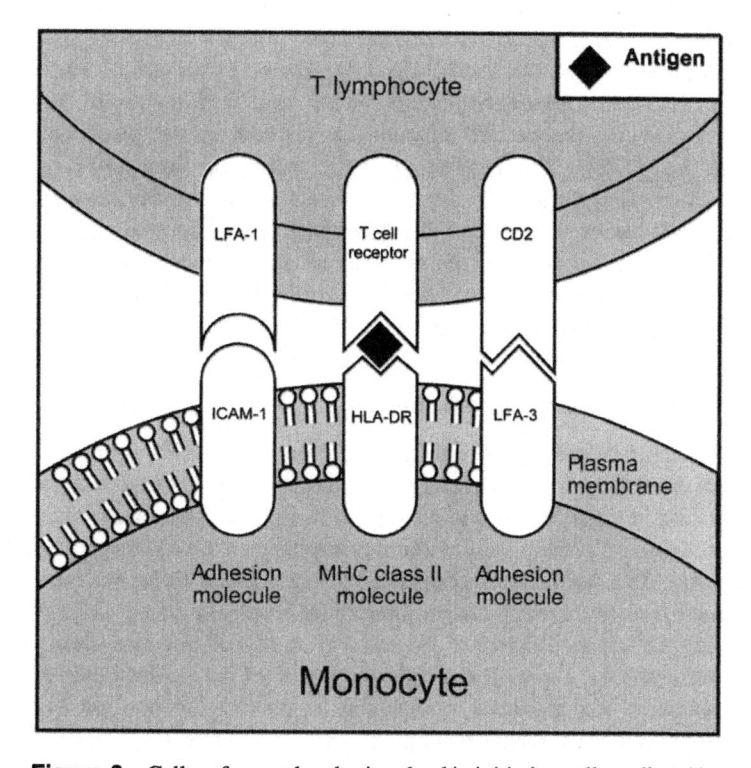

Figure 2 Cell surface molecules involved in initiating cell-mediated immune responses. LFA, leukocyte function-associated antigen; ICAM-1, intercellular adhesion molecule-1; HLA, human leukocyte–associated antigen; MHC, major histocompatibility complex.

adhesion molecule-1 (ICAM-1) leukocyte function-associated antigen (LFA)-1 ligand-receptor pair is also capable of costimulating an immune response (32), enhancing T-cell proliferation and cytokine production.

To assess the effect of β-carotene supplementation on the expression of monocyte surface receptors we undertook a randomized double-blind cross-over study of middle-aged nonsmoking men, who took part in two dietary intervention periods of 26 days, during which they were provided with a daily capsule of either 15 mg β-carotene, a dietary achievable intake (equivalent to 150 g of cooked carrots), or placebo. Following dietary supplementation, there were significant increases in plasma levels of β-carotene and in the percentages of monocytes expressing the MHC class II molecule, HLA-DR, and the adhesion molecules, ICAM-1 and LFA-3 (33). These results suggest that moderate increases in the dietary intake of β-carotene can enhance cell-mediated immune responses in a relatively short period of time, providing a potential mechanism for the anticarcinogenic properties attributed to this compound. The increase in surface molecule expression could also, in part, account for the ability of β-carotene to prevent the reduction in DTH response following exposure to UV radiation, since the latter can inhibit both HLA-DR and ICAM-1 expression in human cell lines.

As well as preventing oxidative damage, it has also been suggested that β-carotene can influence immune cell function by modulating the production of prostaglandin E_2 (PGE_2). This eicosanoid is the major PG synthesized by monocytes and macrophages and is known to possess a number of immunosuppressive properties. It has been suggested that β-carotene might enhance immune responses by altering the activation of the arachidonic acid cascade (from which PGE_2 is derived), since it has been shown to be capable of suppressing the generation of arachidonic acid products in vitro from nonlymphoid tissues (34).

B. Effects of Other Dietary Carotenoids

Very few studies have examined the influence of other carotenoids on human immune function, even though there is strong epidemiological evidence to suggest that lycopene (found in tomatoes) and lutein (found in spinach, peas, watercress, and other vegetables) can protect against the development of prostate and lung cancer, respectively. In addition, tomato intake has been found to be inversely associated with the risk of diarrheal and respiratory infections in young children in the Sudan (35). In order to compare the relative ability of different dietary carotenoids to influence the expression of monocyte surface molecules involved in antigen presentation we undertook comparable studies to the one we had previously carried out with β-carotene, this time providing the same daily intake of lycopene or lutein (15 mg/day) to our middle-aged male volunteers. The results suggest that the latter carotenoids have less of an influence than β-carotene, at least in respect to this particular parameter of immune cell function (36). The less striking effect of either lycopene or lutein supplementation on monocyte surface marker expression that was seen following β-carotene supplementation might be related to the lower plasma levels achieved following supplementation. We previously observed that there might be a threshold effect of plasma β-carotene concentration on the expression of ICAM-1 and LFA-3 (33), and it is possible that the plasma levels of lycopene or lutein achieved following supplementation were not high enough to cause a significant change in the expression of most of the monocyte surface molecules examined. The reason for the difference in plasma levels of these carotenoids following the same level of supplementation is uncertain, but it could reflect differences in their uptake, metabolism, and excretion, or to selective sequestration of different carotenoids to specific sites in the body. It is unlikely that absorption of lycopene from the supplements provided is a problem, since it has recently been shown that the bioavailability of lycopene from tomato juice and dietary supplements is very similar (37). However, lycopene is known to be found in higher concentrations in the prostate (38) than in serum, and this might contribute to the reduced prostate cancer risk associated with the consumption of tomato-based foods (39). Indeed, one possible factor to explain the different effects seen with different carotenoids might be the preferred location of these compounds within the cell and within the body. Carotenoids are lipid soluble; thus, it is thought that most will be concentrated in the lipid-rich membranes of the cell. However, their exact location may influence their effectiveness in modulating specific cellular events. At the whole-body level, it is also possible that not all beneficial effects bestowed by carotenoids might be observed systemically, but only at specific locations in the body, suggesting that there might be "hidden" benefits associated with certain dietary components that we have yet to discover. Carotenoid concentrations vary considerably from tissue to tissue, although the mechanism for this remains poorly understood. For instance, the carotenoids lutein and zeaxanthin are found in high concentrations in the macular region of the eye, suggesting the presence of a binding protein within this specific area of the eye (40).

In another intervention study, we again gave dietary achievable levels of carotenoid supplements, this time to a group of older volunteers (older than 65 years) living in Ireland. We gave these individuals ($n = 52$) either placebo, β-carotene (8.2 mg), or lycopene (13.3 mg) daily for 12 weeks and examined changes in various parameters of cell-mediated immunity. We observed no significant changes in T-cell subset numbers, lectin-stimulated lymphocyte proliferation, or surface molecule expression following any of these interventions (41), in spite of significant increases in the plasma levels of the carotenoids. We concluded that in well-nourished, free-living, healthy individuals, supplementation with relatively low levels of β-carotene or lycopene is not associated with beneficial or detrimental effects on cell-mediated immunity. Another group has also shown recently that enriching the diet with lycopene (by drinking 330 mL of tomato juice daily) for 8 weeks does not appear to modify cell-mediated immune responses in well-nourished elderly men and women (42). These investigators have also shown an apparent opposing effect of lycopene and lutein, in regard to T-lymphocyte proliferation, with lycopene enrichment (by tomato juice) enhancing and lutein enrichment (by spinach powder) inhibiting this activity (43). These results emphasize further that different carotenoids can affect immune cell function in different ways. Therefore, in a diet containing a good mixture of fruits and vegetables, the influence of the combination of carotenoids they contain on immune function may represent the sum total of these different effects and, indeed, the potential for synergistic effects remains to be investigated. The same investigators raised another point of interest in that mononuclear cells obtained from volunteers, following the lycopene supplementation period, had lower endogenous levels of DNA strand breaks, suggesting that tomato juice consumption might induce protective mechanisms in these cells (44). This finding has been also shown by others (45). It raises the question of whether enhanced antioxidative protection of DNA in immune cells is in some way related to the immunomodulatory effects of carotenoids.

IV. CAROTENOID INTAKE, IMMUNE FUNCTION, AND CANCER RISK

The now well-reported failure of three major intervention trials to show a protective effect of β-carotene in the prevention of lung cancer (46–48), with two of the studies showing a statistically significant increase in lung cancer in smokers receiving β-carotene supplementation, was initially a surprising disappointment to study participants, investigators, supplement manufacturers, and researchers in the area. In addition to impacting on the health of smokers involved in these studies, the negative effects have also had an impact on the availability of funds to undertake further studies on the health effects of this compound. The mechanism for the increased lung cancer risk associated with the supplementation is unclear, but several suggestions have been made. Since the participants in these studies could be classified as "high risk" for developing lung cancer (long-term smokers or individuals previously exposed to asbestos), it is possible that many of them had undetected tumors prior to the commencement of supplementation. The stage (or stages) of carcinogenesis against which β-carotene might be effective is unclear, but if the effect is mediated via the immune system it is likely to occur during the promotional stages preceding the formation of a malignant tumor. A recent analysis of the Cancer Prevention Study II, a prospective mortality study of more than 1 million U.S. adults, investigated the effects of supplementation with multivitamins and/or vitamins A, C, and/or E on mortality during a 7-year follow-up period. The use of a multivitamin plus vitamins A, C, and/or E significantly reduced the risk of lung cancer in former smokers and in never-smokers, but increased the risk of lung cancer in persistent smokers in men who had used a multivitamin plus vitamins A, C, and/or E, compared with men who had reported no vitamin supplement use. Interestingly, in this study, no association with smoking was seen in women (49).

A major unresolved dilemma of research into β-carotene is what intake is required to help optimize immune function and provide other health benefits? One of the most likely causes of the failure of the prospective studies is the level of supplementation provided. Most studies of this compound have been undertaken at levels that are not achievable within a normal healthy diet and that are certainly above the intakes associated with benefits in the epidemiological studies. Several authors have suggested that supradietary levels of β-carotene may exhibit pro-oxidant activity, particularly in the presence of high oxygen tensions, as occurs in the lungs (reviewed in 50). It is still unclear whether different intakes are associated with different outcomes or, in mechanistic studies, with different effects on various aspects of immune function. Ongoing clinical trials, such as the Physicians' Health Study II, may provide more insight into the effects of β-carotene supplementation, good or bad.

Of course, the probability remains that the apparent protection of consuming a diet rich in fruits and vegetables is the result of a multifactorial effect of a number of components of these foods. In support of this, two of the prospective studies mentioned above found that higher plasma β-carotene concentrations upon entry into the trials, resulting from dietary consumption as opposed to taking supplements, were associated with a lower risk of lung cancer (51). This emphasizes the need for more studies investigating the effects of enriching the diet with carotenoids in real foodstuffs rather than by supplementation, as is discussed elsewhere in this volume.

V. CONCLUSIONS

Since the immune system is critically dependent on accurate cell–cell communication in order to mount an immune response, immune cell integrity is essential. It is thought that carotenoids might help to maintain this integrity, reducing the damage caused by ROS to cell membranes and their associated receptors, as well as modulating immune cell function by influencing the activity of redox-sensitive transcription factors and the production of cytokines and prostaglandins. However, the results of the prospective studies with β-carotene in smokers remind us that caution must still be taken in making recommendations regarding the taking of supplements that provide a greater intake than can be achieved by eating a diet rich in fruits and vegetables. Further research needs to be undertaken to examine the interaction between different carotenoids, and indeed between combinations of carotenoids and other antioxidant nutrients such as vitamin E and dietary flavonoids, and to establish the levels of intake required to optimize immune responsiveness in different sectors of the population (e.g., the elderly, cigarette smokers). In the "post genomic" era, using the new technologies available in genomics, proteomics, and metabolomics, we can hope to see major advances in our understanding both of the influence of carotenoids on human immune function and of the way that different genotypes within the population respond to dietary intakes of these compounds. In addition, further studies should be undertaken to compare the effects observed following enrichment of the diet with antioxidants via real foodstuffs with those seen following dietary supplementation using pills or capsules, since these real foods undoubtedly contain beneficial compounds that we have yet to discover.

ACKNOWLEDGMENT

This work was supported by the Biotechnology and Biological Sciences Research Council of the United Kingdom.

REFERENCES

1. Drew B, Leeuwenburgh C. Aging and the role of reactive nitrogen species. Ann NY Acad Sci 2002; 959:66–81.
2. Baker KR, Meydani M. Beta-carotene in immunity and cancer. J Optim Nutr 1994; 3:39–50.
3. Gruner S, Volk HD, Falck P, Baehr RV. The influence of phagocytic stimuli on the expression of HLA-DR antigens; role of reactive oxygen intermediates. Eur J Immunol 1986; 16:212–215.
4. Anderson R. Antixidant nutrients and prevention of oxidant-mediated diseases. In: Bendich A, Deckelbaum RJ, eds. Preventive Nutrition. 2d ed. Totowa, NJ: Humana Press, 2001:293–306.
5. Bendich A. Beta-carotene and the immune response. Proc Nutr Soc 1991; 50:263–274.
6. Green HN, Mellanby E. Carotene and vitamin A: the anti-infective action of carotene. Br J Exp Pathol 1930; 11:81–89.
7. Clausen SW. Carotenemia and resistance to infection. Trans Am Pediatr Soc 1931; 43:27–30.
8. Lingen C, Ernster L, Lindberg O. The promoting effect of lycopene on the non specific resistance of animals. Exp Cell Res 1959; 16:384–393.
9. Peto R, Doll R, Buckley JD, Sporn MB. Can dietary beta-carotene materially reduce human cancer rates? Nature 1981; 290:201–208.
10. Bendich A, Shapiro SS. Effect of beta-carotene and canthaxanthin on the immune responses of the rat. J Nutr 1986; 116:2254–2262.

11. Kobayashi T, Iijima K, Mitamura T, Toriizuka K, Cyong JC, Nagasawa H. Effects of lycopene, a carotenoid, on intrathymic T cell differentiation and peripheral CD4/CD8 ratio in a high mammary tumor strain of SHN retired mice. Anticancer Drugs 1996; 7:195–198.

12. Vainio H, Rautalahti M. An international evaluation of the cancer preventive potential of carotenoids. Cancer Epidemiol Biomark Prev 1998; 7:725–728.

13. Fernandes-Carlos T, Riondel J, Glise D, Guiraud P, Favier A. Modulation of natural killer cell functional activity in athymic mice by beta-carotene, oestrone and their association. Anticancer Res 1997; 17:2523–2527.

14. Shklar G, Schwartz J. Tumor necrosis factor in experimental cancer regression with alpha-tocopherol, beta-carotene, canthaxanthin and algae extract. Eur J Cancer Clin Oncol 1988; 24:839–850.

15. Schwartz JL, Shklar G. A cyanobacteria extract and beta-carotene stimulate an antitumor host response against an oral cancer cell. Phytother Res 1989; 3:243–248.

16. Akyon Y. Effect of antioxidants on the immune response of Helicobacter pylori. Clin Microbiol Infect 2002; 8:438–441.

17. Wang X, Willen R, Wadstrom T. Astaxanthin-rich algal meal and vitamin C inhibit Helicobacter pylori infection in BALB/cA mice. Antimicrob Agents Chemother 2000; 44:2452–2457.

18. Lindholm C, Quiding-Jarbrink M, Lonroth H, Hamlet A, Svennerholm AM. Local cytokine response in *Helicobacter pylori*-infected subjects. Infect Immun 1998; 66:5964–5971.

19. Bennedsen M, Wang X, Willen R, Wadstrom T, Andersen LP. Treatment of H. pylori infected mice with antioxidant astaxanthin reduces gastric inflammation, bacterial load and modulates cytokine release by splenocytes. Immunol Lett 1999; 70:185–189.

20. Rivers JK, Norris PG, Murphy GM, Chu AC, Midgley G, Morris J, Morris RW, Young AR, Hawk JL. UVA sunbeds: tanning, photoprotection, acute adverse effects and immunological changes. Br J Dermatol 1989; 120:767–777.

21. Fuller CJ, Faulkner H, Bendich A, Parker RS, Roe DA. Effect of beta-carotene supplementation on photosuppression of delayed-type hypersensitivity in normal young men. Am J Clin Nutr 1992; 56:684–690.

22. Herraiz LA, Hsieh WC, Parker RS, Swanson JE, Bendich A, Roe DA. Effect of UV exposure and beta-carotene supplementation on delayed-type hypersensitivity response in healthy older men. J Am Coll Nutr 1998; 17:617–624.

23. Gollnick PM, Hopfenmuller W, Hemmes C, Chun SC, Schmid C, Sundermeier K, Biesalski HK. Systemic beta-carotene plus topical UV-sunscreen are an optimal protection against harmful effects of natural UV-sunlight: results of the Berlin–Eilath study. Eur J Dermatol 1996; 6:200–205.

24. Lesourd B, Mazari L. Nutrition and immunity in the elderly. Proc Nutr Soc 1999; 58:685–695.

25. Watson RR, Prabhala RH, Plezia PM, Alberts DS. Effect of beta-carotene on lymphocyte subpopulations in elderly humans: evidence for a dose-response relationship. Am J Clin Nutr 1991; 53:90–94.

26. Murata T, Tamai H, Morinobu T, Manago M, Takenaka H, Hayashi K, Mino M. Effect of long-term administration of beta-carotene on lymphocyte subsets in humans. Am J Clin Nutr 1994; 60:597–602.
27. Fryburg DA, Mark RJ, Griffith BP, Askenase PW, Patterson TF. The effect of supplemental beta-carotene on immunological indices in patients with AIDS: a pilot study. Yale J Biol Med 1995; 68:19–23.
28. Santos MS, Leka LS, Ribaya-Mercado JD, Russell RM, Meydani M, Hennekens CH, Gaziano JM, Meydani SN. Short- and long-term beta-carotene supplementation do not influence T cell-mediated immunity in healthy elderly persons. Am J Clin Nutr 1997; 66:917–924.
29. Santos MS, Meydani SN, Leka L, Wu D, Fotouhi N, Meydani M, Hennekens CH, Gaziano JM. Natural killer cell activity in elderly men is enhanced by beta-carotene supplementation. Am J Clin Nutr 1996; 64:772–777.
30. Bach FH. Class II genes and products of the HLA-D region. Immunol Today 1985; 6:89–94.
31. Janeway CA, Bottomly K, Babich J, Conrad P, Conzen S, Jones B, Kaye J, Katz M, McVay L, Murphy DB, Tite J. Quantitative variation in Ia antigen expression plays a central role in immune regulation. Immunol Today 1984; 5:99–104.
32. Springer TA. Adhesion receptors of the immune system. Nature 1990; 346:425–434.
33. Hughes DA, Wright AJA, Finglas PM, Peerless ACJ, Bailey AL, Astley SB, Pinder AC, Southon S. The effect of beta-carotene supplementation on the immune function of blood monocytes from healthy male non-smokers. J Lab Clin Med 1997; 129:309–317.
34. Halevy O, Sklan D. Inhibition of arachidonic acid oxidation by beta-carotene, retinol and alpha-tocopherol. Biochim Biophys Acta 1987; 918:304–307.
35. Fawzi W, Herrera MG, Nestel P. Tomato intake in relation to mortality and morbidity among sudanese children. J Nutr 2000; 130:2537–2542.
36. Hughes DA, Wright AJ, Finglas PM, Polley AC, Bailey AL, Astley SB, Southon S. Effects of lycopene and lutein supplementation on the expression of functionally associated surface molecules on blood monocytes from healthy male nonsmokers. J Infect Dis 2000; 182(suppl 1):S11–S15.
37. Paetau I, Khachik F, Brown ED, Beecher GR, Kramer TR, Chittams J, Clevidence BA. Chronic ingestion of lycopene-rich tomato juice or lycopene supplements significantly increases plasma concentrations of lycopene and related tomato carotenoids in humans. Am J Clin Nutr 1998; 68:1187–1195.
38. Gerster H. The potential role of lycopene for human health. J Am Coll Nutr 1997; 16:109–126.
39. Clinton SK, Emenhiser C, Schwartz SJ, Bostwick DG, Williams AW, Moore BJ, Erdman JW Jr. Cis-trans lycopene isomers, carotenoids, and retinol in the human prostate. Cancer Epidemiol Biomark Prev 1996; 5:823–833.
40. Yemelyanov AY, Katz NB, Bernstein PS. Ligand-binding characterization of xanthophyll carotenoids to solubilized membrane proteins derived from human retina. Exp Eye Res 2001; 72:381–392.
41. Corridan BM, O'Donoghue M, Hughes DA, Morrissey PA. Low-dose supplementation with lycopene or beta-carotene does not enhance cell-mediated immunity in healthy free-living elderly humans. Eur J Clin Nutr 2001; 55:627–635.

42. Watzl B, Bub A, Blockhaus M, Herbert BM, Luhrmann PM, Neuhauser-Berthold M, Rechkemmer G. Prolonged tomato juice consumption has no effect on cell-mediated immunity of well-nourished elderly men and women. J Nutr 2000; 130:1719–1723.

43. Watzl B, Bub A, Brandstetter BR, Rechkemmer G. Modulation of human T-lymphocyte functions by the consumption of carotenoid-rich vegetables. Br J Nutr 1999; 82:383–389.

44. Pool-Zobel BL, Bub A, Muller H, Wollowski I, Rechkemmer G. Consumption of vegetables reduces genetic damage in humans: first results of a human intervention trial with carotenoid-rich foods. Carcinogenesis 1997; 18:1847–1850.

45. Riso P, Pinder A, Santangelo A, Porrini M. Does tomato consumption effectively increase the resistance of lymphocyte DNA to oxidative damage? Am J Clin Nutr 1999; 69:712–718.

46. The Alpha-tocopherol Beta-carotene Cancer Prevention Study Group. The effect of vitamin E and beta-carotene on the incidence of lung cancer and other cancers in male smokers. N Engl J Med 1994; 330:1029–1035.

47. Hennekens CH, Buring JE, Manson JE, Stampfer M, Rosner B, Cook NR, Belanger C, LaMotte F, Gaziano JM, Ridker PM, Willett W, Peto R. Lack of effect of long term supplementation with beta carotene on the incidence of malignant neoplasms and cardiovascular disease. N Engl J Med 1996; 334:1145–1149.

48. Omenn GS, Goodman GE, Thornquist MD, Balmes J, Cullen MR, Glass A, Keogh JP, Meyskens FL, Valanis B, Williams JH, Barnhart S, Hammar S. Effects of a combination of beta carotene and vitamin A on lung cancer and cardiovascular disease. N Engl J Med 1996; 334:1150–1155.

49. Watkins ML, Erickson JD, Thun MJ, Mulinare J, Heath CW, Jr. Multivitamin use and mortality in a large prospective study. Am J Epidemiol 2000; 152:149–162.

50. Palozza P. Prooxidant actions of carotenoids in biological systems. Nutr Rev 1998; 56:257–265.

51. McDermott JH. Antioxidant nutrients: current dietary recommendations and research update. J Am Pharm Assoc 2000; 40:785–799.

24

Therapeutic Uses of Carotenoids in Skin Photosensitivity Diseases

Micheline M. Mathews-Roth
Harvard Medical School and Brigham and Women's Hospital, Boston, Massachusetts, U.S.A.

One of the functions of carotenoid pigments in green plants and photosynthetic microorganisms is to protect these organisms against photosensitization by their own chlorophyll. The author used this protective function of carotenoids to develop a treatment for the photosensitivity associated with the rare genetic disease erythropoietic protoporphyria (EPP). How this treatment was developed, as well as the use of carotenoids in the management of EPP and certain other photosensitivity diseases of the skin, will be reviewed here.

I. STUDIES OF CAROTENOID PROTECTIVE FUNCTIONS IN BACTERIA

Sistrom et al. (1) found that when the wild type of the photosynthetic bacterium, *Rhodospirillum spheriodes*, and a mutant of this bacterium that lacked colored carotenoids were grown in the presence of light and air, the mutant was killed, but the wild type, with its normal component of carotenoid pigments, survived. They showed that the cells' bacteriochlorophyll was responsible for the lethal photosensitization of the mutant, that both oxygen and light were necessary for the destructive reaction to occur, and that the carotenoid pigments were functioning as protective agents against this lethal photosensitization. Their findings that carotenoids can protect against chlorophyll photosensitization have been confirmed in other strains of photosynthetic bacteria, as well as in algae and green plants (2).

The nonphotosynthetic bacterium *Corynebacterium poinsettiae* contains colored carotenoid pigments. Kunisawa and Stanier (3) found that a mutant of this organism that lacked the colored carotenoids is killed in the presence of the exogenous photosensitizer toluidine blue, light, and air, whereas the wild type with its colored pigments was not affected by this exposure. They could not demonstrate the presence of an endogenous photosensitizer in this organism. Sistrom and I (4,5) showed that nonphotosynthetic carotenoid-containing bacteria do indeed contain endogenous photosensitizers. When we exposed the wild type and a colorless mutant of *Sarcina lutea*, another nonphotosynthetic carotenoid-containing organism, to natural sunlight in air for 4 h, we found that, at these high light intensities with no added photosensitizer, the mutant was killed and the wild type was not, and that, here also, oxygen was needed for killing to occur. Other workers have since confirmed the protective function of carotenoid pigments in nonphotosynthetic bacteria (6).

II. A CLINICAL APPLICATION?

Since carotenoid pigments can prevent photosensitization by porphyrins, it seemed to the author that perhaps the administration of carotenoid pigments could prevent photosensitization in patients with diseases in which the photosensitizer had some resemblance to the endogenous photosensitizer in plants, such as those porphyrias characterized with symptoms of light sensitivity, where the excess porphyrins produced by the genetic defect are similar to the porphyrin group of chlorophyll. Preliminary studies in porphyria patients done in the summer of 1961 with Dr. L. C. Harber at New York University School of Medicine suggested that the onset of erythema to artificial light could be delayed by the oral administration of β-carotene. A search of the literature up to that time revealed that Kesten (7) had been able to delay the onset of erythema in a patient with urticaria solare, a disease whose photosensitizer is unknown, with the use of β-carotene.

III. STUDIES IN ANIMALS

It was necessary to develop an animal model to test more thoroughly the hypothesis that carotenoids could protect against photosensitization. Eighteen to 24 h before light exposure, a suspension of 3 mg of β-carotene in Tween-80 (8) or the equivalent volume of Tween-80 alone was administered intraperitoneally to groups of mice. Just prior to light exposure, every mouse in both groups received 1 mg of hematoporphyrin derivative (9) intraperitoneally. Significantly more animals that received β-carotene survived the treatment with hematoporphyrin and light than did those that had not received β-carotene (10). Thus, β-carotene was effective in preventing the lethal photosensitivity induced by injection of hematoporphyrin and exposure to visible light in mice.

IV. CLINICAL STUDIES OF A HUMAN PHOTOSENSITIVITY DISEASE

The successful photoprotection studies in animals suggested that we should determine if the administration of β-carotene could prevent or reduce photosensitivity in patients. The disease chosen for study was EPP. In EPP, ferrochelatase, the enzyme that inserts iron into protoporphyrin to make heme, is defective, resulting in the accumulation of protoporphyrin in blood and other tissues. Leakage of protoporphyrin from blood cells leads to a cascade of reactions resulting in itching, burning, and ulceration of skin on exposure to visible light (11).

The first patient with EPP who was treated, a 10-year-old girl, could tolerate only brief exposures to sunlight. Exposure to a carbon arc lamp (340–640 nm) produced erythema in 2 min. In June 1968, she was given a preparation of concentrated carrot oil in doses approximately equivalent to 30 mg β-carotene per day. After a month of carrot oil ingestion, she could tolerate at least 30 min of carbon arc light and more than 1 h of natural sunlight. By the middle of the summer she could play outdoors in the afternoon without experiencing any symptoms of photosensitivity. In the summer of 1969, she and two other patients were given β-carotene in the form of 10% β-carotene "beadlets" (Hoffman-La Roche). Here also, all three were found to have improved tolerance to sunlight exposure (12,13). In 1970, the author set up a collaborative study to include all the patients of Dr. Harber and those of other physicians who had contacted us concerning the use of β-carotene since the published report of our first three cases. By the summer of 1975, we had treated 133 patients suffering from EPP with β-carotene, using a standard protocol adhered to by all participating physicians (14,15). In July 1975, the U.S. Food and Drug Administration (FDA) approved the use of β-carotene for the management of EPP and we terminated the collaborative study at that time.

In the collaborative study we used the following starting dosage schedule for β-carotene (14,15) and we still recommend it today:

1–4 years of age: 60–90 mg/day
5–8 years of age: 90–120 mg/day
9–12 years of age: 120–140 mg/day
13–15 years of age: 150–180 mg/day
16 years and older: 180 mg/day

The average dose for the patient's age should be administered for 4–6 weeks, and the patient should be instructed not to increase sun exposure either for 4 weeks or until some yellow discoloration of the skin, especially of the palms of the hand, is noted. Then exposure can be increased cautiously and gradually until the patient determines the limits of exposure to light that can be tolerated without the development of symptoms. If the degree of protection is not sufficient, the daily dose of carotene should be increased by 30–60 mg per day for children younger than 16, and up to a total of 300 mg per day for those older than 16. If after 3 months of therapy at these higher doses (blood carotene levels should reach at least 800 μg/dL) no significant increase in tolerance to sunlight exposure has occurred, it can be concluded that β-carotene therapy will not be effective for that patient, and the medication should be discontinued. We found that 84% of the patients increased by a factor of 3 or more their ability to tolerate sunlight exposure without the development of symptoms (14,15). On average, it took between 1 and 2 months for the patients who received benefit from carotene therapy to notice increased tolerance to sun exposure. The majority of patients reported that with β-carotene therapy they could engage in outdoor activities that they were unable to do before therapy started. Children who previous to carotene therapy could not play outdoors to any great extent could now spend hours outside with their friends. Many patients stated that they were able to develop a suntan for the first time in their lives, some feeling that the acquisition of the tan, plus the β-carotene, added to their protection from the sun's effects. The majority of the patients noted that while they were taking β-carotene, reactions from the sun that did occur were less severe in intensity and duration than before therapy, and that they also developed fewer cutaneous lesions during their increased exposure time.

We found that the patients' blood and stool porphyrin levels were not affected by the ingestion of large amounts of β-carotene. Thus, treatment with β-carotene ameliorates photosensitivity in EPP but has no effect on the biochemical lesion in this disease.

Because of the difficulties in the subjective evaluation of therapeutic effect and of setting up a controlled double-blind study in the particular case of β-carotene and EPP, we decided to use phototesting with polychromatic light from 380 to 560 nm (as opposed to monochromatic light) as an objective measure of clinical improvement. Using exposure to xenon arc lamp under the conditions we have developed (14,16), we found that tolerance to xenon arc light exposure increased in those patients who reported benefit from β-carotene therapy, but no increased tolerance to this radiation has been found in patients reporting no improvement. Other workers have also noted increased tolerance to polychromatic xenon arc light after treatment with β-carotene (17,18). Thus, phototesting with polychromatic xenon arc light can serve as an objective method of determining improvement in tolerance to light.

V. CONFIRMATION OF RESULTS

In previous reviews (19–23) I list 63 studies, and here I list two additional studies (24,25) reporting increases in tolerance to sunlight in a majority of patients with EPP treated with high doses of β-carotene, either alone or in combination with canthaxanthin, another naturally occurring carotenoid pigment. In some of these series, as well as in other reports (26–30), there are patients who do not benefit from carotenoid therapy, in spite of adequate pigment dosage. This is most likely due to either poor absorption of pigment, or the use of a β-carotene preparation with low bioavailability, or the patient having markedly elevated blood porphyrin levels. One controlled study of β-carotene therapy in EPP reported little or no improvement in the subjects' photosensitivity (31); unfortunately, these workers used a lower dosage of β-carotene than we had recommended as effective. Later, some of the patients from this unsuccessfully treated study were given higher doses of β-carotene by another investigator, and the patients noted some increased tolerance to sun while taking the higher dose (32). These results emphasize the importance, as mentioned above, of individualizing dosage to each patient and increasing the dose until the patient reports some improvement. The problem of individualizing treatment is especially important to the conduct of a controlled trial and makes double-blinded designs almost impossible. At a minimum, such trials should use a dose of β-carotene large enough to produce amelioration of symptoms in the majority of patients (a minimal period of 3 months' treatment at doses giving blood levels of at least 800 $\mu g/dL$; for adults at least 180 mg/day of β-carotene should be given). As also mentioned, another important factor is the form of β-carotene used; we recommend the use of the Roche 10% β-carotene beadlets (Lumitene, Tishcon), as this preparation has the high level of bioavailability necessary to deliver the elevated blood levels of β-carotene needed for effective photoprotection. In summary, in spite of the occasional treatment failure, from our results and those of the other workers listed above it can be concluded that β-carotene, when administered in sufficiently high doses and using the bioavailable "beadlet" preparation, can be effective in ameliorating photosensitivity in most patients with EPP.

VI. CAROTENOID USE IN OTHER PHOTOSENSITIVITY DISEASES

Since β-carotene appeared to be effective in preventing photosensitivity in EPP, it seemed logical to determine if it could be an effective treatment for other photosensitivity diseases. We reported previously (23) that there have been nine reports of some success in treating with carotenoids patients suffering from congenital porphyria (Gunther's disease). New lesions were significantly decreased in number and severity, and the patients have been somewhat able to increase their sun exposure. In most cases, other treatment modalities, such as transfusions, and meticulous management of skin infections must continue.

As we also reported (23), several groups, including the author's, have used carotenoids to prevent photosensitivity in polymorphic light eruption. Reports of improvement range from one-third to two-thirds of patients tolerating light exposure without developing new lesions. Usually, sunscreens had also to be used to get a beneficial effect from carotenoid intake; sunscreens by themselves did not provide relief for these patients.

Several studies reported that carotenoid treatment was effective in the photosensitivity diseases porphyria cutanea tarda, porphyria variegata, actinic reticuloid, solar urticaria, and hydroa aestivale; however, other studies found carotenoids to be ineffective (23). We would recommend trying β-carotene in these conditions only after the treatment modalities used in these conditions have failed or to enhance their effectiveness if they are having minimal effect.

VII. HOW DO CAROTENOIDS PROTECT AGAINST SKIN PHOTOSENSITIZATION?

Other chapters discuss in detail the various chemical and physical reactions carotenoids can undergo. Some of these are involved in the mechanism of photoprotection. Krinsky (2) suggested four possible ways that carotenoid pigments could exert their protective functions: 1) a filter system in the cell envelope to filter out potentially harmful light; 2) systems that can interact with and quench photosensitizer triplet states; 3) systems that can serve as preferred substrates for photosensitized oxidations; and 4) systems that can stabilize membranes or repair damaged membranes. Since that time, additional evidence has indicated that only the second suggested mechanism, now extended to include quenching of singlet oxygen by carotenoids, seems to be significantly associated with the pigments' protective function (6). Mechanism (a) may have some function in certain plants, although it may not be the sole explanation for the pigments' protective effects in these organisms. This mechanism is also unlikely to be involved in carotenoid protection in humans, as the amounts deposited in skin are not sufficient to act as a physical sunscreen (33,34). In addition, the photoprotective effect of the carotenoids seems to be independent of their absorption spectrum. The findings in photosynthetic organisms that led to the suggestion of mechanism (c) by several groups of workers are thought to be connected with reactions involved with photosynthesis rather than with the protective function of carotenoids (6). The author and Krinsky showed that the presence of carotenoids does not seem to be involved with membrane stability in *Sarcina lutea* (35), thus suggesting that mechanism (d) may not be of wide significance in the protective function of carotenoids.

Thus it would seem that the quenching of excited species is the most widely applicable mechanism for the carotenoids' protective effects. Since the first demonstration of the ability of carotenoids to quench the triplet state of chlorophyll (36) and to quench singlet oxygen (37), many workers, including ourselves, have confirmed that porphyrins form these excited species when illuminated, and that carotenoids can quench them.

Studies on the photoprotective action of carotenoids at the cellular level have also been performed. Using a method of detecting photochemical reactions in epidermis, the author has shown that the carotenoids present in the skin of mice made porphyric by the ingestion of collidine, and also receiving supplementation of either β-carotene or canthaxanthin, could quench photochemical reactions occurring in isolated epidermis (38). In nonporphyric mice supplemented with either of these carotenoids, or with the colorless carotenoid phytoene, the pigments could also quench excited species formed in skin on exposure to UVB (290–320 nm) radiation (39). Although more work needs to be done to determine the actual molecular mechanisms of photosensitization and photoprotection in humans, it is conceivable that carotenoids prevent the porphyrin-induced peroxidation and lipid oxidation of cellular components of endothelial and immune system cells, thereby preventing the release of mediators that give rise to the symptoms associated with photosensitization in EPP and possibly other photosensitivity diseases.

VIII. LACK OF TOXICITY OF CAROTENOIDS IN EPP

The most predominant side effect of carotenoid therapy is carotenodermia, which is most obvious on the palms of the hands and the soles of the feet of people ingesting large amounts of carotenoids, but is only occasionally seen on other parts of the body. This condition disappears within a few weeks after β-carotene intake stops.

We found no abnormalities in blood chemistry or hematology tests that could be attributed to β-carotene intake, nor has it been reported by other workers. A review of the literature found only one instance of any biochemical abnormalities reported from β-carotene use in EPP. Warren and George (40) report that a patient who, starting at age 11 years, was treated with β-carotene alone, then with a mixture of β-carotene and canthaxanthin, and then again with β-carotene alone, was found on routine liver function tests after about 9 years of carotenoid treatment to have an elevated aspartate transaminase (AST) level, but his bilirubin level and other enzyme levels remained within normal limits.

Withdrawal of β-carotene brought the AST back to normal; readministration again caused the AST elevation. Unfortunately, the authors did not state which brand of β-carotene was used at the time the abnormality was found, or if there had been a change in brand used during the period of β-carotene administration, or even if the patient had started taking any other medications, or possibly drinking alcoholic beverages, around the time that the abnormality was discovered. Apparently the β-carotene caused no serious damage, as all liver chemistries including AST remained within normal limits for at least the five years of follow-up covered by this paper (40).

Some patients report gastrointestinal disturbances when they first start taking supplemental β-carotene. Usually these discomforts clear up spontaneously, but some patients require that the dose be lowered. On very rare occasions, a patient may have to stop β-carotene intake to obtain relief.

As discussed elsewhere in this book, carotenoids, including β-carotene, have been investigated for anticancer activity. During the course of two placebo-controlled intervention trials of β-carotene and lung cancer prevention in high-risk individuals (heavy smokers, some of whom were also asbestos workers and heavy drinkers) the group randomized to β-carotene intake had an increase in lung cancer rate as compared with placebo (41,42). However, in another large intervention trial studying β-carotene prevention of all cancers, no increase in any kind of cancer was found in the group taking β-carotene (43). It is possible that alcohol or cigarette smoke may have been a factor in generating some kind of toxic product. Studies by Lieber's group (44) suggest that ethanol reacts with β-carotene and vitamin A (which was also given in one of the cancer studies but not by us), and that smoking can exacerbate this, which may explain why the increase in lung cancers developed in the smokers' study. As we and others have found in EPP patients, β-carotene intake does not seem to pose a risk to people who do not smoke and drink in excess. In fact, people with EPP are warned not to drink, or take medications and hormones, including estrogen and testosterone, which cause cholestasis, as such intake can increase their risk of developing potentially fatal liver disease caused by the excess protoporphyrin which accumulates in their livers.

Canthaxanthin, which has been used in conjunction with β-carotene in Europe, is also effective in preventing photosensitivity, but ingestion of large doses leads to the deposition of pigmented granules in the retinas of some patients, which occasionally may have some effect on night vision (45). The granules have been found to disappear several months after cessation of canthaxanthin ingestion, with return of any visual changes to normal (45). No such granules seem to form from β-carotene ingestion (46). It should be noted that canthaxanthin, although approved by the FDA as a food coloring agent, has not been approved for use as a therapeutic agent for EPP, or for other indications.

IX. SUMMARY

Studies in bacteria, animals, and humans have demonstrated that carotenoid pigments can prevent or reduce skin photosensitivity by endogenous photosensitizers such as chlorophyll or porphyrins, as well as by exogenous photosensitizers such as dyes (e.g., toluidine blue) or porphyrin derivatives. The carotenoids β-carotene and canthaxanthin have been found very effective in the treatment of the photosensitivity associated with EPP and to a lesser extent in the management of certain other photosensitivity diseases. No serious toxicity has been reported as a result their use, although canthaxanthin is not recommended because of its propensity to form retinal granules. The pigments most likely perform their protective function by quenching excited species formed by the interaction of porphyrins or other photosensitizers, light and air, thereby preventing the cellular damage that leads to the symptoms of photosensitivity.

REFERENCES

1. Sistrom WR, Griffiths M, Stanier RY. Biology of a photosynthetic bacterium which lacks colored carotenoids. J Cell Comp Physiol 1957; 48:473–515.
2. Krinsky NI. The protective function of carotenoid pigments. In: Giese AC, ed. Photophysiology, Current Topics. Vol. 3. New York: Academic Press, 1968; 123–195.
3. Kunisawa R, Stanier RY. Studies on the role of carotenoid pigments in a chemoheterotropic bacterium. *Corynebacterium poinsettiae.* Arch Mikrobiol 1958; 31:146–159.
4. Mathews MM, Sistrom WR. Function of carotenoid pigments in non-photosynthetic bacteria. Nature 1959; 184:1892.
5. Mathews MM, Sistrom WR. The function of the carotenoid pigments of *Sarcina lutea.* Arch Mikrobiol 1960; 35:139–146.
6. Krinsky NI. Function. In: Isler O, ed. Carotenoids. Basel: Birkhauser Verlag, 1971:669–706.
7. Kesten BM. Urticaria solare (4,200–4,900 A). Arch Dermatol Syphilol 1951; 64:221–228.
8. Forssberg A, Lingen C, Ernster A, Lindberg O. Modification of x-irradiation syndrome by lycopene. Exptl Cell Res 1959; 16:7–14.
9. Lipson RL, Baldes EJ. Photodynamic properties of a particular hematoporphyrin derivative. Arch Dermatol 1960; 82:508–516.
10. Mathews MM. Protective effect of beta-carotene against lethal photosensitization by hematoporphyrin. Nature 1964; 203:1092.
11. Kappas A, Sassa S, Anderson KE. The porphyrias. In: Stanbury JB, Fredrickson DS, Goldstein JL, Brown MS, eds. The Metabolic Basis of Inherited Disease. New York: McGraw-Hill, 1983:1301–1384.

12. Mathews-Roth MM, Pathak MA, Fitzpatrick TB, Harber LC, Kass EH. Beta-carotene as a photoprotective agent in erythropoietic protoporphyria. Trans Assoc Am Phys 1970; 83:176–184.

13. Mathews-Roth MM, Pathak MA, Fitzpatrick TB, Harber LC, Kass EH. Beta-carotene as a photoprotective agent in erythropoietic protoporphyria. N Engl J Med 1970; 282:1231–1234.

14. Mathews-Roth MM, Pathak MA, Fitzpatrick TB, Harber LC, Kass EH. Beta-carotene as an oral photoprotective agent in erythropoietic protoporphyria. JAMA 1974; 228:1004–1008.

15. Mathews-Roth MM, Pathak MA, Fitzpatrick TB, Harber LC, Kass EH. Beta-carotene therapy for erythropoietic protoporphyria and other photosensitivity diseases. Arch Dermatol 1977; 113:1229–1232.

16. Mathews-Roth MM, Kass EH, Fitzpatrick TB, Pathak MA, Harber LC. Phototesting as an objective measure of improvement in erythropoietic protoporphyria. Arch Dermatol 1979; 115:1381–1382.

17. Krook G, Haeger-Aronson B. Erythrohepatic protoporphyria and its treatment with beta-carotene. Acta Dermatovener 1974; 54:39–44.

18. Wennersten G, Swanbeck G. Treatment of light sensitivity with carotenoids: serum concentrations and light protection. Acta Dermatovener 1974; 54:491–499.

19. Mathews-Roth MM. Beta-carotene therapy for erythropoietic protoporphyria and other photosensitivity diseases. In: Regan JD, Parrish J, eds. The Science of Photomedicine. New York: Raven Press, 1982:409–440.

20. Mathews-Roth MM. Beta-carotene therapy for erythropoietic protoporphyria and other photosensitivity diseases. Biochimie 1986; 68:875–884.

21. Mathews-Roth MM. Carotenoid functions in photoprotection and cancer prevention. J Environ Pathol Toxicol Oncol 1990; 10:181–192.

22. Mathews-Roth MM. Recent progress in the medical applications of carotenoids. Pure Appl Chem 1991; 63:147–156.

23. Mathews-Roth MM. Carotenoids in erythropoietic protoporphyria and other photosensitivity diseases. Ann NY Acad Sci 1993; 691:127–138.

24. Labrouse AL, Salmon-Ehr V, Eschard C, Kalis B, Leonard F, Bernard P. Recurrent painful hand crisis in a four-year-old girl, revealing an erythropoietic protoporphyria. Eur J Dermatol 1998; 8:515–516.

25. Patel GK, Weston J, Derrick EK, Hawk JLM. An unusual case of purpuric erythropoietic protoporphyria. Clin Exp Dermatol 2000; 25:406–408.

26. Smit AFD. Erythropoietic protoporphyria. Br J Dermatol 1980; 102:743.

27. Kuhlwein A, Beykirch W. Das β-carotin als therapeutikum der erythropoetischen protoporphyrie (EPP), nicht der weisheit letzter schluss. Z Hautkr 1980; 55:817–820.

28. Bechtel MA, Bertolone SJ, Hodge SJ. Transfusion therapy in a patient with erythropoietic protoporphyria. Arch Dermatol 1981; 117:99–101.

29. Murphy GM, Hawk JLM, Magnus IA. Late-onset erythropoietic protoporphyria with unusual clinical features. Arch Dermatol 1985; 121:1309–1310.

30. Ross JB, Moss MA. Relief of the photosensitivity of erythropoietic protoporphyria by pyridoxine. J Am Acad Dermatol 1990; 22:340–342.

31. Corbett MF, Herxheimer A, Magnus IA, Ramsay CA, Kobza-Black A. The long-term treatment with beta-carotene in erythropoietic protoporphyria—a controlled trial. Br J Dermatol 1977; 97:655–662.
32. Shafrir A. Comment to Marsden Case Report. Proc R Soc Med 1977; 70:574.
33. Lamola AA, Blumberg W. The effectiveness of beta-carotene and phytoene as systemic sunscreens. Annual Meeting of the American Society for Photobiology. Abstract No. FAM-C4, 1976.
34. Sayre RM, Black HS. Beta-carotene does not act as an optical filter in skin. J Photochem Photobiol B Biol 1992; 12:83–90.
35. Mathews-Roth MM, Krinsky NI. Carotenoid pigments and the stability of the cell membrane of *Sarcina lutea*. Biochim Biophys Acta 1970; 203:357–359.
36. Fugimori E, Tavla M. Light-induced electron transfer between chlorophyll and hydroquinone and the effect of oxygen and beta-carotene. Photochem Photobiol 1966; 5:877–887.
37. Foote CS, Denny RW. Chemistry of singlet oxygen VII. Quenching by beta-carotene. J Am Chem Soc 1968; 90:6233–6235.
38. Mathews-Roth MM. Porphyrin photosensitization and carotenoid protection in mice: in vitro and in vivo studies. Photochem Photobiol 1984; 40:63–67.
39. Mathews-Roth MM. Carotenoids quench evolution of excited species in epidermis exposed to UV-B (290–320 nm) light. Photochem Photobiol 1986; 43:91–93.
40. Warren LJ, George S. Erythropoietic protoporphyria treated with narrow-band (TL-01) phototherapy. Australasian J Derm 1998; 39:179–182.
41. The Alpha-Tocopherol, Beta-carotene Cancer Prevention Study Group. The effect of vitamin E and beta-carotene on the incidence of lung cancer and other cancers in male smokers. N Engl J Med 1994; 330:1029–1035.
42. Omenn GS, Goodman GE, Thornquist MD, Balmes J, Cullen MR, Glass A, Keogh JP, Meyskens FL, Valanis B, Williams JH Jr, Barnhart S, Hammar S. Effects of a combination of beta-carotene and vitamin A on lung cancer and cardiovascular disease. N Engl J Med 1996; 334:1150–1155.
43. Hennekens CH, Buring JE, Manson JE, Stampfer M, Rosner B, Cook NR, Belanger C, LaMotte F, Gaziano JM, Ridker PM, Willett W, Peto R. Lack of effect of long-term supplementation with beta-carotene on the incidence of malignant neoplasms and cardiovascular disease. N Engl J Med 1996; 334:1145–1149.
44. Leo MA, Lieber CS. Alcohol, vitamin A, and beta-carotene: adverse interactions, including hepatotoxicity and carcinogenicity. Am J Clin Nutr 1999; 69:1071–1085.
45. Arden GB, Barker FM. Canthaxanthin and the eye: a critical ocular toxicologic assessment. J Toxicol Cutan Ocular Toxicol 1991; 10:115–155.
46. Poh-Fitzpatrick MB, Barbera L. Absence of crystalline retinopathy after long-term therapy with beta-carotene. J Am Acad Dermatol 1984; 11:111–113.

25

Potential Adverse Effects of β-Carotene Supplementation in Cigarette Smokers and Heavier Drinkers

Demetrius Albanes and Margaret E. Wright
National Cancer Institute, National Institutes of Health, Bethesda, Maryland, U.S.A.

I. INTRODUCTION

As reviewed in detail elsewhere in this volume, abundant epidemiological evidence supports an association between reduced risk of cancer, particularly lung cancer, and higher β-carotene and other carotenoid intake, or higher carotenoid biochemical status. The observed associations are relatively strong and consistent, and led to the initiation and conduct of controlled intervention trials of β-carotene supplementation beginning in the 1980s. The latter studies did not substantiate a protective role for β-carotene supplementation in cancer but instead demonstrated relatively small adverse effects of β-carotene supplementation on cancer incidence and mortality in cigarette smokers. Increased cancer risk was also observed among heavier drinkers in some of the trials. Subsequent experimental evidence supported the trial findings, particularly with respect to a harmful interaction between β-carotene supplementation and tobacco smoke, and provided important leads regarding the biological mechanisms through which β-carotene acted.

This chapter reviews the original controlled trial data regarding the adverse effects of β-carotene supplementation among smokers and heavier drinkers, and outlines the experimental data that may explain the trial findings. As the majority of relevant investigations relate to lung carcinogenesis, we focus on this cancer site and refer to observed interactions with other end points.

II. TRIALS OF β-CAROTENE SUPPLEMENTATION: EVIDENCE OF INTERACTIONS WITH CIGARETTES AND ALCOHOL

The results of several supplementation trials of β-carotene provide evidence for adverse effects in cigarette smokers and heavier drinkers (Table 1). Such effects were apparent in the Skin Cancer Prevention Study that tested β-carotene supplementation (50 mg/day) in 1805 patients with a previous basal cell or squamous cell skin cancer (1). Following 5 years of intervention, the occurrence of first new nonmelanoma skin cancer did not differ significantly by intervention arm [relative risk (RR) for the β-carotene arm = 1.05; 95% confidence interval (CI): 0.91–1.22]. However, evaluation of the intervention effect across subgroups of the population revealed a marginally significant 44% risk elevation for those supplemented with β-carotene who were current smokers, with no β-carotene effect in nonsmokers and former smokers. This finding of a β-carotene–smoking interaction was recently reported by the investigators as being statistically significant ($p = 0.04$) (2).

Adverse interactions between β-carotene supplementation and both cigarette smoking and alcohol consumption in humans were first clearly demonstrated in the Alpha-Tocopherol, Beta-Carotene Cancer Prevention (ATBC) Study. This randomized, double-blind, placebo-controlled trial of 29,133 male cigarette smokers in Finland tested the prevention of lung cancer and other cancers through supplementation with α-tocopherol (50 mg/day) and β-carotene (20 mg/day) for 5–8 years. The ATBC Study Group reported its initial trial intervention findings in 1994 (3) and final lung cancer results in 1996 (4). The data provided no evidence for benefit of β-carotene in the prevention of lung or other cancers, but showed a 16% relative excess of lung cancer for the β-carotene arm (482 versus 412 cases, 95% CI: 2–33% increase in incidence). There were no other statistically significant increases in the incidence of other cancers for the β-carotene arm, although there was a small excess of cases for some sites including prostate and stomach. Overall mortality was also 8% higher in the β-carotene arm (95% CI: 1–16%), and while no adverse interaction was seen with alcohol, most of the excess mortality was observed among men who smoked 20 cigarettes or more daily (RR = 1.11; 95% CI: 1.01–1.16). More detailed subgroup analyses showed that the relative risk of lung cancer for the β-carotene arm was elevated primarily among smokers of 20 cigarettes or more daily (RR = 1.25; 95% CI: 1.07–1.46) compared with lighter smokers in whom no adverse effect was evident (RR = 0.97; 95% CI: 0.76–1.23) (Table 1). There was no further dose–response within the 20+ cigarettes category, and the overall test for trend of the β-carotene intervention effect across smoking categories was not statistically significant ($p = 0.15$) (4). The effect of β-carotene supplementation on lung cancer risk also increased with alcohol consumption. Among men who drank at least 11 grams of ethanol (or slightly less than one

Table 1 Intervention Trials of Supplemental β-Carotene (Alone or in Combination with Other Micronutrients) in Which Modification by Cigarette Smoking and/or Alcohol Consumption Was Observed

Trial	Intervention	End point	Smoking and/or drinking status	Multivariate RR (95% CI)[a]	p interaction
Skin Cancer Prevention Study (1)	β-carotene (50 mg/d) or placebo	Nonmelanoma skin cancer (incidence)	Nonsmoker	0.97 (0.82–1.15)	0.04[b]
			Current smoker	1.44 (0.99–2.09)	
Alpha-Tocopherol, Beta-Carotene Cancer Prevention (ATBC) Study (4)	β-carotene (20 mg/d), alone or in combination with vitamin E, or placebo	Lung cancer (incidence)	5–19 cigs/d	0.97 (0.76–1.23)	0.15
			20–29 cigs/d	1.25 (1.07–1.46)	
			≥30 cigs/d	1.28 (0.97–1.70)	
			<11 g ethanol/d	1.03 (0.85–1.24)	0.05
			≥11 g ethanol/d	1.35 (1.01–1.81)	
Beta-Carotene and Retinol Efficacy Trial (CARET) (6)	β-carotene (30 mg/d) + retinyl palmitate (25,000 IU/d) or placebo	Lung cancer (incidence)	Former smoker[c]	0.80 (0.48–1.31)	0.03
			Current smoker[c]	1.42 (1.07–1.87)	
			Nondrinker	1.07 (0.76–1.51)	0.01
			<Median alcohol	1.71 (0.92–3.17)	
			3rd-quartile alcohol	0.79 (0.50–1.26)	
			4th-quartile alcohol	1.99 (1.28–3.09)	

(continued)

Table 1 *Continued*

Trial	Intervention	End point	Smoking and/or drinking status	Multivariate RR (95% CI)[a]	p interaction
Antioxidant Polyp Prevention Study (2)	β-carotene (25 mg/d), and/or vitamins C and E in combination, or placebo	Colorectal adenoma (recurrence)	Nonsmoker/ nondrinker	0.56 (0.35–0.89)	0.008 (BC × smoke)
			Smoker/nondrinker	1.36 (0.70–2.62)	0.022 (BC × alc)
			Drinker/nonsmoker	1.13 (0.89–1.43)	0.059 (BC × smoke × alc)
			Smoker/drinker	1.33 (0.81–2.17)	
			Smoker/heavy drinker	2.07 (1.39–3.08)	

[a]RR (relative risk) and 95% CI (confidence interval) of active intervention to placebo. In ATBC, RR of β-carotene versus no β-carotene. In Antioxidant Polyp Prevention Study, RR of β-carotene versus placebo, adjusted for supplementation with vitamins C and E.

[b]From Ref. 2.

[c]Non-asbestos-exposed.

drink) daily, the β-carotene intervention relative risk was 1.35 (95% CI: 1.01–1.81), compared to those with lower intake (RR = 1.03; 95% CI: 0.85–1.24; p value for interaction = 0.05). Nondrinkers (11% of the men) showed a reduced risk of lung cancer with β-carotene supplementation, although this was not statistically significant (RR = 0.93; 95% CI: 0.65–1.33). This pattern was suggested for all alcoholic beverage types, and the β-carotene-alcohol interaction was not altered by level of smoking.

The Beta-Carotene and Retinol Efficacy Trial (CARET) studied 18,314 men and women and provided similar evidence for increased lung cancer incidence and total mortality resulting from its daily intervention of β-carotene (30 mg) and retinyl palmitate (25,000 IU) (5). The study was similar to the ATBC Study in that its population was at high risk for lung cancer, being composed of both current (60%) and former (39%) heavy smokers, including asbestos-exposed smokers (22%). After an average of 4 years of intervention, 388 lung cancers developed, with a 28% increase in lung cancer incidence among participants who received the β-carotene/retinyl palmitate combination daily compared with the placebo arm. Overall mortality was also 17% higher in the supplemented group. Subgroup analysis showed higher lung cancer risk elevations among the current smokers (RR = 1.42; 95% CI: 1.07–1.87) and in the highest quartile of alcohol consumption (RR = 1.99; 95% CI: 1.28–3.09), with both results representing statistically significant modifications of the intervention effects (Table 1) (6). The findings in the CARET therefore corroborated those in the ATBC Study, with somewhat greater increases in lung cancer incidence and total mortality in the intervention arm.

Until these results from the CARET were published in early 1996, the ATBC Study findings were viewed cautiously. Thereafter, however, the concordant data from the ATBC Study and CARET represented a striking contradiction to the previous observational epidemiology and provided clear evidence of adverse effects from β-carotene supplementation. Both the ATBC Study and the CARET randomized persons at high risk for lung cancer from cigarette smoking, asbestos exposure, or both, and very high serum concentrations of β-carotene were achieved in response to the daily supplementation. CARET differed from the ATBC Study in that it tested a β-carotene–vitamin A combination and included women and both current and former smokers as well as a large group of workers exposed to asbestos.

The Antioxidant Polyp Prevention Study randomized 864 men and women with a previously removed colorectal adenoma to 25 mg/day of β-carotene (alone or in combination with other micronutrients) or placebo, and showed that the β-carotene intervention conferred no benefit or harm with respect to adenoma recurrence (RR = 1.01; 95% CI: 0.85–1.20) (2,7). Cigarette smoking and alcohol consumption substantially modified the intervention effects for this end point, with a significant 44% reduction in adenoma recurrence in the nonsmoking/nondrinking group, and a greater than twofold increase among smokers who also consumed more than one alcoholic drink daily (Table 1) (2). Nonsignificant increases in risk associated with the β-carotene supplement were also observed in smokers/nondrinkers (RR = 1.36) and drinkers/nonsmokers (RR = 1.13); each of these risk estimates was significantly different from the effects in those who abstained from alcohol use and cigarette smoking (p value for interaction for β-carotene–smoking = 0.008 and for β-carotene–alcohol = 0.02).

In the Carotene Prevention Trial, allocation of 264 patients with first primary head or neck cancer to 50 mg/day of β-carotene or placebo for an average of 4 years did not result in significantly reduced risks of local recurrence and second primary cancers of the head and neck, esophagus, and lung (RR for β-carotene versus placebo = 0.90; 95% CI: 0.56–1.45) (8). Although the intervention did not impact these events or overall mortality, there was significant heterogeneity in survival distributions across four treatment groups defined by intervention assignment and baseline smoking status ($p = 0.03$). However, these differences were largely driven by smoking. Site-specific analyses of second primary tumors revealed an increased, albeit nonsignificant, risk of lung cancer in the intervention group (RR = 1.44; 95% CI: 0.62–3.39), which is consistent with previous trial findings. Stratification of this result by smoking status was not undertaken due to small case numbers.

In contrast to the findings in the ATBC Study and the CARET, the Physicians' Health Study (PHS) of 22,071 male, primarily nonsmoking physicians in the United States showed no difference in lung cancer (or other cancer) incidence after 12 years of supplementation between its β-carotene (50 mg on alternate days) and placebo arms (9). For lung cancer, this was based on only 82 cases versus 88 cases in the two study arms, respectively, and represented a nonsignificant 7% reduction in risk. No adverse or beneficial effects were observed in the β-carotene arm, with the relative overall mortality being 1.01 (nonsignificant), and all the cancer sites showing similarly null results. Furthermore, the PHS demonstrated no intervention arm differences in cancer rates (total, lung, prostate, colon, or nonmelanoma skin incidence) by smoking status or level of alcohol consumption (10,11). For example, the relative risks of lung cancer for the β-carotene arm for nonsmokers, former smokers, and current smokers were 1.0, 0.9, and 1.0, respectively, but only 11% of participants were current smokers. Similar results for total cancer incidence were obtained from the Women's Health Study, whose β-carotene intervention was, because of the aforementioned β-carotene findings, prematurely terminated after up to 3 years, showing neither a significant increase in rates (RR for intervention group = 1.03) nor an interaction with smoking (12).

The Nutrition Intervention Trial (NIT) in Linxian, China tested whether daily supplementation with a combination of β-carotene (15 mg), α-tocopherol (30 mg), and selenium (200 μg) could prevent esophageal and other cancers in a cohort of 29,546 men and women (13). The study showed efficacy for β-carotene supplementation for stomach and overall cancer mortality, and slightly fewer lung cancer deaths based on few cases (11 deaths in the supplemented group versus 20 in the placebo group) who received β-carotene, α-tocopherol, and selenium. However, a companion trial among persons with esophageal dysplasia showed no benefit for daily supplementation with a multiple vitamin–multiple mineral preparation that included β-carotene (15 mg) (14). In these trials of nutritionally at-risk persons who were primarily nonsmokers, no modification of the intervention findings by smoking or alcohol consumption was reported.

Results from these trials provide evidence for a relatively small increase in lung cancer incidence in cigarette smokers and heavier drinkers who were supplemented with β-carotene, and make it unlikely that supplementation with such pharmacological doses of β-carotene for several years is beneficial in the prevention of most cancers. Observations of increased risk of nonmelanoma skin cancer and colon adenomas for smokers and drinkers with β-carotene supplementation suggest that such interactions may not be restricted to lung carcinogenesis. It should be noted that these effects were detectable because of the controlled experimental design of these studies, which minimized or eliminated the impact of confounding. Had these studies not been conducted, interpretation of the observational research would likely have continued in favor of β-carotene being the primary beneficial carotenoid, and the potential downside for higher-dose supplementation in specific high-risk populations may never have been observed or considered. As described below, subsequent experimental investigation of the trial results has led to a greater understanding of the tissue-specific biochemical and molecular effects of carotenoids, particularly with respect to carcinogenesis.

III. EPIDEMIOLOGICAL EVIDENCE FOR INTERACTIONS

Observational studies have shown a range of findings with respect to modification by smoking and alcohol consumption of dietary and biochemical carotenoid associations with cancer. However, few studies are consistent with the controlled trial results outlined above, and most, including many of the trial cohorts reviewed above, show beneficial associations between nonsupplement carotenoid exposure and cancer. For example, from among the prospective studies of lung cancer reviewed in Chapter 17, approximately one-third show stronger *inverse* associations with carotenoids among current smokers, but an equal number show stronger *inverse* associations for never or former smokers, or no differences based on smoking status. Relatively few studies specifically reported effect modification by alcohol consumption, but one occupational cohort of tin miners in China at high risk for lung cancer found increased risk for high serum carotenoid concentrations (including β-carotene, lutein-zeaxanthin, and β-cryptoxanthin) among drinkers and suggested inverse associations among nondrinkers (15). For example, miners who reported consuming alcohol and who were in the high tertiles of serum β-carotene and lutein-zeaxanthin experienced RRs of 7.6 and 2.3, respectively (95% CIs: 3.1–18.6 and 1.2–6.6, and significant dose–response trends). This study did not report subgroup findings for smoking status, possibly because of the high prevalence of smoking within the cohort, but the serum carotenoid–alcohol interaction supports the effect modification of β-carotene supplementation observed in the ATBC Study and the CARET.

IV. EXPERIMENTAL DATA REGARDING β-CAROTENE SUPPLEMENTATION, CIGARETTE SMOKING AND ALCOHOL CONSUMPTION

Toxicities associated with concomitant exposure to cigarette smoke and high doses of β-carotene have been observed not only in large-scale human trials but also in smaller human feeding experiments, in animals, and in in vitro systems. These studies support the clinical trial findings described above and also provide important mechanistic insights into potential cocarcinogenic properties of these exposures. When subgroup analyses from the two major lung cancer prevention trials—the ATBC Study and CARET—were published, Mayne and colleagues advanced several hypotheses to explain the adverse interactions between β-carotene supplementation and cigarette smoking (16). These included β-carotene (a) exerting prooxidant effects at ambient and high (albeit, nonphysiological) oxygen pressures, (b) acting as a tumor promoter and causing progression of latent lung cancers rather than initiating carcinogenesis, and (c) causing adverse effects through its conversion to retinol, which had been postulated to promote carcinogenesis. Another theory proposed that high doses of β-carotene might deplete serum and tissue concentrations of other potentially beneficial substances, such as other carotenoids and vitamin E, making the lung tissue more susceptible to oxidative insults associated with cigarette smoking. For example, two separate human feeding studies demonstrated that ingestion of pharmacological doses of β-carotene in combination with large doses of other carotenoids attenuated absorption and serum concentrations of the latter micronutrients (17,18). However, when the effect of β-carotene supplementation on serum carotenoid levels was examined within the context of several human intervention trials, *increases* in serum levels of α-carotene (19–22), lycopene [in men only; (19)], and β-cryptoxanthin (20), or *no changes* in non-β-carotene carotenoids (23), were observed. Furthermore, in one of these studies, supplementation-related differences in serum carotenoid levels did not differ according to smoking status or the amount of alcohol consumed (20).

A recent series of experiments conducted in ferrets—an animal that absorbs, accumulates, and metabolizes β-carotene similarly to humans—has provided the strongest leads to date regarding the mechanism of interaction between smoking and β-carotene, and has yielded a potential biological explanation for the aforementioned clinical trial findings (Fig. 1). In these studies, animals were supplemented with β-carotene at doses that mimicked those of chemoprevention trials (equivalent to 30 mg/day in humans) and simultaneously exposed to tobacco smoke for several months. Cigarette smoke exposure significantly reduced the elevated levels of β-carotene in both plasma and lung tissue of supplemented animals (24). Levels of β-carotene metabolites (β-apocarotenoids), however, were threefold higher in smoke-exposed versus nonexposed ferrets following incubation of cultured lung tissue fractions with all-*trans* β-carotene (24). These results demonstrated that increased formation of oxidized β-carotene metabolites and concurrent decreases in the parent molecule are likely to occur in the free radical–rich and antioxidant-poor environment of smokers' lungs. In the same study, lower concentrations of retinoic acid—a

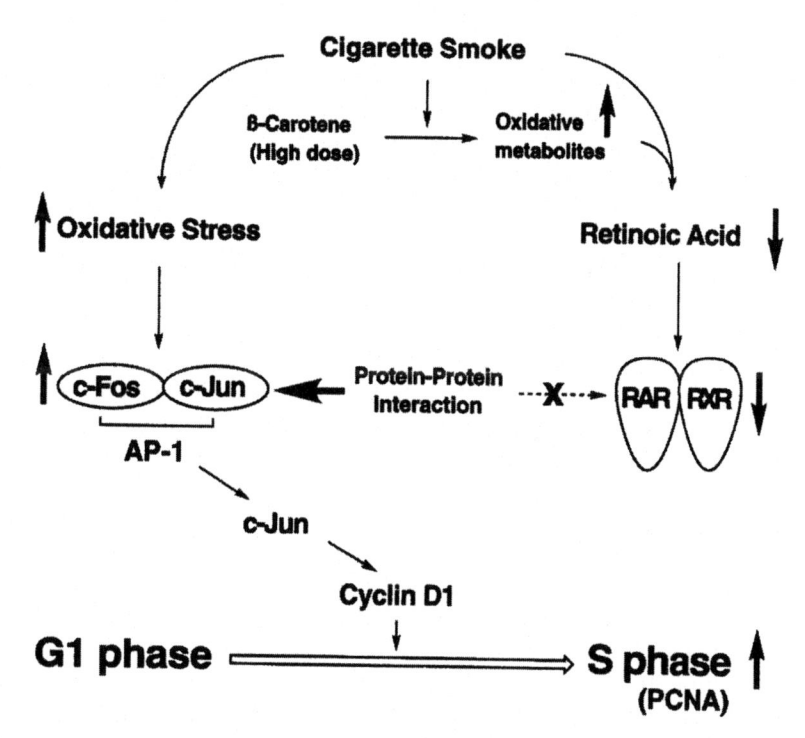

Figure 1 Possible mechanism(s) of effect of cigarette smoke and high-dose β-carotene supplementation on lung cell proliferation. (From Ref. 25.)

compound essential for normal cell growth and regulation—were found in the lung tissues of supplemented ferrets (0.4 ± 0.2 pmol/100 g) compared to controls (1.7 ± 0.7 pmol/100 g) (24). Retinoic acid was not detected in the lungs of the smoke-exposed or smoke-exposed/β-carotene-supplemented groups. Reductions in expression levels of the putative tumor suppressor gene retinoic acid receptor β (RARβ) and increases in markers of activator protein-1 (AP-1) gene expression, which promotes cell proliferation, were also observed in all three treatment groups (24). This was particularly apparent in supplemented ferrets exposed to cigarette smoke (compared to controls, expression of RARβ down-regulated by 73% and expression of AP-1 encoding genes increased threefold to fourfold). Interestingly, in smoke-exposed ferrets consuming doses of β-carotene that more closely approximated physiological concentrations achieved through diet (equivalent to 6 mg/day in humans), much smaller decreases in retinoic acid concentrations and RARβ expression were observed when compared with animals exposed to cigarette smoke and high doses of β-carotene (25). In another experiment, no adverse effects were observed in smoke-exposed ferrets consuming low or high doses of lycopene (equivalent to 15 mg/day and 60 mg/day in humans, respectively) (26). Instead, supplementation with this carotenoid at either dose appeared to exert protective effects against smoke-induced lung carcinogenesis. It should be noted, however, that the lung tissue concentration of β-carotene (26 μmol/kg) achieved with the human equivalent of 30 mg/day supplementation was much greater than the corresponding concentration of lycopene (1.2 μmol/kg, based on the 60 mg/day human equivalent), which may partially explain the divergent findings obtained with these two carotenoids.

Induction of specific cytochrome P450 (CYP) enzymes may provide the link between increased concentrations of β-carotene metabolites, altered retinoic acid profiles in the lungs of supplemented smokers, and enhanced carcinogenesis. β-Carotene and its oxidation products can induce a multitude of CYPs (reviewed in Chapters 8 and 9), whose subsequent activation interferes with normal retinoid signaling (reviewed in Chapter 14). An ancillary study that utilized lung microsomal fractions from the ferrets described above linked cigarette smoke exposure and/or high doses of β-carotene with increased catabolism of retinoic acid by induction of CYP1A1 and CYP1A2 (27). CYPs also have an important role in converting procarcinogens, including those found in cigarette smoke, to their genotoxic forms. Therefore, ingestion of large doses of β-carotene may indirectly enhance the effective exposure of the lung to the carcinogens in tobacco smoke via CYP activation. Increases in oxidative stress, including overproduction of the superoxide anion, have been shown to accompany β-carotene-induced CYP activation in rat lungs (28). These findings offer additional explanations for the increased morbidity and mortality associated with high-dose β-carotene supplementation in smokers.

Simultaneous administration of supplemental β-carotene and ethanol also produces adverse effects in animals and in tissue culture. Since the liver is the primary site of ethanol metabolism, most studies have specifically examined the hepatocellular toxicity associated with coexposure to ethanol and pharmacological doses of β-carotene. However, it is unknown whether the resulting mechanisms can be extrapolated to carcinogenicity in the liver and other organs. Results from an early experiment in which baboons received daily supplements of β-carotene indicated that animals fed extremely high levels of alcohol (50% of total energy) had substantially higher plasma and liver β-carotene levels, slower blood clearance of this carotenoid, and increases in markers of hepatic injury than those not receiving alcohol as part of their diet (29). Increased hepatic β-carotene levels and associated liver injury was also demonstrated in rats consuming β-carotene supplements and ethanol (36% of total energy) (30). The authors postulated that the adverse effects might be due to an ethanol-induced blockage in the conversion of β-carotene to retinol. Accumulation of β-carotene could exacerbate ethanol-induced oxidative stress and/or contribute to localized vitamin A deficiency, both of which may lead to hepatic and extrahepatic carcinogenesis. Since β-carotene and acetaldehyde (a toxic metabolite of ethanol) appear to share a common metabolic pathway, it has also been suggested that each inhibits the other's metabolism via competitive inhibition of relevant enzymes (31). Induction of specific P450 enzymes may also contribute to the toxicity and carcinogenicity associated with coadministration of β-carotene and ethanol. In a recent study, hepatocytes from rats fed β-carotene and ethanol had significantly higher expression levels of CYP2E1 than hepatocytes from animals fed each agent alone (CYP2El content, densitometric units, less than 100 in controls and in β-carotene fed rats, 317 in ethanol-fed rats, and 442 in β-carotene + ethanol-fed rats, p interaction $= 0.012$) (32). Furthermore, consumption of β-carotene independently increased the expression of CYP4A1 in liver microsomes (CYP4A1 content, densitometric units, 158 in controls and 328 in β-carotene fed rats, $p = 0.01$). Induction of both of these P450 enzymes could potentially contribute to carcinogenesis. Although the precise mechanisms underlying the adverse interactions between high-dose β-carotene and ethanol consumption remain less well characterized than corresponding interactions between β-carotene and cigarette smoking, animal and in vitro studies continue to provide important gains in our understanding of this complex process.

V. SUMMARY AND CONCLUSIONS

Given the overwhelming epidemiological data pointing to a beneficial role in many cancers for higher carotenoid intake and status within the normal dietary range, the opposite conclusions derived from two large β-carotene supplementation trials (ATBC Study and CARET) were unanticipated and disappointing. At the same time, they were instrumental in advancing our understanding of the true interrelationships among cancer risk, carotenoid intake (dietary and supplemental) and biochemistry, and vegetable and fruit consumption, and intensified the focus of epidemiological investigations on the range of carotenoids, improved dietary assessment and nutrient data, and increased control of confounders. Data from most other trials and nearly all of the epidemiological studies contradict findings from the two high-risk and some other trial cohorts, which has led to two important conclusions. First, persons at high risk for lung cancer by virtue of cigarette smoking or other high-risk exposures should avoid using β-carotene supplements, as should heavy drinkers, based on the observed interactions. Laboratory studies have substantiated the toxicity resulting from combining high-dose β-carotene supplementation with cigarette smoking or high alcohol intake through direct effects in the lung, liver, and other tissues, including induction of cytochrome P450 enzymes and down-regulation of retinoic acid signaling and RARβ expression. Second, the evidence for a beneficial dietary and biochemical association for β-carotene, lycopene, and other carotenoids remains convincing, and the range of such observed associations continues to be delineated. Whether lower dose carotenoid supplements might afford benefits against cancer or other diseases similar to those derived from higher dietary intake and resulting elevated circulating concentrations remains to be determined through further study.

REFERENCES

1. Greenberg ER, Baron JA, Stukel TA, Stevens MM, Mandel JS, Spencer SK, Elias PM, Lowe N, Nierenberg DW, Bayrd G, Vance JC, Freeman DH Jr, Clendenning WE, Kwan T. A clinical trial of beta carotene to prevent basal-cell and squamous-cell cancers of the skin. The Skin Cancer Prevention Study Group. N Engl J Med 1990; 323:789–795.
2. Baron JA, Cole BF, Mott L, Haile R, Grau M, Church TR, Beck GJ, Greenberg ER. Neoplastic and antineoplastic effects of beta-carotene on colorectal adenoma recurrence: results of a randomized trial. J Natl Cancer Inst 2003; 95:717–722.
3. The effect of vitamin E and beta carotene on the incidence of lung cancer and other cancers in male smokers. The Alpha-Tocopherol, Beta Carotene Cancer Prevention Study Group. N Engl J Med 1994; 330:1029–1035.
4. Albanes D, Heinonen OP, Taylor PR, Virtamo J, Edwards BK, Rautalahti M, Hartman AM, Palmgren J, Freedman LS, Haapakoski J, Barrett MJ, Pietinen P, Malila N, Tala E, Liippo K, Salomaa ER, Tangrea JA, Teppo L, Askin FB, Taskinen E, Erozan Y, Greenwald P, Huttunen JK. Alpha-tocopherol and beta-carotene supplements and lung cancer incidence in the alpha-tocopherol, beta-carotene cancer prevention study: effects of base-line characteristics and study compliance. J Natl Cancer Inst 1996; 88:1560–1570.

5. Omenn GS, Goodman GE, Thornquist MD, Balmes J, Cullen MR, Glass A, Keogh JP, Meyskens FL, Valanis B, Williams JH, Barnhart S, Hammar S. Effects of a combination of beta carotene and vitamin A on lung cancer and cardiovascular disease. N Engl J Med 1996; 334:1150–1155.

6. Omenn GS, Goodman GE, Thornquist MD, Balmes J, Cullen MR, Glass A, Keogh JP, Meyskens FL Jr, Valanis B, Williams JH Jr, Barnhart S, Cherniack MG, Brodkin CA, Hammar S. Risk factors for lung cancer and for intervention effects in CARET, the Beta-Carotene and Retinol Efficacy Trial. J Natl Cancer Inst 1996; 88:1550–1559.

7. Greenberg ER, Baron JA, Tosteson TD, Freeman DH Jr, Beck GJ, Bond JH, Colacchio TA, Coller JA, Frankl HD, Haile RW, Mandel JS, Nierenberg DW, Rothstein R, Snover DC, Stevens MM, Summers RW, van Stolk RU. A clinical trial of antioxidant vitamins to prevent colorectal adenoma. Polyp Prevention Study Group. N Engl J Med 1994; 331: 141–147.

8. Mayne ST, Cartmel B, Baum M, Shor-Posner G, Fallon BG, Briskin K, Bean J, Zheng T, Cooper D, Friedman C, Goodwin WJ Jr. Randomized trial of supplemental beta-carotene to prevent second head and neck cancer. Cancer Res 2001; 61:1457–1463.

9. Hennekens CH, Buring JE, Manson JE, Stampfer M, Rosner B, Cook NR, Belanger C, LaMotte F, Gaziano JM, Ridker PM, Willett W, Peto R. Lack of effect of long-term supplementation with beta carotene on the incidence of malignant neoplasms and cardiovascular disease. N Engl J Med 1996; 334:1145–1149.

10. Cook NR, Le IM, Manson JE, Buring JE, Hennekens CH. Effects of beta-carotene supplementation on cancer incidence by baseline characteristics in the Physicians' Health Study (United States). Cancer Causes Control 2000; 11:617–626.

11. Frieling UM, Schaumberg DA, Kupper TS, Muntwyler J, Hennekens CH. A randomized, 12-year primary-prevention trial of beta carotene supplementation for nonmelanoma skin cancer in the physician's health study. Arch Dermatol 2000; 136:179–184.

12. Lee IM, Cook NR, Manson JE, Buring JE, Hennekens CH. Beta-carotene supplementation and incidence of cancer and cardiovascular disease: the Women's Health Study. J Natl Cancer Inst 1999; 91:2102–2106.

13. Blot WJ, Li JY, Taylor PR, Guo W, Dawsey S, Wang GQ, Yang CS, Zheng SF, Gail M, Li GY, Yu Y, Liu BQ, Tangrea J, Sun YH, Liu FS, Fraumeni JF Jr, Zhang YH, Li B. Nutrition intervention trials in Linxian, China: supplementation with specific vitamin/mineral combinations, cancer incidence, and disease-specific mortality in the general population. J Natl Cancer Inst 1993; 85:1483–1492.

14. Li JY, Taylor PR, Li B, Dawsey SM, Wang GW, Ershow AG, Guo W, Liu SF, Yang CS, Shen Q, Wang W, Mark SD, Zou XN, Greenwald P, Wu YO, Blot WJ. Nutrition intervention trials in Linxian, China: multiple vitamin/mineral supplementation, cancer incidence, and disease-specific mortality among adults with esophageal dysplasia. J Natl Cancer Inst 1993; 85:1492–1498.

15. Ratnasinghe D, Forman MR, Tangrea JA, Qiao Y, Yao SX, Gunter EW, Barrett MJ, Giffen CA, Erozan Y, Tockman MS, Taylor PR. Serum carotenoids are associated with increased lung cancer risk among alcohol drinkers, but not among non-drinkers in a cohort of tin miners. Alc Alcohol 2000; 35:355–360.

16. Mayne ST, Handelman GJ, Beecher G. Beta-carotene and lung cancer promotion in heavy smokers—a plausible relationship? J Natl Cancer Inst 1996; 88:1513–1515.

17. White WS, Stacewicz-Sapuntzakis M, Erdman JW Jr, Bowen PE. Pharmacokinetics of beta-carotene and canthaxanthin after ingestion of individual and combined doses by human subjects. J Am Coll Nutr 1994; 13:665–671.

18. Kostic D, White WS, Olson JA. Intestinal absorption, serum clearance, and interactions between lutein and beta-carotene when administered to human adults in separate or combined oral doses. Am J Clin Nutr 1995; 62:604–610.

19. Wahlqvist ML, Wattanapenpaiboon N, Macrae FA, Lambert JR, MacLennan R, Hsu-Hage BH. Changes in serum carotenoids in subjects with colorectal adenomas after 24 mo of beta-carotene supplementation. Australian Polyp Prevention Project Investigators. Am J Clin Nutr 1994; 60:936–943.

20. Albanes D, Virtamo J, Taylor PR, Rautalahti M, Pietinen P, Heinonen OP. Effects of supplemental beta-carotene, cigarette smoking, and alcohol consumption on serum carotenoids in the Alpha-Tocopherol, Beta-Carotene Cancer Prevention Study. Am J Clin Nutr 1997; 66:366–372.

21. Mayne ST, Cartmel B, Silva F, Kim CS, Fallon BG, Briskin K, Zheng T, Baum M, Shor-Posner G, Goodwin WJ Jr. Effect of supplemental beta-carotene on plasma concentrations of carotenoids, retinol, and alpha-tocopherol in humans. Am J Clin Nutr 1998; 68:642–647.

22. Omenn GS, Goodman GE, Thornquist MD, Rosenstock L, Barnhart S, Gylys-Colwell I, Metch B, Lund B. The Carotene and Retinol Efficacy Trial (CARET) to prevent lung cancer in high-risk populations: pilot study with asbestos-exposed workers. Cancer Epidemiol Biomark Prev 1993; 2:381–387.

23. Nierenberg DW, Dam BJ, Mott LA, Baron JA, Greenberg ER. Effects of 4 y of oral supplementation with beta-carotene on serum concentrations of retinol, tocopherol, and five carotenoids. Am J Clin Nutr 1997; 66:315–319.

24. Wang XD, Liu C, Bronson RT, Smith DE, Krinsky NI, Russell M. Retinoid signaling and activator protein-1 expression in ferrets given beta-carotene supplements and exposed to tobacco smoke. J Natl Cancer Inst 1999; 91:60–66.

25. Liu C, Wang XD, Bronson RT, Smith DE, Krinsky NI, Russell RM. Effects of physiological versus pharmacological beta-carotene supplementation on cell proliferation and histopathological changes in the lungs of cigarette smoke-exposed ferrets. Carcinogenesis 2000; 21:2245–2253.

26. Liu C, Lian F, Smith DE, Russell RM, Wang XD. Lycopene supplementation inhibits lung squamous metaplasia and induces apoptosis via up-regulating insulin-like growth factor-binding protein 3 in cigarette smoke-exposed ferrets. Cancer Res 2003; 63:3138–3144.

27. Liu C, Russell RM, Wang XD. Exposing ferrets to cigarette smoke and a pharmacological dose of beta-carotene supplementation enhance in vitro retinoic acid catabolism in lungs via induction of cytochrome P450 enzymes. J Nutr 2003; 133:173–179.

28. Paolini M, Cantelli-Forti G, P. P, Pedulli GF, Abdel-Rahman SZ, Legator MS. Co-carcinogenic effect of beta-carotene. Nature 1999; 398:760–761.

29. Leo MA, Kim C, Lowe N, Lieber CS. Interaction of ethanol with beta-carotene: delayed blood clearance and enhanced hepatotoxicity. Hepatology 1992; 15:883–891.

30. Leo MA, Aleynik SI, Aleynik MK, Lieber CS. Beta-carotene beadlets potentiate hepatotoxicity of alcohol. Am J Clin Nutr 1997; 66:1461–1469.

31. Ni R, Leo MA, Zhao J, Lieber CS. Toxicity of beta-carotene and its exacerbation by acetaldehyde in HepG2 cells. Alc Alcohol 2001; 36:281–285.

32. Kessova IG, Leo MA, Lieber CS. Effect of beta-carotene on hepatic cytochrome P-450 in ethanol-fed rats. Alcohol Clin Exp Res 2001; 25:1368–1372.

26
Carotenoids: Looking Forward

Norman I. Krinsky
Tufts University, Boston, Massachusetts, U.S.A.

Susan T. Mayne
Yale University School of Medicine, New Haven, Connecticut, U.S.A.

Helmut Sies
Heinriche-Heine-Universität, Düsseldorf, Germany

The preceding twenty-five chapters are comprehensive reviews of the carotenoid literature up to, in many cases, the middle of 2003. Most of these chapters deal with the role that carotenoids may play in human health and disease, including diseases such as cancer, heart disease, eye diseases such as age-related macular degeneration and cataracts, skin photosensitivity diseases, and the impact of carotenoids on the immune system. In several diseases, such as cancer, the available data are ambiguous, but these ambiguities are dealt with and logical explanations are presented.

The ambiguities about carotenoid supplementation in cancer prevention arose when two of the three large scale β-carotene intervention trials evaluating any change in the risk of developing lung cancer in high-risk populations observed an unexpected increase in the incidence of lung cancer (1, 2). The third study, using a relatively healthy population, showed no effect of such treatment, i.e., neither an increase nor a decrease in the incidence of lung cancer (3). The publication of these three studies had a profound effect on our assessment of the role of carotenoids in human health. In the first place, they brought us to a better understanding of the role of individual nutrients in food, as opposed to the effect of whole food. The epidemiological studies published prior to these intervention trials overwhelmingly indicated a positive association between the ingestion of foods rich in β-carotene and a decrease in the incidence of lung cancer. In fact, the effects were frequently strongest among smokers. Based on these observations, along with results of animal studies of beta-carotene and short-term intervention trials in humans, hypotheses were formulated that one of the active ingredients in the diet was β-carotene (4). With the benefit of hindsight, we can now question that hypothesis, but at the time, it seemed reasonable. Then a series of careful studies were carried out, with the results described above. Many people were disappointed with these results, but that is the nature of the scientific enterprise, and should not be construed as "the β-carotene fiasco" (5). Prevention trials are only undertaken when the evidence supporting a benefit of an intervention is supportive but not overwhelming; otherwise, it would be unethical to withhold an agent with acknowledged benefit. Results of clinical trials have opened a new area of carotenoid investigation that involves studying the biological effects of metabolites (other than vitamin A) of β-carotene and other carotenoids.

There are other areas of carotenoid research that will continue to develop, including the use of newer technologies. Research progress in a field is often greatly stimulated by new technologies. One such area involves novel uses of technology for noninvasive determination of carotenoids. The use of resonance Raman spectroscopy for eye carotenoids, and Raman and reflectometric techniques for skin carotenoids, has been described in this volume (6, 7). One may look forward to the day when noninvasive techniques will be able to identify individual carotenoids.

The role of carotenoids as potential antioxidants (8) or prooxidants (9) in vivo is still debatable. Newer assays are being developed that will be able to differentiate the antioxidant capacity of both the lipophilic as well as the aqueous compartments of tissues and body fluids, and thus be able to resolve whether carotenoids have in vivo antioxidant capacity (10). This antioxidant/prooxidant activity may be related to the action of carotenoids on various signal transduction systems (8). As reviewed in this volume (11), carotenoids have been demonstrated to influence various signaling pathways in cell culture systems, and we look forward to studies indicating the importance of these observations in animals and humans.

There are several areas of human nutrition that remain fruitful as far as future advances are concerned. If the reports of nonabsorbers of carotenoids can be carefully validated, this might suggest that carotenoid absorption is not merely a passive process, but may depend on carrier proteins to facilitate their uptake. Such findings would also raise the question as to whether such carrier proteins exhibit *cis-trans* specificity, or structural specificity for the various carotenoids found in the human diet. Another nutritional issue that remains to be resolved is whether, either through selective breeding or by means of genetic modification, new food species can be developed that would increase the availability of provitamin A to nutritionally deprived populations. What comes to mind is the development of golden rice, yellow cauliflower, and other modified foods.

Research on the metabolism of carotenoids is in a renaissance period, with the cloning of the 15, 15'-monooxygenase that converts β-carotene to vitamin A, as described in this volume (12). In addition, there are other monooxygenases that either cleave other carotenoids or cleave at excentric double bonds. All of this leads to the suggestion that these enzymes have been conserved because of the products that they produce, many of which are similar to oxidation products described earlier (13). Again, we can look forward to the characterization of these new products, as well as their potential metabolites, and whatever biological actions they may demonstrate when tested in cells and in animals. Since it has been reported that humans ingest up to 48 different carotenoids in their diet, there will be much work ahead to learn which of these dietary carotenoids serve as substrates for the known monooxygenases or for enzymes still to be found.

This volume has been dedicated to describing the relationships between carotenoids and human diseases. Yet still much remains to be discovered. For example, despite the strength of the epidemiological evidence linking lutein and zeaxanthin to reduced risk of eye diseases such as age-related macular degeneration (14, 15), we still have not uncovered a causal relationship between the onset of this disease and relative lack of these two xanthophylls.

Heart and vascular diseases are in a similar position to age-related macular degeneration. There is overwhelming epidemiological evidence that diets rich in carotenoid sources such as fruits and vegetables are cardioprotective, but when an individual carotenoid such as β-carotene has been studied in intervention trials, the results have been null, i.e., neither a positive nor negative effect (16). This observation would suggest that either β-carotene alone is not the active component in fruits and vegetables, or that some other component(s) of the diet might act in a synergistic fashion with β-carotene, or other carotenoids in the diet, to result in the cardioprotection. Much work remains to be done to resolve this issue.

And then there is cancer and carotenoids. At least in this area, significant cell culture work is being accomplished to warrant a continued interest in the potential for the use of carotenoids or their metabolites either in prevention or treatment of some types of cancer (17). In particular, the work on lycopene and cancers such as prostate cancer holds great promise (18). Much work remains to be done to determine if the cell effects are due to lycopene alone, one of its metabolites, or a combination of products found in tomatoes along with lycopene. So for example, do tomatoes that synthesize primarily other carotenoids such as β-carotene, or have a block in the final steps in lycopene synthesis, also exhibit any biological action in tumor cells grown in culture or in animals used as a model for prostate cancer?

Another area that deserves further investigation is the relationship between inflammatory diseases and carotenoids, particularly with respect to the fact that inflammation produces the same types of oxidizing species that have been shown to oxidize carotenoids to shorter chained molecules. Again, we must identify the biological activities of breakdown products of the dietary carotenoids, in particular β-carotene, α-carotene, β-cryptoxanthin, lutein, and zeaxanthin. These carotenoids constitute the vast bulk of our dietary carotenoids (19), yet with the exception of β-carotene, little is known about their metabolites and whether these metabolites have any biological action. Thus, while it is still too early to make any recommendation regarding the intake of carotenoids, it would be inappropriate to ban the intake of β-carotene as it still supplies a significant portion of the daily intake of vitamin A in many parts of the world. We can look forward to this field expanding rapidly in the near future.

REFERENCES

1. The Alpha Tocopherol Beta Carotene Cancer Prevention Study Group. The effect of vitamin E and beta carotene on the incidence of lung cancer and other cancers in male smokers. New Engl J Med 1994; 330:1029–35.
2. Omenn GS, Goodman GE, Thornquist MD, Balmes J, Cullen MR, Glass A, Keogh JP, Meyskens FL, Jr., Valanis B, Williams JH, Jr., Barnhart S, Hammar S. Effects of a combination of beta carotene and vitamin A on lung cancer and cardiovascular disease. New Engl J Med 1996; 334:1150–5.
3. Hennekens CH, Buring JE, Manson JE, Stampfer M, Rosner B, Cook NR, Belanger C, LaMotte F, Gaziano JM, Ridker PM, Willett W, Peto R. Lack of effect of long-term supplementation with beta carotene on the incidence of malignant neoplasms and cardiovascular disease. New Engl J Med 1996; 334:1145–9.
4. Peto R, Doll RJ, Buckley JD, Sporn MB. Can dietary β-carotene materially reduce human cancer rates? Nature (London) 1981; 290:201–8.
5. Brody J. The nutrient that reddens tomatoes appears to have health benefits. The New York Times. March 12, 1997.
6. Bernstein PS, Gellermann W. Noninvasive assessment of carotenoids in the human eye and skin. In: Krinsky NI, Mayne ST, Sies H, eds. Carotenoids in Health and Disease. Marcel Dekker: New York, 2004:53–84.
7. Stahl W, Sies H. Carotenoids in systemic protection against sunburn. In: Krinsky NI, Mayne ST, Sies H, eds. Carotenoids in Health and Disease. Marcel Dekker: New York, 2004:491–502.
8. Young AJ, Phillip DM, Lowe GM. Carotenoid antioxidant activity. In: Krinsky NI, Mayne ST, Sies H, eds. Carotenoids in Health and Disease. Marcel Dekker: New York, 2004:105–26.
9. Palozza P. Evidence for pro-oxidant effects of carotenoids in vitro and in vivo: implications in health and disease. In: Krinsky NI, Mayne ST, Sies H, eds. Carotenoids in Health and Disease. Marcel Dekker: New York, 2004:127–49.
10. Yeum K-J, Aldini G, Chung H-Y, Krinsky NI, Russell RM. The activities of antioxidant nutrients in human plasma depend on the localization of the attacking radical species. J Nutr 2003; 133:2688–91.

11. Sharoni Y, Danilenko M, Levy J, Stahl W. Anticancer activity of carotenoids: from human studies to cellular processes and gene regulation. In: Krinsky NI, Mayne ST, Sies H, eds. Carotenoids in Health and Disease. Marcel Dekker: New York, 2004:165–96.

12. von Lintig J. Conversion of carotenoids to vitamin A: new insights on the molecular level. In: Krinsky NI, Mayne ST, Sies H, eds. Carotenoids in Health and Disease. Marcel Dekker: New York, 2004:337–56.

13. Wang X-D. Carotenoid oxidative/degradative products and their biological activities. In: Krinsky NI, Mayne ST, Sies H, eds. Carotenoids in Health and Disease. Marcel Dekker: New York, 2004:313–35.

14. Mares JA. Carotenoid and eye disease: epidemiological evidence. In: Krinsky NI, Mayne ST, Sies H, eds. Carotenoids in Health and Disease. Marcel Dekker: New York, 2004:427–44.

15. Landrum JT, Bone RA. Mechanistic evidence for eye diseases and carotenoids. In: Krinsky NI, Mayne ST, Sies H, eds. Carotenoids in Health and Disease. Marcel Dekker: New York, 2004:445–72.

16. Sesso HD, Gaziano JM. Heart and vascular diseases. In: Krinsky NI, Mayne ST, Sies H, eds. Carotenoids in Health and Disease. Marcel Dekker: New York, 2004:473–90.

17. Rock CL. Relationship of carotenoids to cancer. In: Krinsky NI, Mayne ST, Sies H, eds. Carotenoids in Health and Disease. Marcel Dekker: New York, 2004:373–407.

18. Ang E, Miller EC, Clinton SK. Role of lycopene in carcinogenesis. In: Krinsky NI, Mayne ST, Sies H, eds. Carotenoids in Health and Disease. Marcel Dekker: New York, 2004:409–25.

19. Boileau AC, Erdman JW, Jr. Impact of food processing on content and bioavailability of carotenoids. In: Krinsky NI, Mayne ST, Sies H, eds. Carotenoids in Health and Disease. Marcel Dekker: New York, 2004:209–28.

Index